Nutrition and Health

Adrianne Bendich, Ph.D., FACN, FASN, Series Editor

More information about this series at http://www.springer.com/series/7659

Donato F. Romagnolo • Ornella I. Selmin
Editors

Mediterranean Diet

Dietary Guidelines and Impact on Health and Disease

Humana Press

Editors
Donato F. Romagnolo
Room 303
Tucson, AZ, USA

Ornella I. Selmin
Department of Nutritional Sciences
The University of Arizona Cancer Center
Tucson, AZ, USA

Nutrition and Health
ISBN 978-3-319-27967-1 ISBN 978-3-319-27969-5 (eBook)
DOI 10.1007/978-3-319-27969-5

Library of Congress Control Number: 2016931593

Springer Cham Heidelberg New York Dordrecht London

Printed on acid-free paper

Humana Press is a brand of Springer
Springer International Publishing AG Switzerland is part of Springer Science+Business Media
(www.springer.com)

This volume is dedicated to the memories of John Milner, Ph.D., and Mary Frances Picciano, Ph.D., international leaders in nutrition research, who were friends, mentors, coeditors, and inspirational figures to the editors of this volume.

Foreword

The human diet is complex and ever changing (1). We eat hundreds of individual foods, in thousands of wide-ranging combinations, which we prepare and serve using a diverse array of methods, according to markedly different cultural norms (2). To study the effect of diet on human health, nutrition scientists have attempted to isolate the diet's myriad components, individually and in small groups, to examine what effect, if any, they exert on the body. These studies have led to the suggestion that whole foods may have unique effects on health than individual components (3).

Over the past century, nutrition researchers have made many vital, life-saving advances. The discovery of vitamins in the early twentieth century brought about effective treatments for the deficiency diseases, rickets, beriberi, and scurvy. The 1980s and 1990s saw keen interest in naturally occurring plant substances called phytochemicals that display a wide range of health-promoting, disease-fighting potential (4–20).

But these piecemeal advances have bred a piecemeal understanding in the public's mind. Findings on individual dietary components have indirectly led to the demonization of various nutrients and macronutrients, with damaging effects: health fads that promote the near elimination of carbohydrates or that hold up protein as a panacea (21–35). In response to consumer demand, the food industry floods grocery shelves with low-fat potato chips and cookies. And through it all, the slow, steady ballooning of portion sizes, as well as our waistlines, has proceeded apace (36–38).

As our research methods continue to evolve, and our knowledge expands, it's becoming clear that the big picture is what matters most. Recent studies suggest that our usual patterns of dietary intake and physical activity are more important to wellness than our historically narrow focus on consumption of a few individual foods or nutrients can show (39–48). If we are to move the science forward, it's clear that we must take a step back and examine overall patterns of eating and of living.

As Data Mounts, Recommendations Evolve

At the American Institute for Cancer Research (AICR), we've had a front-row seat at the steady accretion of new insights and understanding as the evidence linking diet, physical activity, and weight to cancer risk has grown. This mounting evidence has occasioned a shift in focus from individual nutrients and phytochemicals to overall dietary patterns. In 1981, the first scientific reports to evaluate the evidence linking various dietary components to cancer risk were published. Importantly, both *The Causes of Cancer* by Richard Doll and Richard Peto (1981) (49) and the *US National Academy of Sciences Report Diet, Nutrition and Cancer* (1982) (50) concluded by issuing urgent calls for more and better research, and by the mid-1990s thousands of studies had been published on diet and cancer.

To evaluate and synthesize these new studies, in 1997 AICR and the World Cancer Research Fund published an expert report, *Food, Nutrition, and the Prevention of Cancer: A Global Perspective* (51). The report presented our recommendations for cancer prevention, which reflected the then-current state of the science. By 2007 the sheer amount of new evidence demanded that AICR/WCRF produce a second expert report, *Food, Nutrition, Physical Activity, and the Prevention of Cancer: A Global Perspective* (52), and by now physical activity was rightfully acknowledged as an important component of a healthy lifestyle. The report's recommendations were as follows:

1. Be as lean as possible without becoming underweight.
2. Be physically active for at least 30 min every day.
3. Avoid sugary drinks. Limit consumption of energy-dense foods.
4. Eat more of a variety of vegetables, fruits, whole grains, and legumes such as beans.
5. Limit consumption of red meats (such as beef, pork, and lamb) and avoid processed meats.
6. If consumed at all, limit alcoholic drinks to 2 for men and 1 for women a day.
7. Limit consumption of salty foods and foods processed with salt (sodium).
8. Don't use supplements to protect against cancer.
9. It is best for mothers to breastfeed exclusively for up to 6 months and then add other liquids and foods.
10. After treatment, cancer survivors should follow the recommendations for cancer prevention.

Clearly, science doesn't stand still, so we've instituted a process of ongoing review and analysis that ensures our recommendations for cancer prevention reflect the latest science. We have partnered with WCRF International on the Continuous Update Project (53), which reviews and analyzes the relevant research on a rolling basis, cancer site by cancer site.

A Focus on Meals, Not Micronutrients

AICR's education team has turned our recommendations for cancer prevention into understandable and practical messages for the American public and has created a visual plate-based model for healthy eating, the New American Plate. The appeal of this approach is its simplicity and flexibility as well as its emphasis on whole foods and whole meals. At their core, AICR's New American Plate, the USDA's My Plate, and scores of other similar approaches represent an encouraging trend borne out by the research—a desire to address health research and health messaging by shifting away from a piecemeal focus on individual foods and food components to overall dietary patterns.

Forest for the (Olive) Trees

One such pattern, around which a tremendous amount of research has accrued, is the Mediterranean diet. Many of the recommendations included in the 2007 AICR/WCRF Expert Report overlap with those of the Mediterranean pyramid, which:

- Highlights the importance of regular physical activity and avoiding sugary drinks
- Limits the consumption of energy-dense foods
- Recommends intake of more of a variety of vegetables, fruits, whole grains, and legumes such as beans
- Limits the consumption of red and processed meats and alcohol

It is notable that like the AICR/WCRF recommendations, the Mediterranean diet was included in the Scientific Report of the 2015 Dietary Guidelines submitted to the Department of Human Health Services and US Department of Agriculture (54).

As detailed in this volume, the Mediterranean diet includes a variety of healthy foods in moderate amounts. But it is more than just a checklist of specific foods and beverages. The traditional Mediterranean diet represents a truly holistic approach that combines fresh whole foods and plenty of physical activity. As you read about this fascinating research, you may be struck by how simple and appealing this lifestyle seems, in terms of both its day-to-day pleasures and its many long-term health benefits. The editors, Drs. Donato Romagnolo and Ornella Selmin, nutrition and cancer researchers at the University of Arizona, have invited world-renowned experts to highlight the key aspects of the Mediterranean diet and lifestyle.

The volume opens with *Part I, Mediterranean Diet and Lifestyle in a World Contest.* This chapter introduces the foundational elements of the Mediterranean pyramid for improving natural resources sustainability and prevention of chronic diseases including overweight, obesity, cardiovascular, cancer, and diabetes. A key concept emerges: that prevention of chronic diseases requires approaches that go beyond simple food recommendations but also involve increased accessibility to healthier food and better medical and healthcare.

In *Part II, Historical, Behavioral, and Geographical Perspective on the Mediterranean Diet and Lifestyle,* the volume focuses on the historical and geographical differences and overlaps of diets characteristic of the Mediterranean region. Concerns are expressed that even in Mediterranean countries, departure from local agricultural activities has reduced the availability of traditional healthier foods and increased dependency on large-scale, and possibly not as healthy, processed foods. These changes are modifying dietary patterns and possibly contributing to an increased burden of chronic diseases even in less developed and food-insecure communities.

Part III discusses the role of *Mediterranean Diet and Lifestyle for Health Promotion.* A key component of the Mediterranean diet is olive oil rich in monounsaturated oleic acid. Fish and nuts provide other sources of fats that positively impact the overall fatty acid profile (i.e., more mono- and polyunsaturated fatty acids compared to a Western diet, which is rich in saturated fatty acids). Authors highlight the beneficial effects of compounds present in olive oil against oxidative processes, cardiovascular disease, cancers, and neurodegenerative disorders. The benefits of the Mediterranean diet extend to improved longevity and reduction of inflammatory processes associated with cardiovascular diseases. Also data are discussed linking adherence to a Mediterranean-like diet and lifestyle and reduced risk of metabolic disorders.

In *Part IV, Aging and Cancer Risk,* authors provide evidence of the benefits of foods—and their wide variety of bioactive compounds—commonly present in the Mediterranean diet (i.e., fruits, vegetables, whole grains, unsaturated fatty acids, lean meat) for reducing or slowing the development of conditions associated with aging (i.e., cognitive decline, dementia, Alzheimer's and Parkinson's). Of particular interest to AICR, which focuses on reducing the cancer burden through nutrition, is the emerging evidence that the Mediterranean diet may have protective effects against the development of breast and colon cancer. Progress in these areas can impact on the development of prevention therapies and reduce cancer mortality associated with breast and colorectal malignancies. A chapter on the developing field of epigenetics clearly points out how dietary exposures to foods and bioactives present in the Mediterranean diet can impact gene expression and, possibly, influence gene expression later in life, or even in subsequent generations.

Finally, *Part V, Building a Mediterranean-Like Pyramid* translates the research concepts presented in the opening and health promotion papers into practical suggestions. First, authors highlight the health benefits of physical activity, which is a key component of the Mediterranean pyramid and other lifestyle behaviors. This is a behavioral component that can cut across cultural and geographical differences and contribute to correcting/preventing excessive energy balance and diseases associated with overconsumption. The closing chapters of the volume illustrate selected Mediterranean recipes that include information about ingredients, cooking methods, and nutritional value. In the last chapter, the editors and coauthors have translated the information from each recipe into a week-long dietary plan inspired by the Mediterranean pyramid. The recipe information used to build this dietary plan is an instructional material developed by the editors for the Mediterranean Diet and Health Study Abroad Program. This program is held in Italy every year for students, nutrition professionals, and adults who wish to learn about the health benefits of the Mediterranean diet and lifestyle (55).

In closing, our understanding of diet and health has progressed rapidly. Yet today, we are beset by illnesses related directly to poor diets, inactivity, and soaring obesity rates. We applaud the editors and contributors of this volume, a work that supplies a wider, much-needed perspective on an overall pattern of living.

Washington, DC

Susan Higginbotham, Ph.D., RD.
Glen Weldon

References

1. Antón SC, Potts R, Aiello LC. Human evolution. Evolution of early Homo: an integrated biological perspective. Science. 2014;345(6192):1236828.
2. Lucock MD, Martin CE, Yates ZR, Veysey M. Diet and our genetic legacy in the recent anthropocene: a Darwinian perspective to nutritional health. J Evid Based Complementary Altern Med. 2014;19(1):68–83.
3. Reinwald S, Akabas SR, Weaver CM. Whole versus the piecemeal approach to evaluating soy. J Nutr. 2010;140(12):2335S–43.
4. Liu RH. Potential synergy of phytochemicals in cancer prevention: mechanism of action. J Nutr. 2004;134(12 Suppl):3479S–85.
5. van de Rest O, Berendsen AA, Haveman-Nies A, de Groot LC. Dietary patterns, cognitive decline, and dementia: a systematic review. Adv Nutr. 2015;6(2):154–68.
6. Lu B, Li M, Yin R. Phytochemical content, health benefits, and toxicology of common edible flowers: a review (2000–2015). Crit Rev Food Sci Nutr. 2015 Oct 13:0. [Epub ahead of print] PubMed PMID: 26462418.
7. Hayat K, Iqbal H, Malik U, Bilal U, Mushtaq S. Tea and its consumption: benefits and risks. Crit Rev Food Sci Nutr. 2015;55(7):939–54.
8. Greiner AK, Papineni RV, Umar S. Chemoprevention in gastrointestinal physiology and disease. Natural products and microbiome. Am J Physiol Gastrointest Liver Physiol. 2014 Jul 1;307(1):G1–15.
9. Rebello CJ, Greenway FL, Finley JW. A review of the nutritional value of legumes and their effects on obesity and its related co-morbidities. Obes Rev. 2014;15(5):392–407.
10. Ford NA, Lashinger LM, Allott EH, Hursting SD. Mechanistic targets and phytochemical strategies for breaking the obesity-cancer link. Front Oncol. 2013;3:209.
11. Leiherer A, Mündlein A, Drexel H. Phytochemicals and their impact on adipose tissue inflammation and diabetes. Vascul Pharmacol. 2013;58(1–2):3–20.
12. Vasudeva N, Yadav N, Sharma SK. Natural products: a safest approach for obesity. Chin J Integr Med. 2012 Jun;18(6):473–80.
13. Slavin JL, Lloyd B. Health benefits of fruits and vegetables. Adv Nutr. 2012;3(4):506–16.
14. Boeing H, Bechthold A, Bub A, Ellinger S, Haller D, Kroke A, Leschik-Bonnet E, Müller MJ, Oberritter H, Schulze M, Stehle P, Watzl B. Critical review: vegetables and fruit in the prevention of chronic diseases. Eur J Nutr. 2012;51(6):637–63.
15. Lattimer JM, Haub MD. Effects of dietary fiber and its components on metabolic health. Nutrients. 2010;2(12):1266–89.
16. Andersen C, Rayalam S, Della-Fera MA, Baile CA. Phytochemicals and adipogenesis. Biofactors. 2010;36(6):415–22.
17. McCullough ML, Giovannucci EL. Diet and cancer prevention. Oncogene. 2004;23(38):6349–64.
18. Duncan AM. The role of nutrition in the prevention of breast cancer. AACN Clin Issues. 2004;15(1):119–35.
19. Slavin J. Why whole grains are protective: biological mechanisms. Proc Nutr Soc. 2003;62(1):129–34.
20. Bloch AS. Nutrition for health promotion: phytochemicals, functional foods, and alternative approaches to combat obesity. Dent Clin North Am. 2003;47(2):411–23, viii-ix.

21. Matarese LE, Pories WJ. Adult weight loss diets: metabolic effects and outcomes. Nutr Clin Pract. 2014;29(6):759–67.
22. Kaissi AA, Begun JW. Fads, fashions, and bandwagons in health care strategy. Health Care Manage Rev. 2008;33(2):94–102.
23. Best D, Grainger P. Low-fat or low-carbohydrate diet for cardiovascular health. Can J Cardiovasc Nurs. 2007;17(3):19–26.
24. Volpe SL. Popular weight reduction diets. J Cardiovasc Nurs. 2006;21(1):34–9. Review.
25. Middaugh DJ. Low carb management. Medsurg Nurs. 2005;14(5):348–50.
26. Judge BS, Eisenga BH. Disorders of fuel metabolism: medical complications associated with starvation, eating disorders, dietary fads, and supplements. Emerg Med Clin North Am. 2005;23(3):789–813, ix.
27. Balart LA. Diet options of obesity: fad or famous? Gastroenterol Clin North Am. 2005;34(1):83–90.
28. Cash A, Knehans AW. Low-carbohydrate diets: what should we recommend? J Okla State Med Assoc. 2004;97(10):412–5; quiz 416–7.
29. Baron M. Fighting obesity Part 1: Review of popular low-carb diets. Health Care Food Nutr Focus. 2004;21(10):1,3–6, 11.
30. Halton TL, Hu FB. The effects of high protein diets on thermogenesis, satiety and weight loss: a critical review. J Am Coll Nutr. 2004;23(5):373–85.
31. Acheson KJ. Carbohydrate and weight control: where do we stand? Curr Opin Clin Nutr Metab Care. 2004;7(4):485–92.
32. Roberts DC. Quick weight loss: sorting fad from fact. Med J Aust. 2001;175(11–12):637–40.
33. Moloney M. Dietary treatments of obesity. Proc Nutr Soc. 2000;59(4):601–8.
34. Mishkin B, Mishkin S. Dietary fads and gut mysteries versus nutrition with a grain of common sense. Can J Gastroenterol. 1997;11(4):371–5.
35. Katan MB. Forever fiber. Nutr Rev. 1996;54(8):253–4.
36. Diliberti N, Bordi PL, Conklin MT, Roe LS, Rolls BJ. Increased portion size leads to increased energy intake in a restaurant meal. Obes Res. 2004;12(3):562–8.
37. Bates KJ, Byker Shanks C. Placement of a take-out container during meal influences energy intake. Eat Behav. 2015;19:181–83.
38. Abidin NZ, Mamat M, Dangerfield B, Zulkepli JH, Baten MA, Wibowo A. Combating obesity through healthy eating behavior: a call for system dynamics optimization. PLoS One. 2014;9(12):e114135.
39. Dominguez LJ, Bes-Rastrollo M, Basterra-Gortari FJ, Gea A, Barbagallo M, Martínez-González MA. Association of a dietary Score with incident type 2 diabetes: The Dietary-Based Diabetes-Risk Score (DDS). PLoS One. 2015;10(11):e0141760.
40. Anand SS, Hawkes C, de Souza RJ, Mente A, Dehghan M, Nugent R, Zulyniak MA, Weis T, Bernstein AM, Krauss RM, Kromhout D, Jenkins DJ, Malik V, Martinez-Gonzalez MA, Mozaffarian D, Yusuf S, Willett WC, Popkin BM. Food consumption and its impact on cardiovascular disease: importance of solutions focused on the globalized food system: a report from the workshop convened by the world heart federation. J Am Coll Cardiol. 2015;66(14):1590–614.
41. Rodríguez-Monforte M, Flores-Mateo G, Sánchez E. Dietary patterns and CVD: a systematic review and meta-analysis of observational studies. Br J Nutr. 2015;114(9):1341–59.
42. Andreyeva T, Tripp AS, Schwartz MB. Dietary quality of americans by supplemental nutrition assistance program participation status: a systematic review. Am J Prev Med. 2015;49(4):594–604.
43. Sabaté J, Wien M. A perspective on vegetarian dietary patterns and risk of metabolic syndrome. Br J Nutr. 2015;113 Suppl 2:S136–43.
44. Ríos-Hoyo A, Cortés MJ, Ríos-Ontiveros H, Meaney E, Ceballos G, Gutiérrez-Salmeán G. Obesity, metabolic syndrome, and dietary therapeutical approaches with a special focus on nutraceuticals (Polyphenols): a mini-review. Int J Vitam Nutr Res. 2014;84(3–4):113–23.
45. Shen J, Wilmot KA, Ghasemzadeh N, Molloy DL, Burkman G, Mekonnen G, Gongora MC, Quyyumi AA, Sperling LS. Mediterranean dietary patterns and cardiovascular health. Annu Rev Nutr. 2015;35:425–49.
46. 8: Liese AD, Krebs-Smith SM, Subar AF, George SM, Harmon BE, Neuhouser ML, Boushey CJ, Schap TE, Reedy J. The dietary patterns methods project: synthesis of findings across cohorts and relevance to dietary guidance. J Nutr. 2015;145(3):393–402.
47. Schwingshackl L, Hoffmann G. Diet quality as assessed by the healthy eating index, the alternate healthy eating index, the dietary approaches to stop hypertension score, and health outcomes: a systematic review and meta-analysis of cohort studies. J Acad Nutr Diet. 2015;115(5):780–800:e5.
48. Frazier-Wood AC. Dietary patterns, genes, and health: challenges and obstacles to be overcome. Curr Nutr Rep. 2015;4:82–7.
49. Doll R, Peto R. The causes of cancer: quantitative estimates of avoidable risks of cancer in the United States today. J Natl Cancer Inst. 1981;66(6):1191–308.

50. National Academy of Science. Diet, Nutrition and Cancer. Washington, DC: National Academy Press; 1982.
51. World Cancer Research Fund and American Institute for Cancer Research. Food, nutrition and the prevention of cancer: a global perspective. Washington, DC: American Institute for Cancer Research; 1997.
52. World Cancer Research Fund. Food, nutrition, and the prevention of cancer: a global perspective. Washington, DC: AICR; 2007.
53. http://www.aicr.org/continuous-update-project/. Accessed on 14 Nov 2015.
54. U.S. Department of Agriculture. Scientific Report of the 2015 Dietary Guidelines Advisory Committee to the Secretary of Agriculture and the Secretary of Health and Human Services. http://health.gov/dietaryguidelines/2015-scientific-report. Accessed on 15 Aug 2015.
55. https://global.arizona.edu/study-abroad/program/mediterranean-diet-and-health. Accessed on 14 Nov 14 2015.

Preface

Death incidence attributable to chronic diseases is projected to increase due to the growing and aging population. The rampant increase in the prevalence of overweight and obesity in the USA and other world populations has been attributed to a combination of dietary, socioeconomic, and behavioral causes. These include an imbalance between dietary recommendations and behavior combined with an increasingly sedentary lifestyle. To reduce the burden of chronic diseases, various dietary guidelines are being released by health organizations in the USA and around the world to promote a rebalancing of calories and more physical activity. International efforts are underway to formulate dietary recommendations that prevent chronic diseases and improve quality of life. Unfortunately, socioeconomic constraints contribute to the paradoxical coexistence of noncommunicable diseases with food insecurity.

Various dietary guidelines and patterns emphasize the importance of variety, proportionality, and moderation in food selections. These include the *Mediterranean diet* which, in 2013, was inscribed by UNESCO in the Representative List of the Intangible Cultural Heritage of Humanity. In 2015, the Scientific Report of the Dietary Guidelines for Americans to the US Department of Human Health Services Department of Agriculture recommended the Mediterranean-style pattern among those dietary patterns associated with health promotion. The impetus for developing this volume stems from the wealth of research evidence suggesting that dietary habits and lifestyle characteristic of the Mediterranean region may offer protection against chronic diseases and improve longevity. Contributors have summarized the most up-to-date research evidence related to foods and dietary behaviors that contribute to a healthy Mediterranean diet and lifestyle, the biochemical mechanisms through which bioactive compounds usually found in Mediterranean foods impact on biological processes associated with disease, and opportunities and challenges for implementing a Mediterranean-like dietary pattern in developed and emerging economies. Twenty chapters were assembled by world-renowned experts who conducted a systematic review of the relevant literature and provided an assessment of chronic disease prevention opportunities using diet and food components characteristic of the Mediterranean region. The tone of this text is to establish a "proof of principle" about the importance of the Mediterranean diet and lifestyle approach for disease prevention. The editors regret that because of space limitations not all areas of research related to the Mediterranean diet and lifestyle could be adequately addressed, and acknowledge that geographical differences around the world impose limitations in the choice of foods and dietary customs.

This volume has been organized into five parts to aid in the assimilation of the materials provided. *Part I, Mediterranean Diet and Lifestyle in a World Context*, introduces the challenges and opportunities for maintaining or adopting a Mediterranean-like diet and lifestyle. Emphasis is placed on the realization that sustainability of natural resources is intimately related to agricultural production, food supply, and availability, which in turn impact on dietary behavior and disease risk. Adoption of Mediterranean dietary patterns and lifestyles that have been traditionally associated with reduced incidence of chronic diseases is recommended. Implementation of a Mediterranean-like diet and lifestyle may benefit populations residing in the USA and abroad. Major challenges include globalization of food supplies, food insecurity, and socioeconomic constraints that limit access to healthier foods, affordable education, and medical care.

Part II, Historical, Behavioral, and Geographical Perspective on the Mediterranean Diet and Lifestyle, addresses the historical and behavioral origins of the Mediterranean diet, regional differences in dietary profiles, and the evolution of traditional Mediterranean diet into modern dietary guidelines. The traditional Mediterranean diet reflects the interactions of diverse populations and civilizations that have occupied the Mediterranean basin over thousands of years. In modern times, specific indexes to measure adherence to Mediterranean dietary patterns and their impact on health status have been developed. A key concept that emerges from this section is that food consumption in Mediterranean countries is a cultural element that goes beyond the need to satisfy nutrition needs. Nevertheless, concerns have mounted that modern diet and lifestyle continue to depart from the traditional Mediterranean "Genius loci" as a result of globalization and technological modifications leading to drastic changes in food behavior and increased susceptibility to chronic diseases.

Part III presents evidence of the benefits of the *Mediterranean Diet and Lifestyle for Health Promotion.* In addition to olive oil, which is the main source of fats in the Mediterranean region, this section presents other sources of fats that contribute to the overall profile of fatty acids found in the Mediterranean diet. Authors highlight that micronutrients and microconstituents with antioxidant and other properties are common in vegetable oils used in Mediterranean households. These bioactive compounds protect fatty acids from oxidation and are potentially important for reducing chronic disease risk. Olive oil is convincingly recognized as a food that reduces the risk of cardiovascular diseases, and possibly, certain cancers and neurodegenerative disorders. Research evidence is also presented suggesting that the Mediterranean diet decreases inflammatory parameters and risk of mortality. In Chap. 8, the authors conclude that the coordinated actions of phenolic compounds found in red wine and alcohol exert various health effects including a reduced risk of atherosclerosis. Regular and moderate consumption of red wine, 1–2 drinks a day with meals, is recommended. However, sound clinical judgment is needed to determine if alcohol consumption is appropriate based on age, medical history, gender, and predisposition to dependency. No more than one glass of wine/day is recommended for women and two glasses of wine/day for men. Metabolic syndrome has been recognized as a health concern and clinical challenge. There is general agreement that clinical parameters associated with metabolic syndrome can be greatly improved through adoption of lifestyle and dietary changes characteristic of the Mediterranean diet pattern. For example, research evidence from Mediterranean studies suggested a positive correlation between adherence to diets low in saturated fat, trans-fat, cholesterol, added sugar, and sodium; and high in unsaturated fats, complex unrefined carbohydrates, fruits, vegetables, and fish, with improvement of metabolic abnormalities. Unequivocally, these are dietary features typical of the traditional Mediterranean diet. The adoption of metabolomic approaches may offer new opportunities to monitor the health impact of individual food components and Mediterranean-like diets on metabolic syndrome and chronic disease risk.

Part IV, Aging and Cancer Risk, gives attention to the fact that the Mediterranean diet relies heavily on components such as fruits, vegetables, whole grains, unsaturated fatty acids, and lean meats and offers a regimen of nutrient-dense foods that provide viable, healthy and gradual weight loss while reducing a number of chronic health conditions that are so prevalent in the aging population. Of these, cognitive decline, dementia, and Alzheimer's and Parkinson's disease are age-related conditions that affect mature adults worldwide. Risk factors for cognitive diseases include hypercholesterolemia, obesity, diabetes, and cardiovascular factors, such as hypertension and inflammation. Studies suggest that the Mediterranean diet pattern may be beneficial for preventing and/or attenuating biological processes associated with cognitive impairment. Research data on extra virgin olive oil, the main source of saturated fat in the Mediterranean diet, suggest protective effects of olive oil components on markers of neurodegenerative diseases. Mediterranean-like diet and lifestyle are discussed as options to improve brain mitochondrial functions and for treatment of cognitive impairment and neurodegeneration. Turning to causes impacting cancer death, breast cancer remains the most commonly diagnosed malignancy in women. Epidemiological studies generally recognize the modifying role of diet on breast cancer risk. A Mediterranean dietary pattern and diets high in vegetables, fruit, and fish are associated with a decreased risk of breast cancer. With respect to malignancies of the gastrointestinal tract, mortality rates related to colorectal cancer (CRC) have been declining due to advances in screening and diagnostic technologies. However, CRC remains the third most common cancer diagnosis and fourth leading cause of cancer-related mortality worldwide. Inflammatory bowel diseases (IBD) have been linked to increased risk of CRC. In general, adherence to the Mediterranean dietary pattern has been associated with a decreased risk of IBD and CRC. Mediterranean bioactive food components that modify disease risk include those that affect epigenetic mechanisms and regulate gene expression. Understanding how dietary factors and dietary patterns participate in the regulation of gene expression through epigenetics is a complex task given the wide range of available food choices, diversity of nutrient intakes, individual differences in genetic backgrounds, and intestinal environments where foods are metabolized. Likely, major advances in disease prevention will stem from characterizing the role of numerous enzymes, protein complexes, and factors that participate in epigenetic regulation.

Part V, Building a Mediterranean-like Pyramid, attempts to translate into practice the research concepts presented in the introductory and health promotion chapters. The health benefits of physical activity are undisputed. Regular physical activity mitigates or reverses risk factors commonly associated with chronic diseases including impaired glucose metabolism, dyslipidemia, and low-grade inflammation. Population-based studies document reductions on the order of 30 % or more for incident chronic diseases in active individuals compared to their inactive peers. Physical activity has been associated with improved diet quality and with Mediterranean-like eating patterns in both men and women. This section highlights the need for conservation and improvement of biodiversity to protect and promote in modern era two of the foundational components of the Mediterranean pyramid: biodiversity and conviviality. However, a major challenge remains the implementation of strategies that help populations to transition from dietary practices associated with higher rates of obesity and diabetes to healthier ones. Achieving adherence to healthy eating will require major changes in food behavior and lifestyle. To this end, large-scale efforts are needed involving the coordinated participation of the food and restaurant industries working in collaboration with public health communities and consumers. Overall, the Mediterranean diet emerges as a viable dietary tool to help Americans and other communities around the world to reduce the burden of chronic diseases. However, to make the most of this health promotion opportunity, all stakeholders should participate in a concerted effort and commit to these dietary and lifestyle changes with dispatch.

Chapter 19 presents a compilation of selected recipes from the Mediterranean region. For each recipe, detailed information on the ingredients, quantities, and preparation is presented based on the instructional material developed by the editors for the Mediterranean Diet and Health Study Abroad Program sponsored by the University of Arizona. Recipes are not provided as a medical recommendation, but as examples of dishes that can be prepared without specific culinary training. The closing chapter (Chap. 20) presents estimates of nutrient composition for all recipes discussed in Chap. 19, and their inclusion into a weekly food program using dietary guidelines developed by the Prevención con Dieta Mediterránea (PREDIMED) study to assess adherence to a Mediterranean-like diet. In general, Mediterranean recipes and foods organized into a weekly food pyramid help to meet the requirements for target dietary reference intakes including energy and macronutrients (fat, carbohydrate, protein, and fiber) and for selected minerals (calcium, sodium, and potassium). In the Mediterranean diet, a major contributor to total energy is monounsaturated fatty acids from olive oil and nuts. In this context, concerns have emerged about the quality of olive oil commercially available. For example, in the USA, imported extra virgin olive oil often fails international and US qualitative standards. This suggests that regulatory efforts are needed to inform the consumer about the quality of commercially available olive oil based on standard chemical and biological parameters. Depending on dietary behavior, daily requirements for vitamin D may not be easily met through foods and recipes only.

Thus, endogenous production via skin exposure to sun and/or dietary supplementation may be necessary to achieve minimum vitamin D goals. Strategies useful to alleviate inadequacies in vitamin D include the intake (≥3 times/week) of certain fish-based recipes, adequate sun exposure, and possibly supplemental doses. The usefulness of recipes and food pyramids in meeting nutrient requirements is clearly influenced by physical activity, body weight, height, gender, and age. Nevertheless, great opportunities exist for balancing our plates through adoption of a Mediterranean-like approach.

At the time of the publication of this volume, the US Department of Human and Health Services (HHS) and US Department of Agriculture (USDA) released the 2015–2020 Dietary Guidelines for Americans. As mentioned in various chapters in this volume, the intent of the US Dietary Guidelines for Americans is to translate into practice nutrition recommendations to prevent the incidence and/or reduce the burden of chronic diseases. Given the increased prevalence of overweight, obesity, and diabetes during the last two decades in the USA and other developed countries, and association of these conditions with food insecurity, the timely release of the 2015 Dietary Guidelines is a new opportunity to translate advancements in science into policies that promote health through nutrition. The publication of the Dietary Guidelines followed the submission of recommendations by the 2015 Dietary Guidelines Advisory Committee, which was composed of health and nutrition experts. Reference to these recommendations and a list of areas of investigations and research needs can be found in Chap. 2 and Table 2.1. In general, the Advisory Committee made recommendations for increasing consumption of fruits, vegetables, and whole grains and reducing intake of calories, saturated fat, sodium, refined grains, and added sugars. Moreover, underconsumption of vitamin D, calcium, potassium, and fiber was identified as a public concern for the majority of the US population. Importantly, the 2015 Dietary Guidelines Advisory Committee suggested that sufficient research data were available to model certain dietary patterns, including the Healthy Mediterranean-Style Pattern, and examine their nutritional adequacy. Detailed information about the 2015–2020 Dietary Guidelines for Americans can be found in the Appendix of this volume.

Tucson, AZ, USA

Donato F. Romagnolo, Ph.D., M.Sc.
Ornella I. Selmin, Ph.D.

Series Editor Page

The great success of the *Nutrition and Health Series* is the result of the consistent overriding mission of providing health professionals with texts that are essential because each includes (1) a synthesis of the state of the science; (2) timely in-depth reviews by the leading researchers and clinicians in their respective fields; (3) extensive, up-to-date fully annotated reference lists; (4) a detailed index; (5) relevant tables and figures; (6) identification of paradigm shifts and the consequences; (7) virtually no overlap of information between chapters, but targeted, interchapter referrals; (8) suggestions of areas for future research; and (9) balanced, data-driven answers to patient as well as health professional questions which are based upon the totality of evidence rather than the findings of any single study.

The series volumes are not the outcome of a symposium. Rather, each editor has the potential to examine a chosen area with a broad perspective, both in subject matter and in the choice of chapter authors. The international perspective, especially with regard to public health initiatives, is emphasized where appropriate. The editors, whose trainings are both research and practice oriented, have the opportunity to develop a primary objective for their book, define the scope and focus, and then invite the leading authorities from around the world to be part of their initiative. The authors are encouraged to provide an overview of the field, discuss their own research, and relate the research findings to potential human health consequences. Because each book is developed de novo, the chapters are coordinated so that the resulting volume imparts greater knowledge than the sum of the information contained in the individual chapters.

Mediterranean Diet: Dietary Guidelines and Impact on Health and Disease edited by Donato F. Romagnolo and Ornella Selmin is a very welcome and timely addition to the *Nutrition and Health Series* and fully exemplifies the series' goals. There has been an explosion of clinical research over the last two decades on the associations between the consumption of the Mediterranean diet and reduced risk of several age-related chronic diseases, and these studies alone warrant the development of this 20-chapter tome. However, the volume also includes reviews of the newer indications such as reduced risk of developing allergies in younger aged populations. This unique volume represents the first text to provide an integrated review of the historical basis of this healthful diet, its metabolism, and role in multiple aspects of human health and disease prevention and even treatment. The volume also includes key practice-oriented chapters that provide guidance in the development of the Mediterranean diet pyramid as well as highly relevant recipes and diet plans. The reader is presented with balanced, data-driven discussions of the beneficial effects of the nutrient content of this diet that is also helpful in preventing common nutritional deficiencies such as zinc deficiency. The volume is designed as an important resource for nutritionists and dietitians, research and public health scientists, cardiologists, gastroenterologists, and related physicians and healthcare professionals who interact with clients, patients, and/or family members. The volume provides objective, relevant information for professors and lecturers, advanced undergraduates and graduates, researchers, and clinical investigators who require extensive, up-to-date literature reviews, instructive tables and figures, and excellent references on all aspects of the importance of the Mediterranean diet's role in human health and disease.

The editors of this volume are experts in their respective fields. Donato F. Romagnolo, Ph.D., MSc., is a professor of Nutritional and Cancer Biology and member of the Arizona Cancer and the Toxicology Centers, the BIO5 Institute, and the Southwest Environmental Health Sciences Center at the University of Arizona. He is currently a member of the Executive Committees for the Nutritional Sciences and Cancer Biology Graduate Programs at the University of Arizona. He has served as member and chair for the Advisory Board of the Environmental Gene Expression Group of the Southwest Environmental Health Sciences Center; chair for the Research Frontiers in Nutritional Sciences Conference, Department of Nutritional Sciences; and member and chair of the Internal Advisory Committee for Native American Cancer Prevention Program at the University of Arizona. Dr. Romagnolo is an instructor for undergraduate nutritional biology and graduate metabolic integration at the University of Arizona. As a director and instructor of the Mediterranean Diet and Health Study Abroad Program, Global Studies, at the University of Arizona, he promotes the study of the Mediterranean diet and food compounds for the prevention of chronic diseases. Dr. Romagnolo earned an M.S. and a Ph.D. from Virginia Polytechnic Institute and State University and a B.S. from the University of Padua, Padua, Italy. He has held professional positions as nutritionist for agricultural organizations in Italy and as research manager and consultant for private food industries. He was a postdoctoral fellow at the National Institutes of Environmental Health Sciences, National Institutes of Health. Dr. Romagnolo is a member of several professional organizations, including the American Society for Nutrition and the American Association for Cancer Research. He has published book chapters, monographs, and original research in cancer and nutrition-related scientific journals including *Cancer Research, The Journal of Nutrition, Nutrition and Cancer, Breast Cancer Research, Molecular Carcinogenesis, Environmental and Molecular Mutagenesis, Neoplasia*, and *Experimental Biology and Medicine*. He is a member of the *Journal of Biochemistry Editorial Board*. Dr. Romagnolo has been a member of scientific review panels and received research funding from the National Institutes of Health, the US Department of Breast Cancer Research Program, and the Susan G. Komen Breast Cancer Foundation, the American Institute for Cancer Research, and the Arizona Biomedical Research Commission. In his current position, he promotes research that deals with the role of dietary xenobiotics and natural bioactive compounds as epigenetic regulators of expression of genes involved in cancer and inflammation. Current research focuses primarily on the role of environmental and dietary compounds on epigenetic regulation of breast cancer tumor suppressor and proinflammatory genes and prevention of breast and colorectal tumorigenesis by dietary compounds including those commonly found in the Mediterranean diet. Dr. Romagnolo has coedited with John Milner a volume entitled *Bioactive Compounds and Cancer* that is also part of the *Nutrition and Health Series* published by Springer/Humana Press. Ornella Selmin, Ph.D., is a research associate professor of Nutritional Sciences at the University of Arizona. She is a member and laboratory director at the University of Arizona Cancer Center. Dr. Selmin is a member of the BIO5 Institute and Center for Toxicology at the University of Arizona. She has served as a research grant panelist for the National Science Foundation (NSF), the National Institutes of Health (NIH) Integrated Risk Information System Toxicological Review, the Environmental Protection Agency (EPA), Science Advisory Board, American Heart Association, NIEHS/NIH Superfund Program Grant Review Panel, NIH Minority Biomedical Research Grant Review Panel, and the National Center for Environmental Health/Agency for Toxic Substances and Disease Registry. Dr. Selmin has served as Arizona Assurance Program mentor and member of International Science and Engineering Fair Scientific Review Committee at the University of Arizona. She also has served as a member of the Graduate Program in Microbiology at the University of Arizona. Dr. Selmin received a B.S. in biology and a Ph.D. in molecular and cellular biology at the University of Padua, Italy. She has held various professional positions including visiting fellow at the Laboratory of Developmental Biology and Anomalies, NIDR, NIH, Bethesda, MD; research associate, Laboratory of Developmental Biology, VPI & SU, Blacksburg, VA; and visiting associate, Laboratory of Biochemical Risk Analysis, NIEHS, NIH, Research Triangle Park, North Carolina. Dr. Selmin received the Recordati Industries Research Award for Young Scientist and

Walkabout for Biosafety Excellence Award, vice president for Research at the University of Arizona. Dr. Selmin has published in various environmental, nutrition, and cancer-related journals including *Anti-Cancer Agents in Medicinal Chemistry*, *Advances in Nutrition*, *Molecular Carcinogenesis*, *Journal of Nutritional Gerontology and Geriatrics*, *Journal of Nutritional Biochemistry*, *Cardiovascular Toxicology*, *Cancer Epidemiology*, *Biomarkers & Prevention*, *Cancer Research*, and *Journal of Biochemistry*. Dr. Selmin received research funding from the National Institutes of Health, the US Department of Breast Cancer Research Program, and the Arizona Biomedical Research Commission. Dr. Selmin is the co-instructor of the Mediterranean Diet and Health Study Abroad Program, Global Studies, at the University of Arizona. In her current position at the University of Arizona Cancer Center, she promotes research that deals with the role of environmental xenobiotics and natural bioactive compounds as modulator of genes involved in cardiovascular diseases and breast and colorectal cancer.

The 20 chapters in this comprehensive volume are organized in five parts: Mediterranean Diet and Lifestyle in a World Context; Historical, Behavioral and Geographical Perspective on the Mediterranean and Lifestyle; Mediterranean Diet and Lifestyle for Health; Aging and Cancer Risk; and Building a Mediterranean-Like Pyramid.

Part I: Mediterranean Diet and Lifestyle in a World Context

The two introductory chapters in the first part provide readers with a historical perspective as well as the basics of nutritional aspects of the Mediterranean diet and include discussions of the beneficial environmental impact of this diet especially in the light of the reduction in consumption of red meat. The examination of the nutrient density of the diet and enhanced metabolism of cardioprotective diet components provides the basics of energy balance so that the more clinically related chapters can be easily understood. The first chapter reminds us that the Mediterranean diet reflects the cultural, historical, social, territorial, and environmental heritage that has been transmitted from generation to generation for centuries and is intimately linked to the lifestyles of the Mediterranean people throughout their history. The second chapter reviews the major metabolically related diseases and the importance of the Mediterranean diet compared to other dietary plans and reviews of the global recommendations including that of UNESCO in 2013 that included the diet in the Representative List of the Intangible Cultural Heritage of Humanity and also the diet's inclusion in the Scientific Report of the 2015 US Dietary Guidelines.

Part II: Historical, Behavioral, and Geographical Perspective on the Mediterranean Diet and Lifestyle

Part II contains three chapters that continue the examination of many of the culturally related aspects of the Mediterranean diet and lifestyle. We are reminded, in Chap. 3, that today's version of the Mediterranean diet evolved in the region during a succession of dominant civilizations—Egyptian, Hebrew, Phoenician, Greek, Carthaginian, Roman, Arab, Byzantine, Ottoman, and others. These cultures with varied religious food laws introduced different foods, culinary practices, and food traditions throughout the Mediterranean region. There is a comprehensive review of the relevant diet intake studies and the chapter contains 99 references. The fourth chapter examines the traditional Mediterranean diet that is characterized by a plant-based diet containing legumes, whole grains, fruits and vegetables, nuts, and seeds; olive oil is a main source of fat and there is a low intake of saturated fat, a low-to-moderate intake of dairy products, moderate consumption of fish, and low-to-moderate amounts of wine consumed during meals. This dietary pattern is consumed by people in the 22 countries that border the Mediterranean Sea. The differences between diets in these countries are reviewed and the specific foods are discussed. The chapter also includes a description of the scoring systems currently used to determine the adherence to the Mediterranean diet within survey studies as well as for patient care. This volume has several unique chapters, including Chap. 5 that describes the French diet and food habits that are in many ways comparable to the Mediterranean diet. The main characteristics of the French perspective include the use of olive oil, fresh fruits and vegetables, and fish in addition to little snacking between meals, three meals a day that include a mid-day three-course meal, use of raw or no processed foods, home cooking, eating together, and adherence to cultural foods with reduced use of fast or junk foods.

Part III: Mediterranean Diet and Lifestyle for Health Promotion

The third part of this comprehensive volume examines in depth the key components of the Mediterranean diet and their health consequences. The first chapter reviews the importance of the fat sources and compares and contrasts the fatty acid composition of different oils. The macro- and micronutrient composition and major food sources of the oils are compiled in eight helpful tables. There is a discussion of argan oil used mainly in Morocco; this oil is becoming more popular throughout the Mediterranean region. The major clinical studies that have looked at the association between the fats consumed in Mediterranean diets and health outcomes are also tabulated. Chapter 7 examines the importance of the anti-inflammatory characteristics of the oils consumed in the Mediterranean diet and reviews the role of inflammation in the development of cardiovascular disease. The use of biomarkers of inflammation, including C-reactive protein as an index of cardiovascular risk, is described. The recent evaluation of the anti-inflammatory aspects of the Mediterranean diet has resulted in an expansion of potentially beneficial indications, including cerebrovascular disease, diabetes, and Alzheimer's disease. Chapter 8 reviews the data linking red wine consumption with reduced risk of cardiovascular disease. The authors also discuss the epidemiological data correlating the beneficial effects of red wine on cardiovascular health. The metabolism of red wine is reviewed and the components of red wine that may be responsible for the cardioprotective effects are tabulated. The mechanisms of actions of red wine components on blood vessels and metabolic homeostasis are examined, and the authors conclude that coordinated actions of phenolic compounds and alcohol exert beneficial effects and reduce the risk of atherosclerosis. The next chapter looks at the growing population that is diagnosed with the metabolic syndrome and its consequences. The authors examine the dietary recommendations for lowering this risk and these mirror the major components of the Mediterranean diet. The key characteristics of the metabolic syndrome including obesity, non-insulin-dependent diabetes, hypertension, and dyslipidemia are each examined. The clinical data and recommendations to implement the Mediterranean diet in individuals at risk for the metabolic syndrome are reviewed. Chapter 10, the final chapter in this part, provides the reader with an overview of the relatively new science of metabolomics and examines its uses for determining some of the health effects of the Mediterranean diet.

We learn that the metabolome is defined as the sum of all low molecular weight metabolites or chemicals present in a cell, organ, tissue, biological fluid, or organism. This complex contains lipids, small peptides, carbohydrates, vitamins, and other cofactors derived from both the metabolism of the host and the symbiotic microbiota, and in humans, there are more than 20,000 metabolites. Metabolomics is the study of all of the effects of an exposure on a human and includes environmental exposure as well as the genetic and epigenetic background of that individual. The chapter includes a discussion of important databases including FooDB, the world's largest and most comprehensive resource on food constituents, chemistry, and biology which is part of the Human Metabolome Database and Phenol-Explorer, a comprehensive database on polyphenol content in foods that provides data on polyphenol metabolism and the effects of food processing and cooking. Since the Mediterranean-style eating pattern is rich in bioactive food components that have diverse health effects, metabolomics profiling is an important strategy to examine the systemic effects of its components. The chapter, containing 124 references, reviews the major dietary components of the Mediterranean diet and the studies that have looked at their metabolic effects on health outcomes including blood pressure and colon cancer.

Part IV: Aging and Cancer Risk

The five chapters in this part include in-depth reviews on obesity seen in the elderly, neurological diseases of aging and two of the major cancers of aging, breast, and colon and a last chapter that examines the epigenetic effects of the Mediterranean diet. Chapter 11 describes the physiological changes seen with aging and compares these to similar changes seen with obesity. In particular, both groups have a shift in body composition with an increase in fat and decrease in muscle. There is a review of studies of weight loss in the older population using traditional Western diets compared to studies using the Mediterranean diet; of importance, there appears to be greater retention of lean body mass with the Mediterranean diet even in the face of greater weight loss. The newest intervention research indicates that the Mediterranean diet with olive oil significantly lowers the risk of diabetes in older individuals in a weight loss study. The next chapter, authored by the book's editors and their son, includes a broad-based discussion of the age-related diseases that affect the brain and the neuromuscular system including Alzheimer's disease and Parkinson's disease, as well as some of the forms of dementia that can result in mild cognitive decline or vascular dementia resulting from ischemic or hemorrhagic brain lesions. The chapter contains clear descriptions of the etiology of these diseases and the nutritional factors that have been associated with increased risk including inflammation and the microbiome. Preliminary survey data strongly suggest that the adherence to a Mediterranean diet over a lifetime significantly reduces the risk of developing cognitive and neurological diseases associated with aging. Chapter 13 describes the current state of the evidence evaluating the role of diet patterns in breast cancer prevention with a focus on the Mediterranean diet. The discussion of the current epidemiological evidence and mechanisms supporting a role of the Mediterranean diet including postulated mechanisms of breast cancer protection provided by the individual components within the diet are presented. There is a review of the data from the Women's Health Initiative Dietary Modification Trial with particular insights as the primary author was a principal investigator in this landmark study. Several of the food components of the Mediterranean diet are examined and the major potential mechanisms of action are reviewed; the chapter contains over 100 targeted references. Chapter 14 is authored by the editors and colleagues and describes in detail the molecular mechanisms by which the components of the Mediterranean diet affect the risk of developing irritable bowel disease (IBD) and/or colorectal cancer. Both the genetic and epigenetic effects of olive oil, red wine, low intakes of red meat and the increased intake of omega-3 fatty acids are reviewed and referenced in over 120 citations. The authors propose that the combination of Mediterranean foods, rather than specific ones or bioactive compounds found in the Mediterranean diet, impacts the gut microbiome and contributes to the maintenance of intestinal health and prevention of inflammation and cancer of the colon. The final chapter in this part, Chap. 15, describes the development of epigenetic changes in DNA that have been linked to a number of chronic diseases of aging including cancer. The chapter emphasizes data on genes that retain epigenetic plasticity or flexibility that enables genes to respond to environmental exposures including dietary patterns and specific nutrients/dietary factors such as those found in the Mediterranean diet pattern. Although the majority of research in this area relies on in vitro studies that follow metabolic pathways, the research has been of great value and future studies in populations are warranted.

Part V: Building a Mediterranean-Like Pyramid

The five chapters in Part V describe the great complexity in developing a Mediterranean diet pyramid that includes all aspects of the Mediterranean lifestyle as the cultural aspects of this lifestyle, food preparation, and freshness may be as critical as the food components. The first chapter in this part, Chap. 16, provides an examination of the role of physical activity in the improved health aspects of the Mediterranean diet. The chapter includes a succinct definition of physical activity that is contrasted with the definition of exercise and then reviews and tabulates the relevant studies. The global as well as biochemical markers of improved lipid status, weight management, and other benefits are reviewed and 100 references are included in this comprehensive chapter. Chapter 17 explores the traditional Mediterranean concept of lifestyle; conviviality of routine meals taken together with family and friends; consumption of many different foods, sometimes labeled as biodiversity; and the importance of all of the cultural aspects in addition to the consumption of the foods associated with the Mediterranean diet. The chapter emphasizes the importance of herbs (presented in a comprehensive table that includes medicinal uses of herbs as well as culinary uses) in the preparation of meals and their biological potential to affect the benefits associated with the Mediterranean diet. The final three chapters in this cutting-edge volume provide unique insights into the implementation of the Mediterranean diet by first comparing this diet program to other widely used diet programs and then delving deeply into individual meals and their preparations. Chapter 18 compares and contrasts several healthy eating patterns including the Dietary Approaches to Stop Hypertension (DASH) dietary pattern, the US Department of Agriculture food pattern (USDAFP), and the Mediterranean Diet Pattern (MDP) and the chapter includes over 140 relevant references. The comparisons are tabulated to demonstrate the areas where these three healthful diets are very similar and some of the differences that could be responsible for some of the benefits seen with the Mediterranean diet compared to the two other diet plans. The chapter examines the changes in eating habits of the more urban populations in the Mediterranean nations and how these changes may adversely affect the beneficial effects ascribed when these nations and their populations were more agrarian. Current dietary patterns may result in nutrient deficiencies including calcium, magnesium, and/or dietary fiber; these are reviewed in this insightful chapter. Chapters 19 and 20, authored by the volume's editors, provide the reader with unique recipes that have full nutrient contents and weekly nutrient intakes using the Mediterranean recipes calculated. The figures provide excellent representations of the visual appeal of these meals. The recipes use key foods and their nutrients that are representative of the Mediterranean diet pyramid developed internationally in 2011. It must be said that the volume editors "walk the walk" and have devoted themselves to sharing their Mediterranean culture, food preparation, and its links to a more healthful lifestyle with their professional colleagues and students and now with the readers of these chapters and the entire volume.

The above description of the volume's 20 chapters attests to the depth of information provided by the 37 highly respected chapter authors, many from Mediterranean countries. Each chapter includes complete definitions of terms with the abbreviations fully defined for the reader and consistent use of terms between chapters. Key features of the comprehensive volume include over 80 detailed tables and informative figures; an extensive, detailed index; and more than 1400 up-to-date references that provide the reader with excellent sources of worthwhile practice-oriented information that will be of great value to health providers as well as graduate and medical students.

In conclusion, *Mediterranean Diet: Dietary Guidelines and Impact on Health and Disease* edited by Donato F. Romagnolo and Ornella Selmin provides health professionals in many areas of research and practice with the most up-to-date, well-referenced volume on the importance of this diet and lifestyle in maintaining the overall health of the individual as well as reducing the risk of certain chronic disease conditions. The volume serves the reader as the benchmark for integrating the complex interrelationships between dietary patterns, physical activity, cultural factors, and the individual nutrients and foods, such as wine, olive oil, herbs and spices, bioactive molecules, and other unique dietary constituents that are involved in the maintenance of the body's metabolic integrity. Moreover, the physiological, genetic, and pathological interactions between the dietary components of the Mediterranean diet and the functioning of the endothelium, vascular system, microbiome, and immune cells are clearly delineated so that students as well as practitioners can better understand the complexities of these interactions. Unique chapters examine the evolution of the Mediterranean diet and contrast this diet with that of other nations and also with dietary guidelines that national bodies have recommended. The final chapters of this valuable volume provide hands-on examples of meals that incorporate the essence of the Mediterranean diet and include the recipes as well as the evaluation of the nutrient content of these meals. The editors are applauded for their efforts to develop the most authoritative and unique resource on the Mediterranean diet and its role in health and disease, and this excellent text is a very welcome addition to the *Nutrition and Health Series*.

Adrianne Bendich, Ph.D., F.A.C.N., F.A.S.N.

About the Series Editor

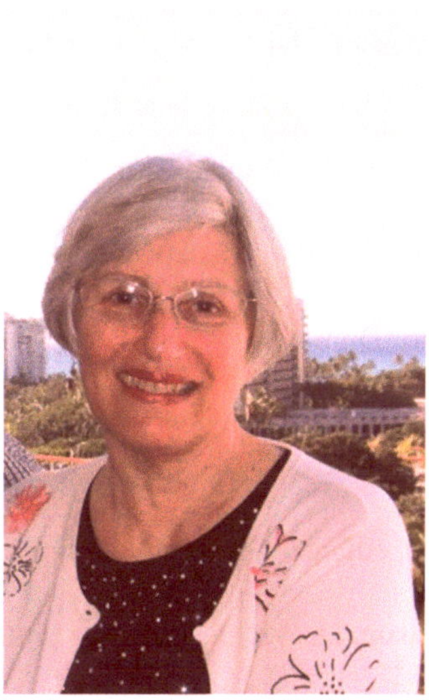

Dr. Adrianne Bendich, Ph.D., F.A.S.N., F.A.C.N., has served as the *Nutrition and Health Series* editor for 20 years and has provided leadership and guidance to more than 200 editors that have developed the 70+ well-respected and highly recommended volumes in the series.

In addition to *Mediterranean Diet: Impact on Health and Disease,* edited by Donato F. Romagnolo and Ornella I. Selmin, major new editions published in 2012–2015 and expected to be published shortly include:

1. *Preventive Nutrition: The Comprehensive Guide For Health Professionals, Fifth Edition,* edited by Adrianne Bendich, Ph.D., and Richard J. Deckelbaum, M.D., 2015
2. *Arginine in Clinical Nutrition*, edited by Rajkumar Rajendram, Vinood Patel, and Victor Preedy, 2016
3. *Beverage Impacts on Health and Nutrition*, *Second Edition*, edited by Ted Wilson, Ph.D., and Norman J. Temple, Ph.D., 2015
4. *Nutrition in Cystic Fibrosis*: *A Guide for Clinicians*, edited by Elizabeth H. Yen, M.D., and Amanda R. Leonard, MPH, RD, CDE, 2015
5. *Glutamine in Clinical Nutrition*, edited by Rajkumar Rajendram, Victor R. Preedy, and Vinood B. Patel, 2015
6. *Nutrition and Bone Health*, *Second Edition*, edited by Michael F. Holick and Jeri W. Nieves, 2015
7. *Branched Chain Amino Acids in Clinical Nutrition*, *Volume 2*, edited by Rajkumar Rajendram, Victor R. Preedy and Vinood B. Patel, 2015
8. *Branched Chain Amino Acids in Clinical Nutrition*, *Volume 1*, edited by Rajkumar Rajendram, Victor R. Preedy, and Vinood B. Patel, 2015
9. *Fructose*, *High Fructose Corn Syrup*, *Sucrose and Health*, edited by James M. Rippe, 2014
10. *Handbook of Clinical Nutrition and Aging*, *Third Edition*, edited by Connie Watkins Bales, Julie L. Locher, and Edward Saltzman, 2014
11. *Nutrition and Pediatric Pulmonary Disease*, edited by Dr. Youngran Chung and Dr. Robert Dumont, 2014
12. *Integrative Weight Management*, edited by Dr. Gerald E. Mullin, Dr. Lawrence J. Cheskin, and Dr. Laura E. Matarese, 2014
13. *Nutrition in Kidney Disease*, *Second Edition*, edited by Dr. Laura D. Byham-Gray, Dr. Jerrilynn D. Burrowes, and Dr. Glenn M. Chertow, 2014

14. *Handbook of Food Fortification and Health, Volume I*, edited by Dr. Victor R. Preedy, Dr. Rajaventhan Srirajaskanthan, and Dr. Vinood B. Patel, 2013
15. *Handbook of Food Fortification and Health, Volume II*, edited by Dr. Victor R. Preedy, Dr. Rajaventhan Srirajaskanthan, and Dr. Vinood B. Patel, 2013
16. *Diet Quality: An Evidence-Based Approach, Volume I*, edited by Dr. Victor R. Preedy, Dr. Lan-Anh Hunter, and Dr. Vinood B. Patel, 2013
17. *Diet Quality: An Evidence-Based Approach, Volume II*, edited by Dr. Victor R. Preedy, Dr. Lan-Anh Hunter, and Dr. Vinood B. Patel, 2013
18. *The Handbook of Clinical Nutrition and Stroke*, edited by Mandy L. Corrigan, MPH, RD; Arlene A. Escuro, MS, RD; and Donald F. Kirby, MD, FACP, FACN, FACG, 2013
19. *Nutrition in Infancy, Volume I*, edited by Dr. Ronald Ross Watson, Dr. George Grimble, Dr. Victor Preedy, and Dr. Sherma Zibadi, 2013
20. *Nutrition in Infancy, Volume II*, edited by Dr. Ronald Ross Watson, Dr. George Grimble, Dr. Victor Preedy, and Dr. Sherma Zibadi, 2013
21. *Carotenoids and Human Health*, edited by Dr. Sherry A. Tanumihardjo, 2013
22. *Bioactive Dietary Factors and Plant Extracts in Dermatology*, edited by Dr. Ronald Ross Watson and Dr. Sherma Zibadi, 2013
23. *Omega 6/3 Fatty Acids*, edited by Dr. Fabien De Meester, Dr. Ronald Ross Watson, and Dr. Sherma Zibadi, 2013
24. *Nutrition in Pediatric Pulmonary Disease*, edited by Dr. Robert Dumont and Dr. Youngran Chung, 2013
25. *Magnesium and Health*, edited by Dr. Ronald Ross Watson and Dr. Victor R. Preedy, 2012
26. *Alcohol, Nutrition and Health Consequences*, edited by Dr. Ronald Ross Watson, Dr. Victor R. Preedy, and Dr. Sherma Zibadi, 2012
27. *Nutritional Health, Strategies for Disease Prevention, Third Edition*, edited by Norman J. Temple, Ted Wilson, and David R. Jacobs, Jr., 2012
28. *Chocolate in Health and Nutrition*, edited by Dr. Ronald Ross Watson, Dr. Victor R. Preedy, and Dr. Sherma Zibadi, 2012
29. *Iron Physiology and Pathophysiology in Humans*, edited by Dr. Gregory J. Anderson and Dr. Gordon D. McLaren, 2012

Earlier books included *Vitamin D, Second Edition*, edited by Dr. Michael Holick; *Dietary Components and Immune Function*, edited by Dr. Ronald Ross Watson, Dr. Sherma Zibadi, and Dr. Victor R. Preedy; *Bioactive Compounds and Cancer*, edited by Dr. John A. Milner and Dr. Donato F. Romagnolo; *Modern Dietary Fat Intakes in Disease Promotion*, edited by Dr. Fabien De Meester, Dr. Sherma Zibadi, and Dr. Ronald Ross Watson; *Iron Deficiency and Overload*, edited by Dr. Shlomo Yehuda and Dr. David Mostofsky; *Nutrition Guide for Physicians*, edited by Dr. Edward Wilson, Dr. George A. Bray, Dr. Norman Temple, and Dr. Mary Struble; *Nutrition and Metabolism*, edited by Dr. Christos Mantzoros; and *Fluid and Electrolytes in Pediatrics*, edited by Leonard Feld and Dr. Frederick Kaskel. Recent volumes include *Handbook of Drug-Nutrient Interactions* edited by Dr. Joseph Boullata and Dr. Vincent Armenti; *Probiotics in Pediatric Medicine* edited by Dr. Sonia Michail and Dr. Philip Sherman; *Handbook of Nutrition and Pregnancy* edited by Dr. Carol Lammi-Keefe, Dr. Sarah Couch, and Dr. Elliot Philipson; *Nutrition and Rheumatic Disease* edited by Dr. Laura Coleman; *Nutrition and Kidney Disease* edited by Dr. Laura Byham-Gray, Dr. Jerrilynn Burrowes, and Dr. Glenn Chertow; *Nutrition and Health in Developing Countries* edited by Dr. Richard Semba and Dr. Martin Bloem; *Calcium in Human Health* edited by Dr. Robert Heaney and Dr. Connie Weaver; and *Nutrition and Bone Health* edited by Dr. Michael Holick and Dr. Bess Dawson-Hughes.

Dr. Bendich is a president of Consultants in Consumer Healthcare LLC and is the editor of ten books including *Preventive Nutrition: The Comprehensive Guide for Health Professionals, Fifth Edition,* coedited with Dr. Richard Deckelbaum (www.springer.com/series/7659). Dr. Bendich serves on the Editorial Boards of the *Journal of Nutrition in Gerontology and Geriatrics, Antioxidants*, and has served as an associate editor for *Nutrition*, the international journal; on the Editorial Board of the *Journal of Women's Health and Gender-Based Medicine*; and on the Board of Directors of the American College of Nutrition.

Dr. Bendich was a director of Medical Affairs at GlaxoSmithKline (GSK) Consumer Healthcare and provided medical leadership for many well-known brands including TUMS and Os-Cal. Dr. Bendich had primary responsibility for GSK's support for the Women's Health Initiative (WHI) intervention study. Prior to joining GSK, Dr. Bendich was at Roche Vitamins Inc. and was involved with the groundbreaking clinical studies showing that folic acid-containing multivitamins significantly reduced major classes of birth defects. Dr. Bendich has coauthored over 100 major clinical research studies in the area of preventive nutrition. She is recognized as a leading authority on antioxidants, nutrition and immunity and pregnancy outcomes, vitamin safety, and the cost-effectiveness of vitamin/mineral supplementation.

Dr. Bendich, who received the Roche Research Award, is a *Tribute to Women and Industry* Awardee and was a recipient of the Burroughs Wellcome Visiting Professorship in Basic Medical Sciences. Dr. Bendich was given the Council for Responsible Nutrition (CRN) Apple Award in recognition of her many contributions to the scientific understanding of dietary supplements. In 2012, she was recognized for her contributions to the field of clinical nutrition by the American Society for Nutrition and was elected a fellow of ASN. Dr Bendich is an adjunct professor at Rutgers University. She is listed in Who's Who in American Women.

About the Editors

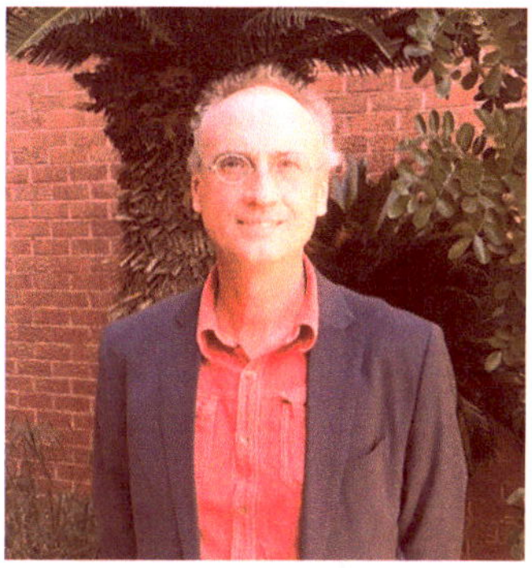

Donato F. Romagnolo, Ph.D., M.Sc., is a professor of Nutritional and Cancer Biology and member of the Arizona Cancer and the Toxicology Centers, the BIO5 Institute, and the Southwest Environmental Health Sciences Center at the University of Arizona. He is currently a member of the Executive Committees for the Nutritional Sciences and Cancer Biology Graduate Programs at the University of Arizona. He has served as a member and chair for the Advisory Board of the Environmental Gene Expression Group of the Southwest Environmental Health Sciences Center; chair for the Research Frontiers in Nutritional Sciences Conference, Department of Nutritional Sciences; and member and chair of the Internal Advisory Committee for Native American Cancer Prevention Program at the University of Arizona. Dr. Romagnolo is an instructor for undergraduate nutritional biology and graduate metabolic integration at the University of Arizona. As a director and instructor of the Mediterranean Diet and Health Study Abroad Program, Global Studies, at the University of Arizona, he promotes the study of Mediterranean diet and food compounds for the prevention of chronic diseases. Dr. Romagnolo earned an M.S. and a Ph.D. from Virginia Polytechnic Institute and State University and a B.S. from the University of Padua, Padua, Italy. He has held professional positions as nutritionist for agricultural organizations in Italy and as research manager and consultant for private food industries. He was a postdoctoral fellow at the National Institutes of Environmental Health Sciences, National Institutes of Health. Dr. Romagnolo is a member of several professional organizations, including the American Society for Nutrition and the American Association for Cancer Research. He has published book chapters, monographs, and original research in cancer and nutrition-related scientific journals including *Cancer Research, The Journal of Nutrition, Nutrition and Cancer, Breast Cancer Research, Molecular Carcinogenesis, Environmental and Molecular Mutagenesis, Neoplasia, and Experimental Biology and Medicine*. He is a member of the *Journal of Biochemistry* Editorial Board. Dr. Romagnolo has been a member of scientific review panels and received research funding from the National Institutes of Health, the US Department Breast Cancer Research Program, the Susan G. Komen Breast Cancer Foundation, the American Institute for Cancer Research, and the Arizona Biomedical Research Commission. In his current position, he promotes research that deals with the role of dietary xenobiotics and natural bioactive compounds as epigenetic regulators of expression of genes involved in cancer and inflammation. Current research focuses primarily on the role of environmental and dietary compounds on epigenetic regulation of breast cancer tumor suppressor and proinflammatory genes and prevention of breast and colorectal tumorigenesis by dietary compounds including those commonly found in the Mediterranean diet. As editor, Dr. Romagnolo coedited with John Milner a volume entitled *Bioactive Compounds and Cancer* for the *Nutrition and Health Series* published by Springer Science+Business Media.

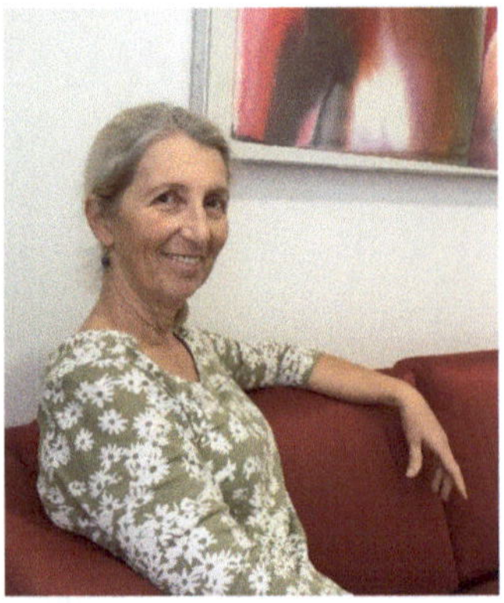

Ornella Selmin, Ph.D. is a research associate professor of Nutritional Sciences at the University of Arizona. She is a member and laboratory director at the University of Arizona Cancer Center. Dr. Selmin is a member of the BIO5 Institute and Center for Toxicology at the University of Arizona. She has served as a research grant panelist for the National Science Foundation (NSF); National Institutes of Health (NIH); Integrated Risk Information System Toxicological Review, the Environmental Protection Agency (EPA), Science Advisory Board; American Heart Association; NIEHS/NIH Superfund Program Grant Review Panel; NIH Minority Biomedical Research Grant Review Panel; and National Center for Environmental Health/Agency for Toxic Substances and Disease Registry. Dr. Selmin has served as Arizona Assurance Program mentor and member of International Science and Engineering Fair Scientific Review Committee, at the University of Arizona. She also has served as a member of the Graduate Program in Microbiology at the University of Arizona. Dr. Selmin received a B.S. in biology and a Ph.D. in molecular and cellular biology at the University of Padua, Italy. She has held various professional positions including visiting fellow at the Laboratory of Developmental Biology and Anomalies, NIDR, NIH, Bethesda, MD; research associate, Laboratory of Developmental Biology, VPI &SU, Blacksburg, VA; and visiting associate, Laboratory of Biochemical Risk Analysis, NIEHS, NIH, Research Triangle Park, North Carolina. Dr. Selmin received the Recordati Industries Research Award for Young Scientist and Walkabout for Biosafety Excellence Award, vice president for Research at the University of Arizona. Dr. Selmin has published in various environmental, nutrition, and cancer-related journals including *Anti-Cancer Agents in Medicinal Chemistry*, *Advances in Nutrition*, *Molecular Carcinogenesis*, *Journal of Nutritional Gerontology and Geriatrics*, *Journal of Nutritional Biochemistry*, *Cardiovascular Toxicology*, *Cancer Epidemiology, Biomarkers & Prevention Cancer Research, and Journal of Biochemistry*. Dr. Selmin received research funding from the National Institutes of Health, the US Department Breast Cancer Research Program, and the Arizona Biomedical Research Commission. Dr. Selmin is a co-instructor of the Mediterranean Diet and Health Study Abroad Program, Global Studies, at the University of Arizona. In her current position at the University of Arizona Cancer Center, she promotes research that deals with the role of environmental xenobiotics and natural bioactive compounds as modulator of genes involved in cardiovascular diseases and breast and colorectal cancer.

Acknowledgments

The editors wish to express their thanks to the US Department of Agriculture for grant support of the 2015 Research Frontiers in Nutritional Sciences on the "*Health Benefits of the Mediterranean Diet: Bringing Science to the Plate*" organized by the Department of Nutritional Sciences and held on January 28–30 on the campus of the University of Arizona, Tucson, AZ. The Conference agenda hosted many of the presentations which have been submitted in the form of chapters to this volume. The editors acknowledge the grant support from the American Institute for Cancer Research, the US Army Breast Cancer Research Program, and the Arizona Biomedical Research Commission. The editors wish to offer special accolades for the efforts of the multiple authors who have contributed to the development of this state-of-the-science text. Special thanks are due to Dr. Adrianne Bendich, *Nutrition and Health Series editor*, for her support through thoughtful comments, suggestions, and encouragements.

Contents

Contributors

Connie W. Bales, Ph.D., R.D. Center for the Study of Aging and Human Development, Duke University Medical Center, Durham, NC, USA

Elliot M. Berry, M.D., F.R.C.P. Department of Human Nutrition and Metabolism, Braun School of Public Health, Hebrew University Hadassah Medical School, Jerusalem, Israel

Michelle A. Briggs, Ph.D., M.S. Department of Biology, Lycoming College, Williamsport, PA, USA

Alessandro Casini, M.D. Department of Experimental and Clinical Medicine, University of Florence, Florence, Italy

Alfredo C. Cordova, M.D. Affinity Surgery/Care New England, Memorial Hospital of Rhode Island, Warren Alpert Medical School of Brown University, Pawtucket, RI, USA

Department of Surgery, Memorial Hospital of Rhode Island, The Warren Alpert Medical School of Brown University, Pawtucket, RI, USA

Maria R. Dalla Francesca, B.S. Fattoria Didattica Altaura, Padova, Italy

Sandro Dernini, Ph.D. Forum on Mediterranean Food Cultures, Rome, Italy

Tom C. Doetschman, Ph.D. Department of Molecular and Cellular Medicine, College of Medicine, The University of Arizona, Tucson, AZ, USA

Micah G. Donovan, B.S. Department of Nutritional Sciences, The University of Arizona, Tucson, AZ, USA

Alessia Fabbri, M.D. Department of Experimental and Clinical Medicine, University of Florence, Florence, Italy

Jennifer A. Fleming, M.S., R.D. Department of Nutritional Sciences, The Pennsylvania State University, University Park, PA, USA

Mariette Gerber, M.D., Ph.D. INSERM-Institut du Cancer de Montpellie, Montpellier, Cedex, France

Scott B. Going, Ph.D. Department of Nutritional Sciences, The University of Arizona, Tucson, AZ, USA

Melanie D. Hingle, Ph.D., M.Ph., R.D. Department of Nutritional Sciences, The University of Arizona, Tucson, AZ, USA

Richard Hoffman, Ph.D., F.R.S.A. School of Life and Medical Sciences, University of Hertfordshire, Hatfield, UK

Kelly A. Jackson, M.S., R.D. Department of Nutritional Sciences, The University of Arizona, Tucson, AZ, USA

Hector C. Keun, Ph.D. Department of Surgery and Cancer, Imperial College, London, UK

Golandam Khayef, M.S., R.D. Department of Nutrition, School of Public Health, Loma Linda University, Loma Linda, CA, USA

Penny M. Kris-Etherton, Ph.D., R.D. Department of Nutritional Sciences, The Pennsylvania State University, University Park, PA, USA

Deepika R. Laddu, Ph.D. Stanford Prevention Research Center, Stanford University School of Medicine, Palo Alto, CA, USA

Jessica A. Martinez, Ph.D. Department of Nutritional Sciences and The University of Arizona Cancer Center, The University of Arizona, Tucson, AZ, USA

Kathryn N. Porter Starr, Ph.D., R.D. Center for the Study of Aging and Human Development, Duke University Medical Center, Durham, NC, USA

Alberto P.G. Romagnolo The University of Arizona Cancer Center, The University of Arizona, Tucson, AZ, USA

Donato F. Romagnolo, Ph.D., M.Sc. Department of Nutritional Sciences, The University of Arizona, Tucson, AZ, USA

Sharon A. Ross, Ph.D., M.P.H. Nutritional Science Research Group, Division of Cancer Prevention, Department of Health and Human Services, National Cancer Institute, National Institutes of Health, Bethesda, MD, USA

Joan Sabaté, M.D., Dr.P.H. Department of Nutrition, School of Public Health, Loma Linda University, Loma Linda, CA, USA

Nadine R. Sahyoun, Ph.D., R.D. Department of Nutrition and Food Science, University of Maryland, College Park, MD, USA

Kavitha Sankavaram, Ph.D. Expanded Food and Nutrition Education Program, University of Maryland, College Park, MD, USA

Ornella I. Selmin, Ph.D. Department of Nutritional Sciences, The University of Arizona, Tucson, AZ, USA

Lluis Serra-Majem, M.D., Ph.D. Research Institute of Biomedical and Health Sciences (IUIBS), University of Las Palmas de Gran Canaria, Las Palmas de Gran Canaria, Spain

International Mediterranean Diet Foundation, London, UK

Alexandros P. Siskos, Ph.D. Department of Surgery and Cancer, Imperial College, London, UK

Francesco Sofi, M.D., Ph.D. Department of Experimental and Clinical Medicine, University of Florence, Florence, Italy

Unit of Clinical Nutrition, University Hospital of Careggi, Florence, Italy

Patricia L. Sparks, Ph.D. Department of Nutritional Sciences, The University of Arizona, Tucson, AZ, USA

Nicole R. Stendell-Hollis, Ph.D., R.D.N. Department of Nutrition, Exercise, and Health Sciences, Central Washington University, Ellensburg, WA, USA

Bauer E. Sumpio, M.D., Ph.D., F.A.C.S. Department of Vascular Surgery, Yale University School of Medicine, New Haven, CT, USA

Brandon J. Sumpio Department of Vascular Surgery, Yale University School of Medicine, New Haven, CT, USA

Cynthia A. Thomson, Ph.D., R.D.N. Health Promotion Sciences Department, The University of Arizona, Tucson, AZ, USA

Antonia Trichopoulou, M.D., Ph.D. WHO Collaborating Center for Nutrition and Health, Athens Medical School, Hellenic Health Foundation, Athens, Greece

Part I
Mediterranean Diet and Lifestyle in a World Context

Chapter 1
Updating the Benefits of the Mediterranean Diet: From the Heart to the Earth

Lluis Serra-Majem and Antonia Trichopoulou

Key Points

- Research has consistently shown that certain dietary patterns, such as the Mediterranean diet (MD), play a role in chronic disease prevention. The MD should be understood not only as a set of foods but also as a cultural model that involves the way foods are selected, produced, processed, and distributed.
- Mediterranean diet interventions showed favorable effects on lipoprotein levels, endothelium vasodilatation, insulin resistance, metabolic syndrome, antioxidant capacity, and myocardial and cardiovascular mortality, and CHD incidence in patients with previous myocardial infarction. Current research is investigating the health impact of the Mediterranean diet against immune and allergic diseases, mental disorders and depression, and quality of life.
- The Mediterranean diet is a cultural, historical, social, territorial, and environmental heritage that has been transmitted from generation to generation for centuries and is intimately linked to the lifestyles of the Mediterranean peoples throughout their history. Compared with current Mediterranean and Western patterns, the traditional MD reduces the water, and to a lower extent, energy resources necessary for the production of meat and dairy products.
- There is a need to reinforce the promotion of the MD in low-income populations and to facilitate the access to key Mediterranean foods to high-risk families, in particular during economic constraints. The Mediterranean diet should be seen for what it is: an extremely healthy and environmentally sustainable food model, as well as an ancient cultural heritage that confers identity and belonging.

Keywords Mediterranean diet • Sustainability • Health benefits • Culture • UNESCO • Environment

L. Serra-Majem, M.D., Ph.D. (✉)
Research Institute of Biomedical and Health Sciences (IUIBS), University of Las Palmas de Gran Canaria, CP 35016 Las Palmas de Gran Canaria, Spain
e-mail: lluis.serra@ulpgc.es

A. Trichopoulou, M.D., Ph.D.
WHO Collaborating Center for Nutrition and Health, Athens Medical School, Hellenic Health Foundation, Alexandroupoleos 23, Athens 11527, Greece
e-mail: atrichopoulou@hhf-greece.gr

D.F. Romagnolo, O.I. Selmin (eds.), *Mediterranean Diet*, Nutrition and Health,
DOI 10.1007/978-3-319-27969-5_1

Introduction

Research has consistently shown that certain dietary patterns, such as the Mediterranean diet (MD), play a role in chronic disease prevention [1–3]. Moreover, the MD has been linked to higher nutrient adequacy in both observational and intervention studies [4, 5]. Thus, the MD, as a plant-centered dietary pattern that does not exclude but admits moderate to low amounts of animal foods, seems to emerge as a dietary pattern that could address both health and environmental concerns [6]. The MD should be understood not only as a set of foods but also as a cultural model that involves the way foods are selected, produced, processed, and distributed [7]. This has been upheld by the fact that the MD was acknowledged by UNESCO as an Intangible Cultural Heritage of Humanity [8]. Unfortunately, current diets in Mediterranean countries are departing from the traditional MD insofar as the quantities and proportions of the food groups are concerned. This is due to the widespread dissemination of Western-type culture, along with the globalization of food production and consumption, which is related to the homogenization of food behavior in the modern era [9]. The aim of the present chapter is to analyze the road map for the MD from its origins circa 1960, and to emphasize the different approaches that have come to light over the last five or six decades: from the heart (public health focus) to the earth (environmental focus).

The Beginnings: Heart Health as the Main Objective

Since its origins, when Ancel Keys initiated his studies on the MD, the principal disease outcome analyzed was cardiovascular disease (CVD) and particularly coronary heart disease (CHD) [10] (Fig. 1.1). Most of the research done was oriented to CVD risk factors and only at the end of the last century were large observational cohorts conducted to increase the evidence regarding the MD and CVD and other disease occurrence. Relevant prospective epidemiological studies and some clinical or community trials, such as the PREDIMED study [2, 11, 12], have exponentially been increasing the level and the quality of the evidence around the MD in the last decades. From the first systematic review of the evidence from MD interventions conducted a few years ago, the MD showed favorable effects on lipoprotein levels, endothelium vasodilatation, insulin resistance, metabolic syndrome, antioxidant capacity, and myocardial and cardiovascular mortality, and CHD incidence in patients with previous myocardial infarction [2]. From the second published systematic review, a meta-analysis of observational cohort studies by Sofi et al. in 2008, revisited in 2010 and 2013 [13] on the evidence of the relationship between the MD and health status, yielded interesting data: a two point increase in the adherence score (or 20 % increase in MD adherence) was significantly associated with a 9 % reduction in overall mortality; 10 % reduction in CVD mortality; 6 % reduction in neoplasm incidence or mortality; and 13 % reduction in the incidence of Parkinson's disease and Alzheimer's disease in the general population.

The epidemiological evidence regarding the relationship between the MD and overweight/obesity is inconsistent. However it reveals that the MD is not related to any increased risk of overweight/obesity and actually points towards a possible role of the MD in preventing overweight/obesity, with physiological mechanisms possibly explaining this protective effect [14]. Furthermore, the PREDIMED trial results pointed out that the MD, especially rich in extra-virgin olive oil, is associated with higher levels of plasma antioxidant capacity. The plasma total antioxidant capacity was related to a reduction in body weight after 3 years of intervention in a high cardiovascular risk population with a Mediterranean-style diet rich in extra-virgin olive oil. Moreover, further PREDIMED results suggested that there was no evidence to sustain the concern that Mediterranean

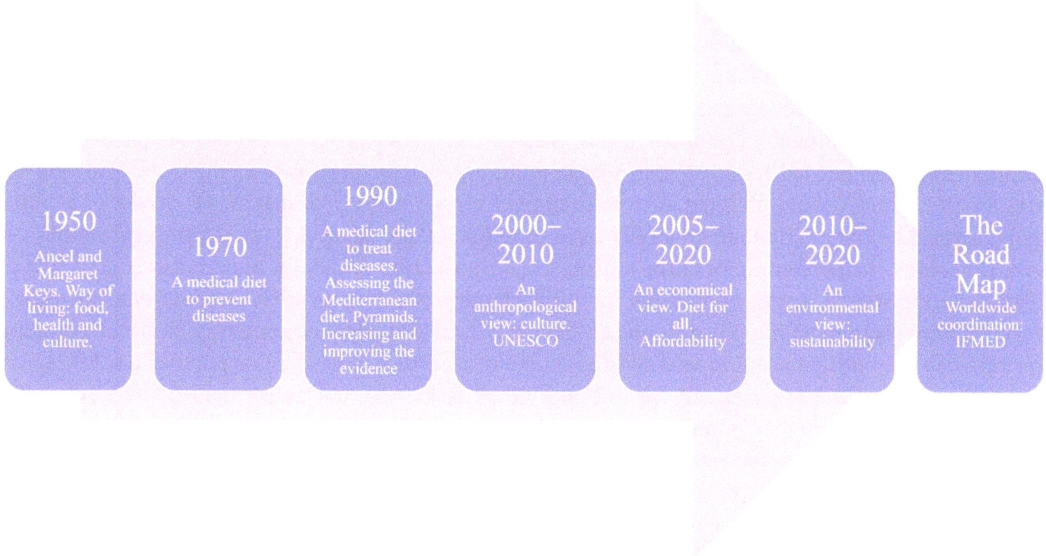

Fig. 1.1 Key steps in the pathway addressing the Mediterranean diet

food items rich in fats of vegetable origin (olive oil or tree nuts) may cause weight gain or be responsible for increased obesity risk, provided that energy intake does not exceed energy expenditure. The MD has also been associated in the PREDIMED study to a lower incidence of type II diabetes, in subjects with higher intake of nuts and extra-virgin olive oil [15]. It should be noted that the role of the MD in the primary prevention of CVD and other cardiovascular conditions has been confirmed by other studies [12, 16].

Greater adherence to the MD has been inversely associated with the glycemic index (GI) and the glycemic load (GL). Nevertheless, further studies are needed to analyze the quality of carbohydrate composition of the MD according to glycemic response so as to increase the scientific evidence underlying the recommendations of the MD as a model of prevention for CVD and diabetes [17]. The relevance of studying the GI and GL mainly relies on the relationship of these indexes with chronic diseases, which have been assessed in several studies. For instance, it has been demonstrated that diets with lower values of GI and GL reduce the risk for diabetes, and its protective action may be similar to whole grain and high fiber intakes. High dietary GI and GL were significantly associated with an increased risk of coronary heart disease events in women. A recent meta-analysis showed that there was a significant association between GI and GL and the risk of colorectal and endometrial cancer, while the relationship with other types of cancer was inconsistent. The mechanisms through which low-GI diets may decrease chronic disease risk are still unknown. After the consumption of a high GI food, a dramatic increase in blood glucose occurs. This is followed by a large insulin response and inhibition of glucagon release. In contrast, low-GI foods produce an attenuated glucose response, due to the prolonged and continued absorption of nutrients from the gastrointestinal tract. Therefore, the resulting hormone responses and their effects are more homeostatic, reducing postprandial hyperglycemia and hyperinsulinemia, and attenuating late postprandial rebounds in circulating non-esterified fatty acids (NEFA). These effects of a low-GI diet could attenuate oxidative stress, which is associated with inflammation and other risk factors for chronic diseases. Although a low GI and GL have been associated with a reduced risk of total mortality and CHD in the PREDIMED study [18, 19], there is still insufficient evidence to warrant the inclusion of dietary recommendations addressing GI and GL for the general population.

Besides the traditionally recognized health benefits against chronic diseases (e.g., CVD, cancer), the MD has other numerous health benefits that are subject of intense research. These include improved immunity and quality of life and prevention against allergic diseases and mental disorders such as depression. Finding a dietary pattern that fulfills the nutritional requirements of a population is a priority to make nutritional recommendations. Nutrient adequacy is defined as the sufficient intake of essential nutrients needed to fulfill nutritional requirements for optimal health. Depending on the criterion of adequacy that is defined, the requirement for a given nutrient may be at a lower or a higher intake level. The criteria that are generally used to define intake adequacy are the prevention of deficiency diseases, the prevention of chronic diseases, the reduction of risk for nutrition-related diseases, subclinical nutritional health conditions identified by specific biochemical or functional measures, and requirements to maintain physiological balance. Nutritional adequacy emerges from the comparison between the nutrient requirement and the intake of a certain individual or population. As neither the real intake nor the requirement for one individual is known, the assessment of nutrient intake adequacy of an individual or population is based on the probability of adequacy [20]. The MD used to be sufficient in calories and rich in vitamins and minerals derived from vegetables, fruits, wholemeal cereals, nuts, virgin olive oil, and fish, which made the risk of deficient micronutrient intakes quite infrequent. This explains why inadequate intakes of the vitamin B group (B1, B2, niacin, B6, folates or B12) were rare in the Mediterranean basin, and why intakes of antioxidant vitamins (vitamins E and C) and carotenes were also high [4, 5]. However, people from Mediterranean countries are changing the traditional MD and include low nutrient-dense foods (such as sweets, bakery products, salted snacks, and sugared soft drinks) or vary their food processing methods (such as refinement of flour) towards a less healthy diet. These changes may have contributed to an increased risk of deficient intakes for certain vitamins, particularly folates, vitamins A and D, as well as inadequate intakes for the rest of the vitamins, especially amongst certain population groups or communities. The MD has been associated with nutritional adequacy in adult population and children. Greater adherence to a MD pattern (MDP) was associated with a higher prevalence of individuals showing adequate intakes of micronutrients [4]. The MDP had similarities with the healthiest patterns defined in non-Mediterranean countries: a positive correlation with intakes of fruits, green leafy vegetables, poultry and fish, and certain lifestyle habits such as nonsmoking and being more physically active. However, when the association of the dietary patterns with their nutrient intake profiles was analyzed, differences arose, especially in relation to fat intake. Prudent and Healthy Diet patterns (HDP) had lower intakes of total and saturated fat, and some studies found even lower intakes of monounsaturated fatty acids (MUFA) [21]. Traditionally, HDP have shown higher percentages of energy coming from proteins and carbohydrate and lower percentages of energy coming from fat when comparing the highest quintile to the lowest. This has always been an argument against the widespread use of olive oil for certain nutritionists who do not support the higher fat in MD and who are in favor of cutting down the total fat intake to less than 20–25 % [22].

Nutritional adequacy may be used to determine the risk of deficiency of the nutrient assessed, in terms of low intakes or high intakes (for instance, the adverse effects of high levels of sodium intake may be applicable to reducing the risk of certain chronic diseases or conditions such as hypertension). However, the complexity of the relationships between dietary intake and the pathology cannot be attributed to a single nutrient but rather to multiple nutrients and associations of foods. Thus, the correct exposure has to be measured to understand such a relationship, and not only nutrients but also foods, and the interaction between them, are of concern for this kind of evaluation. Food pattern analysis, such as the MDP, is then a key issue when investigating the linkages between nutrition and disease. In the last decade there has been growing interest in assessing the relationships between diet and disease through the study of whole dietary pattern (DP) instead of focusing on single nutrients or foods. Besides a priori defined DP, which are based on previous hypotheses (e.g., the MD score), another approach consists of collecting food data and then identifying at a later period the DP followed by the study subjects. This is an a posteriori approach (post hoc) to obtain DP empirically derived from available data through statistical procedures such as principal component analysis. Though several studies have assessed the relationship between a posteriori DP and different health outcomes, to our knowledge little evidence has been collected on post hoc DP and all-cause mortality in Southern European populations. Using factor analysis, Martinez-Gonzalez et al. [23] investigated the association between baseline adherence to an a posteriori defined major DP in a cohort of older Spanish subjects at high cardiovascular risk recruited into the PREDIMED study, a nutritional intervention trial comparing two MDP (enriched with extra-virgin olive oil or nuts) with a low-fat diet for cardiovascular outcomes [23]. Two DPs were uncovered. The baseline Western dietary pattern (WDP) consisted of a higher consumption of processed meats, red meat, refined grains, alcohol, whole-fat dairy products, sauces, eggs, processed meals, commercial bakery, chocolates, and potatoes. In contrast, the baseline MDP was characterized by a higher intake of extra-virgin olive oil, vegetables, fish and seafood, fruits, whole-wheat bread, and nuts. The results showed that a closer baseline adherence to the MDP was associated with a significant 31 % reduction in all-cause mortality, while a higher adherence to the WDP was associated with higher mortality in energy-adjusted analyses. In addition it was observed that within the three intervention groups the protective effect of the MDP or the detrimental effect of the WDP on mortality tended to persist. However the associations were more apparent in the control group. The highest relative risk of mortality was found for participants in the top quartile of the WDP who were allocated to the control (low-fat diet) group.

The MD is the heritage of millennia of exchanges in the Mediterranean basin that have defined and characterized the eating habits of the countries in this region. Unfortunately, it is currently undergoing a steady but rapid transformation as a result of a myriad of factors related to the Western economy including tourism, urbanization, and increased technology as well as the globalization of production and consumption. The Western food culture promotes three elements that may increase health risks: (1) The Western fast food culture based on meat, refined grains, potatoes, ice cream, candies, and beverages high in sugar; (2) The recent (and possibly future) economic crisis which has a higher impact on the most disadvantaged populations and reduces consumption of MD food groups such as fruits, vegetables, virgin olive oil, nuts, and local fish; inversely the consumption of refined grains, potatoes, and sugars is increased; and (3) The promotion of high-protein diets, also prescribed by doctors and specialists, as a tool for weight loss or maintenance, with a major impact on health.

These trends should be countered with actions based on nutrition education, and the commitment that neither cost nor unfounded food choices should be a barrier to the availability of basic foods of the MD, that is olive oil, fruits, vegetables, grains, dairy, nuts, and fish. Governments and nutrition organizations should adopt appropriate actions to preserve this traditional and cultural knowledge base and lead to a diversity of sustainable foods and diets, in addition to fostering short- and-long term health benefits associated with the MD and lifestyle.

The Cultural Approach: UNESCO Recognition

The MD is a cultural, historical, social, territorial, and environmental heritage that has been transmitted from generation to generation for centuries and is intimately linked to the lifestyles of the Mediterranean peoples throughout their history. A legacy passed on within a temporal and spatial constant flow, a living heritage encompassing unique and outstanding cultural spaces and promoting respect for cultural diversity and human creativity. It's an expression of sociability and communication between villages and individuals, a way to reinforce individuals' identities in their places of origin, an integrative element of communities with nature and history, a defense mechanism of agriculture and sustainable rural development, and the landscape and environment of its territory [24].

Since 16 November 2010, the MD has been inscribed into UNESCO's Representative List of Intangible Cultural Heritage of Humanity [8]. The objective of this initiative was to safeguard the immense legacy representing the cultural value of the MD, as well as to share and disseminate its values and benefits internationally. This process was conceived and had been germinating in civil society from the outset and had the privilege of counting on the involvement of national, regional, and local institutions, receiving the unconditional support of the scientific community. It continues to enjoy the support and commitment of all the organizations that for many years had worked in favor of this Mediterranean heritage. Besides, after publicly expressing the wish to present the MD nomination to UNESCO, there was a genuine explosion of enthusiasm and support from institutions and all types of associations, thus consolidating the transversal nature of the project. This elation came to demonstrate that a close bond and genuine identification persisted between the Mediterranean society and its cultural and food heritage.

The Ecological Concern

The environmental consequences of food systems are a main focus of current public debate. How foods are produced, processed, distributed, and consumed have consequences for both human health and the environment [25]. Furthermore, food production is also inevitably a driver of environmental pressures, particularly in relation to climate change, water use, and toxic emissions. Greenhouse gas (GHG) emissions, such as CO_2, CH_4, and N_2O, are responsible for global warming. Agriculture is one of the main contributors to the emissions of the last two gases mentioned while other parts of the food system contribute to CO_2 emissions due to the use of fossil fuels in processing, transportation, retailing, storage, and preparation. Food items differ substantially in their environmental footprints, which can be measured, among many other descriptors, in terms of energy consumption, agriculture land use, water consumption, and GHG emissions [26]. Animal-based foods are by far the most land- and energy-intensive compared with foods of plant origin [27]. Thus, dietary patterns can substantially impact natural resource usage and the environment as well as the health of a given population [26].

In general, there has been substantial literature convergence about the impact of the different food groups on environmental sustainability. Plant-based foods are among those that appear to contribute the least to the environmental footprint. As a result, the traditional MD has a lower impact on water consumption and to a lesser extent energy consumption compared with the current Mediterranean and Western patterns that rely more on meat and dairy products. Plant foods based on vegetables, cereals, and legumes are noteworthy as the food group with the lowest GHG emissions even where processing and substantial transportation is involved [26]. Legumes are clearly an alternative to animal protein foods due to their low environmental impact and long durability [26].

The most relevant dietary distinctions in terms of environmental cost are those that occur between animal-based versus plant-based diets, with an important influence of the various ways foods are grown, processed, and transported. The largest environmental impact of food production from the farm level to consumers is generally associated with primary production. In terms of energy consumption, differences in greenhouse production versus open-air cultivation of certain crops, and canned or frozen produce versus fresh produce are substantial [28]. Besides the energy involved in agricultural production, the amount of energy used in household food storage, preparation, and waste is not negligible [26].

Food policy and dietary guidelines need to develop and move on from the classical approach that only focuses on nutrients and health to one that takes into consideration environmental impact and sustainability. Consumers are becoming more and more concerned about the environment and, even more so, about their personal health and food choices, while cultural culinary traditions are not easy to modify. Some studies suggest that even radical changes in food consumption patterns would provoke quite small environmental benefits [29, 30]. Significantly reducing environmental footprints through a shift from the current non-MD in most European Mediterranean countries towards a MD type would probably not only require substantial changes in consumers' food choices but also imply significant modifications in agrofood-industry practices, public catering supply, and agricultural and trade policies [6, 30]. As for the major producers and exporters of typical Mediterranean products, it would make sense to sustain a MD agricultural production model in Mediterranean countries.

Recently, Sáez-Almendros et al. [31] analyzed the sustainability of the MDP in the context of the Spanish population, whilst also comparing, in terms of their environmental footprints, the current Spanish diet with both the MDP and a typical Western dietary pattern. Studies that assessed food-related environmental impacts of mean food dietary patterns generally concluded that a shift towards less animal-based and more plant-based diets would have both a beneficial effect on climate and on the environment. It was found that the MDP had lower demands on soil, compared to both the Spanish current dietary pattern (SCP) and to WDP, and also on water and energy resources (even though estimates were conservative). In fact, it was observed that a shift towards a MDP would result in a reduction of the Spanish environmental footprint in any of the considered variables from 33 to 72 %. In contrast, a progressive shift towards a WDP would imply an increase in the footprints (12–72 %). These results reinforce the sustainable character of the MDP in an increasingly globalized world [31].

Although legumes are commonly recommended as environmentally friendly meat alternatives, other foods of vegetable origin contribute substantially (along with dairy products as is the case for the MDP and SCP) to either water (vegetable oils in particular, and to some extent nuts) or land usage (cereals and vegetable oils) [31]. In both the SCP and in the WDP, vegetable oils also contribute to a great extent to water and energy consumption footprints. However, animal-based foods were found to cause the highest environmental impact in all dietary patterns considered. As in other studies of the Spanish ecology, meat and dairy foods were the one that most contributed to environmental footprints, although at a much lower absolute level compared to the WDP. As far as GHG emissions and land usage were concerned, undoubtedly meat resulted as the food item that contributed the most compared to other foods, both in the WDP and SCP [31]. It was observed that a reduction in meat consumption decreased GHG emissions, and land usage, subsequently increasing the availability of land for other uses [32]. Even though there is high production variability, which may be as much of 80 % of global agriculture across countries, land use is closely related to livestock production and accounts for more than half of the GHG emissions resulting from agriculture. Meanwhile, dairy products, one of the main sources of animal protein in the MDP, contributed to a great extent in terms of energy consumption in the three dietary patterns. In the MDP, dairy products had the highest impact in all four analyzed footprints. In the MDP, meat had a lower weight compared to the other patterns both in frequency and amount. Regarding GHG emissions, fish showed a remarkable environmental contribution in all the dietary patterns. According to these results, adoption of the MDP in Spain would substantially reduce overall water consumption, despite a possible increase in water consumption from vegetable and fruit groups. Water consumption of certain food groups such as vegetable oils and fats or meat products would still be lower than the WDP.

As a general conclusion, a shift from the current Spanish pattern towards the MDP would be beneficial from both a health and environmental perspective. The MDP presents lower footprints than the current Spanish pattern, and to a much larger extent than the WDP. The MDP results in a lower environmental impact due to the consumption of more plant-derived products and less animal products [31]. The MDP is presented as a cultural, health, and environmentally friendly model. Its adherence in Spain would make a significant contribution to greater sustainability of food production and consumption, in addition to the well-known benefits for public health.

Following the pioneer Keys' initiatives [33], three initial monographies around MD [34–36] drawn a way for further research and policies [37]. The initial focus on the heart survival and medical aspects [38, 39] was followed by a cultural approach and understanding [40–43] that focused on integrating the environmental sustainability and economical concerns [44, 45], particularly in times of financial constraints, with agricultural production [46, 47].

A Look to the Future: Economic Constraints

Improving global nutrition presents several challenges. The rise of obesity has been a rapidly growing problem with severe long-term health and economic consequences. Remarkably, even developed countries lower-income populations tend to be at higher risk for excess body weight. The economic constraints that developed countries are facing, after decades of wealth and development, seem to have paradoxically increased the prevalence of overweight and obesity, which are linked with poor nutrition. This is due to the reduced access to a balanced diet; the loss of traditional diets, such as the MD; and/or lower access to physical activity and sports facilities and resources [46].

Adoption of a specific diet is mainly determined by taste, convenience, and price, and higher adherence to the MD has been associated with higher dietary costs in adults [48]; other healthy dietary patterns are also more expensive than unhealthy choices [49, 50]. This partially explains why low diet quality is more often found in segments of the population with the lowest socioeconomic status (SES). Less is known about the association of monetary diet cost and healthy eating in children and youth, and about the relationship to parental SES. Studies in adult populations have shown that intakes of healthy nutrients and foods are consistently linked to more expensive diets. Adequate intakes of nutrients are paramount, especially for growing children. Therefore, it is of concern that the intake of key nutrients may be considerably lower in the less expensive diets. With this result in mind, it is not surprising that food consumption follows a similar monetary diet cost gradient. In a recent study by Schröder et al. [51, 52], higher consumption of nutrient-rich foods with low to medium energy density such as fruits, vegetables, and fish instead of nutrient-poor, energy-dense foods was more prevalent in high-cost diets and explains the overall lower energy density of these diets. It is of interest to note that energy density was also positively associated with monetary diet cost in German children aged 4–18 years.

A recently published meta-analysis including 27 studies conducted in adult populations showed that high-quality diets cost an average $US 1.54 per 2000 kcal/day more than those with lesser quality [53–55]. The DONALD study, an open cohort study in German children and adolescents, reported a direct association between monetary diet cost and diet quality, but only in those participants with high-quality scores, defined as exceeding the median of the Nutrient Quality Index (NQI) and the Healthy Nutrition Score for Kids and Youth [56]. A study in Swedish children showed that higher diet quality, determined by the 2005 Healthy Eating Index, resulted in higher monetary diet cost [57]. The cost differential of 0.34€ between low and high diet quality found in the Swedish study was comparable with the findings in Spain [51].

Evidence from observational studies carried out in Greece and Spain indicates that higher adherence to the MD by adults is more expensive than higher compliances of westernized diet [48]. The KIDMED index was developed to determine MD adherence in youth [58]. Higher KIDMED scores have been associated with high nutrient adequacy, a healthier food consumption profile, and lower weight and abdominal adiposity [58–61]. In the Schröder et al. study [51], high adherence to the MD, defined as a score more than 8 points on the KIDMED index, was significantly more expensive than low or medium adherence; scoring additional points did not further increase monetary diet cost. In contrast to the results of the DONALD study, this implies an association between increasing the quality of low- and medium-quality diets and higher monetary diet costs that do not apply to further enhancing high-quality diets.

In the Spanish study, the higher cost of the MD was driven by a significantly higher consumption of fish, fruits, and vegetables. In 2000, the average price of 100 g of these foods was 6.58€, 1.51€, and 1.33€, respectively. Prices for pastries, soft drinks, and sweets were considerably lower, but higher consumption of such energy-dense and nutrient-poor foods was strongly related to low MD adherence. Replacing 0.30€/1000 kcal of pastries and sweets with the same monetary cost of low-energy, nutrient-dense foods (specifically fruits, vegetables, and dairy) increased MD adherence by about 1 point [51]. This finding is of importance because even relatively small changes in MD adherence can strongly affect cardiovascular health in adults [62]. The PREDIMED study showed that a 1-point increase in the 14-point MD adherence questionnaire was associated with at least a 12.5 % decrease in CVD incidence [16, 62].

Swedish researchers reported higher monetary diet cost and quality with increasing SES of the parents [57], showing a considerable difference in monetary diet cost and adherence to the MD between extremes of parental education level. At first glance, it seems that 0.50€/2000 kcal/day in monetary diet cost between more and less favorable SES was not that great a difference. However, in a typical 2-child family this difference would total 672€/2000 kcal/year, without counting the parents' food intake. Following dietary recommendations that promote high consumption of low-energy but nutrient-dense foods such as fruits and vegetables and low consumption of nutrient-empty, energy-dense foods will increase diet quality but will also increase the monetary diet cost. This can be a major barrier to opting for healthy food, especially for families with a low SES. Therefore, it is not surprising that increasing monetary diet costs were associated with higher SES, accompanied by a substantial increase in diet quality [51]. However, the traditional MD should be considered the food way of the medium and lower social classes, as has been in the past, instead of a sophysticated and exclusive diet for reach people. Taken together, these considerations emphasize the need to reinforce the promotion of the MD in low-income populations and to facilitate access to key Mediterranean foods to high-risk families, especially during times of economic constraints.

Final Considerations

Governments need to commit themselves to undertake appropriate actions which preserve our traditional and cultural knowledge and lead to the diversity of foods and diets, but not focusing only on the health benefits that could be provided in the short and long term [63]. The recognition by UNESCO, with the consequent increased visibility and acceptance of the MD around the world, along with better and more scientific evidence regarding its benefits and effectiveness on longevity, quality of life, and disease prevention, has taken this dietary pattern to an unprecedented historical moment. This is a favorable situation that could possibly enable the strengthening of the MD around the world, thus potentiating improvements in global health indicators and in a reduction of environmental impact by production and transportation of food resources. To this end, the MD should be seen for what it is: an

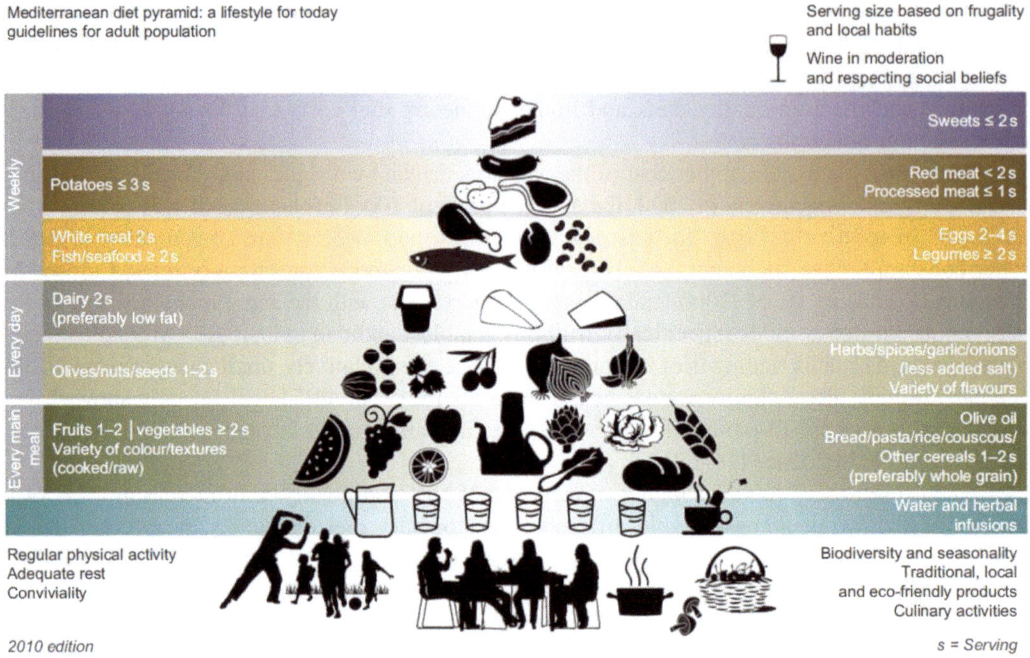

Fig. 1.2 Mediterranean diet pyramid. *Source*: Bach-Faig A, Berry EM, Lairon D, Reguant J, Trichopoulou A, Dernini D, Medina FX, Battino M, Belahsen R, Miranda G, and Serra-Majem L, on behalf of the Mediterranean Diet Foundation Expert Group. Mediterranean diet pyramid today. Science and cultural updates. Public Health Nutr. 2011;14(12A):2274–84 [64]

extremely healthy and environmentally sustainable food model as well as an ancient cultural heritage that confers identity and belonging (Fig. 1.2) [64].

References

1. Trichopoulou A, Martínez-González MA, Tong TY, Forouhi NG, Khandelwal S, Prabhakaran D, et al. Definitions and potential health benefits of the Mediterranean diet: views from experts around the world. BMC Med. 2014;12:112.
2. Serra-Majem L, Roman B, Estruch R. Scientific evidence of interventions using the Mediterranean diet: a systematic review. Nutr Rev. 2006;64(2 Pt 2):S27–47.
3. Sofi F, Abbate R, Gensini GF, Casini A. Accruing evidence on benefits of adherence to the Mediterranean diet on health: an updated systematic review and meta-analysis. Am J Clin Nutr. 2010;92:1189–96.
4. Serra-Majem L, Bes-Rastrollo M, Román B, Pfrimer K, Sánchez-Villegas A, Martínez-González MA. Dietary patterns and nutritional adequacy in a Mediterranean country. Br J Nutr. 2009;101 Suppl 2:S21–8.
5. Castro-Quezada I, Román-Viñas B, Serra-Majem L. The Mediterranean diet and nutritional adequacy: a review. Nutrients. 2014;6(1):231–48.
6. Duchin F. Sustainable consumption of food: a framework for analyzing scenarios about changes in diets. J Ind Ecol. 2005;9:99–114.
7. Serra-Majem L. Nutrición comunitaria y sostenibilidad: concepto y evidencias. Rev Esp Nutr Comunitaria. 2010;16:35–40. Spanish.
8. UNESCO. Representative list of the intangible cultural heritage of humanity. http://www.unesco.org/culture/ich/en/RL/00394. 2010.
9. Da Silva R, Bach-Faig A, Raidó Quintana B, Buckland G, Vaz de Almeida MD, Serra-Majem L. Worldwide variation of adherence to the Mediterranean diet, in 1961–1965 and 2000–2003. Public Health Nutr. 2009;12:1676–84.

10. Keys A, Menotti A, Karoven MI. The diet and the 15-year death rate in the Seven Countries Study. Am J Epidemiol. 1986;124:903–15.
11. Martínez-González MA, Bes-Rastrollo M, Serra-Majem L, Lairon D, Estruch R, Trichopoulou A. Mediterranean food pattern and the primary prevention of chronic disease: recent developments. Nutr Rev. 2009;67:S111–6.
12. Estruch R, Ros E, Salas-Salvadó J, Covas MI, Corella D, Arós F, et al. Primary prevention of cardiovascular disease with a Mediterranean diet. N Engl J Med. 2013;368(14):1279–90.
13. Sofi F, Macchi C, Abbate R, Gensini GF, Casini A. Mediterranean diet and health status: an updated meta-analysis and a proposal for a literature-based adherence score. Public Health Nutr. 2014;17(12):2769–82.
14. Buckland G, Bach A, Serra-Majem L. Obesity and the Mediterranean diet: a systematic review of observational and intervention studies. Obes Rev. 2008;9(6):582–93.
15. Salas-Salvadó J, Bulló M, Estruch R, Ros E, Covas MI, Ibarrola-Jurado N, et al. Prevention of diabetes with Mediterranean diets: a subgroup analysis of a randomized trial. Ann Intern Med. 2014;160(1):1–10.
16. Martínez-González MA, Salas-Salvadó J, Estruch R, Corella D, Fitó M, Ros E, for the PREDIMED Investigators. Benefits of the Mediterranean diet: insights from the PREDIMED study. Prog Cardiovasc Dis. 2015;58(1):50–60.
17. Rodríguez-Rejón AI, Castro-Quezada I, Ruano-Rodríguez C, Ruiz-López MD, Sánchez-Villegas A, Toledo E, et al. Effect of a Mediterranean diet intervention on dietary glycemic load and dietary glycemic index: the PREDIMED study. J Nutr Metab. 2014;2014:985373.
18. Castro-Quezada I, Sánchez-Villegas A, Estruch R, Salas-Salvadó J, Corella D, Schröder H, et al. A high dietary glycemic index increases total mortality in a Mediterranean population at high cardiovascular risk. PLoS One. 2014;9(9):e107968.
19. Castro-Quezada I, Sánchez-Villegas A, Martínez-González MA, Salas-Salvadó J, Corella D, Estruch R, et al. Glycemic index, glycemic load and invasive breast cancer incidence in postmenopausal women: the PREDIMED study. Eur J Cancer Prev. 2015 Dec 1. [Epub ahead of print].
20. Román-Viñas B, Serra-Majem L, Ribas-Barba L, Ngo J, García-Álvarez A, Wijnhoven TMA, et al. Overview of methods used to evaluate the adequacy of nutrient intakes for individuals and populations. Br J Nutr. 2009;101 Suppl 2:S6–11.
21. Bach A, Serra-Majem L, Carrasco JL, Roman B, Ngo J, Bertomeu I, Obrador B. The use of indexes evaluating the adherence to the Mediterranean diet in epidemiological studies: a review. Public Health Nutr. 2006;9(1A):132–46.
22. James WPT, Ferro Luzzi A, Isaksson B, Szostak WB, editors. Healthy nutrition: preventing nutrition related diseases in Europe. Copenhagen, Denmark: WHO Regional Office for Europe; 1988.
23. Martínez-González MA, Zazpe I, Razquin C, Sánchez-Tainta A, Corella D, Salas-Salvadó J, et al. Empirically-derived food patterns and the risk of total mortality and cardiovascular events in the PREDIMED study. Clin Nutr. 2015;34(5):859–67.
24. Serra-Majem L, Medina X. The Mediterranean diet as an intangible and sustainable food culture. In: Preedy VR, Watson RR, editors. The Mediterranean diet. An evidence-based approach. London: Elsevier; 2015. p. 37–46.
25. Gussow JD, Clancy KL. Dietary guidelines for sustainability. J Nutr Educ. 1986;18:1–5.
26. Carlsson-Kanyama A, González AD. Potential contributions of food consumption patterns to climate change. Am J Clin Nutr. 2009;89(Suppl):S1704–9.
27. Baroni L, Cenci L, Tettamanti M, Berati M. Evaluating the environmental impact of various dietary patterns combined with different food production systems. Eur J Clin Nutr. 2007;61:279–86.
28. Reijnders L, Soret S. Quantification of the environmental impact of different dietary protein choices. Am J Clin Nutr. 2003;78 Suppl 3:S664–8.
29. Tukker A, Goldbohm RA, De Koning A, Verheijden M, Kleijn R, Wolf O, et al. Environmental impacts of changes to healthier diets in Europe. Ecol Econ. 2011;70:1776–88.
30. Wallén A, Brandt N, Wennersten R. Does the Swedish consumer's choice of food influence greenhouse gas emissions? Environ Sci Policy. 2004;7:525–35.
31. Sáez-Almendros S, Obrador B, Bach-Faig A, Serra-Majem L. Environmental footprints of Mediterranean versus Western dietary patterns: beyond the health benefits of the Mediterranean diet. Environ Health. 2013;12:118.
32. Stehfest E, Bouwman L, van Vuuren DP, den Elze MGJ, Eickhout B, Kabat P. Climate benefits of changing diet. Clim Change. 2009;95:83–102.
33. Keys A, Keys M. Eat well & stay well. New York: Doubleday & Company, Inc; 1959.
34. Helsing E, Trichopoulou A, editors. The Mediterranean diet and food culture—a symposium. London, U.K. Eur J Clin Nutr. 1989;43:1–92.
35. Serra-Majem L, Helsing E, editors. Changing patterns of fat intake in Mediterranean countries. London, U.K. Eur J Clin Nutr. 1993;47:1–100.
36. Nestlé M, editor. Mediterranean diets: science and policy implications. California, U.S.A. Am J Clin Nutr. 1995;61:1313–427.
37. Serra-Majem L, Ferro-Luzzi A, Bellizzi M, Salleras L. Nutrition policies in Mediterranean Europe. Nutr Rev. 1997;55(11 Pt 2):S42–57.
38. Trichopoulou A, Kouris-Blazos A, Wahlqvist ML, Gnardellis C, Lagiou P, Polychronopoulos E, et al. Diet and overall survival in elderly people. BMJ. 1995;311(7018):1457–60.

39. Trichopoulou A, Bamia C, Trichopoulos D. Anatomy of health effects of Mediterranean diet: Greek EPIC prospective cohort study. BMJ. 2009;338:b2337.
40. Trichopoulou A, Lagiou P. Healthy traditional Mediterranean diet: an expression of culture, history, and lifestyle. Nutr Rev. 1997;55(11 Pt 1):383–9.
41. Willett WC, Sacks F, Trichopoulou A, Drescher G, Ferro-Luzzi A, Helsing E, Trichopoulos D. Mediterranean diet pyramid: a cultural model for healthy eating. Am J Clin Nutr. 1995;61 Suppl 6:S1402–6.
42. Serra-Majem L, Bach-Faig A, Raidó-Quintana B. Nutritional and cultural aspects of the Mediterranean diet. Int J Vitam Nutr Res. 2012;82(3):157–62.
43. Serra-Majem L, Trichopoulou A, Ngo de la Cruz J, Cervera P, García Alvarez A, La Vecchia C, et al. International task force on the Mediterranean diet. Does the definition of the Mediterranean diet need to be updated? Public Health Nutr. 2004;7(7):927–9.
44. Serra-Majem L, Bach-Faig A, Miranda G, Clapes-Badrinas C. Foreword: Mediterranean diet and climatic change. Public Health Nutr. 2011;14(12A):2271–3.
45. Germani A, Vitiello V, Giusti AM, Pinto A, Donini LM, del Balzo V. Environmental and economic sustainability of the Mediterranean Diet. Int J Food Sci Nutr. 2014;65(8):1008–12.
46. Bonaccio M, Di Castelnuovo A, Bonanni A, Costanzo S, De Lucia F, Persichillo M, et al. Decline of the Mediterranean diet at a time of economic crisis. Results from the Moli-sani study. Nutr Metab Cardiovasc Dis. 2014;24(8):853–60.
47. Shapira N. 'Health-oriented agriculture' for nutritional security versus climate change risks in the Mediterranean Basin. World Rev Nutr Diet. 2011;102:201–11.
48. Schröder H, Marrugat J, Covas MI. High monetary costs of dietary patterns associated with lower body mass index: a population-based study. Int J Obes. 2006;30:1574–9.
49. Drewnowski A, Eichelsdoerfer P. The Mediterranean diet: does it have to cost more? Public Health Nutr. 2009;12(9A):1621–8.
50. Lopez CN, Martinez-Gonzalez MA, Sanchez-Villegas A, Alonso A, Pimenta AM, Bes-Rastrollo M. Costs of Mediterranean and western dietary patterns in a Spanish cohort and their relationship with prospective weight change. J Epidemiol Community Health. 2009;63(11):920–7.
51. Schröder H, Gomez SF, Ribas-Barba L, Pérez-Rodrigo C, Bawaked RA, Fitó M, Serra-Majem L. Monetary diet cost, diet quality, and parental socioeconomic status in Spanish youth. Br J Nutr. 2015 (in press).
52. Schröder H, Vila J, Marrugat J, Covas MI. Low energy density diets are associated with favorable nutrient intake profile and adequacy in free-living elderly men and women. J Nutr. 2008;138(8):1476–81.
53. Saulle R, Semyonov L, La Torre G. Cost and cost-effectiveness of the Mediterranean diet: results of a systematic review. Nutrients. 2013;5(11):4566–86.
54. Abdullah MM, Jones JP, Jones PJ. Economic benefits of the Mediterranean-style diet consumption in Canada and the United States. Food Nutr Res. 2015;59:27541.
55. Rao M, Afshin A, Singh G, Mozaffarian D. Do healthier foods and diet patterns cost more than less healthy options? A systematic review and meta-analysis. BMJ Open. 2013;3(12):e004277.
56. Alexy U, Schwager V, Kersting M. Diet quality and diet costs in German children and adolescents. Eur J Clin Nutr. 2014;68(10):1175–6.
57. Ryden PJ, Hagfors L. Diet cost, diet quality and socio-economic position: how are they related and what contributes to differences in diet costs? Public Health Nutr. 2011;14(9):1680–92.
58. Serra-Majem L, Ribas L, Garcia A, Perez-Rodrigo C, Aranceta J. Nutrient adequacy and Mediterranean Diet in Spanish school children and adolescents. Eur J Clin Nutr. 2003;57 Suppl 1:S35–9.
59. Schroder H, Mendez MA, Ribas L, Funtikova AN, Gomez SF, Fito M, et al. Caloric beverage drinking patterns are differentially associated with diet quality and adiposity among Spanish girls and boys. Eur J Pediatr. 2014;173(9):1169–77.
60. Schroder H, Mendez MA, Ribas-Barba L, Covas MI, Serra-Majem L. Mediterranean diet and waist circumference in a representative national sample of young Spaniards. Int J Pediatr Obes. 2010;5(6):516–9.
61. Schroder H, Mendez MA, Gomez SF, Fito M, Ribas L, Aranceta J, et al. Energy density, diet quality, and central body fat in a nationwide survey of young Spaniards. Nutrition. 2013;29(11–12):1350–5.
62. Schroder H, Salas-Salvado J, Martinez-Gonzalez MA, Fito M, Corella D, Estruch R, Ros E. Baseline adherence to the Mediterranean diet and major cardiovascular events: Prevencion con Dieta Mediterranea trial. JAMA Intern Med. 2014;174(10):1690–2.
63. Piscopo S. The Mediterranean diet as a nutrition education, health promotion and disease prevention tool. Public Health Nutr. 2009;12(9A):1648–55.
64. Bach-Faig A, Berry EM, Lairon D, Reguant J, Trichopoulou A, Dernini S, et al. Mediterranean Diet Foundation Expert Group. Mediterranean diet pyramid today. Science and cultural updates. Public Health Nutr. 2011;14(12A):2274–84.

Chapter 2
Mediterranean Diet and Lifestyle in a Modern World Context

Donato F. Romagnolo and Ornella I. Selmin

Key Points

- Nutrition and lifestyle have been shown to impact the etiology of major causes of death including heart, malignant neoplasms, chronic lower respiratory, cerebrovascular, Alzheimer's, and diabetes diseases. The death incidence attributable to these causes is projected to increase due to the growing and aging population. Socioeconomic constraints contribute to the coexistence of non-communicable diseases with food insecurity.
- The rampant increase in the prevalence of overweight and obesity in the US and world populations have been attributed to a combination of dietary, socioeconomic, and behavioral causes. These include increases in calories consumed; greater average carbohydrate intake, larger portion sizes, greater food quantity and calories per meal; and transition to a more sedentary lifestyle. During the last three decades, various graphical representation (pyramids, plates) have been adopted by US, international, and world health organizations to promote better food selections and lifestyles.
- An imbalance between recommendations and dietary behavior combined with an increasingly sedentary lifestyle likely contribute, along with socioeconomic factors, to the overweight and obesity epidemic in the USA and other countries.
- Recently dietary guidelines in the USA and abroad promote the idea of rebalancing calories with more physical activity to manage weight and reduce the burden of chronic diseases.
- Research evidence suggests that dietary habits and lifestyle of populations residing in Mediterranean countries may offer protection against chronic diseases and improve longevity. The Scientific Report of the 2015 Dietary Guidelines to the DHHS and USDA included the Mediterranean-style Pattern among those associated with health benefits.

Keywords Chronic diseases • Diet • Lifestyle • Food pyramid • Mediterranean diet • Prevention • Health

D.F. Romagnolo, Ph.D., M.Sc. (✉) • O.I. Selmin, Ph.D.
Department of Nutritional Sciences, Shantz Bldg, The University of Arizona,
Tucson, AZ 85721, USA
e-mail: donato@u.arizona.edu; selmin@u.arizona.edu

D.F. Romagnolo, O.I. Selmin (eds.), *Mediterranean Diet*, Nutrition and Health,
DOI 10.1007/978-3-319-27969-5_2

Introduction

Health Trends in the USA and the World

Major causes of death in the USA include heart, malignant neoplasms, chronic lower respiratory, cerebrovascular, Alzheimer's, and diabetes diseases [1] (Fig. 2.1). Unfortunately, coupled to improved longevity are projections suggesting that chronic disease burden will increase markedly with the growing and aging population. For example, whereas US total life expectancy increased by 0.1 year from 78.7 years in 2011 [2], cancer incidence is projected to increase for US populations ranging from 65 to 74 years of age and to a larger degree for subjects 75 year of age and older [3]. Nutrition and lifestyle have been shown to impact the etiology of chronic diseases. For example, it has been estimated that a healthy diet may reduce ~30 % of all cancers [4]. Healthy diet can reduce heart disease by 80 %, and stroke and some cancers by 70 %. Importantly, evidence that there is a 20–30 years lag-period between initial insult and death for most types of cancer suggests that vast opportunities may exist for cancer prevention. Similarly, dietary efforts to reduce the burden of cardiovascular disease have focused on limiting the intake of refined carbohydrates and excess adiposity [5].

Overweight and Obesity

The prevalence of combined overweight and obesity in US adults (≥20 years of age) is ~155 million, which in 2010, represent ~68 % of this group (Fig. 2.2). Fully, ~36 % of US adults are obese. Men and women of all race/ethnic groups in the population appear to be affected by the epidemic of overweight and obesity [6]. Obesity (body mass index, BMI ≥30 kg/m^2, or about 30 lb overweight for 5′4″ person) is associated with marked excess mortality in the USA. Even more concerning is the excess

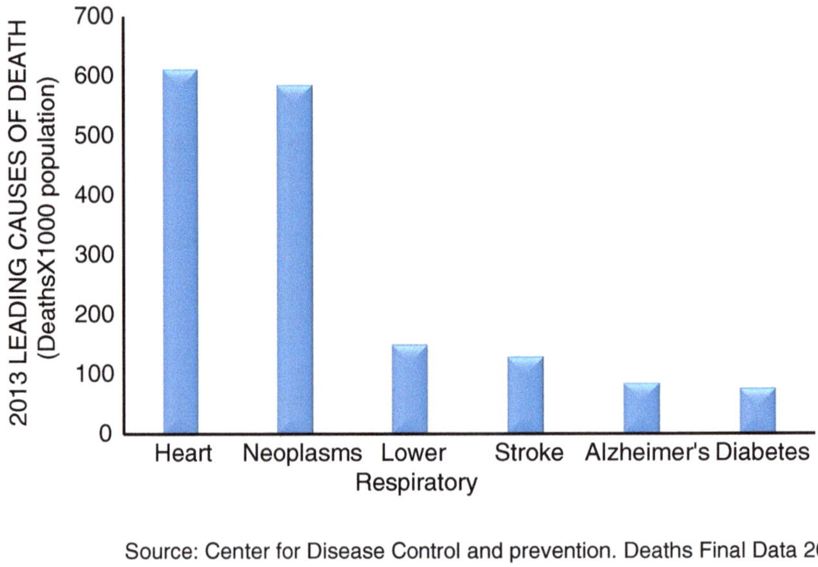

Fig. 2.1 Leading causes of death in the USA. *Bars* represent numbers of deaths × 1000 population in 2013 for various chronic diseases [1]

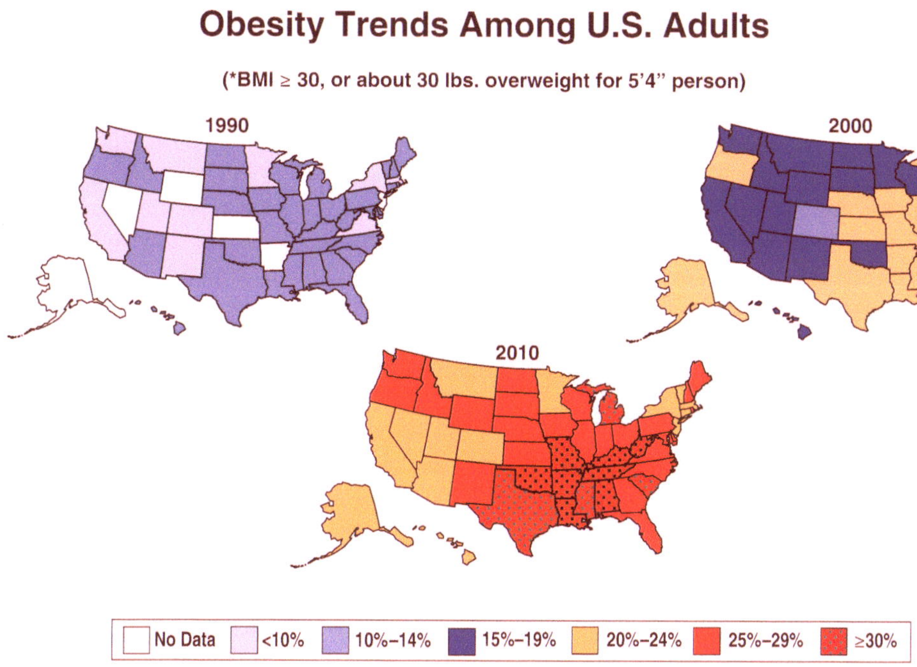

Source: Behavioral Risk Factors Surveillance System, Center for Disease Control and Prevention.

Fig. 2.2 Obesity trends among US adults. Diagrams represent obesity trends in 1990, 2000, 2010 [6]

morbidity associated with overweight and obesity in terms of risk factor development and incidence of diabetes mellitus, cardiovascular end points (including coronary heart disease, stroke, and heart failure), and various health conditions such as asthma, cancer, end-stage renal disease, and degenerative joint disease. Obesity and overweight account for ~15–20 % of cancer deaths in the USA [7]. Among children 2–19 years of age, ~32 % are overweight and obese (which represents ~24 million children) and ~17.0 % are obese (12.7 million children). According to the National Center for Health Statistics (NCHS), the prevalence of obesity among US children and adolescents aged 2–19 during the last three decades (1963–1965 through 2007–2012) has nearly tripled [8]. Although the prevalence of obesity among children aged 2–5 years decreased significantly from 13.9 % in 2003–2004 to 8.4 % in 2011–2012, race-specific and socioeconomic factors contribute to some disparities in the prevalence of obesity. For example, obesity is higher for Black (~50 %) and Hispanic (~39 %) compared to White (34 %) Americans. Mexican American boys and girls and African American girls are disproportionately affected with higher incidence rates of obesity compared to other ethnic groups.

Obesity Epidemic and Food Insecurity

The shift from rural food-producing to urbanized lifestyle coupled with economic constraints has contributed to the paradoxical coexistence of obesity with food insecurity [9]. Population studies suggested that food insecurity was a problem with nearly 15 % of American households unable to secure adequate food to meet their nutrition needs [10]. Remarkably, the highest incidence of obesity occurs among poor and least educated groups for which an inverse relationship between energy density and cost favor the consumption of low-cost energy-dense foods (i.e., refined grains, added sugars, and fats) [11] over healthier and more expensive ones (i.e., fish, fruits, and vegetables). As a result, any food-assistance and recommendation program aimed at reducing the incidence of obesity and related chronic diseases may not achieve its full potential until changes in socioeconomic variables occur, i.e., adequate foods, lifestyle, education, and medical care become accessible to under-privileged communities. These societal needs are in stark contrast with the fact that ~15 % of US adults have used a weight-loss dietary supplement at some point in their lives, with more women reporting use (20.6 %) than men (9.7 %). To lose weight is one of the top 20 reasons why people take dietary supplements. Approximately $2 billion a year are spent on weight-loss dietary supplements in pill form (e.g., tablets, capsules, and softgels) [12].

Global comparisons of obesity prevalence showed that among developed countries the USA ranked first (~33 %) followed by Canada, Australia, and the UK (~28 %) (Fig. 2.1) [13]. High prevalence ranging from 33 to 42 % was also found in North African countries including Kuwait, Lybia, Qatar, and Saudi Arabia. Intermediate prevalence was observed in Central (Mexico, 28 %), South America (20–26 %), Russia and France (~24 %), Italy and Sweden (~21 %). Significantly lower prevalence was found in China (7 %) and India (5 %). Estimates from WHO indicated that worldwide obesity more than doubled since 1980. In 2014, more than 1.9 billion adults, 18 years and older, were overweight. Of these people, over 600 million were obese. In 2014, about 39 % of world adults aged 18 years and over were estimated to be overweight, and 13 % were likely obese. Remarkably, in countries where most of the world's population lives, overweight and obesity conditions contribute to mortality more than underweight and malnutrition. It was estimated that 42 million children under the age of 5 were overweight or obese in 2013. Strikingly, the rate of increase of childhood overweight and obesity has been higher in developing countries with emerging economies compared to that of developed nations.

The rampant increase in the prevalence of overweight and obesity in the US and world populations have been attributed to a combination of dietary, socioeconomic, and behavioral causes. These include increases in calories consumed; greater average carbohydrate intake, in particular, of starches, refined grains, and sugars; larger portion sizes, greater food quantity and calories per meal; increased consumption of sugar-sweetened beverages, snacks, commercially prepared meals, and higher energy-density foods; food insecurity and transition to a more sedentary lifestyle [14]. Data from the US National Health and Nutrition Examination Survey [15] indicated that between 1971 and 2000, the average total energy consumption among US adults increased by 22 % in women (from 1542 to 1886 kcal/d) and by 10 % in men (from 2450 to 2693 kcal/d). During the same period, higher prevalence in overweight and obesity in the USA have occurred in spite of an overall reduction in dietary fat intake as a percentage of caloric intake [16, 17]. In support of this, epidemiological studies showed that a reduction in saturated fatty acid intake below ~10 % of total energy intake was not associated with a lower risk of cardiovascular diseases and may actually favor carbohydrates intake [5]. These cumulative data point to excessive carbohydrates, rather than fat, as a contributing cause for the obesity epidemic and likely worsening of metabolic states characterized by increased triglycerides and reduced HDL cholesterol.

Diabetes

Obesity is a condition that predisposes to the development of diabetes. Epidemiological studies of diabetes suggest it is a major cause of stroke and heart disease [18]. In the USA, the number of subjects diagnosed with diabetes has increased steadily since early 1990s. In 2012, 29.1 million Americans, or ~9.5 % of the population, had diabetes. Of these, approximately 1.25 million American children and adults (~5 % of total cases) have type 1 diabetes whereas type 2 diabetes is the prevalent form. The prevalence of diabetes in the USA varies with race and ethnicity with Mexican Americans and non-Hispanic Blacks contributing ~13 % of diagnosed diabetes cases from 2007 to 2009 compared to a lower ~7–8 % for non-Hispanic Whites and Asian Americans. Mexican Americans residing in the USA have a 50 % lifetime risk of diabetes [19]. Although the prevalence of diabetes in senior Americans (age 65 and older) remains relatively high (~26 %) recent statistics suggested that the estimated number of new cases of diagnosed diabetes was the highest among younger adults (45–64 years of age) [18] compared to older groups. This is particularly troubling considering that in subject with diabetes the mortality related to cardiovascular diseases nearly doubles [20]. The dramatic incidence of diabetes in younger adults clearly points to poor dietary and lifestyle practices as major targets for prevention.

Food Recommendations

Food Groups and Pyramids

Evidence of dietary guidelines in the USA trace back to more than hundred years ago when in 1894 the US Department of Agriculture (USDA) emphasized the importance of variety, proportionality and moderation in food selection [21] (Fig. 2.3). From the early- to mid-1900s, the USDA issued various recommendations based on food group guidelines which remained in use until the 1970s. It was not until 1970s that the focus of recommendations shifted from securing adequate nutrition to prevention of chronic diseases due over consumption. In 1980, the first edition of the Dietary Guidelines highlighted recommendations for five major groups including the bread, cereal, rice and pasta group; the vegetable group; the fruit group, the dairy (milk, yogurt, and cheese); the protein (meat, poultry, fish, dry beans, eggs) and nuts group; and the fats, oils, and sweets group. Since 1980, the USDA and Department of Human Health Services (DHHS) released Dietary Guidelines that in 1990 included percent targets for total fat (30 % of calories) and saturated fat (less than 10 % of calories) [22]. In 1992, the USDA released the first Food Pyramid to help Americans to choose healthy diets [23] (Fig. 2.3). The term pyramid, which derives from the Greek "pyramis," refers to pointy structures characterized by a quadrilateral base and a rising triangular top. It is commonly associated with ancient tombs of Egyptian pharaohs [24] and other civilizations in Mesoamerica [25] and India [26]. The concept of pyramid has often been used in sociology and economics to represent inequities by including at the base the poorest groups with fewer resources and power, and at the top, the more affluent and smaller groups [27]. Based on this stratification, the graphical representation of the pyramid was adopted by the USDA to place on top oils and sweets to suggest that they should be used sparingly. Then, below and in increasing order of consumption, the pyramid included horizontal sections representing the dairy group (milk, yogurt, and cheese); protein (meat, poultry, fish, eggs, dry beans) and nuts group; vegetable and fruit group; and at the bottom of the pyramid, to suggest larger consumption, the bread, cereal, rice and pasta group (Fig. 2.3). Unfortunately, the fact that Americans consumed fewer servings for the grain, vegetable, and fruit groups, and nearly triple the recommended added sugars [28] revealed a disconnect between food pyramid recommendations and consumer knowledge and behavior [29]. This imbalance between recommendations and dietary behavior combined with an increasingly sedentary lifestyle are at the basis, among other factors, of the overweight and obesity epidemic in the USA, and possibly other communities leaving abroad but under similar socioeconomic conditions. A subject of concern regarding the 1992 Food Pyramid was its replacement of fats without discriminating bad vs. good ones (i.e., saturated vs mono and polyunsaturated) thus likely favoring increase intakes of other food sources (i.e., carbohydrates) to meet energy needs [30].

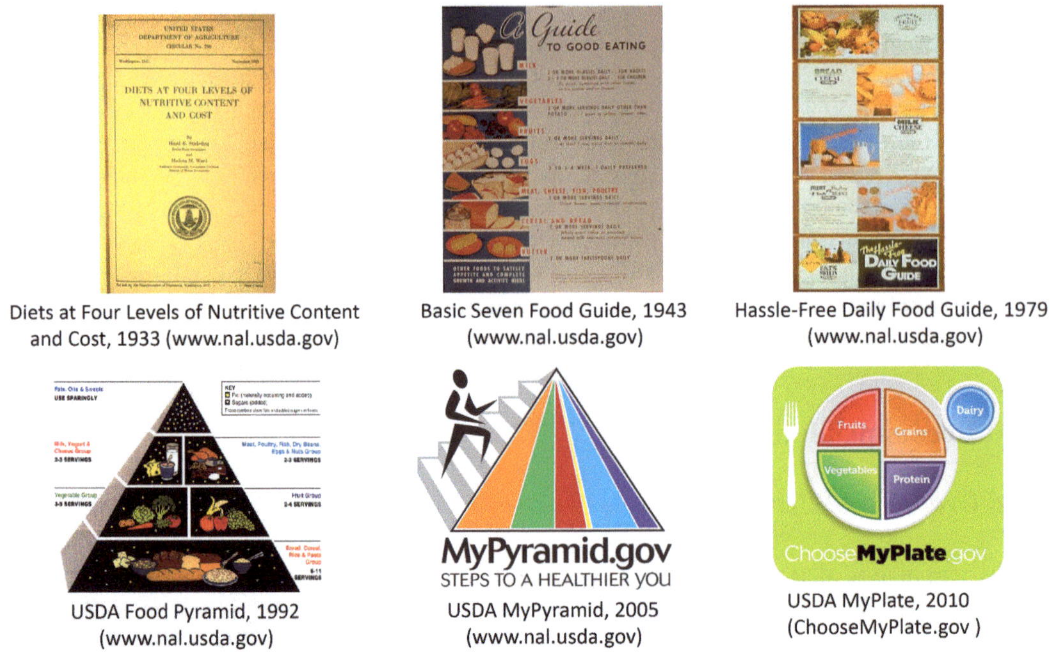

Fig. 2.3 Selected US food guides and pyramids. Pictures represent graphical representations of selected food guides and pyramids published by the US Department of Agriculture [50]. The current food guide for Americans is MyPlate issued in 2010 [36]

In 2004, the World Health Organization (WHO) released the Global Strategy on Diet, Physical Activity and Health (GSDPAH) [31] to address the needs for promoting healthy diets and regular physical activity, and to prevent non-communicable diseases. A central tenet of this initiative was evidence that unhealthy diets and physical inactivity were among the leading causes of major non-communicable diseases, such as cardiovascular disease, type 2 diabetes, and certain types of cancer, and contributed substantially to the global burden of disease, death and disability in the world. Moreover, the WHO-GSDPAH recognized that patterns of unhealthy behavior and the non-communicable diseases associated with them clustered with poor communities and hampered their social and economic development. Also, in the poorest countries, where infectious diseases and undernutrition were found to dominate disease burden, the prevalence of overweight and obesity paralleled the increasing trends of overweight and obesity of low-income groups in developed countries.

In 2005, the USDA launched "MyPyramid," which compared to the 1992 food pyramid, adopted colored vertical, rather than horizontal, stripes of different size to depict the contribution of each food group [21]. In addition, the "MyPyramid" logo included a stair to highlight the importance of physical activity. Specific recommendations were to limit fat intake (20–35 % energy) to vegetable oils, and energy intake. Early reviews recognized that the 2005 food pyramid provided improved guidelines for less energy and more adequate nutrient intake, but also anticipated that without discretionary energy restriction Americans would be at risk of excessive energy intake [32]. Also, concerns were raised over the high recommended intakes of red meat, dairy products, and refined starches [30] and the overall promotion of a low-fat diet. As a result, alternative health eating indexes [33] and pyramids [34] were proposed to better predict risk of diseases and encourage a reduction in the intake of saturated fats, refined starches, and exclude trans-fatty acids.

From Pyramids to Plates

The 2010 Dietary Guidelines were designed to help people choose a healthier diet [35]. It reinforced the idea of balancing calories with physical activity to manage weight; consuming more fruits, vegetables, whole grains, vegetable oils (MUFA and PUFA), fat-free and low-fat dairy products, and seafood; and consuming fewer foods with sodium (salt), saturated and trans-fats, cholesterol, added sugars, and refined grains. The USDA replaced the graphical concept of pyramid with “MyPlate” illustrating on a plate the five food groups that should be the building blocks for a healthy diet [36]. In light of the burgeoning of overweight and obesity among people residing in the USA concerns persist about difficulties to promote and define proper adherence to healthier dietary patterns. The fact that people may continue to eat more of certain, but not healthier, foods (e.g., solid fats and added sugars) as in the past is a major challenge against the fight on overweight and obesity and prevention of related chronic diseases [37].

Mediterranean Diet and Lifestyle

Scientific Report of the 2015 Dietary Guidelines to the DHHS and USDA

In its Scientific Report of the 2015 Dietary Guidelines to the DHHS and USDA [38], the Advisory Committee recognized that dietary patterns of the American public are suboptimal and casually related to poor individual and population health, higher chronic disease rates, whereas a significant portion of the households suffers from food insecurity. Suggested targets for dietary recommendations included increasing consumption of fruits, vegetables, and whole grains; reduce intake of calories, saturated fat, sodium, refined grains, and added sugars. Moreover, under consumption of vitamin D, calcium, potassium, and fiber were identified as of public concern for the majority of the US population. At the time of preparation of this volume, the 2015 Scientific Report to the DHHS and USDA is being translated into the 2015 Dietary Guidelines for Americans. In its summary statement, the Advisory Committee concluded that it had enough descriptive information, from existing research and data, to model three dietary patterns and examine their nutritional adequacy. These included the Healthy US-Style Pattern, the Healthy Mediterranean-Style Pattern, and the Healthy Vegetarian Pattern based on the evidence they included the food and components of a dietary pattern associated with health benefits.

Research evidence suggests that dietary habits and lifestyle of populations residing in Mediterranean countries may offer protection against chronic diseases, i.e., cardiovascular diseases [39] and improve longevity [40]. Some of the health protective effects of the Mediterranean diet and lifestyle have been attributed to high levels of polyphenols which are abundant in fruits and vegetables. Interestingly, the lower rates of coronary heart disease in the Mediterranean region were found [41, 42] where fat intake was relatively high (35–40 %), but mostly from olive oil (70–80 % of the MUFA oleic acid). These data of fat consumption in Mediterranean populations raise the provocative question whether or not recommending diets low in fat, and the widespread availability of zero- or low-fat foods, may be compensated with higher intakes of refined starches and sugars, and actually contribute to the burden of chronic diseases (e.g., overweight, obesity). For example, controlled feeding studies showed that compared to carbohydrates, both monounsaturated (MUFA) and polyunsaturated (PUFA) fats in Mediterranean diets reduced LDL and triglycerides and increase HDL cholesterol [43]. Importantly, these metabolic effects were greater in subjects with underlying insulin resistance. Earlier studies showed that a total fat intake of ~35–40 % energy, with mono and polyunsaturated fatty acids and saturated fatty acids contributing ~20–30 % and 9 % energy, respectively, reduced the risk of cardiovascular diseases [44, 45]. Therefore, the question dietary prescription of further reducing saturated fatty acids (i.e., below ~10 %) may not be beneficial and actually increase the proportion of carbohydrates while reducing the potential health benefits of fatty acids found in dairy products (i.e., conjugated linoleic acid). Thus, specific contributions of various dietary fatty acids need to be taken into consideration when making recommendations about dietary fat intake. For example, the predominant unsaturated fatty acids present in olive oil (18:1) and fish (EPA, DHA) cannot be equated to those in soy and corn that are rich in linoleic acid (18:2) and for which some evidence of obesogenic and diabetogenic effects have been observed in preclinical studies compared to coconut oil rich in saturated fatty acid [46]. Other examples of beneficial bioactive compounds commonly present in Mediterranean diets include fiber (whole grains) and polyphenols (fruits, vegetables, wine and berries). For example, studies showed that wine in moderation has a positive effect; however, too much has a negative effect on mortality due to all causes and cardiovascular diseases [39]. A diet that includes moderate alcohol consumption, primarily with meals and physical activity are central components of the Mediterranean lifestyle.

During the last decade, the health effects of foods and bioactive food components present in Mediterranean diets have been the subject of intense investigations. Figure 2.4 depicts the number of publications appeared in PubMed since 1995 and cited in two time periods, from 1995 to 2004 and from 2005 to 2015, for Mediterranean diet and each disease. Not surprisingly, studies of cardiovascular diseases contributed the highest number of citations during both periods, but clearly there has been a marked increase in research publications for all five chronic diseases in conjunction with the increased incidence of overweight and obesity. The Mediterranean Diet was inscribed by UNESCO in 2013 [47] in the Representative List of the Intangible Cultural Heritage of Humanity. The editors and contributors of this volume recognize that other dietary patterns and lifestyles can promote health and protect against chronic diseases [48, 49]. However, due to the vast literature and limited space, the

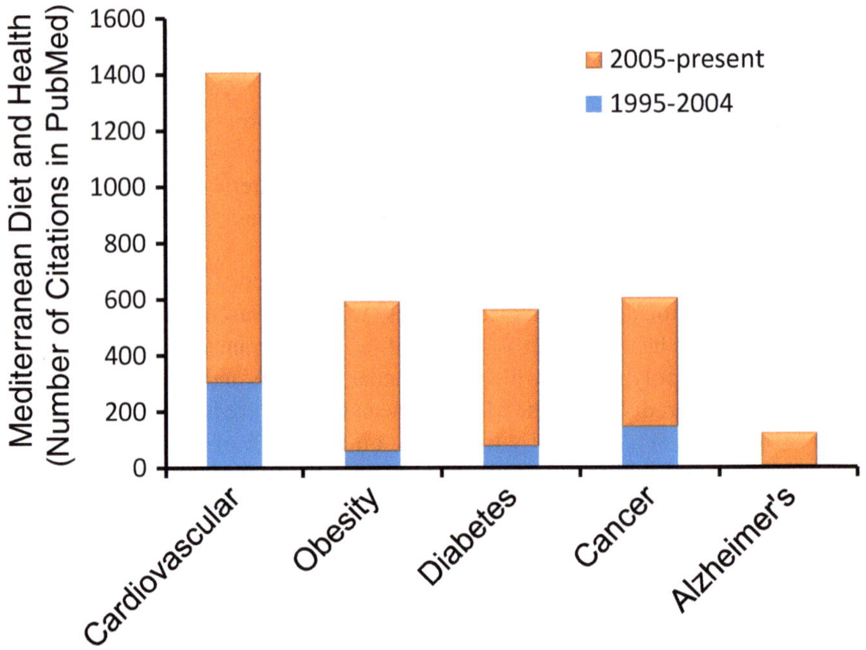

Fig. 2.4 Publications on Mediterranean diet and health during the last 20 years. *Bars* represent number of citations in PubMed for two time periods (1995–2004 and 2005–present) for combinations of Mediterranean diet and specific chronic diseases

main focus of this volume is to summarize the most up-to-date evidence related to the potential benefits of foods and dietary behaviors that are characteristic of the Mediterranean region with special emphasis on socioeconomics and practices that contribute to the Mediterranean diet and lifestyle; the mechanisms through which bioactive compounds usually found in Mediterranean diets and foods impact on biological process; and opportunities and challenges for implementation of a Mediterranean-like dietary pattern in developed and emerging economies. The volume closes with a chapter presenting example of recipes and their nutritional composition.

Summary and Conclusions

In the USA and the world the establishment of dietary guidance based on food groups finds its roots in traditions concerning agricultural production, culinary activities and healthy eating, and community development [50]. Ethnic and cultural guidelines [51] have been the focus of intense study during the last two decades because of the causative role of diet and behavior on the development of major chronic non-communicable diseases. In spite of intense efforts by various US, international, and World Health Organization there appear to be little or no progress on the fight against overweight and obesity and related chronic diseases (i.e., cancer, diabetes, cardiovascular). Major research efforts and lifestyle changes are needed to reverse these trends in the USA and communities abroad but affected by similar health burdens (Table 2.1). Adoption of dietary patterns and lifestyles that have been traditionally associated with reduced incidence of chronic diseases are recommended. Implementation of these changes, such as a Mediterranean diet and lifestyle may offer some benefits to populations residing in the USA and abroad [52]. Major challenges include Westernization of food supplies [53], and lifestyle and socioeconomic constraints that limit access to healthier foods, affordable education, and medical care.

Table 2.1 Areas of investigation and specific research needs[a]

1. *Food and nutrient intakes and health*
– Include more respondents from race/ethnic minorities and non-US born residents
– Include higher proportion of older Americans and pregnant women
– Conduct research on early-life nutrition and dietary patterns
– Increase the quantity and quality of food composition databases and develop new biomarkers of intake and nutritional status
– Evaluate effects of fortification strategies and supplement use and their doses (i.e., Ca, Fe, vitamin D, K, fiber)
– Develop research definition for meals and snacks
– Develop concept of dietary patterns and approaches to quantify nutrients, foods, and food groups in population-based studies
– Conduct surveillance on the prevalence and trends of nutrition-related chronic diseases
2. *Dietary patterns, foods and nutrients, and health outcomes*
– Study dietary patterns research for other health outcomes beyond cardiovascular disease and body weight in relation to ethnic backgrounds and life course stages
– Develop modeling of food patterns
– Study long-term cardio-metabolic effects of the various dietary patterns
3. *Individual diet and physical activity behavior*
– Collect and characterize types of eating venues (i.e., eating out vs eating at home) and longitudinal impact
– Assess sedentary behaviors and activities and impact on variables of health (i.e., overweight, obesity) across the life span

(continued)

Table 2.1 (continued)

– Assess types, modalities, and frequencies of self-monitoring and counseling on weight loss intervention and maintenance in various ethnic/racial groups and minorities
– Examine effects of mobile health technologies on dietary and weight outcomes
– Establish impact of current, and needs for novel, food labeling across various settings (i.e., home, restaurants, etc.)
– Establish impact of socioeconomic constraints on food insecurity on health parameters
– Determine the impact of acculturation on dietary intake, sedentary behaviors, body weight, and chronic disease outcomes
– Investigate the relationships dietary and energy intake, and energy expenditure on sleep patterns and body weight outcomes
4. *Food environment*
– Measure all aspects of the food environment increasing healthy food access
– Implement better research methods in obesity intervention research and in child care settings
– Improve knowledge regarding food procurement and practices
– Study daily food behavior of children at school in relation to food policies and outside of school
– Study long term health impact of food interventions and to increase vegetables consumption
– Assess worksite interventions across racially/ethnically diverse populations
5. *Food sustainability and safety*
– Determine affordability and accessibility of foods to various sectors of the population
– Perform analyses of US domestic dietary patterns and sustainability
– Study how agricultural production and consumer behaviors influence sustainability of food practices and economic benefits and challenges
– Improve nutrient profiles of high- and of low-trophic farmed seafood and production efficiency
– Develop methods to ensure control of contaminant levels in all seafood
– Examine effect of low and high levels of coffee on health outcomes (pregnancy, sleep, cancer, cognitive, cardiovascular, diabetes) and in children and adults
– Examine the risks of aspartame related to some cancers
6. *Cross-cutting public health topics*
– Design studies with sufficient power
– Assess efficacy of methodologies for sample collections (e.g., 24-h urine collections)
– Link behavioral interventions to adherence to sodium intake recommendations (i.e., low vs. high, portion size)
– Impact of substitution of saturated fats with different carbohydrates (e.g., refined vs. whole grains) or various polyunsaturated fats and oils on cardiovascular disease
– Examine gene–nutrient interactions
– Assess levels of sugars and low-calorie sweeteners and link to health outcomes in general population and subgroups, and policies to reduce their intakes
– Asses implementation of front-of-package labeling
7. *Physical activity*
– Assess best practices to reduce sedentary life and increase physical activity (duration, frequency, type)
– Establish health impact of physical activity for children, older adults and population at large across the lifespan

[a]*Source*: US Department of Agriculture, Scientific Report of the 2015 Dietary Guidelines for Americans, Appendix E1 [38]

References

1. Center for Disease Control and Prevention. Detailed tables for the national vital statistics report (NVSR); deaths: final data for 2013. http://www.cdc.gov/nchs/fastats/deaths.htm. Accessed 10 Sep 2015.
2. Xu J, Kochanek KD, Murphy SL, Arias E. Mortality in the United States, U.S. Department of Health and Human Services, Centers for Disease Control and Prevention. NCHS Data Brief No. 2012;128:1–7.
3. Cancer Trends Progress Report, National Cancer Institute, NIH, DHHS, Bethesda, MD, March 2015. http://progressreport.cancer.gov. Accessed 10 Sep 2015.
4. World Cancer Research Fund/American Institute for Cancer Research. Food, nutrition, physical activity, and the prevention of cancer: a global perspective. Washington, DC: AICR; 2007.
5. Siri-Tarino PW, Sun Q, Hu FB, Krauss RM. Saturated fat, carbohydrate, and cardiovascular disease. Am J Clin Nutr. 2010;91:502–9.
6. U.S. Department of Health and Human Services, National Institute of Diabetes and Digestive and Kidney Diseases. Overweight and obesity statistics. http://www.niddk.nih.gov/health-information/health-statistics/Pages/overweight-obesity-statistics.aspx. Accessed 10 Sep 2015.
7. Alberts DS, Lluria-Prevatt M. Foreword. In: Milner JA, Romagnolo DF, editors. Bioactive compounds and cancer. New York, NY: Humana Press-Springer Science; 2013.
8. Center for Disease Control and Prevention, National Center for Health Statistics, Childhood obesity facts. http://www.cdc.gov/obesity/data/childhood.html. Accessed 10 Sep 2015.
9. Hruschka DJ. Do economic constraints on food choice make people fat? A critical review of two hypotheses for the poverty-obesity paradox. Am J Hum Biol. 2012;24:277–85.
10. Gooze RA, Hughes CC, Finkelstein DM, Whitaker RC. Obesity and food insecurity at the same table: how head start programs respond. Prev Chronic Dis. 2012;9, E132.
11. Drewnowski A, Specter SE. Poverty and obesity: the role of energy density and energy costs. Am J Clin Nutr. 2004;79:6–16.
12. U.S. Department of Health and Human Services, National Institutes of Health, Office of Dietary Supplements. Dietary supplements for weight loss. https://ods.od.nih.gov/factsheets/WeightLoss-HealthProfessional. Accessed 10 Sep 2015.
13. World Health Statistics. World Health Organization. Organization, 2015. http://www.who.int/gho/publications/world_health_statistics/2015/en/. Accessed 10 Sep 2015.
14. U.S. Department of Health and Human Services, National Institute of Diabetes and Digestive and Kidney Diseases. Understanding adult overweight and obesity. http://www.niddk.nih.gov/health-information/health-topics/weight-control. Accessed 7 Sep 2015.
15. Center for Disease Control and Prevention. Trends in intake of energy and macronutrients, United States, 1971-2000, Morbidity Mortality Weekly Report. 53(4), February 6, 2004. http://www.cdc.gov/mmwr/preview/mmwrhtml/mm5304a3.htm. Accessed 1 Sep 2015.
16. Chanmugam P, Guthrie JF, Cecilio S, Morton JF, Basiotis PP, Anand R. Did fat intake in the United States really decline between 1989-1991 and 1994-1996? J Am Diet Assoc. 2003;103(7):867–72.
17. Willett WC. Is dietary fat a major determinant of body fat? Am J Clin Nutr. 1998;67(3 Suppl):556S–62S. Review. Erratum in: Am J Clin Nutr 1999;70(2):304.
18. Centers for Disease Control and Prevention. National diabetes statistics report: estimates of diabetes and its burden in the United States. Atlanta, GA: U.S. Department of Health and Human Services; 2014.
19. Fisher-Hoch SP, Vatcheva KP, Rahbar MH, McCormick JB. Undiagnosed diabetes and pre-diabetes in health disparities. PLoS One. 2015;10(7):e0133135. doi:10.1371/journal.pone.0133135.
20. Gregg EW, Cheng YJ, Saydah S, Cowie C, Garfield S, Geiss L, Barker L. Trends in death rates among U.S. adults with and without diabetes between 1997 and 2006: findings from the National Health Interview Survey. Diabetes Care. 2010;35:1252–7.
21. Davis C, Saltos E. Dietary recommendations and how they have changed over time. In: America's eating habits, United States Department of Agriculture, Agriculture Information Bulletin No. (AIB-750). 1999:33–50. http://www.ers.usda.gov/publications/aib-agricultural-information-bulletin/aib750.aspx. Accessed 7 Sep 2015.
22. U.S. Department of Agriculture and U.S. Department of Health and Human Services: dietary guidelines for Americans, 2005. 6th ed. Washington, DC: US Government Printing Office; 2005. www.dietaryguidelines.com. Accessed 10 Sep 2015.
23. U.S. Department of Agriculture Food Pyramid. 1992. http://www.nal.usda.gov/fnic/Fpyr/pymid.gif.
24. National Geographic: Egypt—Great Pyramid of Khufu at Giza. http://nationalgeographic.com. Accessed 1 Sep 2015.
25. Harner M. The Enigma of Aztec sacrifice. Natural History. 1977;86(4):46–51.
26. UNESCO, World Heritage Convention, World Heritage Committee. Evaluation of cultural properties, International Council on Monuments and Sites. June 28–July 2004, Suzhou, China. http://whc.unesco.org/archive/2004/whc04-28com-inf14ae.pdf. Accessed 8 Sep 2015.

27. Krieger N. Ladders, pyramids and champagne: the iconography of health inequities. J Epidemiol Community Health. 2008;62:1098–104.
28. Putnam J, Allshouse J, Kantor LS. U.S. per capita food supply trends: more calories, refined carbohydrates and fats. Food Rev. 2002;25:2–15.
29. Goldberg JP, Belury MA, Elam P, Finn SC, Hayes D, Lyle R, St Jeor S, Warren M, Hellwig JP. The obesity crisis: don't blame it on the pyramid. J Am Diet Assoc. 2004;104:1141–7.
30. Chiuve SE, Willett WC. The 2005 Food Guide Pyramid: an opportunity lost? Nat Clin Pract Cardiovasc Med. 2007;4(11):610–20.
31. World Health Assembly 57.17. Global strategy on diet and physical activity. Geneva: World Health Organization; 2004.
32. Gao X, Wilde PE, Lichtenstein AH, Tucker KL. The 2005 USDA Food Guide Pyramid is associated with more adequate nutrient intakes within energy constraints than the 1992 Pyramid. J Nutr. 2006;136(5):1341–6.
33. Willett WC, McCullough ML. Dietary pattern analysis for the evaluation of dietary guidelines. Asia Pac J Clin Nutr. 2008;17 Suppl 1:75–8.
34. Willett W. Eat, drink and be healthy. New York: Simon and Schuster; 2005.
35. U.S. Department of Agriculture and U.S. Department of Health and Human Services: dietary guidelines for Americans, 2010. 7th ed. Washington, DC: US Government Printing Office; 2010. www.dietaryguidelines.com. Accessed 8 Sep 2015.
36. U.S. Department of Agriculture. ChooseMyPlate. http://www.choosemyplate.gov.
37. Jahns L, Kranz S. High proportions of foods recommended for consumption by United States Dietary Guidance contain solid fats and added sugar: results from the National Health and Nutrition Examination Survey (2007-2008). Nutr J. 2014;20:13–23.
38. U.S. Department of Agriculture. Scientific report of the 2015 Dietary Guidelines Advisory Committee to the Secretary of Agriculture and the Secretary of Health and Human Services. http://health.gov/dietaryguidelines/2015-scientific-report. Accessed 15 Aug 2015.
39. Cordova AC, Sumpio BJ, Sumpio BE. Perfecting the plate: adding cardioprotective compounds to the diet. J Am Coll Surg. 2012;214:97–114.
40. Trichopoulou A, Kouris-Blazos A, Wahlqvist ML, Gnardellis C, Lagiou P, Polychronopoulos E, Vassilakou T, Lipworth L, Trichopoulos D. Diet and overall survival in elderly people. BMJ. 1995;311(7018):1457–60.
41. Covas MI, et al. Perfecting the plate: adding cardioprotective compounds to the diet. Ann Intern Med. 2006;145:333–41.
42. De Lorgeril M, Salen P, Martin JL, Mamelle N, Monjaud I, Touboul P, Delaye J. Effect of a mediterranean type of diet on the rate of cardiovascular complications in patients with coronary artery disease. Insights into the cardioprotective effect of certain nutriments. J Am Coll Cardiol. 1996;28:1103–8.
43. Willett WC. The Mediterranean diet: science and practice. Public Health Nutr. 2006;9:105–10.
44. Dayton S, Pearce ML, Hashmoto S, Dixon WJ, Tomiyasu U. A controlled clinical trial of a diet high in unsaturated fat in preventing complications of atherosclerosis. Circulation. 1969;39–40 Suppl 2:1–63.
45. Leren P. The Oslo Diet-Heart Study. Circulation. 1970;42:935–42.
46. Deol P, Evans JR, Dhahbi J, Chellappa K, Han DS, Spindler S, Sladek FM. Soybean oil is more obesogenic and diabetogenic than coconut oil and fructose in mouse: potential role for the liver. PLoS One. 2015;10(7), e0132672.
47. UNESCO. Representative list of the intangible cultural heritage of humanity. 2013. http://www.unesco.org/culture. Accessed Sep 2015.
48. National Heart, Lung, and Blood Institute. Your guide to lowering your blood pressure with DASH. NIH Publication no. 06-4082. Bethesda, MD: NIH, National Heart, Lung, and Blood Institute; 2006.
49. Tangney CC. DASH and Mediterranean-type dietary patterns to maintain cognitive health. Curr Nutr Rep. 2014;3(1):51–61.
50. A brief history of USDA food guides. http://fnic.nal.usda.gov/dietary-guidance/dietary-guidelines/historical-dietary-guidance. Accessed 6 Sep 2015.
51. U.S. Department of Agriculture, Ethnic/Cultural Food Pyramids. http://fnic.nal.usda.gov/dietary-guidance/past-food-pyramid-materials/ethniccultural-food-pyramids. Accessed 6 Sep 2015.
52. Bach-Faig A, Berry EM, Lairon D, Reguant J, Trichopoulou A, Dernini S, Medina FX, Battino M, Belahsen R, Miranda G, Serra-Majem L, Mediterranean Diet Foundation Expert Group. Mediterranean diet pyramid today. Science and cultural updates. Public Health Nutr. 2011;14:2274–84.
53. Garcia-Closas R, Berenguer A, González CA. Changes in food supply in Mediterranean countries from 1961 to 2001. Public Health Nutr. 2006;9:53–60.

Part II
Historical, Behavioral, and Geographical Perspective on the Mediterranean Diet and Lifestyle

Chapter 3
Historical and Behavioral Perspectives of the Mediterranean Diet

Sandro Dernini and Elliot M. Berry

Key Points

- Mediterranean diet (MD) patterns have developed over the past 5000 or more years spreading from the Fertile Crescent and influenced by the conquests of many different civilizations. As a result the MD is in continuous evolution. There is not one single MD, but rather a number of variations on a basic theme adapted to individual country's cultures. The MD is more than just a diet; it represents a lifestyle, a social cultural expression of the different Mediterranean food cultures.
- Current data suggest that adherence is decreasing because of multifactorial influences including: lifestyle changes, food globalization, economic and sociocultural factors. In this chapter we present the evolution of the MD from an historical and behavioral perspective, moving from the 1950s model of a healthy diet, which reduced morbidity and mortality, to a model of a sustainable diet, which also lessens the overall impact on the human ecosystem, and finally as an intangible cultural heritage, acknowledged by UNESCO.
- As background for more detailed discussions of such questions, this chapter presents an overview of the historical antecedents and recent interest in the MD, and identifies future challenges related to the current status of the MD.
- The challenge for public health nutrition is to reverse such trends especially since the MD and lifestyle (as opposed to single nutrients) has a proven beneficial health profile as well as being sustainable and eco-friendly.

Keywords Mediterranean diet • Lifestyle • History • Culture • Food behavior • Evolution • Sustainability

S. Dernini, Ph.D.
Forum on Mediterranean Food Cultures, Via Giovanni da Castel Bolognese, 89, 00153 Rome, Italy
e-mail: Sandro.Dernini@fao.org

E.M. Berry, M.D., F.R.C.P. (✉)
Department of Human Nutrition and Metabolism, Braun School of Public Health, Hebrew University Hadassah Medical School, Jerusalem 91120, Israel
e-mail: elliotb@ekmd.huji.ac.il

D.F. Romagnolo, O.I. Selmin (eds.), *Mediterranean Diet*, Nutrition and Health,
DOI 10.1007/978-3-319-27969-5_3

Introduction

The Mediterranean Diet (MD) is the expression of the evolution of the millennial history of the Mediterranean made by a peculiar geographic mosaic and climate and a complex of different ancient civilizations, cultures, food traditions and lifestyles, with continuous interactions, additions and exchanges inside and outside the region. This unique natural Mediterranean cultural environment has generated a variety of food systems that, throughout the centuries, were at the crossroads of different food sources and food habits. These varied fundamentally among themselves under the influence of thedietary rules of the three main Mediterranean monotheistic religions: Judaism, Christianity, and Islam. As a result, over the course of time Mediterranean dietary patterns have shown numerous variations and have been subject to many transformations.Dietary patterns among Mediterranean populations have neither been static nor homogeneous; indeed, they expressed the continuous vicissitudes throughout the centuries that changed the overall Mediterranean environment, reflecting also the long history of food insecurity that made frugality a fundamental characteristic of the MD.

The dietary and lifestyle patterns embraced by the Mediterranean people over the centuries are also the result of a number of factors: food production availability, seasonality, the use of small-scale technologies, the wide variety of local cultivars used, the freshness of the food consumed, their homemade preparation, the frugality and the conviviality of meals, and a physically active lifestyle. Diets of the Mediterranean populations have been a subject of interest since antiquity [1–3]. In the absence of written records, data on ancient diets must be adduced from whatever evidence is available. In the case of MD, such evidence is copious [4–8]. The geographic and evolutionary origins of the MD encompass the history of Western civilization. The rise of agriculture (domestication of crops) and animal husbandry took place from 10000 to 4000 B.C., while the wheel, metallurgy, writing, and city states arose from 4000 to 1000 B.C. These essential developments in the evolution of civilization originated in the fertile crescent—from Mesopotamia, the ancient near East, Canaan, and Egypt [9].

This dynamic evolving context was a result of a succession of dominant civilizations—Egyptian, Hebrew, Phoenician, Greek, Carthaginian, Roman, Arab, Byzantine, Ottoman, and more. They introduced and/or diffused different foods, culinary practices, and food traditions throughout the Mediterranean region. The MD became, in time, with its shared basic food elements, the multifaceted expression of the various food cultures representing the different lifestyles of the Mediterranean peoples, their religions and cultural practices [9].

Historical Perspective of the Evolution of the MD: From a Healthy Dietary Pattern to a Sustainable Diet and an Intangible Cultural Heritage

Concept of the MediterraneanPyramid

The concept of the MD began to be studied in the 1950s as a model of a healthy diet [10] which reduced morbidity and mortality. This notion developed in the 2000s to a model of sustainable diet [11] which also considers the overall impact on the ecosystem [12], and was then recognized as an intangible cultural heritage acknowledged by UNESCO [13].

Figure 3.1 traces the historical development of the MD. What has emerged is the evolution of the MD from a healthy dietary pattern of specific foods to a comprehensive Mediterranean lifestyle, an intangible cultural heritage, in which food, health, culture, people, and sustainability all interact into a new model of a sustainable diet [14]. The term "MD" implies the existence of some common dietary characteristics in Mediterranean countries such as: high amounts olive oil and olives, fruits,

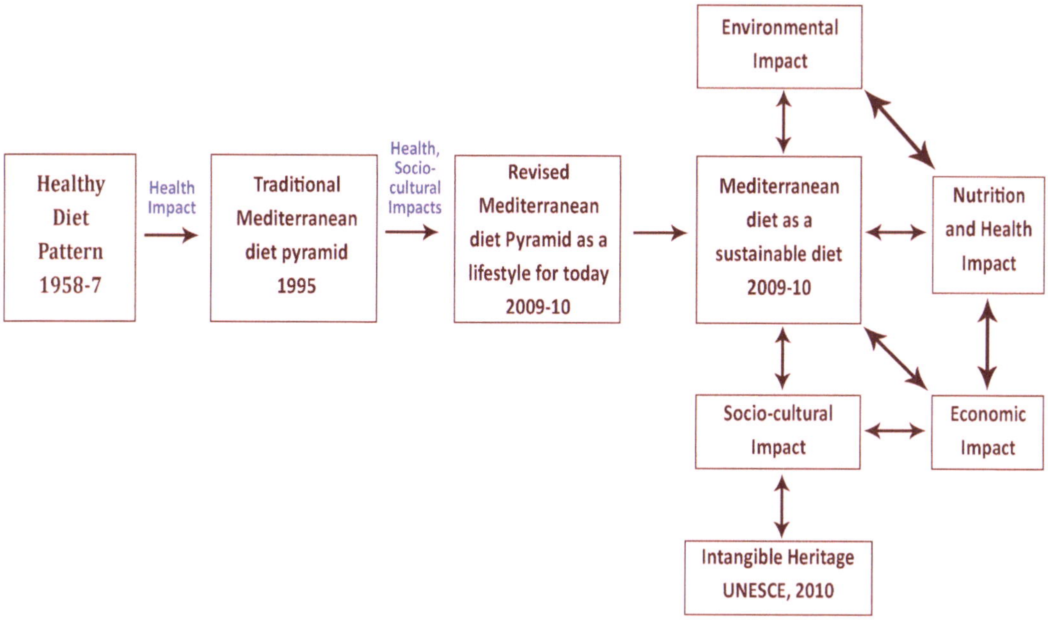

Fig. 3.1 The evolution of concepts surrounding the Mediterranean diet

vegetables, cereals (mostly unrefined), legumes, nuts, and fish, moderate amounts of dairy products (preferably cheese and yogurt), and low quantities of meat and meat products. Wine in moderation is acceptable when it is not contradictory to religious and social norms [15–17].

The Recent Historical and Conceptual Development of the MD

The MD has been recognized as being one of the healthiest diets in the world [18–22]. Indeed, numerous recent studies have confirmed that better adherence to a traditional MD is consistently associated with a markedly reduced risk of cardiovascular events and mortality [23–28]; a lower incidence of the metabolic syndrome [29–32]; a lower risk for cancer [33–35]; and prevention of noncommunicable diseases (NCD) [36]. The first systematic investigation on dietary intakes in the Mediterranean region took place in 1948 in the island of Crete, with a major epidemiologic study conducted by Lei and Allbaugh, to determine how best to raise the population's standard of living [37]. In the early 1960s, the famous Seven Countries Study was conducted in the USA, Japan, Italy, Greece, the Netherlands, Finland, and Yugoslavia. The outcomes of this study were published by Ancel Keys, in "Coronary Heart Disease in Seven Countries" [10] and in "How to Eat Well and Stay Well: the Mediterranean Way" [38], and in "Seven Countries: A Multivariate Analysis of Death and Coronary Heart Disease" [39]. These studies initiated the scientific interest on the health benefits of the MD.

Ancel Keys summarized his major contribution to the concept of the MD thus: "My concern about diet as a public health problem began in the early 1950s in Naples, where we observed very low incidences of coronary heart disease associated with what we later came to call the good MD." The heart of this diet is mainly vegetarian, and differs from American and Northern European diets in that it was much lower in meat and dairy products and uses fruit for dessert. These observations led to the subsequent research in the "Seven Countries Study," in which it was demonstrated that "saturated fat was the major dietary villain" [40].

In the 1960s, a large-scale Eurotom study [41] showed that diets in the Mediterranean region were characterized by a much greater intake of cereals, vegetables, fruit, and fish; a much smaller intake of potatoes, meat and dairy foods, eggs, and sweets, but with a high intake of olive oil as the principal source of monounsaturated fat. In the 1980s, the European MONICA research project [42] confirmed the relationship between dietary habits and cardiovascular health, with much reduced mortality rates for persons following a Mediterranean-type dietary pattern.

In 1988, in Delphi, Greece, a symposium was held on "The MD and food culture" by the Association of Schools of Public Health in the European Region and the European Regional Office of WHO [43]. In 1992, in Barcelona, a seminar was held on the "*Changing patterns of fat intake in Mediterranean countries*" by the Catalonian Department of Health, in collaboration with the European Office of the World Health Organization,[44]. Both these meetings raised the awareness among the scientific community on the healthy benefits of the Mediterranean dietary patterns. This led to the International Conference "*The Diets of the Mediterranean*," held in 1993, in Cambridge, at Harvard School of Public Health, organized by Oldways Preservation & Exchange Trust and the WHO/FAO Collaborating Center in Nutritional Epidemiology, linking the MD to the improved health and longevity of populations consuming it [2]. The MD was represented graphically as a pyramid [15] and referred to the food patterns typical of Crete and Southern Italy in the early 1960s.

In 1996, in Barcelona, the first International Congress on the MD was convened by the Foundation for the Advancement of the MD. In 2000, in London, an International Conference on the MD was held by the International Task Force for Prevention on Coronary Heart Disease which proposed a "*Consensus statement*: *dietary fat, the MD, and lifelong good health*" in which was highlighted the increasing scientific evidence of the positive health effects of the traditional MD [45]. In 2002, in Barcelona, an International Task Force on the MD was established by the Foundation for the Advancement of the MD. This recognized the need to redefine and update the traditional MD in light of the changes in this model that had occurred over the past 40 years or that may come about in the future [46]. Also in 2002, in Lametia Terme, Italy, the redefinition of the MD continued with the first Forum on Mediterranean Food Cultures "Feeding minds—fighting hunger: dialogues among Mediterranean civilizations," where nutritionists, anthropologists, educators, rural development experts, representatives of FAO and UNESCO reached a new joint understanding of the MD as an expression of the diversity of the food cultures present in the Mediterranean area. Until then, the perception of the MD was associated primarily with its health benefits, the consumption of a balanced amount of nutrients, distributed according to a pyramidal structure, instead of being more properly associated with a daily lifestyle, where "food" had, as well as a health role, also cultural, social, religious, economic, and environmental functions.

From 2003 to 2005, in Rome, Barcelona, and Athens, this interdisciplinary and multicultural discussion on redefining the MD continued, leading to the Third Forum on Mediterranean Food Cultures, held in 2005 at the Sapienza University of Rome, with the issue of "*The 2005 Rome Call for a Common Action on Food in the Mediterranean*" [47]. In this forum, participants agreed on a shared definition of the MD by recalling that the ancient Greek word δίαιτα meant "equilibrium," "lifestyle," and the MD was defined more than just a diet—rather as a whole lifestyle pattern with physical activity playing an important role. It was stressed that the uniqueness of the Mediterranean dietary pattern was not related only to a list of foods (some traditional) but also in their sustainability (mostly fresh, seasonally and locally grown), their preparation, and the way and context in which these foods are consumed. All these aspects were, and still are, key components of the MD.

Alarmed by the increasing erosion of the MD [2, 44, 48–50], all participants supported the process for recognition of the MD by UNESCO as an intangible cultural heritage of humanity. In 2007, to this end, the governments of Greece, Italy, Morocco and Spain submitted a transnational application to UNESCO [51]. In 2009, as a continuation of the 2005 Rome Call, the Forum on Mediterranean Food Cultures and the Foundation for the Advancement of the MD started a dialogue to reach a consensus among the international MD scientific community for a new revised, updated, and unpatented Mediterranean pyramid, as well as on the MD as a model of a sustainable diet [12, 17, 52]. In November 2009, in Parma, Italy, the third CIISCAM Conference on "The MD Today: A Model of Sustainable Diet" discussed a number of issues. Although there was a consensus on the identity of the traditional MD pattern, questions were raised about the need to update the current recommendations considering the new lifestyle, and dietary, environmental, and health challenges facing the new generations, different countries and sectors of the population [53]. It was emphasized that the importance of the MD for the rest of the world lay not in its specific foods and nutrients, but in the methods used to characterize/analyze it and the philosophy of sustainability at its core. These same methods could be used to define sustainable diets in other eco- and food-systems [54]. Also, a consensus was reached on a number of issues including a simple graphic mainframe to be adapted thereafter to the specific characteristics of each Mediterranean country (Fig. 3.2a, b) [14].

The MD, linked to theMediterranean cultural and natural environment, was presented as a resource of sustainable development as well as an intangible cultural heritage to be safeguarded and enhanced. Reaching this first consensus was the result of continuous negotiations and sometimes uneasy confrontation/dialogue among all participants [14]. Then, in March 2010, in Barcelona, at the 8th International Congress on the MD, this consensus position was again revised by the International Scientific Committee of the MD Foundation and finalized with a new revised pyramid (Fig. 3.3), in which the concept of sustainability was represented through the inclusion in the graph of references to biodiversity, seasonality, and "eco-friendly" products [17].

In 2010, FAO and Bioversity International organized a technical workshop and an international scientific symposium on "biodiversity and sustainable diets," in which MD emerged as a case study for the assessment of sustainable diet in different agro-ecological zones [55]. Its purpose was to mainstream, as a common path, biodiversity, nutrition and sustainable diets, as central to sustainable development. As one of the symposium's major outcomes, a consensus position was reached on the following definition of sustainable diets: "Sustainable diets are those diets with low environmental impacts which contribute to food and nutrition security and to healthy life for present and future generations. Sustainable diets are protective and respectful of biodiversity and ecosystems, culturally acceptable, accessible, economically fair and affordable; nutritionally adequate, safe and healthy; while optimizing natural and human resources" [56].

At the end of 2010, the inscription of the MD in the UNESCO Representative List of the Intangible Cultural Heritage of Humanity, was approved as follows: "The MD constitutes a set of skills, knowledge, practices and traditions ranging from the landscape to the table, including the crops, harvesting, fishing, conservation, processing, preparation and, particularly, consumption of food. The MD encompasses more than just food rather a social cultural expression of the different food cultures Mediterranean. It promotes social interaction, since communal meals are the cornerstone of social customs and "festive events" [13].

The inscription of the MD in theUNESCO Intangible Cultural Heritage List raised the requirement of sustainability as a safeguarding measure as well as the utmost critical need to identify an inventory of this "intangible heritage". This inventory is both a complex process and indispensable tool to evaluate and decide what, and how, the intangible cultural heritage of the MD should be protected and transmitted [51]. However, some 4 years later, it seems that there is an impasse, especially at the level of governments and public policies, to act practically in relation to safeguarding the MD, which is sorely needed [57]. In the last decade, the MD has become the object of increasing studies on its sustainability, particularly on its lower environmental impact [58–61]. However, there is still a need of further cross-cuttinginterdisciplinary approaches to define the most appropriate metrics to assess the sustainability of the MD by taking into account all its sustainability dimensions of health/nutrition, environment, economic, and sociocultural [13].

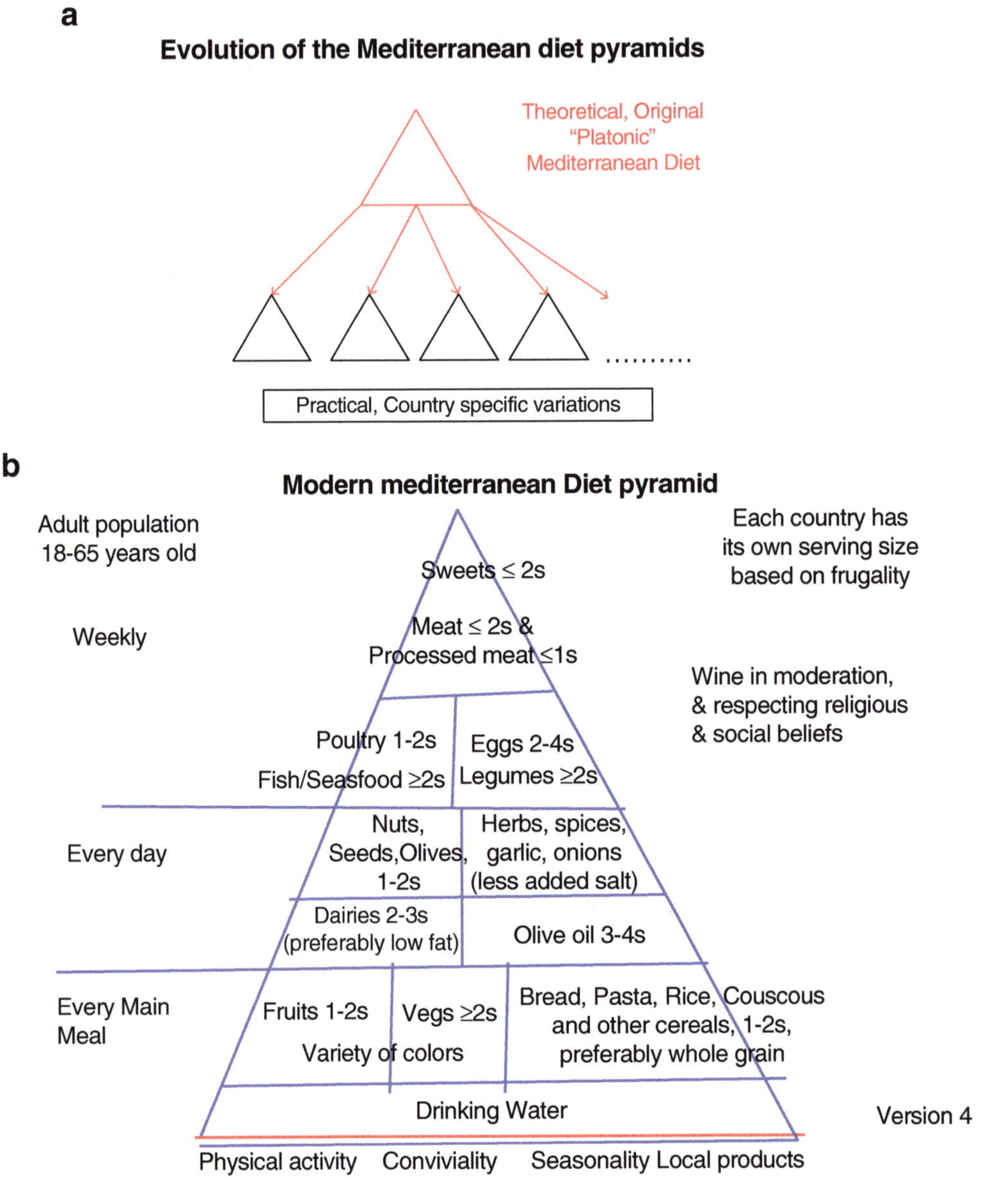

Fig. 3.2 Evolution of the Mediterranean pyramids. (**a**) The diagram shows the mainframe scheme for the evolution of the Mediterranean pyramid; (**b**) Elements of the modern Mediterranean pyramid

Changes of Behavior and Adherence

Historic Modifications of the MD

The MD, as it was defined since and after Ancel Keys' first study, is closely related to the evolution of the Mediterranean lifestyles, and deeply influenced bycultural and economic modifications during the last decades. Despite its increasing popularity worldwide, the MD is today endangered in all

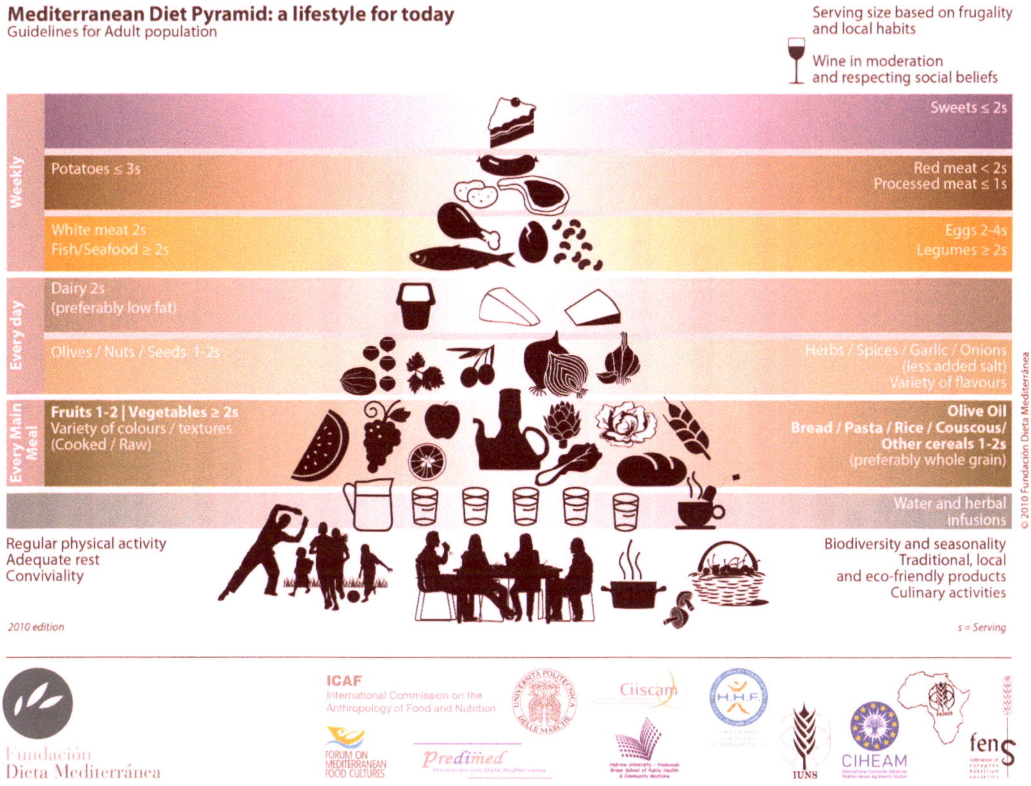
Mediterranean Diet Pyramid: a lifestyle for today
Guidelines for Adult population
Serving size based on frugality and local habits
Wine in moderation and respecting social beliefs
Weekly
Sweets ≤ 2s
Potatoes ≤ 3s
Red meat < 2s
Processed meat ≤ 1s
White meat 2s
Fish/Seafood ≥ 2s
Eggs 2-4s
Legumes ≥ 2s
Every day
Dairy 2s
(preferably low fat)
Olives / Nuts / Seeds 1-2s
Herbs / Spices / Garlic / Onions
(less added salt)
Variety of flavours
Every Main Meal
Fruits 1-2 | Vegetables ≥ 2s
Variety of colours / textures
(Cooked / Raw)
Olive Oil
Bread / Pasta / Rice / Couscous/
Other cereals 1-2s
(preferably whole grain)
Water and herbal infusions
Regular physical activity
Adequate rest
Conviviality
Biodiversity and seasonality
Traditional, local
and eco-friendly products
Culinary activities
2010 edition
s = Serving
© 2010 Fundación Dieta Mediterránea
The use and promotion of this pyramid is recommended without any restriction
Fundación Dieta Mediterránea
ICAF
International Commission on the Anthropology of Food and Nutrition
FORUM ON MEDITERRANEAN FOOD CULTURES
Predimed
Ciiscam
H.H.F.
IUNS
CIHEAM
fens

Fig. 3.3 Revised Mediterranean pyramid

countries of the Mediterranean area. Investigations in the early 1990s already showed that dietary patterns throughout the Mediterranean countries, were moving away increasingly from those collected by Keys in the 1960s [44, 62, 63] and, thus, the MD was considered to be at risk of becoming an "endangered species" [2]. Moreover, recent data have confirmed that in many Mediterranean countries this loss of adherence to the MD is continuing [64–70]. Various dietary scores of adherence to the MD have been developed and extensively reviewed [20, 45–50, 71–76]. In the decline of the adherence to the MD, there are two major concerns: an increase in the consumption of lipids (e.g., meat, dairy products) (Fig. 3.4) and a decrease in the consumption of complex carbohydrates (e.g., cereals and legumes) [77].

Changes of diets and consumption patterns in the Mediterranean region are the result of population growth [79]; globalization [57, 80, 81]; urbanization [80]. According to UNEP/MAP [82], the Mediterranean agricultural and rural models, including the Mediterranean dietary model, are under increasing threat from the predominance of imported consumption patterns.

Nutritional investigations point out that the longer survival benefit associated with the MD could be partly attributed to Mediterranean traditional foods, which are critical components of this diet [83, 84]. The scenario for the expected impacts of trade liberalization, climate change, and the lack of efficient rural policies offers a gloomy picture in some Southern and Eastern Mediterranean countries, with the prospect of aggravated regional imbalances, deeper ecological degradation, and persistent or accrued social instability [85]. The Mediterranean area is passing through a "*nutritional transition*" in which, in the Southern and Eastern Mediterranean countries, problems of undernutrition coexist with overweight, obesity (Table 3.1), and food-related chronic diseases [86].

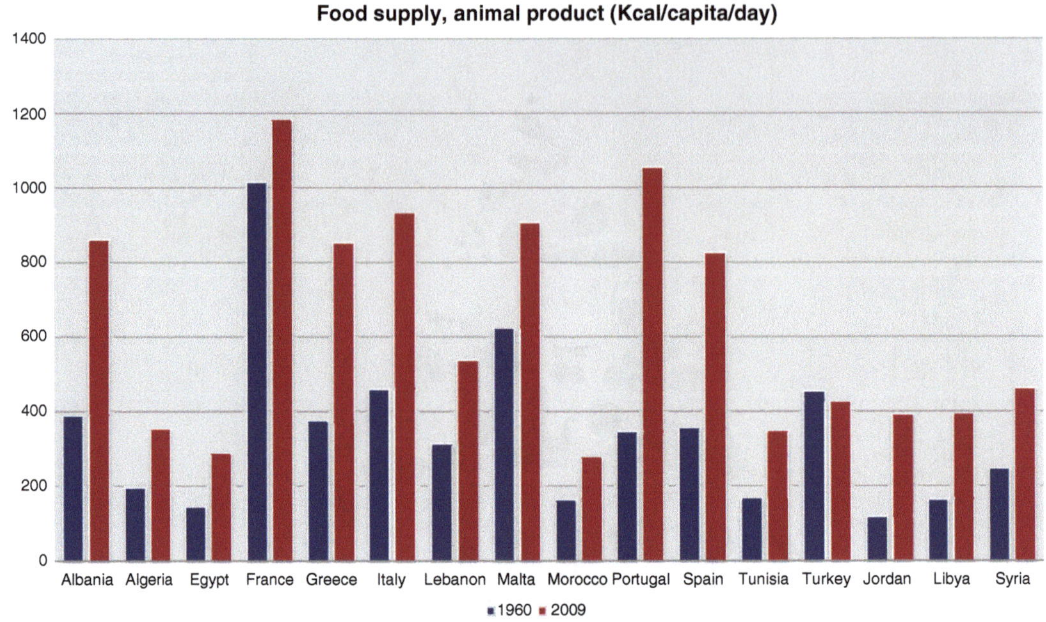

Fig. 3.4 Supply of animal-based products in the Mediterranean countries (*Source*: [78])

Determinants of Adherence to the MD

The abandonment of traditional healthy habits and the emergence of new lifestyles associated with socioeconomic changes are causing an increasing cultural erosion process that poses important threats to the preservation and transmission of the MD to future generations [87].

Changes inintergenerational and gender relations, the role of women in society and interrelations with the rest of the world (tourism and migrations) are having erosive effects on Mediterranean lifestyles and, consequently, on the increasing westernization of food consumption patterns in the Mediterranean area. These changes are influenced to a large extent by urbanization, organization of working time, growing participation of women in economic life, fewer household members, fewer generations living together, a surge of supermarkets, and a dissocialized collective environment [17, 88–91].

A number of studies have recently been published to explore the determinants of adherence to the MD in Greece, Spain, and Italy in both the youth and adults. Costarelli et al. [92] looked at the relationship to health-related quality of life in 359 Greek adolescents. All components were significant especially the level of maternal education and the number of meals per day eaten with the family. The ZOOM8 study [93] looked at adherence to the MD in 1740 Italian school children aged 8–9 years. Only 5.0 % were high and 62.2 % were average adherers, with no relation to gender or BMI. Factors associated with better adherence included: higher maternal (but not paternal) education, having breakfast with the family, having and liking lunch at school, no free access to food, availability of fruit and pulses and liking vegetables, lower TV (videogame, computer, etc.) time, and a low population size of the place of residence.

Concerning adults, in the Moli-sani study from Italy [94] based on 744 subjects mean age 52.1 years, the odds of increased adherence to the MD and also a lower prevalence of obesity were significantly related to greater nutrition knowledge, evaluated by a 92 multiple choice questionnaire. Data from the PREDIMED trial in Spain on 7305 participants (55–80 years of age) [95] showed that greater adherence to the MD was positively related to education, activity, and better health profiles

Table 3.1 Obesity, overweight, and malnutrition (undernourishment) in selected Mediterranean countries

Specification	Overweight 2011 (%) (WHO, 2011)	Obesity 2011 (%) (WHO, 2011)	Undernourishment 2010–2012 (%) (FAO, WFP, and IFAD; 2012)
Albania	54.4	21.3	–
Algeria	45.5	16.0	<5
Egypt	67.9	33.1	<5
Iraq	62.3	27.0	26.0
Israel	60.9	26.2	–
Jordan	64.1	30.0	<5
Lebanon	61.8	27.4	<5
Libya	61.9	27.8	<5
Morocco	46.8	16.4	5.5
Syria	61.2	27.1	<5
Tunisia	53.7	22.3	<5
Turkey	61.9	27.8	<5

Source: CIHEAM-Bari's elaboration using data from WHO 2011 and FAO-WFP-IFAD 2012 [99]

concerning glucose tolerance, lower waist to height ratios, and non-smoking. It is not clear if the health benefits were causal for promoting adherence or secondary to the diet itself. The answer is probably both.

These studies suggest areas for possible interventions to improve adherence patterns. The atmosphere and lifestyle habits at home are crucial, in particular the role of the mother in determining family meal composition and food choices. The role of school meals is also an important determinant of peer-group eating habits which, if properly integrated, may continue into adulthood. Other influences that might help improve lifestyle are the use of role models—sportsmen for boys and media stars for girls; media campaigns (TV advertising bans on food at peak viewing times) and family outdoor activities. Removing vending machines for sweet drinks at schools and their environs is another program used to combat obesity. However, positive carrots are to be preferred to negative sticks, as eating should be a fun and a pleasurable experience rather than a (legal) menu list of do's and don'ts [96]. There are no simple or simplistic solutions to improving adherence. Bottom (family) up and top (Government) down programs are both needed.

The population in the Southern Mediterranean is mainly young. By 2020, 36 % of the population in the South will still be under 20 years of age compared to 20 % in the North. It is a well-known fact that young people, who are going through the phase of a break between generations ("adolescent revolt") are more open to media influences and fashion trends, and that they cultivate a certain degree of ambiguity between modern food which has a social identity appeal and traditional food [81]. Our relationship with food is constantly evolving, as it depends on various factors (age, social position, sociotype, etc.) [89]. And, more generally, lifestyles in the second half of the last century have undergone profound changes, due not only to economic developments, but also to the changing structure of the family and the advancement of food technologies. Eating habits and organization of meals have changed, incorporating foods which previously had only been infrequently eaten because of higher costs and lower availability. Drewnowski and Eichelsdorfer [97] tested whether the MD could be an affordable low-energy-density model for dietary change in helping combat the obesity epidemic in the U.S. Their results were inconclusive since they depended on finding the right balance between good nutrition, affordability and acceptable social norms, all of which required further study and consumer education. However, a recent systematic review found that the health benefits of adopting Mediterranean dietary patterns could lead to an increased life expectancy and a reduction in total lifetime health costs [98].

Conclusions

The MD is recognized as being one of the healthiest diets in the world. However, there is currently an increasing erosion of its adherence among Mediterranean populations which undermines their identity since food traditions are intimately linked to the diversity of their cultures.

The interaction between cultural and economic aspects, together with the introduction of more advanced technologies, has rapidly and profoundly changed original consumption patterns, with a considerable increase in the consumption of beef, condiments made from vegetable fats other than olive oil, and drinks over-sweetened with simple sugars. This type of diet leads to an increase in daily caloric intake that would be compatible only with an active lifestyle like that of the Mediterranean farmer, but is certainly excessive in relation to the sedentary habits of a student or an employee who lives and works in the city. From here, it is but a short step to overweight and obesity. The emergence of new lifestyles associated with socioeconomic changes pose significant threats to the preservation and transmission of the MD to future generations. Therefore, the increased scientific interest in the MD as a model of sustainability should be also seen as part of the safeguarding measures for the MD, as requested for its UNESCO acknowledgment as an intangible cultural heritage.

The complexity of the multi-dimensions of sustainability, within the radical transformation of the contemporary global scenario and the changes of its food consumption and production patterns [99], requires new forms of dialogue, at different levels. Connecting the nutritional well-being of the individual and the community to the sustainability of our everyday living is the current challenge for the MD for the benefit of present and future generations.

References

1. Fidanza F. Diets and dietary recommendations in ancient Greece and Rome and the school of Salerno. Prog Food Nutr Sci. 1979;3:79–99.
2. Nestle M. MDs: historical and research overview. Am J Clin Nutr. 1995;61(Suppl):1313S–20S.
3. Haber B. The MD: a view from history. Am J Clin Nutr. 1997;66(suppl):1053S–7.
4. Seymour TD. Life in the Homeric age. New York: The Macmillan Co; 1907. p. 208–34.
5. Yonge CD, editor. The Deipnosophists or banquet of the learned of Athenaeus, vol. 1–3. London: George Bell & Sons; 1909.
6. Darby WJ, Ghalioungui P, Grivetti L, editors. Food: the gift of Osiris, vol. 1, 2. London: Academic Press; 1977.
7. Vermeule E. Greece in the bronze age. Chicago: University of Chicago Press; 1964.
8. Vickery KF. Food in early Greece. Illinois Stud Soc Sci. 1936;20:1–97.
9. Berry E, Arnoni Y, Aviram M. The Middle Eastern & Biblical origins of the MD. Public Health Nutr. 2011;14(12A):2288–95.
10. Keys AB. Coronary heart disease in seven countries. Circulation. 1970;51–52 Suppl.
11. Gussow JD. MDs: are they environmentally responsible? Am J Clin Nutr. 1995;61(Suppl):1383S–9.
12. Burlingame B, Dernini S. Sustainable diets: the MD example. Public Health Nutr. 2011;14(12A):2285–7.
13. UNESCO. Representative list of the intangible cultural heritage of humanity. 2010.
14. Dernini S, Berry EM, Bach-Faig A, Belahsen R, Donini LM, Lairon D, et al. A dietary model constructed by scientists: The MD. Mediterra 2012. The MD for sustainable regional development. Paris: CIHEAM, Presses de Sciences Po; 2012. p. 71–88
15. Willett W, Sacks F, Trichopoulou A, Drescher G, Ferro-Luzzi A, Helsing E, et al. MD pyramid: a cultural model for healthy eating. Am J Clin Nutr. 1995;61:1402S–6.
16. Trichopoulou A, Lagiou P. Healthy traditional MD: an expression of culture, history and lifestyle. Nutr Rev. 1997;55:383–9.
17. Bach-Faig A, Berry EM, Lairon D, Reguant J, Trichopoulou A, Dernini S, et al. MD pyramid today. Science and cultural updates. Public Health Nutr. 2011;14(12A):2274–84.
18. de Lorgeril M, Renaud S, Mamelle N, et al. Mediterranean alpha-linolenic acid-rich diet in secondary prevention of coronary heart disease (Erratum. Lancet 1995;345:738). Lancet. 1994;343:1454–9.

19. Menotti A, Kromhout D, Blackburn H, Fidanza F, Buzina R, Nissinen A. Food intake patterns and 25-year mortality from coronary heart disease: cross-cultural correlations in the Seven Countries Study. The Seven Countries Study Research Group. Eur J Epidemiol. 1999;15(6):507–15.
20. Martínez-González MA, Fernandez-Jarne E, Serrano-Martinez M, et al. MD and reduction in the risk of a first acute myocardial infarction. An operational healthy dietary score. Eur J Nutr. 2002;41:153–60.
21. Trichopoulou A, Costacou T, Bamia C, Trichopoulou D. Adherence to a MD and survival in a Greek population. N Engl J Med. 2003;348:2599–608.
22. Mendez MA, Popkin BM, Jakszyn P, Berenguer A, Tormo MJ, Sanchez MJ, et al. Adherence to a MD is associated with reduced 3-year incidence of obesity. J Nutr. 2006;136:2934–8.
23. Estruch R, Ros E, Salas-Salvadó J, Covas MI, Corell D, Arós F, et al. Primary prevention of cardiovascular disease with a MD. N Engl J Med. 2013;368:1279–90.
24. Trichopoulou A, Bamia C, Trichopoulos D. Anatomy of health effects of MD: Greek EPIC prospective cohort study. BMJ. 2009;338:b2337.
25. Martínez-González MA, Bes-Rastrollo M, Serra-Majem L, Lairon D, Estruch R, Trichopoulou A. Mediterranean food pattern and the primary prevention of chronic disease: recent developments. Nutr Rev. 2009;67 suppl 1:S111–6.
26. Buckland G, González CA, Agudo A, et al. Adherence to the MD and risk of coronary heart disease in the Spanish EPIC cohort study. Am J Epidemiol. 2009;170(12):1518–29.
27. Buckland G, Bach A, Serra-Majem L. Obesity and the MD: a systematic review of observational and intervention studies. Obes Rev. 2008;9:582–93.
28. Sofi F, Cesari F, Abbate R, Gensini GF, Casini A. Adherence to MD and health status: meta-analysis. BMJ. 2008;337:a1344.
29. Tortosa A, Bes-Rastrollo M, Sanchez-Villegas A, Basterra-Gortari FJ, Nunez-Cordoba JM, Martinez-Gonzalez MA. MD inversely associated with the incidence of metabolic syndrome: the SUN prospective cohort. Diabetes Care. 2007;30(11):2957–9.
30. Babio N, Bullo M, Basora J, Martinez-Gonzalez MA, Fernandez-Ballart J, Marquez-Sandoval F, et al. Adherence to the MD and risk of metabolic syndrome and its components. Nutr Metab Cardiovasc Dis. 2009;19(8):563–70.
31. Kastorini CM, Milionis HJ, Esposito K, Giugliano D, Goudevenos JA, Panagiotakos DB. The effect of MD on metabolic syndrome and its components a meta-analysis of 50 studies and 534,906 individuals. J Am Coll Cardiol. 2011;57(11):1299–313.
32. Kesse-Guyot E, Fezeu L, Hercberg S, Ahluwalia N, Lairon D. Adherence to MD reduces the risk of metabolic syndrome: a prospective study. Nutr Metab Cardiovasc Dis. 2012;142(5):909–15.
33. La Vecchia C. MD and cancer. Public Health Nutr. 2004;7(7):965–8.
34. Bosetti C, Pelucchi C, La Vecchia C. Diet and cancer in Mediterranean countries: carbohydrates and fats. Public Health Nutr. 2009;12(9A):1595–600.
35. Vernele L, Bach-Faig A, Buckland G, Serra-Majem L. Association between the MD and cancer risk: a review of observational studies. Nutr Cancer. 2010;62(7):860–70.
36. Serra-Majem L, Roman B, Estruch R. Scientific evidence of interventions using the MD: a systematic review. Nutr Rev. 2006;64:S27–47.
37. Allbaugh LG. Crete: a case study of an underdeveloped area. Princeton, NJ: Princeton University Press; 1953.
38. Keys AB, Keys M, editors. How to eat well and stay well the Mediterranean way. Garden City, NY: Doubleday; 1975.
39. Keys A (ed). (1980) Seven countries: a multivariate analysis of death and coronary heart disease. Keys ABe, editor: Harvard University Press, Cambridge, MA.
40. Keys AB. MD and public health: personal reflections. Am J Clin Nutr. 1995;61(Suppl):1321S–23S.
41. Cresta M, Ledermann S, Garnier A, et al. Étude des consommations alimentaires des population de onze régions de la Communauté européenne en vue de la détermination des niveaux de contamination radioactive: rapport, Centre d'étude nucléaire de Fontenay-aux-Roses; 1969
42. Stewart AW, Kuulasmaa K, Beaglehole R, for the WHO MONICA Project. Ecological analysis of the association between mortality and major risk factors of cardiovascular disease. Int J Epidemiol. 1994;23:505–16.
43. Trichopoulou A, Helsing E, editors. The Mediterranean diet and food culture, a symposium. Eur J Clin Nutr. 1989;43 Suppl 2.
44. Serra-Majem L, Helsing E, editors. Changing patterns of fat intake in Mediterranean countries. Eur J Clin Nutr. 1993;47 Suppl 1.
45. International Task Force for Prevention of Coronary Heart Disease Website. Consensus statement: dietary fat, the MD and lifelong good health, 2000; 2000.
46. Serra-Majem L, Trichopoulou A, Ngo de la Cruz J, Cervera P, Garcia Alvarez A, La Vecchia C, et al. Does the definition of the MD need to be updated? Public Health Nutr. 2004;7(7):927–9.
47. Dernini S. Transmitting Mediterranean food culture through art: a creative inter-disciplinary approach. Public Health Nutr. 2006;9(8A):1141–3.

48. Gerber M. Qualitative methods to evaluate MD in adults. Public Health Nutr. 2006;9(1A):147–51.
49. Bach A, Serra-Majem L, Carrasco JL, Roman B, Ngo J, Bertomeu I, et al. The use of indexes evaluating the adherence to the MD in epidemiological studies: a review. Public Health Nutr. 2006;9(1A):132–46.
50. Kourlaba G, Panagiotakos DB. Dietary quality indices and human health: a review. Maturitas. 2009;62:1–8.
51. Reguant-Aleix J, Sensat F. The MD, intangible cultural heritage of humanity. Mediterra 2012. Paris: CIHEAM, Sciences Po Les Presses; 2012. p. 465–84.
52. Medina FX. Food consumption and civil society: MD as a sustainable resource for the Mediterranean area. Public Health Nutr. 2011;14(12A):2346–9.
53. Lairon D, Berry EM. The need for a revised MD pyramid. The MD today: a model of sustainable diet, 3rd CIISCAM International Conference. Parma2009.
54. Burlingame B, Dernini S. MD as a model of a sustainable diet. The MD today: a model of sustainable diet, 3rd CIISCAM International Conference. Parma 2009.
55. Keys B, Dernini S, editors. Sustainable diets and biodiversity. Directions and solutions for policy, research and action. Rome: FAO/Bioversity International; 2012.
56. FAO/Bioversity. Report of the international symposium on Biodiversity and Sustainable Diets. Rome; 2010.
57. González Turmo I. The MD: consumption, cuisine and food habits. Mediterra 2012. The MD for sustainable regional development. Paris: CIHEAM, Presses de Sciences Po; 2012. p. 115–32.
58. Duchin F. Sustainable consumption of food: a framework for analyzing scenarios about changes in diets. J Ind Ecol. 2005;9(1-2):99–114.
59. van Dooren C, Marinussen M, Blonk H, Aiking H, Vellinga P. Exploring dietary guidelines based on ecological and nutritional values: a comparison of six dietary patterns. Food Policy. 2014;44:36–46.
60. Dernini S, Meybeck A, Burlingame B, Gitz G, Lacirignola C, Debs P, et al. Developing a methodological approach for assessing the sustainability of diets: the MD as a case study. New Medit. 2013;12(3):28–36.
61. Baroni L, Cenci L, Tettamanti M, Berati M. Evaluating the environmental impact of various dietary patterns combined with different food production systems. Eur J Clin Nutr. 2007;61(2):279–86.
62. Kafatos A, Kouroumalis I, Vlachonikolis I, Theodorou C, Labadarios D. Coronary-heart-disease risk-factor status of the Cretan urban population in the 1980s. Am J Clin Nutr. 1991;54:591–8.
63. Ferro-Luzzi A, Branca F. MD, Italian-style: prototype of a healthy diet. Am J Clin Nutr. 1995;61(Suppl):1338S–45.
64. IOTF. EU platform on diet, physical activity and health. Briefing paper. London, UK: International Association for the Study of Obesity; 2005.
65. Garcia-Closas R, Berenguer A, Gonzalez C. Changes in food supply in Mediterranean countries from 1961 to 2001. Public Health Nutr. 2006;9(1):53–60.
66. Belahsen R, Rguibi M. Population health and MD in southern Mediterranean countries. Public Health Nutr. 2006;9(8A):1130–5.
67. Alexandratos N. The MD, in a world context. Public Health Nutr. 2006;9(1A):111–7.
68. da Silva R, Bach-Faig A, Quintana BR, Buckland G, Vaz de Almeida MD, Serra-Majem L. Worldwide variation of adherence to the MD in 1961-1965 and 2000-2005. Public Health Nutr. 2009;12(9A):1676–84.
69. Vareiro D, Bach-Faig A, Raidó Quintana B, Bertomeu I, Buckland G, Vaz de Almeida MD, et al. Availability of Mediterranean and non-Mediterranean foods during the last four decades: comparison of several geographical areas. Public Health Nutr. 2009;12(9A):1667–75.
70. León-Muñoz LM, Guallar-Castillón P, Graciani A, López-García E, Mesas AE, Aguilera MT, et al. Adherence to the MD pattern has declined in Spanish adults. J Nutr. 2012;142(10):1843–50.
71. Trichopoulou A, Kouris-Blazos A, Wahlqvist ML, Gnardellis C, Lagiou P, Polychronopoulos E, et al. Diet and overall survival in elderly people. BMJ. 1995;311:1457–61.
72. Alberti-Fidanza A, Fidanza F, Chiuchiu M, Verducci G, Fruttini D. Dietary studies on two rural Italian population groups of the Seven Countries Study. 3. Trend of food and nutrient intake from 1960 to 1991. Eur J Clin Nutr. 1999;53:854–60.
73. Fidanza F, Alberti A, Lanti M, Menotti A. Mediterranean Adequacy Index: correlation with 25-year mortality from coronary heart disease in the Seven Countries Study. Nutr Metab Cardiovasc Dis. 2004;14:254–8.
74. Sanchez-Villegas A, Martinez J, de Irala J, Martınez-Gonzalez M. Determinants of the adherence to an a priori defined Mediterranean dietary pattern. Eur J Nutr. 2002;41:249–57.
75. Serra-Majem L, Ribas L, Ngo J, Ortega RM, Garcıa A, Perez-Rodrigo C, et al. Food, youth and the MD in Spain. Development of KIDMED, MD Quality Index in children and adolescents. Public Health Nutr. 2004;7(7):931–5.
76. Sofi F, Macchi C, Abbate R, Gensin GF, Casini A. MD and health status: an updated meta-analysis and a proposal for a literature-based adherence score. Public Health Nutr. 2014;17(12):2769–82.
77. Maillot M, Issa C, Vieux F, Lairon D, Darmon N. The shortest way to reach nutritional goals is to adopt Mediterranean food choices. Evidence from computer-generated personalized diets. Am J Clin Nutr. 2011;94(4):1127–37.
78. FAO. Food balance sheets; 2012.
79. Bleu P. 20 Years of sustainable development in the Mediterranean: review and outlook. Blue Plan Notes. 2012;22.

80. Florensa S, Aragall X. Mutations in Mediterranean societies. Mediterra 2012. The MD for sustainable regional development. Paris: CIHEAM, Presses de Sciences Po; 2012. p. 91–113
81. Padilla M. Dietary patterns and trends in consumption. Mediterra 2008: the future of agriculture and food in Mediterranean countries. Paris: CIHEAM, Presses de Sciences Po; 2008. p. 149–70
82. UNEP/MAP. Mediterranean strategy for sustainable development: a framework for environmental sustainability and shared prosperity. Tenth meeting of the Mediterranean commission on sustainable development (MCSD). Athens; 2005.
83. Trichopoulou A, Vasilopoulou E, Georga K, Soukara S, Dilis V. Traditional foods: why and how to sustain them. Trends Food Sci Technol. 2006;17:498–504.
84. Trichopoulou A. Diversity v. globalization: traditional foods at the epicentre. Public Health Nutr. 2012;15(6):951–4.
85. Medina FX. MD, culture and heritage: challenges for a new conception. Public Health Nutr. 2009;12:1618–20.
86. Aounallah-Skhiri H, Traissac P, El Ati J, Eymard-Duvernay S, Landais E, Achour N, et al. Nutrition transition among adolescents of a south-Mediterranean country: dietary patterns, association with socio-economic factors, overweight and blood pressure. A cross-sectional study in Tunisia. Nutr J. 2011;10:38.
87. Dernini S. The erosion and the renaissance of the MD: a sustainable cultural resource. Quaderns de la Mediterrania. 2011;16:75–82.
88. Kearney J. Food consumption trends and drivers. Philos Trans R Soc. 2010;365:2793–807.
89. Berry EM, DeGeest S. Tell me what you eat and I will tell you your sociotype: coping with diabesity. Rambam Maimonides Med J. 2012;3(2):e0010.
90. Padilla M. Evolution of MD: facts, causes, effects. Proceedings cost action 916 conference on "Bioactive micro-nutrients in MD and health". Rome; 2000. p. 263–71.
91. Padilla M, Capone R, Palma G. Sustainability of the food chain from field to plate: case of the MD. Sustainable diets and biodiversity: united against hunger. Rome: FAO/Bioversity International; 2012. p. 230–41.
92. Costarelli V, Koretsi E, Geotgitsogianni E. Health-related quality of life of Greek adolescents: the role of the MD. Qual Life Res. 2012;22(5):951–6.
93. Roccaldo R, Censi L, D'Addezio L, Toti E, Martone D, D'Addesa D, et al. Adherence to the MD in Italian school children (The ZOOM8 Study). Food Sci Nutr. 2014;Early Online:1–8.
94. Bonaccio M, Di Castelnuovo A, Costanzo S, De Lucia F, Olivieri M, Donati MB, et al. Nutrition knowledge is associated with higher adherence to MD and lower prevalence of obesity. Results from the Moli-sani study. Appetite. 2013;68:139–46.
95. Hu EA, Toledo E, Diez-Espino J, Estruch R, Corella D, Salas-Salvado J, et al. Lifestyles and risk factors associated with adherence to the MD: a baseline assessment of the PREDIMED trial. PLoS One. 2013;8:e60166.
96. Eisenberg M, Atallah R, Grandi SM, Windle SB, Berry EM. Legislative approaches to tackling the obesity epidemic in Canada. CMAJ. 2011;183(13):1496–500.
97. Drewnowski A, Eichelsdoerfer P. The MD: does it have to cost more? Public Health Nutr. 2009;12(9A):1621–8.
98. Saulle R, Semyonov L, La Torre G. Cost and cost-effectiveness of the MD: results of a systematic review. Nutrients. 2013;5:4566–86.
99. FAO, WFP, IFAD. The state of food insecurity in the World 2012. Economic growth is necessary but not sufficient to accelerate reduction of hunger and malnutrition. Rome: FAO; 2012

Chapter 4
Historical origins of the Mediterranean Diet, Regional Dietary Profiles, and the Development of the Dietary Guidelines

Nadine R. Sahyoun and Kavitha Sankavaram

Key Points

- The diet of the Mediterranean basin (22 countries located within Europe, Africa, and Asia) is abundant in foods of plant origin such as legumes, whole grains, fruits and vegetables, nuts and seeds, and olive oil as a main source of fat and contains low amounts of saturated fat. There are a few regional differences in dietary patterns around the Mediterranean Sea but also many similarities. The diet's origins reflect the interactions of diverse populations and civilizations over thousands of years.
- The Mediterranean diet has sparked interest among researchers for its positive effects on health outcomes, including lower mortality rates from cardiovascular disease, some cancers, and, generally, rates of chronic diseases that are among the lowest in the world.
- Since 1993, experts on diet, nutrition, and health have convened a series of conferences to review research on the composition and health implications of Mediterranean diets, resulting in a Mediterranean food guide pyramid which suggests healthy food choices. This is accompanied by messages about healthy diet selection and healthy lifestyle practices. Indexes to measure adherence to the Mediterranean dietary patterns and its impact on health status have also been developed.
- However, the Mediterranean diet continues to evolve as a result of globalization and technological advances resulting in changes to the traditional diet.

Keywords Mediterranean diet origins • Regional dietary patterns • Mediterranean dietary pyramid • Mediterranean diet indexes • Mediterranean lifestyle

---

N.R. Sahyoun, Ph.D., R.D. (✉)
Department of Nutrition and Food Science, University of Maryland,
0112 Skinner Building, College Park, MD 20742, USA
e-mail: nsahyoun@umd.edu

K. Sankavaram, Ph.D.
Expanded Food and Nutrition Education Program, University of Maryland,
College Park, MD 20742-7521, USA
e-mail: kavitha@umd.edu

D.F. Romagnolo, O.I. Selmin (eds.), *Mediterranean Diet*, Nutrition and Health,
DOI 10.1007/978-3-319-27969-5_4

Introduction

The diet of countries surrounding the Mediterranean basin has been a subject of great interest over the past 50 years. This interest stems from results of studies that showed that adults consuming a Mediterranean diet had the lowest rates of chronic diseases in the world and the highest longevity [1, 2]. Since these positive health outcomes could not be attributed to higher educational levels or health expenditures, they were, therefore, linked to a healthy diet and a particular lifestyle. This has resulted in ongoing research efforts to identify and characterize the Mediterranean diet and its health benefits.

Traditional Mediterranean Diet (MD) is characterized by a diet abundant in foods of plant origin such as legumes, whole grains, fruits and vegetables, nuts and seeds, and olive oil as a main source of fat; a low intake of saturated fat; a low-to-moderate intake of dairy products; moderate consumption of fish; and low-to-moderate amounts of wine during meals [3]. This dietary pattern is consumed by people in countries bordering the Mediterranean Sea [3–5]. There are currently 22 countries on the shores of the Mediterranean Sea, located within three continents (Europe, Africa, Asia) as seen in Fig. 4.1 [6]. These countries starting from Spain and in a clockwise direction include Spain, France, Monaco, Italy, Slovenia, Croatia, Bosnia-Herzegovina, Montenegro, Albania, Greece, Turkey, Syria, Lebanon, Israel, Palestinian territories, Egypt, Libya, Tunisia, Algeria, Morocco, and the islands of Cyprus and Malta. Although there are many similarities in foods consumed in the Mediterranean countries, the definition of "Mediterranean diet" varies by region of the Mediterranean basin and by countries [7]. Dietary intake may also vary within individual countries since eating patterns are influenced by traditions, culture, religion, and the economy [7, 8]. In this chapter, we review the historical origins of the MD, regional differences in food patterns, dietary guidelines, and the most commonly used dietary indexes used to evaluate adherence to the MD.

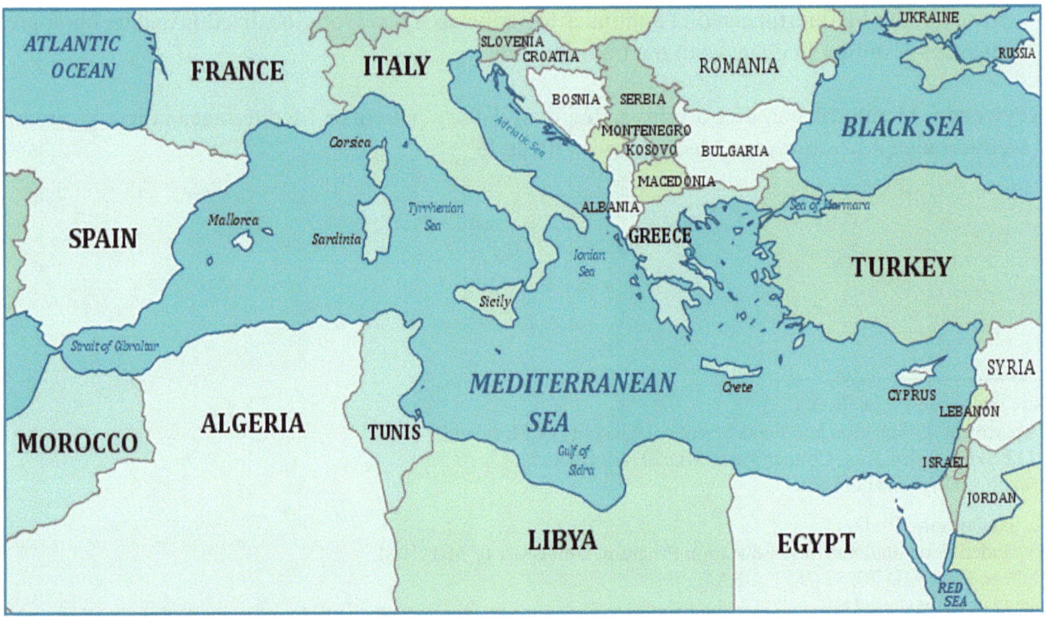

Fig. 4.1 Countries surrounding the Mediterranean Sea. *Source*: Owl & Mouse Educational Maps [6]

Recognition of the MD and Its Health Benefits

The first investigation into the Mediterranean dietary pattern took place in 1948. The government of Greece concerned about improving the economic, social, and health conditions of its population post-World War II invited the Rockefeller Foundation to conduct an epidemiologic study on the island of Crete. In response, epidemiologist Leland Allbaugh conducted a comprehensive survey of the demographic, social, economic, and dietary characteristics of the population. The results showed that 61 % of total energy from the Cretan diet came from plant foods, such as cereals, pulses, fruits, and vegetables. Only 7 % of calories were from animal foods such as meat, fish, eggs, and dairy products. Additionally, data from the food balance for all of Greece showed that the food supply contributed about 74 % of total energy from plant-based foods and 7 % from animal foods. In contrast, the US food supply contributed only 37 % of energy from foods of plant origin and 33 % from animal foods [9]. The Cretan diet also derived about 38 % calories from fat similar to the percentage in the US food supply. However, in the Cretan diet, table fat came predominately from foods of plant origin such as olives and olive oil. The researchers observed few nutritional problems in Crete and concluded that the diets were generally nutritionally adequate. However, some study participants expressed dissatisfaction with their diet listing meat as a food that was lacking in their diet. Ironically, in response to these comments Allbaugh observed that the Cretan food could be improved by incorporating more foods of animal origin [9].

In 1952, Ancel Keys initiated a series of studies known as the Seven Countries Study to examine the relationship between diet and health in Italy, Greece, the USA, Japan, Finland, the Netherlands, and Yugoslavia. This study, which lasted for nearly three decades and included about 12,000 men ages 40–59 years, was one of the first studies that associated MD with health [10]. The results showed strong evidence linking dietary intake with serum cholesterol levels and cardiovascular disease whereby lower rates of cardiovascular diseases were observed among participants with low consumption of saturated fats [9, 11].

Another study led by the European Atomic Energy Commission (EURATOM) from 1963 to 1965 also obtained exhaustive data on the quality and quantity of food consumed by families in 11 regions of 6 European countries. The study compared dietary patterns of nine regions in Northern Europe and two regions in Southern Europe. Although no absolute differences in fat intake were seen in north-south regions, the types of fat and the foods contributing to total fat intake was quite different. The consumption of butter was higher in the northern regions whereas olive oil was the main source of fat in southern regions. Margarine was not consumed by southern regions and less meat and more cereals, fruits, and vegetables were consumed [9]. Following these studies, the beneficial effects of MD in reducing chronic diseases became widely accepted.

Historical Origins of the MD

The regions surrounding the Mediterranean basin have seen the rise and fall of many great civilizations. The history, traditions, and cultures of the different Mediterranean countries reflect the interactions of its diverse populations over thousands of years as this was an area of transport, trade, and cultural exchanges which, naturally, included exchange of food and shaped dietary eating patterns. Current dietary patterns of the communities in that region reflect that common history.

The origin of the MD dates back to the early ninth millennium BC. Archaeological and botanical evidence indicate a dietary pattern with high quantities of cereals and leguminous vegetables [8, 12]. These cereals and legumes were produced in the areas of Syria, Palestine, and Southern Turkey. Pigs, sheep, and cattle were also domesticated at that time, and it is known that all these crops and products had spread to Greece and southern regions of Italy and Spain in early 6000–4000 BC [12]. Evidence of olives, figs, and vines existed from the fourth millennium on, and the Greeks and Phoenicians, a great civilization which originated on the Eastern Mediterranean coast and centered in the area of modern Lebanon and Syria, spread these products to other regions of the Mediterranean in the first millennium BC. Olives, wheat, and vines were established everywhere on the shores of the Mediterranean Sea by the middle of the first millennium BC and came to represent the identity and character of the MD. Olive oil was used as cooking fat or in soups and as a spread on bread but also as soap, medicine, and lubricant [8].

Cereals were the main food for Carthaginians, another important civilization in the Southern part of the Mediterranean located in the area of present Tunis, and also for Phoenicians who consumed them mainly as bread, porridge (*puls punica*), or as biscuit (*punicum*). Breads were made using special earthenware bread ovens (*tabounas*) and are still used in several countries especially, Morocco and Tunisia. Numerous fruits and nuts such as pomegranates, dates, figs, almonds, and pistachio nuts, were available and consumed fresh or dried. Although little is known about the history of vegetables, fruits, and nuts, a wide range was consumed in the Mediterranean region by the time of the Roman Empire. Livestock was used to produce milk and dairy products but rarely used as meat. Evidence also shows consumption of fish by the Carthaginians which included shellfish and crustaceans [8].

Later in the period of the Roman Empire between the seventh and third centuries BC, Roman colonization changed the food patterns of the regions that they governed. Romans modernized agriculture and with the spread of the irrigation system, some of the regions of Roman Africa, which included defeated Carthage in Tunisia, Algeria and Libya were transformed into the bread basket of the peninsula. Romans also spread the growth of a variety of vegetables including onions, leeks, lettuce, carrots, asparagus, pulses, and fruits such as apples, pears, plums, along with indigenous fruits from China and India, such as peaches and apricots. Roman colonization played a significant role in the establishment of the MD since they occupied areas with Mediterranean climatic type for over 750 years [12].

In the seventh century AD, the Arabs expanded along the North African coast and into Spain. They invented new farming methods and introduced new foods, including spinach, chard, and mallow; aubergine from India; and okra from Ethiopia [8]. The Arabs also introduced rice, sugarcane, and sweet oranges from China and India. These crops were later expanded to Italy, Spain, and Sicily [12]. Production in vineyards was reduced due to the religious beliefs of Arabs, who only consumed fruits and unfermented grape juice. The cultivation of aromatic, medicinal, and coloring plants such as cumin, caraway, and anise also increased and so did consumption of dates. With exploration of the Americas, new crops were introduced into the Mediterranean region by the Andalusian traders in the seventeenth century. For example, potatoes were introduced via Portugal, maize via Turkey, and tomatoes and peppers through Italy [8].

Over time, a dietary pattern composed largely of vegetables, fruits, legumes, and nuts with lower rates of meat consumption consolidated in the Mediterranean region and sparked interest among researchers for its positive effects on health outcomes, including lower mortality rates from cardiovascular disease, some cancers and, generally, rates of chronic diseases that are among the lowest in the world [9]. In addition, scientists from around the world who have studied the benefits of this food pattern have recognized the importance of the MD not only as food but also as an integral component of the Mediterranean culture and identity [13].

Similarities and Differences of Mediterranean Dietary Patterns

Mediterranean regional dietary patterns share many common attributes but also some noticeable differences. For example, some of these differences include the amount and type of fat, vegetables, and fruit in the diet and the consumption of whole grains [4, 14]. Noah and Truswell explored those similarities and differences by interviewing women who immigrated to Australia from Spain, southern

France, Italy, Malta, Croatia, Bosnia, Albania, Greece, Cyprus, Turkey, Syria, Lebanon, Egypt, Libya, Tunisia, Algeria, and Morocco. These researchers observed the women's methods of food shopping and preparation, and reviewed recipes in cookbooks. They grouped dietary patterns into four different regions based on the food habits that are similar among neighboring countries [4]. These groups (described below) include Western, Adriatic, Eastern, and North African dietary patterns.

Western Mediterranean Groups

Western groups include Spain, France, Italy, and Malta. The populations of these countries consume high amounts of cereal products such as bread and pasta, mostly made from white flour and semolina. Rice and potatoes are also part of their diet. Dairy consumption is predominantly from cheese and butter. Pulses are eaten in varied quantities depending on the country, with France consuming the most. Vegetables are consumed in high amounts with tomatoes eaten daily and garlic, parsley, basil, and oregano used extensively. Artichoke, broccoli, and eggplant are used moderately. Apples and citrus fruit are also moderately consumed. Olive oil is the main source of oil especially in Italy and Spain while France uses more butter than the rest of the countries in that region. Animal proteins are mainly from pork and preserved meats but other protein sources such as chicken, veal, lamb, beef, fish and fish products are also moderately consumed. Alcohol consumption is very high [4, 14].

Adriatic Mediterranean Groups

Adriatic groups include Croatia, Bosnia, and Albania. These countries consume bread and white wheat flour and rice. However, the consumption of rice is only moderate compared to the western Mediterranean countries. Dairy product consumption is high and mainly in the form of butter and buttermilk. Ricotta and cottage cheese, sour cream, and clotted cream are also consumed very often. Dried pulses are not a major part of the diet as in other regions, especially in the Eastern Mediterranean countries. The main vegetables include okra and eggplant. Vine and cabbage leaves are stuffed with rice and ground beef, a practice quite similar to dishes eaten in most of the Eastern Mediterranean countries. Apples and citrus fruit are eaten most frequently by this group. Olive oil consumption is relatively low and clarified butter is often used in cooking. Beef and chicken are the most common meats consumed. Alcohol consumption is low depending on the country and its religious affiliation. Turkish coffee is consumed daily [4].

Eastern Mediterranean Groups

Eastern Mediterranean groups include Greece, Lebanon, Cyprus, Turkey, and Egypt. These countries consume white wheat flour bread and rice. Burghul (Bulgur), crushed wheat berries, is exclusively consumed within this group of countries. Dairy product consumption is high and mainly in the form of yogurt and cheese. Pulses such as lentils are frequently consumed, while dried broad beans are most common in the Egyptian cuisine. There is a high consumption of vegetables in stews and salads and several of these, such as zucchini, eggplants, vine, and cabbage leaves, are stuffed with rice and ground meat. The common herbs used in this group are dill, parsley, coriander, and oregano. There is moderate consumption of fruit. Fresh and dried dates are consumed mainly in Egypt. The use of olive oil varies from negligible (Egypt) to high (Greece). Clarified butter is often used. Chicken consumption is high with moderate levels of beef, lamb, pigeon, and preserved meats. Nuts are prominent in

Lebanon and Turkey. Alcohol consumption is moderate except in Egypt where it is low due to religious beliefs. Turkish (also known as Greek) coffee is consumed daily [4, 14]. Tea is very common in Egypt.

North African Mediterranean Groups

These include Libya, Algeria, Morocco, and Tunisia. Bread and white wheat flour products are highly consumed but use of rice is very minimal. Breads made out of whole meal and barley flour are also common. Couscous, made out of granules of wheat flour, is consumed more than rice. There is moderate intake of dairy products such as cheese, clotted cream, and buttermilk as a drink. Vegetables are frequently consumed in stews with tomatoes, pumpkin, potatoes, and chickpeas most specific to this group. Allspice and turmeric are often used in cooking. Fruits are eaten in moderate to large amounts and dates and date molasses are essential in the diet. Olive oil consumption ranges from high (Libya) to low (Morocco). Lamb is the meat most commonly eaten. Alcohol is not consumed. Tea drinking also varies from high (Libya and Morocco) to low (Algeria) [4].

Development of the Mediterranean Dietary Guidance

In 1993, in the first of a series of conferences entitled "Public Health Implications of Traditional Diets," a group of experts on diet, nutrition, and health met to review research on the composition and health implications of MDs. Modeled on the USDA food guide pyramid, a MD pyramid was developed, based on the dietary patterns observed in the countries surrounding the Mediterranean basin in the early 1960s [15]. The pyramid was designed to reflect healthy food choices rather than recommendations. The Mediterranean pyramid indicated relative frequencies of certain food groups although the particular foods remained nonspecific in order to underline the potential variation of the food groups regionally. The pyramid described a diet that was considerably high in foods from plant sources—fruits and vegetables, breads and grains, legumes, nuts, and seeds—compared to the dietary pattern suggested in the USDA food guide pyramid. The foundation of the Mediterranean food guide pyramid consisted of a variety of wheat and other grain products and potatoes. The next level from the base of the pyramid included distinct categories for vegetables, fruits, beans, legumes, and nuts. The next levels of the pyramid included olive oil, cheese, and yogurt and to a lesser extent other foods. The tip of the pyramid included foods such as red meat and sweets recommended to be consumed sparingly and on a monthly basis. The pyramid also suggested moderate consumption of wine and most consumption of the fat from olive oil, which is rich in monounsaturated fatty acid. In addition, the traditional MD pyramid emphasized the importance of regular physical activity.

Subsequent to the 1993 meeting, the International Congress on the MD was convened in Barcelona in 1996 and this led to the signing of the "*Declaration of Barcelona on the Mediterranean Diet*" whose main objective was to preserve the traditional Mediterranean dietary habits and high quality of food production. The proceedings from this meeting emphasized the healthy eating aspects of the diet and included cultural and historical aspects to the diet. From then on the meetings were held every 2 years and proceedings were published in special editions of the journal *Public Health Nutrition* [16]. In the conference held in 1998, a consensus statement on dietary fat and overall dietary pattern was released which emphasized that restriction of total fat was not needed as long as calories were not consumed in excess. The statement also recommended a diet low in saturated fats and hydrogenated oils and an increase in the consumption of fruits, vegetables, whole grains, fish, nuts, and low-fat dairy products. Details of the accomplishments at the various meetings of the congress are available at the website of Fundaci6n Dieta Mediterránea [17].

In 2002, at the Barcelona conference, the International Task Force on the MD discussed redefining and updating the MD. Additionally, it was agreed that any positive dietary changes that may have occurred over the past 40 years be recognized, acknowledged, and addressed within the food guide model [18]. The updated version of the Mediterranean pyramid was released in 2010 and in contrast to the previous version included quantification of food by addressing proportions and frequency of servings. The updated visual representation of the pyramid follows the previous pattern. The base of the pyramid is comprised of foods that should sustain the diet. Foods to be eaten in moderate or limited amounts are included at the upper levels. The graphic was accompanied by messages that incorporate lifestyle factors in addition to food habits (Fig. 4.2, Table 4.1) [19, 20].

In the USA, the dietary guidelines are visually represented by MyPlate which replaced the US food guide pyramid in 2011. There are only a few similarities between the two visuals. In the USA, the food guide was simplified and does not have visuals of foods. It shows proportionality of recommended food groups through relative size on a plate. The website for MyPlate provides guidance regarding food plans and worksheets, health messages, and recommendations for physical activity [21]. There is a recommendation to minimize intake of saturated fat but does not specify the consumption of olive oil, which occupies the central portion of the Mediterranean diet pyramid. MyPlate also does not incorporate religious, social, or cultural beliefs.

In 2002, the forum on Mediterranean Food Cultures held its first meeting in Italy to preserve and acknowledge the cultural heritage of the Mediterranean population and represent its dietary patterns [16, 22]. In the subsequent forum meetings, a process was initiated to request that UNESCO recognize the MD as an intangible cultural heritage which represents a way of life. A document was released

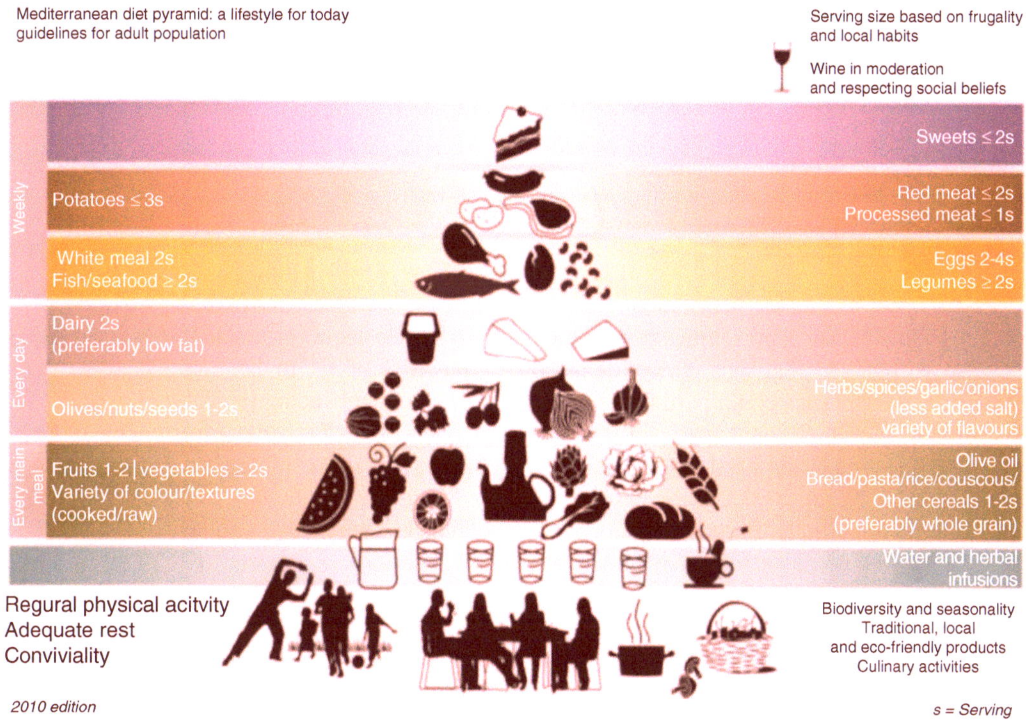

Fig. 4.2 Mediterranean Diet Pyramid updated. Eighth international congress on the Mediterranean Diet, Barcelona 2010. *Source*: Adapted from: [19, 20]

Table 4.1 Key Mediterranean pyramid messages

•	The traditional Mediterranean Diet (MD) pyramid has evolved to adopt the new way of life.
•	At the base, the pyramid includes foods that should sustain the diet and, at the upper levels, foods to be eaten in moderate amounts.
•	The pyramid includes social and cultural elements characteristic of the Mediterranean way of life. It also reflects the composition and number of servings of meals.
•	The Mediterranean Pyramid pattern addresses healthy adult populations and should be adapted to the specific needs of children, pregnant women, and other health conditions.
•	The pyramid places at the base foods of plant origin. They provide key nutrients and other protective substances that contribute to general well-being, maintain a balanced diet; and should be consumed in greater proportion and frequency than foods located at the central and upper levels of the pyramid.
•	*Every day*:
–	(1) Cereals. One or two servings per meal in the form of bread, pasta, rice, couscous, and others. Preferably whole grain; (2) Vegetables. For lunch and dinner; two servings per meal, at least one of the serving should be raw. Choose a variety of colors and textures for best antioxidant protection; (3) Fruits. One or two servings per meal. Should be chosen most frequently as dessert.
–	Maintain good hydration with water and herbal infusions, reduce salt content.
–	Prefer low-fat yogurt and cheese.
–	Olive oil is the main source of fat.
–	Consume spices, herbs, garlic, and onions to introduce flavor and palatability to dishes. Include olives, nuts, and seeds.
–	Recommends moderate consumption of wine, if acceptable, during meals and other fermented beverages.
•	*Weekly*:
–	Fish (two or more servings), white meat (two serving), and eggs as good sources of animal protein. Fish and shellfish as good sources of healthy fats.
–	Consume small quantities of red meat (less than two servings weekly).
–	Consume legumes (more than two servings/week) and cereals as healthy protein and lipid sources. Potatoes (~three servings/week) preferably fresh, as part of traditional recipes with meat and fish.
•	*Occasionally*:
–	Sugars, candies, and pastries, soft drinks.
–	Elements of lifestyle: moderation, socialization, cooking, seasonality, biodiversity, eco-friendliness, traditional and local food products, physical activity, rest.

Source: Bach-Faig A, 2011 [19].

to highlight the MD as representing more than just food but also equilibrium and lifestyle [16, 23]. It was also recognized that a common definition of the MD needs to be established so that all Mediterranean countries could participate in safeguarding and enhancing its diet and way of life. In the year 2007, a transnational application was submitted to UNESCO by the governments of Greece, Italy, Morocco, and Spain for the recognition of the MD as part of the intangible cultural heritage of humankind [16, 24]. In 2013 UNESCO recognized the Mediterranean dietary pattern as an intangible Cultural Heritage of Italy, Portugal, Spain, Morocco, Greece, Cyprus, and Croatia.

Indexes for Measuring Adherence to the Mediterranean Dietary Pattern

In order to further define and refine the composition of the MD and its recommendations, it is essential to expand our understanding of the relationship between dietary pattern and health. To accomplish this, indexes were developed based on current nutrition knowledge and predefined dietary patterns to measureadherence of individuals and populations to the MD [25, 26]. These diet scores or indexes were used to examine associations between the consumption of Mediterranean dietary patterns and chronic disease outcomes. There are over ten different Mediterranean diet scoring indexes. They differ by the food or food group items included, the scoring method, and the score cut-off values. In this chapter, we focus on three indexes that have been used most frequently to determine adherence to the Mediterranean dietary pattern. These include Mediterranean Diet Score (MDS), Diet Score (MedDietScore), and Mediterranean Adequacy Index (MAI).

Mediterranean Diet Score (MDS)

Trichopoulou and colleagues developed the Mediterranean Diet Score (MDS) to measure individuals' adherence to a traditional Greek style Mediterranean Diet Pattern using an 8-point measure of diet quality [27]. The score includes eight components: (1) High ratio of MUFAs to SF, (2) Moderate alcohol consumption, (3) High legume consumption, (4) High consumption of cereals including bread and potatoes, (5) High consumption of fruits, (6) High consumption of vegetables, (7) Low consumption of milk and dairy products, and (8) Low consumption of meat and meat products [27]. A high MDS score indicates good diet quality. The scoring system consists of assigning 1 point to intakes above median intake of the study subjects; all other intakes receive 0 points. So, if consumption of vegetables, legumes, fruits, cereals, and fish (which are considered beneficial) is consumed in quantities below median intake, then a zero is assigned, otherwise one point is assigned. Food groups such as meat and dairy products that are recommended in moderate amounts are given a value of one if consumption is below the median, otherwise a value of zero is assigned. A value of one is given for alcohol consumption in men (10 g to less than 50 g of ethanol/day) and women (5 g to less than 25 g of ethanol/day). For the consumption of fat, the ratio of monounsaturated fatty acids (MUFAs) to saturate fatty acid (SFAs) is calculated. Adherence to MD can have a diet score ranging from 0 to 8. A score of 4 and above shows good adherence to the MD and has been associated with positive health outcomes [26, 27]. The MDS scoring pattern is illustrated in Table 4.2.

Several variations to the MDS index were developed to evaluate dietary pattern and associations to health outcomes. Examples of such variations include scoring fish separately from meat products [28–31], or combining starchy roots with vegetables rather than with cereals as in the MDS index [32]. Also, a new scoring was developed based on tertile consumption of food groups (except for red

Table 4.2 Scoring system of the Mediterranean Diet Score (MDS) index

Nutrients or food groups	Scoring	
MUFA:SFA	>Median	1 (else: 0)
Legumes	>Median	1 (else: 0)
Cereals (including breads and potatoes)	>Median	1 (else: 0)
Cereals (including breads and potatoes)	>Median	1 (else: 0)
Fruits and Nuts	>Median	1 (else: 0)
Vegetables	>Median	1 (else: 0)
Fish, meat, and meat products	<Median	1 (else: 0)
Milk and dairy products	<Median	1 (else: 0)
Alcohol	Men (10 g to less than 50 g of ethanol/day) and women (5 g to less than 25 g of ethanol/day)	1 (else: 0)

Source: Adapted from Trichopoulou et al. 1995 [27]

wine) resulting in values ranging from 9 to 27 [33]. Additionally, to allow the score to be applied to non-Mediterranean populations that consume minimal amounts of monounsaturated fat from olive oil, intake of polyunsaturated fatty acids (PUFAs) was included along with monounsaturated fatty acids in the numerator [30].

An alternative Mediterranean diet score (aMED) was created based on the MDS index of Trichopoulou et al. [34]. This aMED score includes a few modifications such as excluding potato products from the vegetable group, separating fruit and nuts into two groups, eliminating the dairy group, including whole grain products only, including only red and processed meats for the meat group, and assigning alcohol intake between 5 and 15 g/day for 1 point. Possible scores on the aMED range from 0 to 9 [34].

Diet Score (MedDietScore)

Panagiotakos and colleagues developed a MD index based on an individual's adherence to Greek Mediterranean diet . This MedDietScore is based on 11 components (non-refined cereals, fruits, vegetables, potatoes, legumes, olive oil, fish, red meat, poultry, full fat dairy products, and alcohol) [35, 36]. Each component is assigned a score ranging from 0 to 5 depending on intake. But red meat, poultry, and full fat dairy products are scored on a reverse scale since they are not typical of a MD. Potatoes were included as a separate group although potatoes are not included in the Mediterranean diet pyramid. The score ranges from 0 to 55 points with the higher values indicating greater adherence to the MD. This index was inversely associated with several health indicators such as hypertension, hypercholesterolemia, diabetes, obesity and cardiovascular disease risk [36–39]. Panagiotakos and colleagues developed a computer program which automatically calculates the MedDietScore from a food frequency questionnaire. This scoring system is shown in Table 4.3 [35].

Table 4.3 Scoring system of the Diet Score (MedDietScore) index

	Frequency of consumption (servings/month)					
How often do you consume	Never	1–4	5–8	9–12	13–18	>18
Non-refined cereals (whole grain bread, pasta, rice, etc.)	0	1	2	3	4	5
Potatoes	0	1	2	3	4	5
Fruits	0	1	2	3	4	5
Vegetables	0	1	2	3	4	5
Legumes	0	1	2	3	4	5
Fish	0	1	2	3	4	5
Red meat and products	5	4	3	2	1	0
Poultry	5	4	3	2	1	0
Full fat dairy products (cheese, yogurt, milk)	5	4	3	2	1	0
	Never	Rare	<1	1–3	3–5	Daily
Olive oil (use in cooking, times/week)	0	1	2	3	4	5
	<300	300	400	500	600	>700 or 0
Alcoholic beverages (ml/day, 100 ml = 12 g ethanol)	5	4	3	2	1	0

Source: Panagiotakos DB, 2006 [35].

Mediterranean Adequacy Index (MAI)

MAI was developed to compare the dietary intake of a free-living population to the traditional Italian style Mediterranean dietary pattern. This traditional dietary pattern was determined by researchers to be the one consumed by men in Nicotera, one of the rural southern areas of Italy included as part of the Seven Countries Study conducted by Ancel Keys. The Nicotera diet became the reference diet and known as the *Healthy Reference Italian Mediterranean diet* (HRIMD) because of the very low prevalence of coronary heart disease, diabetes, obesity, and hypertension of the population in that region [40, 41].

MAI is calculated by dividing the sum of the percentage of the total energy from ten typical Mediterranean foods (bread, cereals, legumes, potatoes, vegetables, fruits, fish, vegetable oils, and red wine) by the sum of the percentage of the total energy from eight non-typical Mediterranean foods (milk, cheese, meat, eggs, animal fats, margarines, cakes, pies, cookies, and sugar). The food groups determined to be typical Mediterranean foods were obtained from the reference diet or HRIMD. MAI is calculated using the following formula:

$$\frac{\left(\begin{array}{c}\%\mathrm{encereals} + \mathrm{legumes} + \mathrm{potatoes} + \mathrm{vegetables} + \\ \mathrm{fruitsfreshanddry} + \mathrm{fish} + \mathrm{wine} + \mathrm{virginoliveoil}\end{array}\right)}{\left(\begin{array}{c}\%\mathrm{energymilk} + \mathrm{cheese} + \mathrm{meat} + \mathrm{eggs} + \mathrm{animalfatsandmargarines} + \\ \mathrm{sweetbeverages} + \mathrm{cakes} / \mathrm{pies} + \mathrm{cookies}\end{array}\right)}$$

The higher the MAI score the greater the source of energy from Mediterranean foods. The median MAI of the HRIMD is between 4.0 and 8.5 [42].

Another method of computing MAI is by expressing intakes of the 18 food groups as grams/day. In this calculation a sum of the ten typical Mediterranean foods or food groups expressed as grams/day is divided by the sum of the eight less typical Mediterranean food groups expressed as grams/day. The average MAI of the HRIMD using this method is between 4.6 and 10.1 [42]. However, using grams instead of percent of calories has its limitations because of the different energy densities of foods that are not accounted for in using gram values.

The MAI was validated at the population level by looking at associations between intake using the MAI and 25-year total mortality and mortality from coronary heart disease in populations of different cultures [40, 42]. The MAI of some countries is shown in Table 4.4 for two time periods: 1961–1965 and 2000–2003 [3].

Changes in Dietary and Lifestyle Patterns Over Time

A main purpose of the indexes is to measure current dietary patterns and their impact on health status as compared to the dietary patterns of certain regions of Greece and Italy in the 1960s. In fact, it was to preserve the healthy food patterns of the Mediterranean regions and the accompanying lifestyle that Mediterranean dietary guidelines were developed and updated with messages that include both dietary and lifestyle recommendations. This is important because the Mediterranean diet continues to evolve. The changes observed over the last decades are outcomes of technological developments that affect people's way of life and lead to closer interactions and exchanges with different parts of the world. Globalization has led to the availability of more processed and convenience foods, a decrease in whole grain cereals, and a rise in animal sources of food and fat. Fats from animal products increased significantly in Greece, Spain, and Italy from 1960 to 2001 [43]. These same changes were also observed in the Southern Mediterranean region [44]. Table 4.3 shows the change in MAI ranking of Mediterranean

Table 4.4 Ranking of countries by the Mediterranean adequacy index (MAI) in two time periods

	1961–1965		2000–2003	
Countries	Ranking	MAI	Ranking	MAI
Greece	1	5.54	10	2.04
Albania	2	5.07	7	2.51
Turkey	3	5.03	5	2.80
Egypt	4	4.81	1	4.09
Tunisia	5	4.57	6	2.65
Japan	6	4.11	16	1.51
Romania	7	3.89	11	2.02
Libya	8	3.81	9	2.09
Algeria	9	3.61	4	2.81
Portugal	10	3.39	18	1.27
Morocco	11	3.37	3	3.25
Syria	12	3.35	8	2.25
Spain	13	3.35	21	1.19
Italy	14	3.30	15	1.62
Yugoslavia	15	3.13	22	1.15
Iran	16	2.87	2	3.65
Mauritania	17	2.87	13	1.77
Lebanon	18	2.70	14	1.72
Bulgaria	19	2.68	20	1.20
Cyprus	20	2.39	27	0.96
Chile	21	2.24	19	1.27
South Africa	22	1.87	12	1.78
Poland	23	1.84	23	1.12
Israel	24	1.62	24	1.09
Malta	25	1.56	17	1.42
Hungary	26	1.48	37	0.73
France	27	1.28	32	0.82
Argentina	28	1.13	25	0.97
Czechoslovakia	29	1.10	30	0.83
Finland	30	1.04	29	0.87
Austria	31	0.98	38	0.73
Ireland	32	0.97	33	0.80
Norway	33	0.88	26	0.97
Switzerland	34	0.88	39	0.72
Germany	35	0.82	34	0.76
Sweden	36	0.72	31	0.82
Canada	37	0.71	36	0.75
Australia	38	0.68	40	0.70
United Kingdom	39	0.68	28	0.87
Denmark	40	0.67	35	0.76
U.S.	41	0.63	41	0.64

Source: da Silva, 2009 [3]

and non-Mediterranean countries from 1961–1965 to 2000–2003. The rise in intake of calories and particularly of low nutrients, energy dense foods, and the parallel decrease in physical exertion, has led to an increase in the prevalence of overweight and obesity.

Conclusions

The positive health outcomes as observed by Ancel Keys in the 1960s may be attributable to lifestyle factors in addition to dietary intake. These habits included a physically active life, and fixed-meal patterns limiting eating to particular times of the day, with lunchtime followed by a siesta of variable duration. Socialization is another component of meal consumption where major social-familial contacts occur. This is accompanied by environmental characteristics such as sun and sea [45]. Some of these lifestyle factors have also changed in recent years so that the main meal shifted from noon to the evening. This shift may be due to work schedules, continuous working days, and the increasing distance between the work site and home. Although in many countries people still enjoy the leisurely mealtimes and more relaxed lifestyle, these are also changing. With these changes and a better understanding of the relationship between dietary patterns and health status, periodic updating of the Mediterranean guidelines will be necessary, as occurs with the US Dietary guidelines.

References

1. Sofi F, Cesari F, Abbate R, Gensini GF, Casini A. Adherence to Mediterranean diet and health status: meta-analysis. BMJ. 2008;337:a1344.
2. Serra-Majem L, Roman B, Estruch R. Scientific evidence of interventions using the Mediterranean diet: a systematic review. Nutr Rev. 2006;64(2 Pt 2):S27–47.
3. da Silva R, Bach-Faig A, Raidó QB, Buckland G, Vaz de Almeida MD, Serra-Majem L. Worldwide variation of adherence to the Mediterranean diet, in 1961-1965 and 2000-2003. Public Health Nutr. 2009;12(9A):1676–84.
4. Noah A, Truswell AS. There are many Mediterranean diets. Asia Pac J Clin Nutr. 2001;10(1):2–9.
5. Karamanos B, Thanopoulou A, Angelico F, et al. Nutritional habits in the Mediterranean Basin. The macronutrient composition of diet and its relation with the traditional Mediterranean diet. Multi-centre study of the Mediterranean Group for the Study of Diabetes (MGSD). Eur J Clin Nutr. 2002;56(10):983–91.
6. Owl & Mouse Educational Maps (2014). Retrieved 29 July 2014 from http://www.yourchildlearns.com/online-atlas/mediterranean-map-print.htm.
7. Simopoulos AP. The Mediterranean diets: what is so special about the diet of Greece? The scientific evidence. J Nutr. 2001;131(11 Suppl):3065s–73s.
8. Essid MY. History of Mediterranean food. In *Medi*terra: The Mediterranean diet for sustainable regional development, 1st ed. Presses de Sciences Po; 2012. p. 51–69.
9. Nestle M. Mediterranean diets: historical and research overview. Am J Clin Nutr. 1995;61(6 Suppl):1313S–20.
10. Keys AE. Seven countries: a multivariate analysis of death and coronary heart disease. Cambridge, MA: Harvard University Press; 1980.
11. Trichopoulou A, Lagiou P. Healthy traditional Mediterranean diet: an expression of culture, history, and lifestyle. Nutr Rev. 1997;55(11 Pt 1):383–9.
12. Grigg D. Food consumption in the Mediterranean region. Tijdschrift voor economische en sociale geografie. 1999;90(4):391–409.
13. Reguant-Aleix J. The Mediterranean Diet: Designed for the future. In *Medi*Terra: The Mediterranean diet for sustainable regional development, 1st ed. Presses de Sciences Po; 2012. p. 504.
14. Rivera D, Obón C, Heinrich M, Inocencio C, Verde A, Fajardo J. Gathered Mediterranean food plants—ethnobotanical investigations and historical development. Forum Nutr. 2006;59:18–74.
15. Willett WC, Sacks F, Trichopoulou A, et al. Mediterranean diet pyramid: a cultural model for healthy eating. Am J Clin Nutr. 1995;61(6 Suppl):1402S–6.
16. Dernini S, Berry EM, Bach-Faig A, Belahsen R, Donini LM, Lairon D, Serra-Majem L, Cannella C. A dietary model constructed by scientists. In *Medi*Terra: The Mediterranean diet for sustainable regional development, 1st ed. Presses de Sciences Po; 2012. p. 71–88.

17. Fundación Dieta Mediterránea. Proceedings of International Congress. Retrieved 29 July 2014 from http://dieta-mediterranea.com/en/whatwedo/events/mediterranean-diet-congress/.
18. Serra-Majem L, Trichopoulou A, Ngo de la Cruz J, et al. Does the definition of the Mediterranean diet need to be updated? Public Health Nutr. 2004;7(7):927–9.
19. Bach-Faig A, Berry EM, Lairon D, et al. Mediterranean diet pyramid today. Science and cultural updates. Public Health Nutr. 2011;14(12A):2274–84.
20. Fundación Dieta Mediterránea. Mediterranean diet pyramid. Retrieved 29 July 2014 from http://dietamediterranea.com/dietamed/piramide_INGLES.pdf.
21. US Department of Agriculture. Choose MyPlate. Retrieved 19 March 2014 from www.choosemyplate.gov.
22. Dernini S. Towards the advancement of the Mediterranean food cultures. Public Health Nutr. 2006;9(1A):103–4.
23. Dernini S. Transmitting Mediterranean food culture through art: a creative interdisciplinary approach. Public Health Nutr. 2006;9(8A):1141–3.
24. Reguant-Aleix J, Arbore MR, Bach-Faig A, Serra-Majem L. Mediterranean heritage: an intangible cultural heritage. Public Health Nutr. 2009;12(9A):1591–4.
25. Milà-Villarroel R, Bach-Faig A, Puig J, et al. Comparison and evaluation of the reliability of indexes of adherence to the Mediterranean diet. Public Health Nutr. 2011;14(12A):2338–45.
26. Bach A, Serra-Majem L, Carrasco JL, et al. The use of indexes evaluating the adherence to the Mediterranean diet in epidemiological studies: a review. Public Health Nutr. 2006;9(1A):132–46.
27. Trichopoulou A, Kouris-Blazos A, Wahlqvist ML, et al. Diet and overall survival in elderly people. BMJ. 1995;311(7018):1457–60.
28. Trichopoulou A, Costacou T, Bamia C, Trichopoulos D. Adherence to a Mediterranean diet and survival in a Greek population. N Engl J Med. 2003;348(26):2599–608.
29. Trichopoulou A, Bamia C, Trichopoulos D. Mediterranean diet and survival among patients with coronary heart disease in Greece. Arch Intern Med. 2005;165(8):929–35.
30. Trichopoulou A, Orfanos P, Norat T, et al. Modified Mediterranean diet and survival: EPIC-elderly prospective cohort study. BMJ. 2005;330(7498):991.
31. Psaltopoulou T, Naska A, Orfanos P, Trichopoulos D, Mountokalakis T, Trichopoulou A. Olive oil, the Mediterranean diet, and arterial blood pressure: the Greek European Prospective Investigation into Cancer and Nutrition (EPIC) study. Am J Clin Nutr. 2004;80(4):1012–8.
32. Osler M, Schroll M. Diet and mortality in a cohort of elderly people in a north European community. Int J Epidemiol. 1997;26(1):155–9.
33. Schröder H, Marrugat J, Vila J, Covas MI, Elosua R. Adherence to the traditional Mediterranean diet is inversely associated with body mass index and obesity in a Spanish population. J Nutr. 2004;134(12):3355–61.
34. Fung TT, McCullough ML, Newby PK, et al. Diet-quality scores and plasma concentrations of markers of inflammation and endothelial dysfunction. Am J Clin Nutr. 2005;82(1):163–73.
35. Panagiotakos DB, Milias GA, Pitsavos C, Stefanadis C. MedDietScore: a computer program that evaluates the adherence to the Mediterranean dietary pattern and its relation to cardiovascular disease risk. Comput Methods Programs Biomed. 2006;83(1):73–7.
36. Panagiotakos DB, Pitsavos C, Arvaniti F, Stefanadis C. Adherence to the Mediterranean food pattern predicts the prevalence of hypertension, hypercholesterolemia, diabetes and obesity, among healthy adults; the accuracy of the MedDietScore. Prev Med. 2007;44(4):335–40.
37. Panagiotakos DB, Chrysohoou C, Pitsavos C, Stefanadis C. Association between the prevalence of obesity and adherence to the Mediterranean diet: the ATTICA study. Nutrition. 2006;22(5):449–56.
38. Panagiotakos DB, Tzima N, Pitsavos C, et al. The association between adherence to the Mediterranean diet and fasting indices of glucose homoeostasis: the ATTICA Study. J Am Coll Nutr. 2007;26(1):32–8.
39. Panagiotakos DB, Pitsavos C, Stefanadis C. Dietary patterns: a Mediterranean diet score and its relation to clinical and biological markers of cardiovascular disease risk. Nutr Metab Cardiovasc Dis. 2006;16(8):559–68.
40. Alberti A, Fruttini D, Fidanza F. The Mediterranean Adequacy Index: further confirming results of validity. Nutr Metab Cardiovasc Dis. 2009;19(1):61–6.
41. Alberti-Fidanza A, Fidanza F. Mediterranean Adequacy Index of Italian diets. Public Health Nutr. 2004;7(7):937–41.
42. Fidanza F, Alberti A, Lanti M, Menotti A. Mediterranean Adequacy Index: correlation with 25-year mortality from coronary heart disease in the Seven Countries Study. Nutr Metab Cardiovasc Dis. 2004;14(5):254–8.
43. Alexandratos N. The Mediterranean diet in a world context. Public Health Nutr. 2006;9(1A):111–7.
44. Belahsen R, Rguibi M. Population health and Mediterranean diet in southern Mediterranean countries. Public Health Nutr. 2006;9(8a):1130–5.
45. Bellisle F. Infrequently asked questions about the Mediterranean diet. Public Health Nutr. 2009;12(9A):1644–7.

Chapter 5
Implementing the Mediterranean Diet: A French Perspective and Comparisons with Other Mediterranean Countries

Mariette Gerber

Key Points

- The French population displays favorable figures in terms of overweight and obesity compared to other European populations, developed countries and even some developing countries. The French population, because of their adherence to traditional food and gastronomy, has better resisted the "westernization" of eating habits compared to other Mediterranean countries in Europe.
- The structure and temporal organization of meals during the day, without snacking, is the main nutritional aspect. Adding fast/junk food to the Mediterranean diet might deteriorate its health benefits.
- Considering food as a pleasure and healthy habit to share, and as part of the due respect for the environment, not simply as a physiological need, is the main cultural change that needs to be encouraged.

Keywords Mediterranean diet • French culture and gastronomy • Food habits • Meals structure and organization

Introduction

We first have to explain why it is worth considering the French perspective and its implementation into the Mediterranean diet. The two main reasons belong to different domains: health and culture. The first aspect is a clearly demonstrable argument, and easy to spread in populations, whereas the second one is founded on long-lasting eating behaviors and a renowned gastronomy. To spread this culture will require a change in eating behaviors. Even with strong evidence about the good health provided by a dietary pattern, cultural and behavioral habits might be stronger. It is enough to think about the attachment to tobacco. It is the responsibility of the nutritionist to decipher the most relevant

M. Gerber, M.D., Ph.D. (✉)
Expert at ANSES, France; INSERM-Institut du Cancer de Montpellier,
34298 Montpellier Cedex 5, France
e-mail: mariette.gerber@sfr.fr

D.F. Romagnolo, O.I. Selmin (eds.), *Mediterranean Diet*, Nutrition and Health,
DOI 10.1007/978-3-319-27969-5_5

traits, and of the Public Health actors to work on the implementation of a healthy and agreeable dietary pattern. Thus, after a description of these two points in relation to the main principles of the French eating culture, participation to the Mediterranean diet will be covered, and an example of French Mediterranean dietary pattern will be provided.

Health

Differences in Overweight and Obesity Across Mediterranean Countries

The main health indicator that characterizes France is its prevalence of obesity. Despite variations in measurements methods [1–3], France is the country with the lowest prevalence of overweight and obese persons among developed countries. In 2012, 32.3 % of French people >18 years old were overweight and 15 % were obese [4]. However, this favorable figure hides strong regional disparities: in Northern France the obesity prevalence is 21.8 %, whereas in the Mediterranean regions it is 13.2 % [4]. Of course, eating habits are not the only cause of overweight and obesity. Physical activity is another factor, as are socioeconomic differences. This last aspect is demonstrated even within the French Mediterranean regions since the western Languedoc-Roussillon, a region with a high unemployment rate, has a prevalence of 14.4 % obesity, whereas in the wealthier eastern part, Provence-Alpes-Côte d'Azur, obesity prevalence is only 12.5 % [4]. Besides, some other traits such as "how it is eaten" rather than "what is eaten" might play a role in the lower percentage of obesity in some French regions who are not strictly Mediterranean (South-East and West, parts of France, 13.4 % and 13.2 % respectively). These observations may suggest an effect of the French cultural habits on obesity prevalence. Nevertheless, in 2008, the Mediterranean regions of France reported lowered prevalence of obesity than their immediate Mediterranean neighbors, Italy with 17.2 %, and Spain with 24.1 % [1]. This is even more striking for children: in France, 14.9 % of girls and 13.1 % of boys are overweight or obese, whereas 34.7 % of girls and 37.1 % of boys are overweight or obese in Italy, and 29.5 % of girls and 32.3 % of boys are overweight or obese in Spain [2].

In Crete, the model for the Mediterranean diet, children had higher mean BMI than similar American cohorts. Compared to their American counterparts, Cretans had higher proportions of overweight in both genders across all ages tested [5]. This discrepancy is also observed in the evolution of the prevalence of overweight, as shown in Fig. 5.1. Thus, France not only shows a lower prevalence of obesity and overweight than the other developed countries, but also lowers rates than in Mediterranean countries. It seems that Mediterranean countries have not resisted the Westernization of their eating habits as well as France. We can find an explanation for this observation in the culture of eating in France.

Culture

Sticking to Tradition

Attachment and interest to food has developed over centuries in France, giving rise to French gastronomy, which although highly sophisticated still retains the importance of the quality of the ingredients, the use of genuine basic components and foods, and also the pleasure of well-prepared dishes. The UNESCO has registered the French gastronomy on the list of the "immaterial patrimony of humanity" in 2010 for all its components: good quality products, preferably grown locally, which are

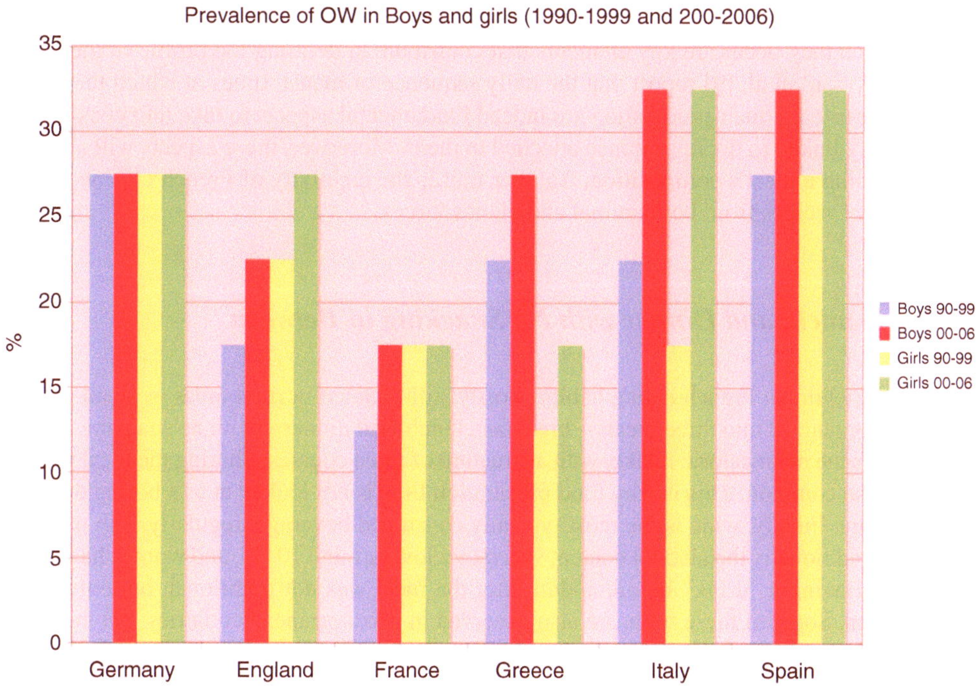

Fig. 5.1 Evolution of the prevalence of overweight in boys and girls from West-European countries (IASO 2008 [2])

organized in the meal along their taste; careful selection of the dishes reflecting the diversity of the French regions organized along a ritual sequential "menu" of 3 or 4 dishes; conversations, part of the commensality with conviviality; harmonious combination of dishes and wines; esthetics of the table setting . This recognition reinforced the attachment of France to its food culture [6]. This excellence made French gastronomy famous all over the world, and this pride is accompanied by a solid contempt for the type of food not respecting these characteristics of quality, meal organization and conviviality, namely the fast-food type, energy dense food that you can eat in the street. This feeling is a likely explanation for the resistance to change. Another explanation is that French cuisine is strongly anchored in family life, and all the family is immersed in an interest for food, thus maintaining the French eating habits. Daughters (and more recently sons) receive most of their mothers' recipes because cooking most of the meals is also a French habit. Tradition is strong in this domain for several reasons, one being that recipes require freshness and quality of products, but also because shopping in markets and specialized stores (butcher's, bakery, and cheese shops) is a pleasure, as well as treating family and friends, that makes the cook and the tablemates happy! All this gives the French people a lot of opportunities to talk about food and wonderful meals, demonstrating the importance they attach to eating. This is not just a physiological act, but a social interaction.

How can French eating culture be related to the Mediterranean diet? The Mediterranean diet is characterized not only by its food pattern with use of olive oil, but also by other traits related to the organization of the meals and to their chronology through the day. This has been shown in a study comparing a Mediterranean island where the traditional habits were lost, namely Malta, to another one where the traditional habits were well maintained, Sardinia (Italy) [6]. These characteristics were traditionally present all over France, since meal patterns, structure, and rituals are fundamental aspects in French eating habits, and, even if partly modified by modern life, they remain largely routine [7]. The act of eating involves a set of rituals, described by Poulain [8] as the "space of food consumption habits." The number of occasions when food is consumed, their structure, the time and the social context in which they occur are key elements that contribute to defining the profile of the total daily food intake. Aymard et al. [9] report that the daily sequence of meals, times at which they are taken and the time devoted to their preparation are indeed fundamental aspects to take into consideration as they are directly linked to the importance attached to them. Moreover, these aspects will also contribute to determining a meal's composition. Another trait is the creativity of French cuisine, ensuring a high diversity of recipes from both animal and plant sources.

Breakfast, Lunch, and Dinner with No Snacking in Between

In the typical traditional French eating habits, mostly still retained in rural areas or small cities, [10], food intake is organized into three meals—breakfast, lunch, and dinner—with no snacking in between. Lunch provides the main caloric intake, with a structure of three courses. Sharing the meal with family or friends is also common. This is why food preparation time is not looked at as a boring duty but as a pleasure to share. Finally, wine is the most typically consumed beverage, regularly with meals and in moderation. Traditionally the alcohol content was rather low (around 10 %), and women had a very low consumption. Having a "drink" before and/or after the meal was not traditional, but only to mark a special occasion. Some of these traits are also observed in Mediterranean countries, but they are reinforced by the French food culture, and thus could better resist "Westernization" of eating habits.

Relationship Between Health and the French Eating Habits

Dietary Patterns and Behavior

The dietary pattern in many regions of France, especially south of the Loire river, is close to the traditional Mediterranean diet of Greece or Italy, where the principal dietary components are whole grain cereals for energy, many fruits and vegetables (raw and cooked, fresh and preserved), olive oil for salad dressing and cooking, and moderate amounts of meat and dairy. This diet is now universally recognized as favorable to health [11]. This Mediterranean diet is of course largely present in the regions along the Mediterranean coast: Languedoc-Roussillon [10] and Provence-Alpes-Côte d'Azur. But it is also present in parts of Rhône-Alpes, Aquitaine, and Midi-Pyrénées [12], where fruit, vegetables, and fish are consumed in quantities comparable to the French Mediterranean regions, the only difference being that other vegetable oils (sunflower and grape seed oils) are used as well as olive oil.

The three-meal structure is an important aspect of the relationship of French and Mediterranean diets with health. Snacking is known to be a factor contributing to weight gain, because most of the time the caloric intake just adds to that of the previous and following meals [13]. It has been shown in a Mediterranean country that snacking significantly increases (by 34 %) the risk of a weight gain of ~3.0 kg/year [14]. Eating in front of a TV, especially alone, is strongly related to obesity risk. This behavior is not only an obvious factor of a sedentary lifestyle, but it is accompanied by a dysregulation of energy intake, favoring an over-intake [15–17].

Diversity of Foods

The diversity of foods and recipes in French and Mediterranean cuisines provide a large range of micronutrients and microconstituents known for their health benefits. In addition, the three-course lunch is the best way to achieve the recommended intake of fruit and vegetables, and to consume a high nutrient density meal with sufficient energy.

Eating the main intake of calories at noon allows time to expend the energy during the rest of the day, instead of going to sleep soon after. This is compensated in some cultures where early dinner might be followed by practicing some sports. Especially for elderly people who need time for a high intake of protein to be absorbed, the main meal at noon is a must [18]. Sharing meals with family and/or friends also prevents rapid consumption, which is deleterious to digestion, and is also part of maintaining social links, which are important for slowing down cognitive decline.

Wine consumption is a subject of much discussion with regard to Public Health. It intrinsically belongs to the Northern shores of the Mediterranean,[1] and has been shown to significantly and convincingly decrease the risk of CVD, with a statistically significant reduction of 22 % for a moderate intake (26.0 g) of two to three drinks a day [20]. For diabetes the relation is probable, with a significant decrease of 34 % for an intake of 12–24 g/day [21, 22]. Alcohol contributes to the pleasure of the meal and its conviviality. However, it significantly increases the risk of cancers of the upper digestive tract, by 3 %/drink/week, and of colon cancer, by 7 % for 1 drink/day, or 10 g alcohol, and of 38 % for consumption of 5 drinks/day, or 50 g of alcohol [23]. Alcohol also linearly increases risk of breast cancer. The dose-response meta-analysis of the continuously updated project of the WCRF [24] showed that consumption of 10.0 g of ethanol/day was associated with statistically significant increased risk for all ER-positive (ER+) tumors (12 %), but not ER-negative tumors. A more recent study by Chen et al. [25] confirms that 5–10 g of alcohol/day significantly increases breast cancer risk by 15 %. Women are more vulnerable to the effects of alcoholic beverages, and it is wise for Mediterranean women to consume low amounts of alcoholic beverages.

One of the last reports of the large European EPIC study on the life-time use of alcohol, and overall and cause-specific mortality showed a significant association when comparing extreme drinkers (≥30 g/day in women and ≥60 g/day in men) to moderate drinkers (0.1–4.9 g/day), with an increase in risk of overall mortality of 27 % in men and 53 % in women [26]. However, the analysis of cause-specific mortality showed no association of cardiovascular mortality with these intakes of alcohol. Moreover, it takes twice as much wine as beer to show a 15 % risk of overall mortality in women and four times as much in men. These observations should not be taken as an encouragement, but rather to underline that moderate wine drinking in the context of a pleasant meal shared with family or friends, will not negatively weigh on our health. Moderation has to be kept as an objective, and wine should remain a part of the pleasure enjoyed during a good meal.

Finally, we mention earlier the contempt for fast/junk food which keeps away most of the French from the fast food places. This is not anecdotal because we have some indications that unhealthy food deteriorates the benefits of Mediterranean diet. Martin-Gonzalez et al. analyzed the relationship between cardiovascular diseases and Mediterranean diet in a Spanish cohort using both an a priori and an a posteriori dietary patterns [27]. As expected, the patients with the highest Med score showed a significant risk reduction for cardiovascular disease (HR = 0.41, 0.18–0.95). The principal component analysis conducted on the cohort identified two *a posteriori* patterns "Western" and "Mediterranean." The "Western" was associated with a significant increased risk (HR = 2.10, 1.06–4.18) whereas the "Mediterranean" did not show any risk reduction (HR = 1.14, 0.54–2.39). Interestingly, a higher consumption of meat was recorded in the highest quantile of the pattern (184 g/day) compared to the lower (173 g/day). And meat showed a high factor loading in the "Western" pattern, which was associated to an increased risk.

In the same line, but investigating the association of a posteriori dietary patterns with breast cancer, the E3N study identified a Western/alcohol dietary pattern associated with an increased risk of breast cancer (HR = 1.20, 1.03–1.38) and a Mediterranean/healthy dietary pattern associated with a decreased risk (HR = 0.85, 0.75–0.95) [28]. However, there was no association with this pattern for the women

[1]The traditional beverage in the Southern Mediterranean is tea, rich in catechins like wine. If alcohol represents a limit to wine consumption, the added sugar in tea is likely a problem with regard to obesity [19].

with energy intake >2000 kcal/day. This increase in energy was due to unhealthy foods also found in the Western/alcohol dietary pattern (French fries, processed meats, sandwiches, cakes) while intakes of healthy foods (fruit, raw and cooked vegetables, olive oil, sunflower oil, fish) was higher in women with an energy intake ≤2000 kcal. The contempt for unhealthy food (generally high energy-density and low micronutrient density food, fast-food, junk food) which is part of the French food culture might play a role in the French lower obesity prevalence.

How to Incorporate the French Perspective in the Mediterranean Diet?

The main traits of the French similarity and/or contribution to the Mediterranean diet are indicated in Table 5.1, together with their corresponding potential health benefits.

No Snacking, 3 Meals a Day, 3-Course Meal

Except for children (the traditional tasty snack of bread and chocolate) and maybe for very elderly people who cannot get enough food in one meal because of dental or gastrointestinal troubles (the afternoon dessert "entremet" made of cooked fruit or milk), snacking has to be forgotten and food intake organized instead into three meals a day: breakfast, lunch, and dinner. Below are some suggestions for adults.

Breakfast

Since the nineteenth century, the French breakfast was traditionally made of bread, butter, jam and milk, consumed with coffee. Jam was an ersatz for fruit in winter (at my grandparents' home we had jam for dessert in winter). Obviously this has to be adapted to today's life and increased food accessibility. Seasonal fruit will be the essential part (to initiate the daily acquisition of vitamin C); cereals will provide energy in the form of whole bread, accompanied with fresh cheese (cottage cheese might be fine); if other types of cereals with milk are chosen, they should be without added sugar, processing and various added vitamins and minerals. Tea or coffee will accompany this breakfast. However, those who cannot live without bread and butter ("tartines") may eat them with homemade jam from time to time.

Table 5.1 French similarity and/or contribution to Mediterranean diet with the corresponding potential health effect

Behavior	Health outcome
No snacking	Decreases the risk of weight gain
3-course meal	Permits a sufficient and high quality intake of micronutrients and microconstituents
Seasonal foods	
Food and recipe diversity	
Main caloric intake at noon	Decreases the risk of weight gain
Cooking at home	Avoids salt or sugar excess found in processed food, and contaminants from packaging, possibly responsible for weight gain
Moderate (1–2 glasses/day for women; 2–3 glasses/day for men) and regular intake of wine with meals	Contributes to risk reduction of CVD, and eventually of diabetes without jeopardizing health status if kept in moderate amounts
Commensality	Increases time spent in meal to favor digestion
	Develops social links and slow cognitive declines

Lunch: The Three-Course Meal

Lunch is the meal providing the highest energy intake. The *first course* is an "entrée,"[3]most of the time consisting of raw vegetables (carrots, cucumber, tomatoes, red or Chinese cabbage, beets, etc.), dressed with extra virgin olive oil and lemon juice or wine vinegar. Raw vegetables ("crudités"), because of their vitamin C (ascorbic acid) content, tend to lower gastric pH, decreasing the likelihood of metabolizing nitrates and nitrites to carcinogenic nitrosamines. In addition to vitamin C, microconstituents, such as carotenoids and phenols, will be provided by this first course. From time to time, and according to the season, one can propose cooked vegetables (leaks, asparagus, artichokes). One can also add some kind of seafood or "charcuterie" (traditional and home processed pork meat), although no more than once a week, and better if less. The *second course* is the main dish, high in protein (mainly for growing children and adolescents, but also for aged persons who less efficiently assimilate protein and need to avoid sarcopenia). It might be from animal source (fish at least twice a week, red meat or poultry once or twice a week at most, eggs, once a week) or a plant source (legumes combined with cereals and/or small amount of meat).

Leafy vegetables (Italian cuisine has a wonderful variety of them, see the variety and qualities in Hoffman and Gerber, [27]), turnips, cabbages, or the summer vegetables eggplants, tomatoes, zucchini, squashes, will be served with the protein dish, alternatively with whole cereals, rice, bulgur, pasta made of hard wheat. I intentionally mentioned *summer* vegetables: eggplants, tomatoes, zucchini, and others if grown in winter are much less rich in micronutrients and microconstituents, especially phenols, and it is an aberration to use them instead of other winter vegetables, full of necessary vitamins, minerals, and microconstituents, just to make believe that you are eating "Mediterranean." There are no eggplants, tomatoes, or zucchini in winter in Mediterranean countries. Besides, preserved tomatoes with olive oil and herbs are richer in carotenoids and phenols than raw summer ones. Cooking in winter with tomato sauce is an excellent way to cut down on fat and calories and to take advantage of a lot of micronutrients and microconstituents. Fruit will constitute the *third course*, the dessert. Cheese might be present if there is no animal protein in the second course. Once or twice a week we can indulge ourselves with sweets. One can prioritize sweets with fruit, almonds, or bitter chocolate. A moderate amount of wine (as described above) will accompany this meal, which might be followed by coffee or tea.

Dinner

This is made essentially of a vegetable-based dish: soups, pies, or salads. Twice or three times a week cheese will enrich this meal, and goat or ewe cheese are preferred (please see chapter in this volume on oils and fats in Mediterranean diet). On the remaining days, nuts will be very welcome, and once or twice a week biscuits could be added to the meal, with a fresh fruit present every evening. As a drink, one glass of wine or herb tea (thyme, rosemary, verbena) can be chosen. From time to time, a large evening dinner with friends characterized by successive courses interrupted by long chats, will help to keep a balanced food intake.

A scheme of this organization and structure of meals over a week is shown in Fig. 5.2. Such a scheme might look "rigid" as mentioned by the American sociologist Daniel Lerner in 1956 (quoted in 7), but what is within the scheme might be and has to be varied, to result different and enticing. To combine a pleasant way of eating together with a well-balanced diet demands a diversity of food sources and recipes and an interest in eating well for both health and pleasure. After practicing for some time, this simply becomes a habit. Once the basic principles are understood, one can vary with suggestions found in several books [28]. The diet described in this book has been successfully tested in a nutritional intervention with positive effects observed on risk factors for CVD [29, 30]. The proposed meal organization is necessary for keeping the main caloric intake at noon. Its duration over

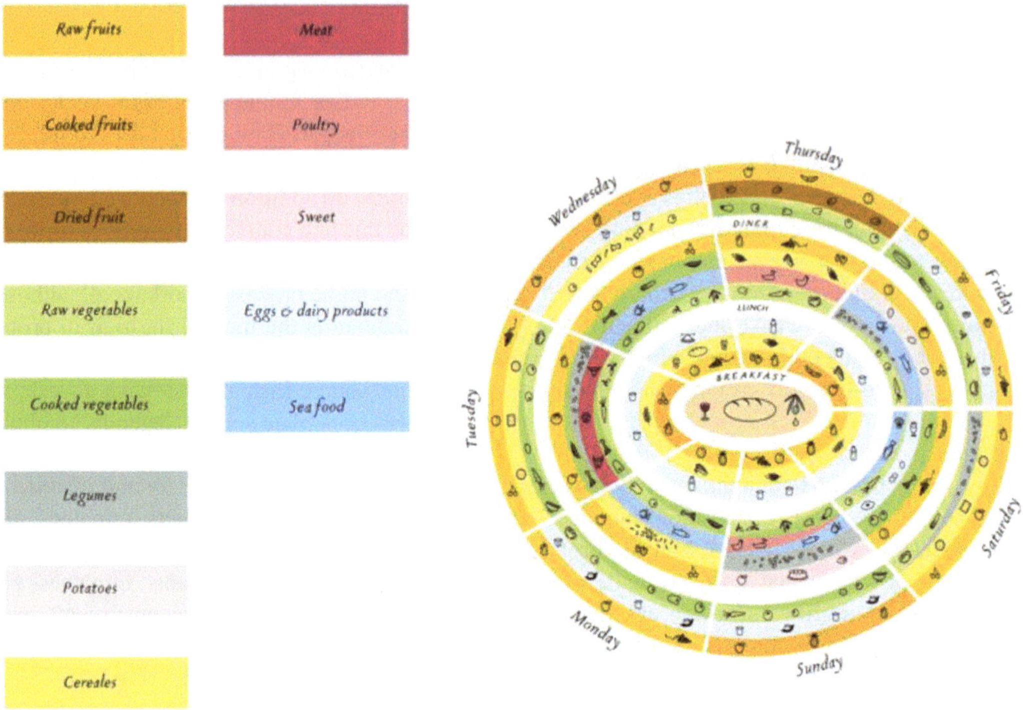

Fig. 5.2 Illustration of the implementation of the Mediterranean diet-French style over a week period. In the center, foods used every day: whole bread at the three meals; a glass of wine at lunch and/or dinner; olive oil for cooking and salad dressing. Then three rings for breakfast; four for lunch; and three for dinner

three courses, and the social exchange with partners during the meal, avoids feeling "over full" in the afternoon. If wine makes you sleepy, wine can be kept for the evening meal, and water will be the preferred beverage at noon. Sodas are to be avoided, since they are known to contribute to weight gain [31] and unhealthy fast/junk foods, which could deteriorate the benefits of Mediterranean diet.

Such a meal organization would demand a disruption for many people in their normal life. However, this can be adapted. Many companies have their own cafeterias where it is possible to have a full lunch, and the 30–45 min it lasts can be shared with colleagues, to exchange ideas on many subjects, creating a relaxed atmosphere at work. These companies' cafeterias, as well as school and university cafeterias, generally propose a choice of dishes. In some cultures individual choice is important and represents a major motivation in eating habits [7]. The choice in the same food group is clearly an advantage for an informed consumer, but may result in repetitive choices in some people, and especially children, forgetting the necessary variety of food sources. This repetition might ultimately be deleterious, depending upon the choice. It is worth remembering that the first experience of food for children is in the family, where traditionally meals are cooked at home with one menu for all. In public catering, where one has to consider ethnic differences, it might be interesting to get close to traditional familial practices in order to maintain a food culture.

In some situations, lunch can be simplified in order to be taken at the workplace, as long as the nutritional principles are maintained, including sharing this time with friends or colleagues, which is always beneficial. A special room might be dedicated for lunches in office spaces.

Conviviality applies also to breakfast and dinner, generally shared with the family.

Another important point is the habit to cook at home and to treat family and friends with a home-cooked meal. Cooking at home allows the cook to become skilled with the quality of foods

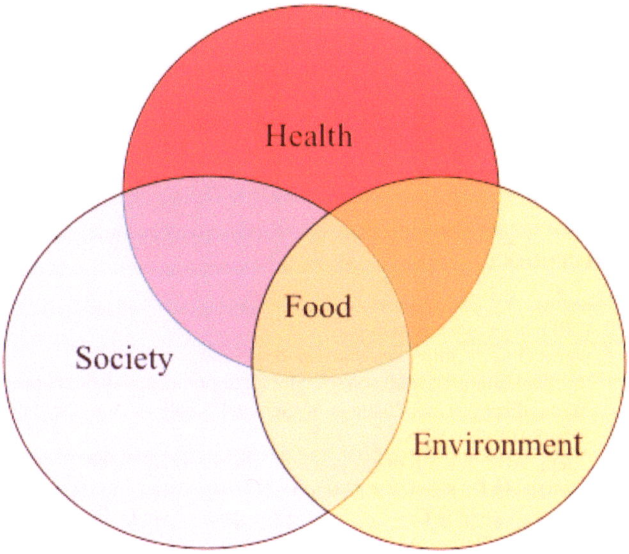

Fig. 5.3 Illustration of how food is a meeting point. Interacting entities include health and prevention of non-transmissible diseases; society with conviviality and transmission of culture; and environment with requirement for improved food security and quality in agriculture and food industry

and with various ingredients. It might seem difficult within the time-tight schedule of a working life; however, some recipes are easily realized, and others can be prepared in advance and just warmed up for the meal [28].

When buying processed food, one is dependent upon the technical and commercial choices of the food company, which might be reasonable, or might not. When cooking at home, it is possible to know the origin of the various ingredients in the meals. Substances used in packaging, such as phthalates and bisphenol A, especially harmful to pregnant women and newborns and also associated with negative effects on male fertility [32, 33], are then avoided. Buying fresh food and ingredients, as near as possible to the source of production, without or a limited amount of processing and packaging is a healthy improvement to our daily diet. This aspect might look time-consuming, but nowadays it is possible, even through the web, to get meat and vegetables directly from the producers. Thus, the whole act of eating will develop local production activities, benefiting society, and improving or reducing environmental contamination. This central aspect of dietary choices is illustrated in Fig. 5.3. The Food industry is encouraged by Public Health recommendations to improve their processes and packaging practices in order to minimize exposure to toxic compounds for the consumer.

Conclusions

In this chapter, we have discussed the main characteristics of the French perspective to the Mediterranean diet: no snacking, three meals a day, a three course meal, buying raw or no processed foods, home cooking, the main meal at midday, eating together, and adherence to cultural foods with reluctance for fast/junk foods. Some of these aspects (regular food intakes, buying, cooking) might look somewhat tedious, but they represent the best way to personalize the act of eating, transform it into an important part of our life, with positive implications on our own health, our family and friends, our well-being and also our environment. These aspects can be adapted to our actual lifestyle, taking advantage of the technology to facilitate buying, cooking and preserving food. When making dietary choices, these are some the factors that may influence our health: maintain quality and diversity of foods; stress the importance of the participation of plant foods (vegetables, fruit, whole cereals, legumes, oils with olive oil to be preferred); consume moderate amounts of animal products (meat, dairy) and wine; pay attention to the structure and organization of the meals; do not forget about the pleasure of eating and sharing meals with others. Thus, beyond these practical suggestions, it is an attitude to food intake that is to be implemented: eating is not an ancillary act but a responsible one with major implications for ourselves and for society.

References

1. WHO. http://www.who.int/.
2. World Obesity. http://www.worldobesity.org.
3. Ng M, Fleming T, Robinson M. Global, regional, and national prevalence of overweight and obesity in children and adults during 1980-2013: a systematic analysis for the Global Burden of Disease Study 2013. Lancet. 2014;S0140:60460–8.
4. Obepi. 2012. www.roche.fr/content/dam/corporate/roche_fr/doc/obepi_2012.pdf.
5. Mamalakis G, Kafatos A, Manios Y, Anagnostopoulou T, Apostolaki I. Obesity indices in a cohort of primary school children in Crete: a six year prospective study. Int J Obes Relat Metab Disord. 2000;24:765–71.
6. Tessier S, Gerber M. Comparison between Sardinia and Malta: the Mediterranean diet revisited. Appetite. 2005;45:121–6.
7. Fischler C, Masson E. Manger. Français, Européens et Américains face à l'alimentation. Odile Jacob, Paris; 2008.
8. Poulain JP. Sociologies de l'alimentation Presses. Paris: Universitaires de France; 2002.
9. Aymard M, Grignon C, Sabban F. A la recherche du temps social. In: Aymard M, Grignon C, Sabban F, editors. Le temps de manger, Alimentation, emploi du temps et rythmes sociaux. Paris: Ed, Institut National de la Recherche Agronomique, de la Maison des sciences de l'homme; 1993.
10. Scali J, Richard A, Gerber M. Diet profiles in a population sample from Mediterranean Southern France. Public Health Nutr. 2001;4:173–82.
11. Estruch R, Ros E, Salas-Salvado J, et al. Primary prevention of cardiovascular disease with a Mediterranean diet. N Engl J Med. 2013;368:1279–90.
12. Perrin AE, Dallongeville J, Ducimetière P, et al. Interactions between traditional regional determinants and socio-economic status on dietary patterns in a sample of French men. Br J Nutr. 2005;93:109–14.
13. Cohen DA, Sturm R, Lara M, Gilbert M, Gee S. Discretionary calorie intake a priority for obesity prevention: results of rapid participatory approaches in low-income US communities. J Public Health (Oxf). 2010;32:379–86.
14. Bes-Rastrollo M, Sanchez-Villegas A, Basterra-Gortari FJ, et al. Prospective study of self-reported usual snacking and weight gain in a Mediterranean cohort: the SUN project. Clin Nutr. 2010;29:323–30.
15. Braude L, Stevenson RJ. Watching television while eating increases energy intake. Examining the mechanisms in female participants. Appetite. 2014;76C:9–16.
16. Chaput JP, Klingenberg L, Astrup A, Sjodin AM. Modern sedentary activities promote overconsumption of food in our current obesogenic environment. Obes Rev. 2011;12:e12–20.
17. Marsh S, Ni MC, Maddison R. The non-advertising effects of screen-based sedentary activities on acute eating behaviours in children, adolescents, and young adults. A systematic review. Appetite. 2013;71:259–73.
18. Walrand S, Short KR, Bigelow ML, et al. Functional impact of high protein intake on healthy elderly people. Am J Physiol Endocrinol Metab. 2008;295:E921–8.
19. Issa C, Darmon N, Salameh P, et al. Mediterranean diet pattern with low consumption of liquid sweets and refined cereals is negatively associated with adiposity in adults from rural Lebanon. Int J Obes (Lond). 2011;35:251–8.
20. Costanzo S, Di Castelnuovo A, Donati MB, Iacoviello L, de Gaetano G. Wine, beer or spirit drinking in relation to fatal and non-fatal cardiovascular events: a meta-analysis. Eur J Epidemiol. 2011;26:833–50.
21. Koppes LL, Dekker JM, Hendriks HF, Bouter LM, Heine RJ. Moderate alcohol consumption lowers the risk of type 2 diabetes: a meta-analysis of prospective observational studies. Diabetes Care. 2005;28:719–25.
22. Mekary RA, Rimm EB, Giovannucci E, et al. Joint association of glycemic load and alcohol intake with type 2 diabetes incidence in women. Am J Clin Nutr. 2011;94:1525–32.
23. Fedirko V, Tramacere I, Bagnardi V, et al. Alcohol drinking and colorectal cancer risk: an overall and dose-response meta-analysis of published studies. Ann Oncol. 2011;22:1958–72.
24. World Cancer Research Fund. 2010. http://www.dietandcancerreport.org/cancer_resource_center/downloads/cu/Breast-Cancer-2010-Report.pdf.
25. Chen WY, Rosner B, Hankinson SE, Colditz GA, Willett WC. Moderate alcohol consumption during adult life, drinking patterns, and breast cancer risk. JAMA. 2011;306:1884–90.

26. Ferrari P, Licaj I, Muller DC, et al. Lifetime alcohol use and overall and cause-specific mortality in the European Prospective Investigation into Cancer and nutrition (EPIC) study. BMJ Open. 2014;4:e005245. doi:10.1136/bmjopen-2014-005245.
27. Hoffman R, Gerber M. The Mediterranean diet Health and Science. UK: Wiley-Blackwell; 2012.
28. Gerber M. Santé et alimentation Méditerranéenne au quotidien. France: Edisud; 2004.
29. Vincent S, Gerber M, Bernard MC, et al. The Medi-RIVAGE study Mediterranean diet, cardiovascular risks and gene polymorphisms rationale, recruitment, design, dietary intervention and baseline characteristics of participants. Public Health Nutr. 2004;7:531–42.
30. Vincent-Baudry S, Defoort C, Gerber M, et al. The Medi-RIVAGE study: reduction of cardiovascular risk factors after 3 month-intervention with a Mediterranean-type diet or a low-fat diet. Am J Clin Nutr. 2005;82:964–71.
31. Malik VS, Pan A, Willett WC, Hu FB. Sugar-sweetened beverages and weight gain in children and adults: a systematic review and meta-analysis. Am J Clin Nutr. 2013;98:1084–102.
32. Grob K, Biedermann M, Scherbaum E, Roth M, Rieger K. Food contamination with organic materials in perspective: packaging materials as the largest and least controlled source? A view focusing on the European situation. Crit Rev Food Sci Nutr. 2006;46:529–35.
33. Harley KG, Aguilar Schall R, Chevrier J, et al. Prenatal and postnatal bisphenol A exposure and body mass index in childhood in the CHAMACOS cohort. Environ Health Perspect. 2013;121:514–20.

Part III
Mediterranean Diet and Lifestyle for Health Promotion

Chapter 6
Mediterranean Oils and Fats, and Disease Risk

Mariette Gerber and Richard Hoffman

Key Points

- Fat intake and the proportions of fatty acids in the Mediterranean diet are in agreement with international recommendations. In addition to olive oil—the main source of fats in the Mediterranean diet—other sources of fats contribute to important differences in the overall fatty acid profile compared to a Western diet.
- Micronutrients and microconstituents with antioxidant and other properties are present in oils in the Mediterranean diet. They protect fatty acids from oxidation and are potentially important for reducing disease risk.
- Olive oil is convincingly associated with a reduced risk of cardiovascular disease, and with possible risk reductions for cancers and neurodegenerative disorders.

Keywords Mediterranean diet • Olive oil • Medium chain fatty acids • Fish • Nuts

Introduction

Since the work of Ancel Keys, fats in the Mediterranean diet (MD) were recognized as being different from those in the Western diet and for being responsible for the good health markers of the Mediterranean countries, despite a rather high fat intake. In the Seven Countries study, Ancel Keys noted that Crete had a rate of coronary heart disease (CHD) almost 32 times lower than East Finland, although the overall fat intake in Crete was not much lower than in East Finland (36.1 % of total energy intake (TEI) and 38.5 % TEI, respectively) [1]. However, the saturated fatty acids (SFA) contributed 23.7 % of total calories in East Finland compared to 7.7 % in Crete. This observation suggested that overall dietary fat consumption was not a major determinant of risk for CHD, and it is now

M. Gerber, M.D., Ph.D. (✉)
Expert at ANSES, INSERM-Institut du Cancer de Montpellier, France,
34298 Montpellier cedex 5, France
e-mail: mariette.gerber@sfr.fr

R. Hoffman, Ph.D., R.F.S.A.
School of Life and Medical Sciences, University of Hertfordshire,
Hatfield AL10 9AB, UK
e-mail: r.hoffman@herts.ac.uk

D.F. Romagnolo, O.I. Selmin (eds.), *Mediterranean Diet*, Nutrition and Health,
DOI 10.1007/978-3-319-27969-5_6

recognized that protection against CHD is related more to the types of fats that are consumed rather than to overall fat consumption.

In addition to monounsaturated fatty acids (MUFA), it appeared that polyunsaturated fatty acids (PUFA), especially *n*-3 PUFA, also played a role in the beneficial effects of this diet. Also important in the MD is the source of fatty acids, the main one being olive oil and preferably extra virgin olive oil (EVOO), which is associated with a reduction in mortality and the incidence of the main nontransmissible diseases. Other oils, namely argan and grape-seed, are limited to some regions, and may protect against aging of the skin. Animal fats in the MD are noted for their sources, which are mainly goats and sheep, and for the presence of medium chain fatty acids (≤10 C), which are less atherogenic and potentially less obesogenic than longer chain fatty acids (≥12 C). Fish and plant sources are also important in the MD. Nuts are sources of PUFA, (*n*-6 PUFA and *n*-3 PUFA depending upon the nut variety) together with micronutrients, minerals and microconstituents. Greens, such as purslane and kale, also provide α-linolenic acid, an essential FA, and the precursor of eicosapentaenoic acid (EPA). This mix of fatty acids is a characteristic of the MD and contributes to the observed health effects of this diet, even though olive oil is the predominant source readily available to the consumer.

The specificity of the Mediterranean diet (MD) relates not only to added fats, namely oils, but also to certain foods as sources of fatty acids. In this chapter, after a general review of total fat intake in Mediterranean countries, we will discuss the oils consumed in these countries, their production, consumption, and relation to diseases. Olive oil is almost exclusively used for cooking and salad dressing, and two other oils used more locally, namely argan and grape seed oils, will also be described. The principal food sources of fats in the MD will also be described.

Total Fat in MD

The benchmark studies on Mediterranean diets with regard to the recognized beneficial effects on cardiovascular diseases (CVD) are the prospective Seven Countries study [1] and the PREDIMED intervention study [2]. In the Cretan cohort in the Seven Countries study, the total fat content was 36.1 % of TEI, with 7.7 % from SFA, 25.8 % from MUFA and 2.5 % from total PUFA. In the PREDIMED study one group consumed an MD enriched with EVOO and the other an MD enriched with nuts, and these were compared with a low-fat control diet. For the MD+EVOO group, total fat, SFA, MUFA, and PUFA intake were 41.2 %, 9.4 %, 22.1 % and 6.1 %, of TEI, respectively. Thus, a typical MD, as modelled by nutritionists, is approximately 36–40 % total fat, 7–10 % SFA, 19–25 % MUFA and 3–6 % PUFA. The source of MUFA is almost exclusively olive oil, and for PUFA, long chain *n*-3 PUFA (LC *n*-3 PUFA) intake was 0.37 % of TEI in the PREDIMED study [2] (no data in [1]).

A comparison can be made between the current MD in the twenty first century in Mediterranean countries and the diet in the U.S. (Table 6.1) [3–7]. The total fat content of the current MD is generally

Table 6.1 Dietary estimates of fat intake (as % total energy intake) in Mediterranean diets and the US diet (around 2000) compared to a model Mediterranean diet

	Med diet model	Crete [6]	Greece [5]	Spain [7]	Southern Italy [3]	USA [4]
Total fat	36–40	39.3±1.3	40.9±0.2	39.3±6.8	34.7±7.7	32.9±0.4
SFA	7–10	11.4±0.5	12.1±0.1	11.8±2.6	10.2±2.9	11.0±0.2
MUFA	19–25	18.9±1.2	20.6±0.1	18.8±4.3	20.5±5.1	12.4±0.2
PUFA	3–6	4.9±0.4	5.3±0.1	6.0±1.7	4[a]	6.9±0.1
LC *n*-3 PUFA	0.37	NA	NA	NA	NA	NA

SFA saturated fatty acids, *MUFA* monounsaturated fatty acids, *PUFA* polyunsaturated fatty acids, *LC n-3 PUFA* long chain polyunsaturated fatty acids, *NA* not available

[a]By subtraction

higher than that of the U.S. The MD and U.S. diets have comparable levels of SFA, and it is the higher content of MUFA in the MD that is responsible for the differences between total fat content. This is mainly attributable to the high consumption of olive oil, which is rich in the MUFA oleic acid. In the Western diet, MUFA are mostly from animal origin. PUFA intake tends to be higher in the U.S, and in Mediterranean countries only Spain has PUFA intake almost as high as the U.S. However, the specificity of the sources has to be considered. A large part of the PUFAs in Spain are from marine origin—Spain is characterized by the highest consumption of fish in Europe: mean 54.0 g/day/subject of the Spanish cohort (Q1: 5.16; Q2: 19.12; Q3: 30.78 Q4: 48.42; Q5: 91.85) [8], whereas fish consumption in the U.S. is much lower (15.6 g/day/person; CI 14.67–16.63 [9]). By contrast, seed oils generally rich in linoleic acid, such as sunflower, safflower, soybean, are common in the U.S., but they are seldom used in Mediterranean countries. Data for the years 2005–2006, calculated by two different methods, report linoleic acid (*n*-6) as 7.2 % and 6.2 % of TEI and LC *n*-3 PUFA as ~0.04 % and ~0.06 % of TEI [10], whereas the baseline consumption of LC *n*-3 PUFA in the 2003–2004 PREDIMED cohort was 0.32 % TEI, almost ten times more than in the U.S. [2]. Thus, there are differences between Mediterranean countries and the U.S. not only in the quantity and the source of MUFA but also in the quantity of LC *n*-3 PUFA.

Because the MD avoids the consumption of industrialized processed foods, it will be low in industrial *trans* fatty acids. The MD does contain ruminant-derived *trans* fatty acids, but, unlike industrial *trans* fatty acids, there is no evidence that the levels of ruminant *trans* fatty acids consumed in the MD are harmful [11].

Dietary Sources of Fat in the MD

The main sources of dietary fat in Mediterranean countries are olive oil, dairy products, and meat, with smaller contribution from seafood, nuts, and other plant foods. Although the relative contributions of these will vary between countries, most Mediterranean populations following a traditional MD have high olive oil consumption, moderate consumption of dairy products and low consumption of meat. Data from the European Prospective Investigation into Cancer and Nutrition (EPIC) study [5] found that oil (mostly olive oil) was the principal source of added fat in the Greek, Spanish (Granada), and Sicilian (Southern Italy) diet compared to margarine and butter in the UK General Population group (Table 6.2). However—mainly for economic reasons—other oils are now increasingly replacing olive oil, especially in Greece. Dairy was the second major contributor to fats in these countries, and was mostly from cheese in the Greek and Sicilian diets, although milk also made a significant contribution in the Spanish diet.

Table 6.2 Contribution of food groups to dietary fat intake in the EPIC study [5]

Country	Mean contribution of major food groups (and selected subgroups) to total dietary fat intake (%)			
	Added fats and oils	Dairy produce	Meat and meat products	Other
Greece	48 (93 % oils)	19 (67 % cheese)	9 (21 % processed)[a]	
Spain (Granada)	39 (90 % oils)	17 (43 % cheese; 48 % milk)	15 (63 % processed)[a]	
Sicily	30 (96 % oils)	17 (83 % cheese)	14 (53 % processed)[a]	15 (condiments and sauces)
UK	27 (43 % margarine, 26 % butter)	16 (37 % milk; 39 % cheese)	12 (53 % processed)	14 (cakes)

[a]Processed food in Mediterranean countries and in France is traditionally a small-scale way of preservation

Oils

Olive Oil

Olive trees have been part of Mediterranean agriculture for thousands of years, as shown by their representation on the tombs of ancient Egypt. Oil production is restricted to the zones of olive tree culture. However, this is not restricted to Mediterranean countries on the Northern and Southern shores of the Mediterranean, since olive trees are also cultivated in California, several South American countries, and Australia. The oil quality depends on the methods used for its production and the way it is preserved.

Production

The origin and production of olive oil are thoroughly detailed in Hoffman and Gerber [12]. Briefly, olive oil is either made from olives when they turn from green to purple (e.g. in Tuscany), or in regions such as Corsica from fully ripe olives, that is to say black olives. The olives are treated as soon as possible after harvest, and in conditions that avoid fermentation. First, the juice is extracted from the pulp, and then the aqueous phase is separated from the lipid phase. Only mechanical steps are used to obtain the final product (crushing at temperatures ≤29 °C, or, for EVOO, by pressure or centrifugation), and this step is largely responsible for the quality of the oil, and consequently for the qualification of extra-virgin, virgin, or ordinary. The degradation of oleic acid triglycerides to free fatty acids, resulting in acidity, is an indicator of quality, together with organoleptic properties. These are categorized from 1 to 10 by a council of experts from the olive tree growers (Table 6.3). Non-virgin olive oils are extracted by solvent and have an acidity ≤2 %. There are also mixtures of refined or pulp residues, and ordinary or virgin oils, generally with low acidity but no organoleptic qualification.

Composition and CVD Risk

Composition in relationship to diseases is briefly mentioned here. The saponifiable part of olive oil is made up of fatty acids, among them the MUFA oleic acid, and the relationship of MUFA to metabolic disorders and cardiovascular diseases will be discussed. The properties of the unsaponifiable fraction, i.e., triterpenes, sterols, tocopherols, carotenoids, and phenolics (tyrosol and hydroxytyrosol; flavonoids and lignans) are also increasingly attracting the attention of scientists, first for their antioxidant properties, which preserve the oil from oxidation, and also for other properties potentially implicated in chronic degenerative diseases. For example, a health benefit for hydroxytyrosol has been recognized by the European Food Safety Agency [13].

Various studies have assessed the health benefits of olive oil. Several expert committees have described the basis for making a robust judgement for a causal relationship between a nutrient or food

Table 6.3 Categories of virgin olive oil

Type of olive oil	Organoleptic properties (1–10)	Acidity (%)	Extraction pressure (atm)	Temperature (°C)
Extra virgin olive oil	>6.5	≤0.8	1	<27
Virgin olive oil	>5.5	≤2	2–3	≤29
Ordinary virgin olive oil	>3.5	≤3.3	>3	≤29
Lampante	<3.5	>3.3	>3	≤29

and disease risk [14, 15]. Consistency between several observational studies is necessary, and prospective studies are favored over case-control studies. When available, there should be randomized controlled trials (RCT) of sufficient size and duration, with more weight being given to disease incidence as an endpoint rather than to biological markers. Experimental studies, both in vivo and in vitro, can provide biological plausibility. We followed these guidelines for assessing the health benefits of olive oil. Many epidemiological studies, including RCT, have shown that a Mediterranean dietary pattern that includes olive oil is convincingly associated with a reduced risk of CVD, and is probably associated with a reduced risk of certain cancers and neurodegenerative diseases (reviewed in [16] and also discussed in one chapter in this volume). Only a few of these epidemiological studies have focused on the specific effect of olive oil. We will report on these specific studies.

Ancel Keys, the pioneer advocate of the MD, first proposed that it was the ratio of MUFA:SFA that was the key component for the health benefits of the MD [1]. Although this suggested that the importance of olive oil was to provide MUFA, later on it was established that MUFA from sources other than olive oil (animal fat contains 40–45 % MUFA) did not have the same beneficial effect [12, 17]. Consequently, more recent studies have been undertaken to decipher the specific effects of olive oil on CVD mortality and morbidity (Table 6.4).

In an analysis conducted on the EPIC population in Spain, a high intake of olive oil decreased the risk of overall mortality by 26 % and deaths due to CVD by 44 % [18]. In a study from Spain, there was a reduction of CVD incidence of 7 % for each 10 g increase of olive oil per 8.4 MJ ingested, and this effect was greater for EVOO (risk reduction 14 %) [19]. In the Italian-EPIC cohort [20], women with a high level of olive oil consumption had a reduced risk of nonfatal and fatal myocardial infarction (MI) although it should be noted that this study has been criticized because the relative risks (RR) were not adjusted for age. But the post-menopausal women subgroup might be considered as homogeneous enough with regard to age since CHD increases only of 3–4 U/1000 between the ages 55–64 years and 65–74 years. Thus, it is possible to accept the observed significant risk reduction of 45 % for a consumption of 31 g versus 15 g/day of olive oil. In the Three-City Study, those with intensive use of olive oil had a lower risk of stroke compared to those who never used olive oil [21].

A recent meta-analysis by Martinez-Gonzalez et al. [22] found a nonsignificant relationship between CHD and olive oil intake in three case-control studies and five prospective studies, but there were strong heterogeneities in both types of analysis, which were not explained by sensitivity studies. A significant risk reduction was observed in the analysis of three cohorts for the relationship between olive oil and stroke: summarized risk estimates were 0.82 (CI 0.67–0.86), also with a high heterogeneity. A significant risk reduction was also observed for the overall analysis 0.82 (CI 0.70–0.96), but again the high heterogeneity limits the conclusions that can be drawn from this meta-analysis.

Two analyses from the PREDIMED study report new data supporting the evidence of a superior benefit for EVOO versus non-virgin olive oil. The first analysis was an observational study derived from the prospective analysis of the whole cohort, and was based on baseline consumption of olive oil prior to randomisation into groups. In individuals with high cardiovascular risk, there was a statistically significant reduction in total cardiovascular risk and stroke (but not MI) for total olive oil consumption or for consumption of EVOO, but not for consumption of non-virgin OO [23]. These results were confirmed after adjusting for adherence to an MD (Table 6.4). The second analysis was performed on the randomized trial protocol [24]. There were 6705 participants in this analysis. During a median follow-up of 4.7 years there were 246 cases of atrial fibrillation: 72 in the MD+EVOO group, 82 in the MD+nuts group, and 92 in the control. The group with the diet enriched with EVOO had a significant risk reduction of 38 % for atrial fibrillation (RR 0.62; CI 0.45–0.85). This significant risk reduction was not observed in the group with the diet enriched with nuts reinforcing the superiority of EVOO over nuts in reducing mortality, which was also observed in the PREDIMED study [2].

These results highlight the possible important contribution of minor components in EVOO for cardiovascular protection. Short-term studies with cardiovascular risk factors as end-points also suggest that phenolic compounds are important for the cardiovascular benefits of virgin olive oil.

Table 6.4 Epidemiological studies on the health effects of olive oil[a]

Study	Disease outcome	Study design	Number of subjects/cases age range	Olive oil type	Exposure measurement	Statistical adjustments	Intake categorisation	Relative risk (95 % CI)	Trend
Martinez-Gonzalez et al. [24] Spain	Atrial fibrillation (AF)	Intervention Predimed Follow-up 4.7 years	6705 in 3 groups	EVOO	MD+EVOO MD+Nuts Control low-fat	Time-dependent Cox model; known predictors of AF; baseline adherence to MD	Diet enriched in EVOO 1 L/week versus Control Low fat Increment EVOO/5 % energy	0.62 (0.45, 0.88) 0.90 (0.84, 0.96)	0.002
Bendinelli et al. [20] (EPICOR study, Italy)	Myocardial infarction	Prospective Follow-up average 7.85 years	29,689/144 Women 35–74 years	Total OO	Validated EPIC FFQ	Cox models: 1. Energy; 2. Education, fruit, vegetables, meat, smoking, alcohol body weight, and waist circumference	≥31.2 g/day versus ≤15.9 g/day	0.56 (0.31, 0.99)	0.04
Buckland et al, [18] (EPIC-Spain)	Overall and CVD mortality	Prospective Follow-up 8–12 years	40,622/1 915 deaths/416 CVD Women 29–69 years	Total OO	Validated dietary history questionnaire 600 items	Cox models: 1. Age, sex, study center; 2. Non-nutritional factors: BMI, waist circumference smoking; alcohol; PA 3- Foods of the Med diet score	29.4 g/day /8.4 MJ versus < 14.9 g/day /8.4 MJ	Overall mortality: 0.74 (0.64, 0.87); CVD mortality 0.56 (0.40, 0.79)	<0.001 <0.001
Buckland et al. [19] (EPIC-Spain)	CHD incidence	Prospective Follow-up 8–12 years	40,142/587 29–69 years (38 % males)	Total OO EVOO	Validated dietary history questionnaire 600 items	Cox models: 1. Age, sex, study center; 2. Non-nutritional factors: BMI, waist circumference, smoking, alcohol, PA 3. Foods of the Med diet score, excluding olive oil and alcohol 4- Goldberg exclusions	≥28.9 g versus <10 g	0.78 (0.59, 1.03)	0.079
Guasch-Ferré et al. [23] (PREDIMEDSpain)	CVD events and mortality	Prospective Follow-up 4.8 years	7216 subjects at risk for CVD/227 events/323 deaths; 67 ± 6 (42 % males)	Total OO, non-virgin OO, EVOO	Validated dietary history questionnaire 137 items	Cox models: 1. Age, sex, intervention group; 2. Non-nutritional factors: BMI, waist circumference, smoking, alcohol; PA, markers of risk factors; 3. Med diet score, excluding olive oil and alcohol	Total OO: 56.9 ± 10 versus 21.4 ± 8 g/day EVOO/34.6 ± 27.4 versus 9.1 ± 11 g/day Non virgin OO: 21.7 ± 25.1 versus 12.1 ± 11.7 g/day	CV event total OO; 0.65 (0.47, 0.91) EVOO 0.61 (0.44, 0.85) Non-virgin OO: NS *CV mortality* total OO 0.52 (0.73, 0.96) EVOO:NS OO: NS	0.01 <0.01 0.04

Buckland et al. [32] Spain, Italy, Greece	Breast cancer	Prospective 9-year follow-up	62,284/1 256 cases	Total OO	Validated FFQ	Cox models: Age, education, reproductive factors, fruit, vegetables, meat , smoking, alcohol body weight	30.1 g/day versus 11.1 g/day	0.77 (0.48, 1.26)	
Berr et al. [35] (Three-City study, France)	Cognitive decline	Prospective Median follow-up 4 years	6924 65–≥80 years (39.7 % males)	Total OO	Frequency of broad categories food and preferred added fat	Cox models: 0-Age, sex, education, center, baseline cognitive; 1. Health behaviors and health status 2. smoking and dietary habits	No use versus intensive use	Visual memory: 0.83 (0.69, 0.99); Verbal fluency 0.85 (0.70, 1.03)	0.01
Martinez-Lapiscina et al. [36] Spain	Mild cognitive impairment	Prospective in Predimed-Navarra trial	285, 95/group intervention	EVOO		Multivariate logistic regression analysis[b]	Diet enriched in EVOO 1 L/week versus Control Low fat	0.34 (0.12, 0.97)	
Garcia-Arenzana et al. [34] Spain	Mammographic density	Cross-sectional	3548 women aged 45–69	OO	FFQ 117 items	Proportional odds-model: Age, BMI, parity, menopause, alcohol, smoking; Test for multiple testing	Increment/ 22 g	0.86 (0.76, 0.96)	0.009
Valls-Pedret et al. [37] Spain	Cognitive decline	Cross-sectional in Predimed trial	447, 52 % women 55–80 year	OO VOO	Validated FFQ 137 items ml/day: Total OO: mean: 38 (0–75) VOO: median: 4 (0–70)	Multiple linear regression models adjusted for various food groups (energy adjusted, BMI, alcohol, tobacco, age, gender)	OO and VOO/10 g/day	Regression coefficient Immediate memory: 0.755 (0.15, 1.358) delayed memory: 0.163 (0.010, 0.316)	0.014* 0.037*

[a]*OO* olive oil, *VOO* virgin olive oil, *EVOO* extra virgin olive oil, *PA* physical activity, *BMI* body mass index, *CV* cardiovascular, *TG* triglyceridemia, *FFQ* food frequency questionnaire, Goldberg exclusion, exclusion of participants with poor concordance of energy intake to energy expenditure identified using Goldberg criteria

[b]Adjustments for sex, age, education, apoE, genotype, family history of cognitive impairment/dementia, smoking, physical activity, body mass index, hypertension, dyslipidemia, diabetes, alcohol, and total energy intake

*p for significance of the regression coefficient

For example, the EUROLIVE study, comparing olive oil high and low in phenolic compound, found a linear increase in HDL cholesterol levels for low-, medium-, and high-polyphenol olive oil, and a linear decrease in oxidized LDL levels [25]. A reduction in LDL oxidation by EVOO with a minimum hydroxytyrosol content is the basis for a recent health claim issued by the European Food Safety Authority for the benefits of EVOO [13].

Cancers

A beneficial effect of adherence to an MD (as assessed by a Mediterranean diet score) and reduced cancer risk is found to be greater in Mediterranean than in non-Mediterranean, populations [12]. The overall cancer mortality in the Spanish study quoted above showed a RR <1 but was not significant [18]. In the PREDIMED study, no statistically significant associations were found for consumption of any type of olive oil and mortality from all types of cancer [23]. However, different cancer sites are characterized by different risk factors and for some types of cancer there are indications of a specific effect of olive oil, and this is supported by several in vitro and in vivo experimental studies [26]. A review of 25 studies reported risk reduction for upper digestive and respiratory tract cancers, breast and, possibly, colorectal, and other cancer sites [27], but this study was limited because of the low number of cases per cancer site, most of the studies were case-controls, and because of the absence of a pertinent meta-analysis technique. *A posteriori* dietary patterns analysis has also demonstrated a greater risk reduction in breast cancer when olive oil was present as part of the diet [28–31]. A few studies have addressed the question of the specific effect of olive oil on cancers. In a study of olive oil and breast cancer in the Mediterranean countries of the EPIC study, there was a nonsignificant risk reduction for estrogen receptor negative (ER-), progesterone receptor negative (PR-) breast cancers with a high olive oil intake [32]. These cancers are known to be different from ER+ breast cancers in terms of risk factors, but they represent only 25–30 % of all breast cancers and the lack of statistical power might explain the large CI (see Table 6.4). This observation, nevertheless, is supported by an experimental model showing that the olive oil phytochemical oleuropein is more cytotoxic for basal-like ER- MDA-MB-231 cells than for luminal ER+ MCF-7 cells [33]. In addition, a recent large cross-sectional multicenter Spanish study suggested that olive oil could reduce mammographic density, a risk factor for breast cancer, even though calorie intake was associated with an increase in mammographic density [34].

Neurodegenerative Diseases

In the prospective Three City Study, olive oil was associated with a decrease in cognitive impairment [35] (Table 6.4). In the PREDIMED-Navarra trial, better post-trial cognitive performance was observed for the 95 participants allocated to the MedDiet+EVOO group versus control in all cognitive domains, and significantly better performance across fluency and memory [36]. This group also showed lower mild cognitive impairment compared with the control group. Participants assigned to the MD+nuts group did not differ from controls. In a cross-sectional analysis of participants of the PREDIMED study, consumption of some foods was independently associated with better cognitive function. Among these foods, total olive oil positively correlated with immediate verbal memory and virgin olive oil with delayed verbal memory (Table 6.4) [37].

Antioxidant and anti-inflammatory phenolic compounds in EVOO may contribute to these beneficial effects since oxidative stress and inflammation are associated with neurodegeneration in experimental models. In subjects of the SUVIMAX cohort, consumption of MUFA from olive oil significantly reduced the severity of skin photo-aging. Only MUFA from olive oil was effective, suggesting that it might be the phenolic compounds or squalene in olive oil that are actually responsible for the beneficial effect on skin photo-aging [38].

Argan Oil

For a long time, use of argan oil was restricted to the MD of Morocco, mainly because there was only local craft production. But due to its interesting composition, it is now used more widely not only for its organoleptic qualities, but also, and maybe more so, for its use in cosmetics [39].

Production

Argan oil is essentially produced in Morocco, in the region of Essaouira and in the Southern desert area. The source is the fruit of a small thorny arborescent bush (*Argania spinosa, fam. Sapotaceae*). Like almonds, this fruit is protected by two envelopes, a soft green one and a woody one, and inside are two or three seeds from which oil is produced. Traditionally, because of the thorns, it could not be collected by hand, and the harvest was from fruits that had fallen, either spontaneously or by using a pole, or the seeds were collected from the excrements of goats, which climb on the tree to eat the fruits, digest the tender envelop and reject the seeds in the woody envelope. This envelope is manually removed and the seeds may be softly warmed or not before being milled. The resulting paste is again worked by hand and the oil is obtained by decanting. Nowadays, most of the steps are done mechanically, except for the rupture of the woody envelop, which is mainly done by women in cooperatives. This semi-industrialized process produces virgin argan oil: extra virgin <1 g/100 g of free oleic acid; pure virgin <2 g/100 g of free oleic acid; ordinary virgin <3.3 g/100 g of free oleic acid. There is also a solvent extraction process, and the resulting oil is only used for industry or cosmetic use.

Composition

The saponifiable fraction of argan oil includes fatty acids whose profile is given in Table 6.5. The proportion of α-linolenic acid (ALA) is highly variable depending upon the terrain, the state of the plant and the method of extraction. There is a higher proportion of PUFA and a lower content of MUFA in argan oil than in olive oil. The unsaponifiable fraction represents microconstituents (~1 to 1.5 % of the oil) and essentially consists of tocopherols, phenolic compounds, triterpenes, and sterols. These microconstituents are characterized by a high antioxidant activity and increase the stability of the oil. The content of microconstituents varies with the preparation method (temperature and duration of seed grilling) and traces of metal or organic material. Table 6.6 shows estimates of the major components from 16 determinations. Of note are the particular microconstituents found in argan oil that differ compared to other oils and to olive oil (except for squalene), and the high variability in levels of constituents, mostly dependent on the type of preparation.

Table 6.5 Fatty acid compositions of argan oil and grape seed oil

	Argan oil (% total fatty acids)	Grape seed oil (% total fatty acids)
Total SFA	20	12.8
• Palmitic acid	12–14	7.1
• Stearic acid	5–8	5.1
Total MUFA	45	16.4
• Oleic acid	37–48	15.8
Total PUFA	35	70.9
• Linoleic acid	31–40	70.6
• α-Linolenic acid	0.09–2.63	0.3

Table 6.6 Microconstituents of argan oil

	Content (mg/kg)
Tocopherols[a]	50–200
Phenolics	
• Ferulic acid and syringic acid	4–152
Triterpenes	2950 ± 2000
• Squalene	3000–3200
Sterols	
• Scotenol	1420 ± 1100
• Spinasterol	1150 ± 700

[a]85 % γ-tocopherol

Argan Oil and Disease Risk

The conclusion of a recent review on argan oil was that "There are still no strong clinical data available that provide evidence of the efficacy of argan oil in humans. That argan oil constituents have pharmacological properties *in vitro* is not sufficient to ascertain the clinical potential of whole argan oil. More studies are necessary to determine its impact on human health" [40]. Most of the arguments for a health effect of argan oil are based on *in vitro* studies that have analyzed the biological effect of each microconstituent. The strongest evidence concerns the hypo-cholesterolemic effect of argan oil and an effect on the potential risk reduction of cardiovascular diseases. A few human studies support this hypothesis. In a cross-sectional study of 96 subjects, of whom 62 subjects were regular argan oil consumers and the others not, Drissi et al. [41] showed that the regular consumers had lower plasma LDL cholesterol levels (12.7 %, $p<0.05$) and Lp (a) (25.3 %, $p<0.05$) compared with the nonconsumers. In an intervention study, 39 dyslipidemic patients (79 % women) were recruited and randomly assigned to the two following groups: the argan group (25 ml/day of argan oil at breakfast for 3 weeks), and the control group (butter 20 g/day) [42]. After 3 weeks, blood total cholesterol was significantly lower in the argan oil group ($p=0.04$), as was LDL cholesterol (23.8 % and 25.6 % lower, respectively $p=0.02$). HDL cholesterol levels had increased in the argan oil group by 26 % at the end of the intervention period compared to baseline ($p=0.01$). Thrombin-induced platelet aggregation was lower in the argan oil group ($p<0.05$), and oxidative status was enhanced as a result of lower platelet malondialdehyde and higher glutathione peroxidase activities ($p<0.05$). The LDL-cholesterol-lowering and the HDL-cholesterol-raising effects might be explained by the subtle balance between SFA and PUFA in argan oil, and the anti-aggregating action by the phenolic extracts [43].

Only *in vitro* studies have investigated anticarcinogenic activity of argan oil, especially on prostate cancer lines [44]. Another often advertised quality of argan oil concerns skin: argan oil has now become a standard ingredient in shampoos, body care products as well as in moisturizers due to its moisturizing effect. A clinical study using topical application showed some benefit [45]. However, it could also be orally efficient: Cosgrove et al. [46] reported that, among other nutrients, a higher linoleic intake was associated with a lower senile dryness (OR 0.75; CI 0.64–0.88) and skin atrophy (OR 0.78; CI 0.65, 0.95) [47]. Linoleic acid is incorporated into the ceramides of epidermal cement and principally that of the ceramide 1 subclass, which plays a key role in the organization of the stratum corneum lipids [47]. The beneficial effect on skin could also be due to squalene.

Thus, supported by a few human studies, composition and biological plausibility, one can assume that argan oil may have a preventive effect for cardiovascular disease. Its beneficial effect on skin is possible but data are insufficient. Even though the efficiency of production and the capacity for distribution of argan oil are rather limited, it remains an interesting product for the health, economy, and culture of Morocco.

Grape Seed Oil

This oil was extracted from grape seeds for the first time in the seventeenth century. In France, it was cultivated and produced for trading in 1800 around the city of Albi, South-Western France, by the agronomist Jean-Baptisite Rougier de la Bergerie.

Production and Composition

The production of grape seed oil is associated with the vine culture, which is common on the North shores of the Mediterranean. Grape seeds are a by-product of the wine industry. The oil is obtained by crushing the seeds, followed by solvent extraction, with an efficiency of about 12–13 %. The main producer is Italy (20,000 tons) followed by France (2,000 tons). The oil is used locally mainly for salad dressing.

The main fatty acid composition of grape seed oil is shown in Table 6.5 [48]. Grape seed oil has a very high content of linoleic acid, and only safflower oil shows a comparable content. However, grape seed oil has almost twice the content of tocopherols—410 mg/kg versus 267 mg/kg, and 132.8 mg/kg versus 87 mg/kg of α-tocopherol. α-Tocopherol will protect against peroxidation of the high content in PUFA. The unsaponifiable fraction is modest. Because they are not fat-soluble, none of the phenolic compounds present in the seed are found in the oil. The main microconstituents are sterols and tocopherols with 3 g/kg of total sterols, comprising 69 % β-sitosterol, and 410 mg/kg of total tocopherols, comprising 32 % α-tocopherol (133 mg/kg).

Grape Seed oil and Disease Risk

Several studies with grape seeds have analyzed the effects of the catechins and proanthocyanidins, but these phenolics are not present in the oil. There are no epidemiological studies investigating the relationship of grape seed oil and health. One interesting group of compounds are the policosanols (PC), which are suspected to decrease LDL-cholesterol and increase HDL-cholesterol, but this assertion is still controversial. Grape seed oil was found to contain high quantities of PC (245.15 mg/kg oil) [49]. Hexacosanol is the most abundant PC in grape seed oil, followed by octacosanol, tetracosanol, and triacontanol in decreasing order.

Based on epidemiological studies [17], a good way to decrease the risk of CHD in populations characterized by a high intake of SFA is to increase PUFA intake. This is illustrated in the South-West of France, where the rather high intake of duck and goose meat and fat is accompanied with a high intake of fish, vegetables, and the use of grape seed oil for salads. This region has a lower incidence of CHD than most European countries (with the exception of Barcelona, which is characterized by an MD with olive oil), and it was the lowest in France [50].

Another quality of grape seed oil, and one promoted by cosmetic companies, is its beneficial effect on skin. Because of the high proportion of linoleic acid, this product is comparable to argan oil, maybe with the added benefit of the high content of vitamin E.

Thus grape seed oil may be of benefit if the dietary pattern is rich in animal sources of fat, but it cannot replace olive oil and its multiple nutritional advantages. As a by-product of the wine production, the use of grape seed oil in cosmetic use is of interest.

Fats in Foods

Fats in foods contribute to the overall consumption of dietary fat and specific fatty acids. Animal foods generally contribute more than plant foods to this intake. Among animal foods, mammals should be considered separately from fish, and among plant foods nuts are of particular importance.

Each of these foods will be successively covered and characterized with regard to disease risk specifically in relation to their fat content and fatty acid composition.

Animal Foods

Dairy Products and Meats

Intake of dairy products and meats is moderate in the MD, and lower than in the Western diet [51]. The main sources are small livestock, namely goats and sheep. A notable difference in the SFA composition of milk from goats and sheep versus cow milk is the far higher levels of the medium chain fatty acids (MCFA) caproic (C6:0), caprylic (C8:0), and capric (C10:0) in triglycerides of ovine milk (Table 6.7). For example, goat milk typically contains 15–18 % MCFA compared to 5–9 % in cow milk (Table 6.8) [52, 53]. In the MD, milk from goats and sheep is mainly processed into cheese or yogurt, rather than being consumed raw or converted into butter. Lipolysis during cheese maturation can increase free MCFA several fold [54]. In Mediterranean countries, goats and sheep spend most of the time grazing in the wild and consequently the ALA content in their meat and milk is higher than for beef with 2.5 % of total fatty acids in lamb meat compared to 1.3 % in beef [55].

Fatty Acids in Meats and Dairy Products and Disease Risk

Even though there are no epidemiological studies comparing dietary patterns that include either beef or lamb, there are data suggesting that the differences in fatty acid compositions between small livestock and cattle are significant. In a nutritional analysis of the Nurse's Health Study [56] in relation to CVD, it was found that only the sum of C12:0 to C18:0 increased the risk of CVD (RR 1.29; CI 1.00–1.66, by an increment of 5 % of energy), the main contributors being hard cheese and beef. Obviously, these fatty acids raise LDL-cholesterol more than unsaturated fatty acids [57], but you cannot make cheese with sunflower oil. Of more relevance is an intervention study that was conducted on 41 healthy adults with initial plasma cholesterol concentration between 4.8 and 7.8 mmol/L

Table 6.7 Main medium chain fatty acids in milks (% fatty acid methyl ester) [51, 52]

Fatty acids	Goat	Sheep	Cow
Caproic (C 6:0)	2.9	2.4	1.6
Caprylic (C8:0)	2.6	2.7	1.3
Capric (C10:0)	7.8	10.0	3.0

Table 6.8 Total fat and fatty acids in various nuts [70]

	Total fat (/100 g)	SFA (/100 g)	MUFA[a] (/100 g)	PUFA (/100 g)	
				α-Linolenic acid	Linoleic acid
Almonds	52.8	4.0	33.7	0.0	12.6
Hazelnuts	62.4	4.5	46.6	0.1	8.4
Peanuts	49.7	6.9	24.6	0.0	15.7
Pistachios	46.0	5.6	24.2	0.3	13.6
Walnuts (English)	65.2	6.1	8.9	9.1	38.1

[a]As oleic acid

receiving in a cross-over design an iso-energetic diet with 50 g/day of cow's milk or sheep's milk [58]. Replacing cows' with sheep's dairy fat led to a 0.33 mmol/L (CI 0.11–0.56) decrease (i.e. 6 %) in total plasma cholesterol concentration, decreasing from 5.53 mmol/L (s.d. = 0.90) to 5.20 mmol/L (s.d. = 0.90). The decrease was higher for LDL-cholesterol (0.18 mmol/L; CI 0.02–0.33) than for HDL-cholesterol (0.11 mmol/L; CI 0.02–0.20).

Beside their probable hypocholesterolemic effect, MCFAs are also rapidly oxidized and so can be less obesogenic than longer chain SFA [59]. This is because metabolism of MCFA in the body is distinct from longer chain FAs. MCFA can be hydrolyzed from triglycerides in the stomach and duodenum by lipases. Most MCFAs in goat and sheep milk triglycerides are esterified at the *sn-3* position of the glycerol moiety [60], the preferred position for hydrolysis by gastric lipase [61]. Free MCFAs, either from the action of lipases in the gut or preformed due to lipolysis during cheese maturation, are absorbed directly in the intestine without re-esterification, and then transported, mainly via the portal vein, to the liver, where they are rapidly oxidized.

Fish

Fish and other seafood are not only popular dishes in some regions close to the Mediterranean shore but fish is also eaten in the hinterland, which brings a strong tradition of salting, marinating, and smoking fillets from fatty fish. Fish is the main dietary source of eicosapentaenoic acid (EPA) and docosahexaenoic acid (DHA). Although ALA can theoretically act as a precursor of LC-PUFA, conversion is poor (<8 % to EPA and <4 % to DHA). LC-PUFAs occur predominantly in fatty fish, and good sources in the Mediterranean are sardines, anchovies, and mackerel. Levels of EPA and DHA in preserved anchovies have been estimated at 466 and 886 mg/100 g, respectively, with even higher levels of EPA and DHA in fresh mackerel (662 and 886 mg/100 g, respectively) and fresh sardines (638 and 1269 mg/100 g respectively) [62].

The EPA and DHA contents of oily fish are dependent on their diet since oily fish are themselves poor converters of ALA into EPA and DHA. Phytoplankton, on the other hand, are good converters, and hence oily fish will contain high levels of EPA and DHA if they have consumed a diet rich in plankton, or if they have consumed other fish [63]. A study found that oily fish from the warm waters of the Mediterranean contained lower levels of LC *n*-3 PUFA than fish from colder, more northerly waters [64]. However, the season and stage of the reproductive cycle of the fish are probably more important factors that influence fatty acid content [65]. Farmed fish will only contain significant amounts EPA and DHA if their feed contains these fatty acids [66]. Because declining fish resources have to be considered, it is important to use recommended feeding guidelines [66] and to follow a plant-based diet for the fish in the last 3 months before selling in order to provide the consumer with the required EPA and DHA [67].

Fatty Acids of Fish and Disease Risk

LC *n*-3 PUFA are essential fatty acids, and fish are the major source. The necessity of LC *n*-3 PUFAs is recognized by the international agencies WHO and FAO [68]. Recommendations are established with a convincing level of evidence for fetal, infant, and child development, for pregnant and lactating women, and with a probable level of evidence for the prevention of chronic disease. Meta-analyses of recent studies looking at the relationship between fish intake and measurements of blood concentrations of LC *n*-3 PUFA with diabetes, reported an increased risk associated with an increased proportion of LC *n*-3 PUFAs in the serum [69]. However, these meta-analyses displayed high heterogeneity, and the risk was restricted to North-American populations suggesting a confounding factor either related to cooking practices or to other food-related factors, or to an unknown contaminant in the fish consumed in North America, the first hypothesis being the more likely [70].

Plant Foods

The contribution of plant foods to fat intake is rather modest. Nuts are the main contributors and provide SFA, MUFA, *n*-3 PUFA, and *n*-6 PUFA. Some greens contain significant amounts of ALA.

Nuts

Nuts are an important source of fats in the MD. Nuts contain a favorable fatty acid composition: they are low in SFA (4–16 %), and in most nuts about half of the total fat content is MUFA (oleic acid). Nuts contain variable amounts of PUFA, and walnuts are noteworthy for their high ALA content (Table 6.8) [71]. Nuts also contain a wide variety of fat-soluble antioxidants, tocopherols, and phytosterols. Almonds are especially rich in α-tocopherol, whereas walnuts contain significant amounts of γ-tocopherol.

Fatty Acids of Nuts and Disease Risk

It was demonstrated two decades ago that the subtle balance of fatty acids in almonds and walnuts could decrease cholesterol levels when replacing SFA [72]. The high proportion of ALA in walnuts may have another benefit since this fatty acid is known to be a precursor of LC *n*-3 PUFA. However, the efficiency of conversion is rather low, around 10 % for EPA, and almost zero for DHA. However, EPA is important for prevention of CHD, and hence ALA may be of benefit [73]. Although fatty acids play a central role in mediating the health properties of nuts, fiber, antioxidant phenolic compounds in the pellicle (skin) and minerals also have important roles. This has been demonstrated in data from the nut cohort of the PREDIMED study [2].

Vegetables

Because vegetable consumption is high in the traditional MD, vegetables constitute an important source of certain fatty acids, and in particular ALA—"the plant *n*-3 fatty acid." Some commonly consumed green leafy vegetables such as spinach and kale are excellent sources of ALA (121 mg/100 g and 180 mg/100 g respectively) [74]. Purslane, the emblematic green of the Cretan diet, is the richest source of ALA of any green leafy vegetable, the leaves containing 300–400 mg ALA/100 g [75]. Wild greens, still commonly collected in many rural Mediterranean regions, constitute another important source of ALA [76]. Among the commonly consumed pulses in the MD (chickpeas, lentils, and white beans), chickpeas are exceptionally rich in fat, particularly linoleic acid, although they contain relatively low quantities of ALA. However, some pulses, such as small white beans and white lupines, were found in a study from Greece to be exceptional sources of ALA (529 mg/100 g and 484 mg/100 g respectively) [77].

The previous discussions of ALA apply also to vegetables, and even though their contribution is modest they may play a role in CVD prevention when fish is absent from the diet.

Conclusions

Olive oil has for a long time been the almost exclusive added fat in the Mediterranean diet and was to a large extent probably responsible for the good health indicators of the countries around the Mediterranean Sea. Because olive oil has to be cultivated and produced with great care, it is rather expensive. However the price is justifiable, and price should not be a barrier to its wider use, and supportive economic policies could help in widening its consumption.

Food sources of PUFAs will complete the lipid intake, and among these LC n-3 PUFA are required for optimal infant and child development and for the prevention of chronic diseases. Even though nuts and some greens can provide PUFA, and especially ALA, the precursor of EPA, this is not in sufficient quantity, therefore DHA will not be synthesized. Fish are the almost exclusive source, and their exploitation has to be regulated in order to protect resources. Fish farming may be a solution if sustainable conditions are used. Thus, economic and environmental considerations play a part in the context of food, and this requires the involvement of nutritionists in order to guide recommendations for better health.

References

1. Keys A, Menotti A, Karvonen MJ, Aravanis C, Blackburn H, et al. The diet and 15-year death rate in the seven countries study. Am J Epidemiol. 1986;124(6):903–15.
2. Estruch R, Ros E, Salas-Salvado J, Covas MI, Corella D, et al. Primary prevention of cardiovascular disease with a Mediterranean diet. N Engl J Med. 2013;368(14):1279–90.
3. Barbagallo CM, Cavera G, Sapienza M, Noto D, Cefalu AB, et al. Nutritional characteristics of a rural Southern Italy population: the Ventimiglia di Sicilia Project. J Am Coll Nutr. 2002;21(6):523–9.
4. Ford ES, Capewell S. Trends in total and low-density lipoprotein cholesterol among U.S. adults: contributions of changes in dietary fat intake and use of cholesterol-lowering medications. PLoS One. 2013;8(5), e65228.
5. Linseisen J, Welch AA, Ocke M, Amiano P, Agnoli C, et al. Dietary fat intake in the European Prospective Investigation into Cancer and Nutrition: results from the 24-h dietary recalls. Eur J Clin Nutr. 2009;63 Suppl 4:S61–80.
6. Sarri KO, Linardakis MK, Bervanaki FN, Tzanakis NE, Kafatos AG. Greek Orthodox fasting rituals: a hidden characteristic of the Mediterranean diet of Crete. Br J Nutr. 2004;92(2):277–84.
7. Valdes J, Grau M, Subirana I, Marrugat J, Covas MI, et al. Secular trends in energy intake and diet quality in a Mediterranean population. Ann Nutr Metab. 2009;54(3):177–83.
8. Engeset D, Alsaker E, Lund E, Welch A, Khaw KT, et al. Fish consumption and breast cancer risk. The European Prospective Investigation into Cancer and Nutrition (EPIC). Int J Cancer. 2006;119(1):175–82.
9. Jacobs HL, Kahn HD, Stralka KA, Phan DB. Estimates of per capita fish consumption in the U.S. based on the continuing survey of food intake by individuals (CSFII). Risk Anal. 1998;18(3):283–91.
10. Blasbalg TL, Hibbeln JR, Ramsden CE, Majchrzak SF, Rawlings RR. Changes in consumption of omega-3 and omega-6 fatty acids in the United States during the 20th century. Am J Clin Nutr. 2011;93(5):950–62.
11. Motard-Belanger A, Charest A, Grenier G, Paquin P, Chouinard Y, et al. Study of the effect of trans fatty acids from ruminants on blood lipids and other risk factors for cardiovascular disease. Am J Clin Nutr. 2008;87(3):593–9.
12. Hoffman R, Gerber M. Evaluating and adapting the Mediterranean diet for non-Mediterranean populations: A critical appraisal. Nutr Rev. 2013;71(9):573–84.
13. EFSA Scientific Opinion on the substantiation of health claims related to polyphenols in olive and protection of LDL particles from oxidative damage, maintenance of normal blood HDL cholesterol concentrations, maintenance of normal blood pressure, "anti-inflammatory properties" "contributes to the upper respiratory tract health" "can help to maintain a normal function of gastrointestinal tract" and "contributes to body defences against external agents." EFSA J 2011;9:2033–57
14. WHO Diet, nutrition and the prevention of chronic diseases. World Health Organization Technical Report Series no. 0512-3054 (Print 2013) 2003.
15. World Cancer Research Fund/American Institute for Cancer Research Food, Nutrition, Physical Activity, and the Prevention of Cancer: a Global Perspective. 2007.
16. Hoffman R, Gerber M. The Mediterranean diet: health & science. Oxford: Wiley-Blackwell; 2012.
17. Jakobsen MU, O'Reilly EJ, Heitmann BL, Pereira MA, Balter K, et al. Major types of dietary fat and risk of coronary heart disease: a pooled analysis of 11 cohort studies. Am J Clin Nutr. 2009;89(5):1425–32.
18. Buckland G, Mayen AL, Agudo A, Travier N, Navarro C, et al. Olive oil intake and mortality within the Spanish population (EPIC-Spain). Am J Clin Nutr. 2012;96(1):142–9.
19. Buckland G, Travier N, Barricarte A, Ardanaz E, Moreno-Iribas C, et al. Olive oil intake and CHD in the European Prospective Investigation into Cancer and Nutrition Spanish cohort. Br J Nutr. 2012;108(11):2075–82.

20. Bendinelli B, Masala G, Saieva C, Salvini S, Calonico C, et al. Fruit, vegetables, and olive oil and risk of coronary heart disease in Italian women: the EPICOR Study. Am J Clin Nutr. 2011;93(2):275–83.
21. Samieri C, Feart C, Proust-Lima C, Peuchant E, Tzourio C, et al. Olive oil consumption, plasma oleic acid, and stroke incidence: the Three-City Study. Neurology. 2011;77(5):418–25.
22. Martinez-Gonzalez MA, Dominguez LJ, Delgado-Rodriguez M. Olive oil consumption and risk of CHD and/or stroke: a meta-analysis of case-control, cohort and intervention studies. Br J Nutr. 2014;112(2):248–59.
23. Guasch-Ferre M, Hu FB, Martinez-Gonzalez MA, Fito M, Bullo M, et al. Olive oil intake and risk of cardiovascular disease and mortality in the PREDIMED Study. BMC Med. 2014;12:78.
24. Martinez-Gonzalez MA, Toledo E, Aros F, Fiol M, Corella D, et al. Extravirgin olive oil consumption reduces risk of atrial fibrillation: the PREDIMED (Prevencion con Dieta Mediterranea) trial. Circulation. 2014;130(1):18–26.
25. Covas MI, Nyyssonen K, Poulsen HE, Kaikkonen J, Zunft HJ, et al. The effect of polyphenols in olive oil on heart disease risk factors: a randomized trial. Ann Intern Med. 2006;145(5):333–41.
26. Casaburi I, Puoci F, Chimento A, Sirianni R, Ruggiero C, et al. Potential of olive oil phenols as chemopreventive and therapeutic agents against cancer: a review of in vitro studies. Mol Nutr Food Res. 2013;57(1):71–83.
27. Pelucchi C, Bosetti C, Negri E, Lipworth L, La Vecchia C. Olive oil and cancer risk: an update of epidemiological findings through 2010. Curr Pharm Des. 2011;17(8):805–12.
28. Bessaoud F, Daures JP, Gerber M. Dietary factors and breast cancer risk: a case control study among a population in Southern France. Nutr Cancer. 2008;60(2):177–87.
29. Cottet V, Touvier M, Fournier A, Touillaud MS, Lafay L, et al. Postmenopausal breast cancer risk and dietary patterns in the E3N-EPIC prospective cohort study. Am J Epidemiol. 2009;170(10):1257–67.
30. Mourouti N, Papavagelis C, Plytzanopoulou P, Kontogianni M, Vassilakou T, et al. Dietary patterns and breast cancer: a case-control study in women. Eur J Nutr. 2015;54(4):609–17.
31. Siari S, Scali J, Richard A, Tretarre B, Daures JP, et al. Subregional variations of dietary consumption and incidences of cancer in Southern France. Nutrition and lifestyle: opportunities for cancer prevention. Oxford: International Agency for Research on Cancer; 2002. Oxford University Press [distributor], Lyon.
32. Buckland G, Travier N, Agudo A, Fonseca-Nunes A, Navarro C, et al. Olive oil intake and breast cancer risk in the Mediterranean countries of the European Prospective Investigation into Cancer and Nutrition study. Int J Cancer. 2012;131(10):2465–9.
33. Elamin MH, Daghestani MH, Omer SA, Elobeid MA, Virk P, et al. Olive oil oleuropein has anti-breast cancer properties with higher efficiency on ER-negative cells. Food Chem Toxicol. 2013;53:310–6.
34. Garcia-Arenzana N, Navarrete-Munoz EM, Lope V, Moreo P, Vidal C, et al. Calorie intake, olive oil consumption and mammographic density among Spanish women. Int J Cancer. 2014;134(8):1916–25.
35. Berr C, Portet F, Carriere I, Akbaraly TN, Feart C, et al. Olive oil and cognition: results from the three-city study. Dement Geriatr Cogn Disord. 2009;28(4):357–64.
36. Martinez-Lapiscina EH, Clavero P, Toledo E, San JB, Sanchez-Tainta A, et al. Virgin olive oil supplementation and long-term cognition: the PREDIMED-NAVARRA randomized, trial. J Nutr, Health Aging. 2013;17(6):544–52.
37. Valls-Pedret C, Lamuela-Raventos RM, Medina-Remon A, Quintana M, Corella D, et al. Polyphenol-rich foods in the Mediterranean diet are associated with better cognitive function in elderly subjects at high cardiovascular risk. J Alzheimers Dis. 2012;29(4):773–82.
38. Latreille J, Kesse-Guyot E, Malvy D, Andreeva V, Galan P, et al. Dietary monounsaturated fatty acids intake and risk of skin photoaging. PLoS One. 2012;7(9), e44490.
39. Marfil NR, Cabrera VC, Gimenez MR, et al. Importancia nutriciona, economica y cultural des aceite de argan. Fundacion Euroarabe des Altas Estudias. Granada, Spain: Cordoba. Alianza Grupo genero; 2009.
40. Monfalouti HE, Guillaume D, Denhez C, Charrouf Z. Therapeutic potential of argan oil: a review. J Pharm Pharmacol. 2010;62(12):1669–75.
41. Drissi A, Girona J, Cherki M, Godas G, Derouiche A, et al. Evidence of hypolipemiant and antioxidant properties of argan oil derived from the argan tree (Argania spinosa). Clin Nutr. 2004;23(5):1159–66.
42. Haimeur A, Messaouri H, Ulmann L, Mimouni V, Masrar A, et al. Argan oil prevents prothrombotic complications by lowering lipid levels and platelet aggregation, enhancing oxidative status in dyslipidemic patients from the area of Rabat (Morocco). Lipids Health Dis. 2013;12:107.
43. Berrougui H, Cloutier M, Isabelle M, Khalil A. Phenolic-extract from argan oil (Argania spinosa L.) inhibits human low-density lipoprotein (LDL) oxidation and enhances cholesterol efflux from human THP-1 macrophages. Atherosclerosis. 2006;184(2):389–96.
44. Drissi A, Bennani H, Giton F, Charrouf Z, Fiet J, et al. Tocopherols and saponins derived from Argania spinosa exert, an antiproliferative effect on human prostate cancer. Cancer Investig. 2006;24(6):588–92.
45. Derouiche A, Cherki M, Drissi A, Bamou Y, El Messal M, et al. Nutritional intervention study with argan oil in man: effects on lipids and apolipoproteins. Ann Nutr Metab. 2005;49(3):196–201.

46. Cosgrove MC, Franco OH, Granger SP, Murray PG, Mayes AE. Dietary nutrient intakes and skin-aging appearance among middle-aged American women. Am J Clin Nutr. 2007;86(4):1225–31.
47. Bouwstra JA, Gooris GS, Dubbelaar FE, Weerheim AM, Ijzerman AP, et al. Role of ceramide 1 in the molecular organization of the stratum corneum lipids. J Lipid Res. 1998;39(1):186–96.
48. Feinberg M, Favier JC, Ireland-Ripert J. épertoire général des aliments/Table de composition des corps gras TEC DOC Lavoisier/Ciqual-Regal, 1987.
49. Jung DM, Lee MJ, Yoon SH, Jung MY. A gas chromatography-tandem quadrupole mass spectrometric analysis of policosanols in commercial vegetable oils. J Food Sci. 2011;76(6):C891–9.
50. Tunstall-Pedoe H. MONICA Monograph and Multimedia Sourcebook. Geneva: World Health Organization; 2003.
51. Marangoni F, Martiello A, Galli C. Dietary fat intake of European countries in the Mediterranean area: An update. World Rev Nutr Diet. 2007;97:67–84.
52. Park YW, Juarez M, Ramos M, Haenlein GFW. Physico-chemical characteristics of goat and sheep milk. Small Rumin Res. 2007;68(1-2):88–113.
53. German JB, Dillard CJ. Composition, structure and absorption of milk lipids: a source of energy, fat-soluble nutrients and bioactive molecules. Crit Rev Food Sci Nutr. 2006;46(1):57–92.
54. Collins YF, McSweeney PLH, Wilkinson MG. Lipolysis and free fatty acid catabolism in cheese: a review of current knowledge. Int Dairy J. 2003;13(11):841–66.
55. McCance RA, Widdowson EM, Paul AA, Southgate DAT. McCance and Widdowson's The composition of foods. 4th revised and extended ed./by A.A. Paul and D.A.T. Southgate/[for the] Ministry of Agriculture, Fisheries and Food [and the] Medical Research Council. edn. H.M.S.O. ; Amsterdam ; Oxford : Elsevier/North-Holland Biomedical Press, London; 1978.
56. Hu FB, Stampfer MJ, Manson JE, Ascherio A, Colditz GA, et al. Dietary saturated fats and their food sources in relation to the risk of coronary heart disease in women. Am J Clin Nutr. 1999;70(6):1001–8.
57. Tholstrup T, Ehnholm C, Jauhiainen M, Petersen M, Hoy CE, et al. Effects of medium-chain fatty acids and oleic acid on blood lipids, lipoproteins, glucose, insulin, and lipid transfer protein activities. Am J Clin Nutr. 2004;79(4):564–9.
58. Skeaff CM, Williscroft K, Mann J, Chisholm A. Replacing cows' with sheep's dairy fat lowers plasma cholesterol concentration in participants consuming dairy fat-rich diets. Eur J Clin Nutr. 2004;58(2):250–7.
59. Legrand P, Rioux V. The complex and important cellular and metabolic functions of saturated fatty acids. Lipids. 2010;45(10):941–6.
60. Tziboula-Clarke A. Goat milk. Encyclopedia of dairy sciences. Amsterdam: Academic Press; 2003.
61. Rogalska E, Ransac S, Verger R. Stereoselectivity of lipases. II Stereoselective hydrolysis of triglycerides by gastric and pancreatic lipases. J Biol Chem. 1990;265(33):20271–6.
62. Sirot V, Oseredczuk M, Bemrah-Aouachria N, Volatier J-L, Leblanc J-C. Lipid and fatty acid composition of fish and seafood consumed in France: CALIPSO study. J Food Comp Anal. 2008;21:8–16.
63. Sargent JR. Fish oils and human diet. Br J Nutr. 1997;78 Suppl 1:S5–13.
64. Tornaritis M, Peraki E, Georgulli M, et al. Fatty acid composition and total fat content of eight species of Mediterranean fish. Int J Food Sci Nutr. 1993;45:135–9.
65. Bandarra N, Batista I, Nunes M, Empis J, Christie W. Seasonal Changes in Lipid Composition of Sardine (Sardina pilchardus). J Food Sci. 1997;62(1):40–2.
66. Anses Rapport: Consommation des poissons, mollusques et crustacés 2010.
67. Geurden I, Borchert P, Balasubramanian MN, Schrama JW, Dupont-Nivet M, et al. The positive impact of the early-feeding of a plant-based diet on its future acceptance and utilisation in rainbow trout. PLoS One. 2013;8(12), e83162.
68. FAO. Fats and fatty acids in human nutrition. Report of an expert consultation; 2010.
69. Wallin A, Di Giuseppe D, Orsini N, Patel PS, Forouhi NG, et al. Fish consumption, dietary long-chain n-3 fatty acids, and risk of type 2 diabetes: systematic review and meta-analysis of prospective studies. Diabetes Care. 2012;35(4):918–29.
70. Mozaffarian D, Shi P, Morris JS, Grandjean P, Siscovick DS, et al. Methylmercury exposure and incident diabetes in U.S. men and women in two prospective cohorts. Diabetes Care. 2013;36(11):3578–84.
71. Ros E, Mataix J. Fatty acid composition of nuts--implications for cardiovascular health. Br J Nutr. 2006;96 Suppl 2:S29–35.
72. Abbey M, Noakes M, Belling GB, Nestel PJ. Partial replacement of saturated fatty acids with almonds or walnuts lowers total plasma cholesterol and low-density-lipoprotein cholesterol. Am J Clin Nutr. 1994;59(5):995–9.
73. Mozaffarian D, Ascherio A, Hu FB, Stampfer MJ, Willett WC, et al. Interplay between different polyunsaturated fatty acids and risk of coronary heart disease in men. Circulation. 2005;111(2):157–64.

74. USDA. USDA National Nutrient Database for Standard Reference Release 26. doi:http://www.ars.usda.gov/nutrientdata; 2013.
75. Simopoulos AP, Tan DX, Manchester LC, Reiter RJ. Purslane: a plant source of omega-3 fatty acids and melatonin. J Pineal Res. 2005;39(3):331–2.
76. Vardavas CI, Majchrzak D, Wagner KH, Elmadfa I, Kafatos A. Lipid concentrations of wild edible greens in Crete. Food Chem. 2006;99(4):822–34.
77. Kalogeropoulos N, Chiou A, Ioannou M, Karathanos VT, Hassapidou M, et al. Nutritional evaluation and bioactive microconstituents (phytosterols, tocopherols, polyphenols, triterpenic acids) in cooked dry legumes usually consumed in the Mediterranean countries. Food Chem 2010;121(3):682–90.

Chapter 7
Inflammation and Cardiovascular Disease and Protection by the Mediterranean Diet

Francesco Sofi, Alessia Fabbri, and Alessandro Casini

Key Points

- Cardiovascular disease is the first cause of death and disability all over the world.
- Inflammation plays an essential role in the initiation and progression of the atherosclerotic process, the main cause of cardiovascular disease.
- A consensus about the role of diet in preventing cardiovascular disease has gradually emerged. The appropriate dietary profile to reduce cardiovascular risk burden in the general population diseases remains a challenging and a highly relevant issue.
- Mediterranean diet has been extensively reported to be the optimal dietary profile for reducing cardiovascular risk profile in the general population.

Keywords Diet • Mediterranean diet • Nutrition • Cardiovascular disease • Inflammation • Cytokines • Atherosclerosis • Prevention

Introduction

The relationship between nutrition pattern and health has been studied intensively for over than half a century. Since first results coming from one of the landmark studies in this field, the Seven Countries' Study, the effect of nutrition on human health has been amply reported by many case–control, prospective cohort and randomised clinical trials, providing evidence that diet may significantly affect the health state of the population [1, 2]. A correct dietary intake, associated with a correct lifestyle, may

F. Sofi, M.D., Ph.D. (✉)
Department of Experimental and Clinical Medicine, University of Florence, Italy 2 Don Carlo Gnocchi Foundation, Onlus IRCCS, Florence, Italy, 50134 Florence, Italy

Unit of Clinical Nutrition, University Hospital of Careggi, Florence, Italy
e-mail: francesco.sofi@unifi.it

A. Fabbri, M.D. • A. Casini, M.D.
Department of Experimental and Clinical Medicine, University of Florence, Italy 2 Don Carlo Gnocchi Foundation, Onlus IRCCS, Florence, Italy, 50134 Florence, Italy
e-mail: alessia.fabbri83@gmail.com

D.F. Romagnolo, O.I. Selmin (eds.), *Mediterranean Diet*, Nutrition and Health,
DOI 10.1007/978-3-319-27969-5_7

in fact contribute to the maintenance of a healthy status. Conversely, wrong dietary habits may favour the incidence of different chronic diseases such as cardiovascular, neoplastic, and neurodegenerative diseases as well as different disease states such as obesity, diabetes, alteration of blood lipid profile, and hypertension, the combination of which may lead to the metabolic syndrome.

Over the last few years, major scientific associations strongly addressed their preventive strategies to the reduction of the global risk burden and, in this scenario, a great importance was attributed to issues related to nutrition. To date, the famous aphorism "we are what we eat" seems to be more pertinent than ever, since scientific evidence has demonstrated that dietary quality and quantity are important determinants of health status. However, despite a wide consensus on the goals of nutritional habits required to prevent cardiovascular disease, many concerns are expressed on the ideal diet for its prevention.

Inflammation and Cardiovascular Disease

Cardiovascular disease is the major cause of disability and premature death throughout the world, and contributes substantially to the escalating costs of health care. The underlying pathology is atherosclerosis, which develops over many years and is usually advanced by the time symptoms occur, generally in middle age. Actually, atherosclerosis has long been considered the result of lipid accumulation in the artery wall, but there is currently compelling evidence that inflammation plays a key role at all stages of the disease [3]. Early phases of atherosclerosis involve the recruitment of inflammatory cells from the circulation, their adhesion to the endothelium and finally migration to sub-endothelial space, a complex process mediated by inflammatory stimuli, which involves cytokine production and upregulation of adhesion molecules on endothelial cells and leucocytes. Moreover, inflammation is also crucial in the development of instability and rupture of atheromatous plaques and the subsequent appearance of ischemic events in advanced stages of the disease. Traditional risk factors of cardiovascular disease such as age, sex, hypertension, dyslipidemia, diabetes, and smoking have been the pillars of cardiovascular risk assessment for the past several decades. However, many cardiovascular events occur in patients without traditional risk factors and emerging biomarkers have been investigated to improve identification of at-risk asymptomatic patients [4].

Indeed, with the recognition that atherosclerosis is an inflammatory process several plasma markers of inflammation have also been evaluated as potential tools for prediction of the risk of coronary events. One of the most relevant inflammatory parameters is certainly the C-reactive protein (CRP) [5]. It is a non-specific marker of inflammation produced mainly in hepatocytes in response to several cytokines. CRP participates in the plaque deposition exerting proatherogenic effects in many cells involved in atherosclerosis, but also induces monocyte adhesion and transmigration into the vessel wall, macrophage polarisation and infiltration of both adipose tissue and atherosclerotic lesions. In addition, CRP binds highly atherogenic oxidized Low-Density Lipoprotein Cholesterol and it is able to inhibit endothelial nitric oxide synthase by inducing impaired vasoreactivity. Large observational studies have reported that CRP is a strong and independent predictor of adverse cardiovascular events, including myocardial infarction, ischemic stroke, and sudden cardiac death.

Together with CRP, other inflammatory markers and mediators have been reported to play a role in the pathogenic pathway of atherosclerosis such as interleukin IL-6, which is generally accepted as an acute phase inflammatory reactive protein produced upon stimulation by tumour necrosis factor-alpha and a known trigger of CRP synthesis [4]. In fact, chronic elevation of IL-6 levels has been shown to be associated with increased cardiovascular risk.

In addition, increasing interest has been demonstrated also for the CD40 ligand, which plays an important role in the progression of atherosclerotic lesion [6]. In fact, a large number of cells involved in the atherosclerotic process such as endothelial cells, T cells, macrophages, smooth muscle cells, and platelet express on their surface this proinflammatory cytokine and its receptor. The CD40–CD40 ligand system is a pathway associated with both prothrombotic and proinflammatory effects and ligation of CD40 to all these types of cells triggers the expression of various proinflammatory mediators.

Mediterranean Diet

Over the last few years a large body of evidence on the relationship between nutrition and chronic degenerative diseases has led researchers to search for the feeding pattern most suitable to the maintenance of an optimal health status. Different types of diet were imposed to public attention, but the one that got the greatest interest is certainly the Mediterranean diet (MD) [7].

The concept of the MD dates back to the 1960s', when Ancel Keys coined the term following the results of an epidemiological study, which demonstrated that populations (Italian and Greek) that overlooked the Mediterranean Sea had a reduced incidence of cardiovascular disease and cancer in comparison to other populations [1]. In this study, known as the "Seven Countries' Study", dietary behaviour, lifestyles and health status of 12,763 subjects aged between 40 and 59 years residing in different countries of the world were analysed: the USA, Finland, the Netherlands, Italy, Greece, the former Yugoslavia, and Japan. The first results were surprising because lower rates of mortality and incidence of cardiovascular disease in the countries bordering the Mediterranean basin were showed in comparison to the other countries covered by the study [1].

Following studies have confirmed these results, and the MD with its specific foods has spread throughout the world as synonymous of healthy diet, effective against cardiovascular disease [7]. Nowadays, all the most important and influential scientific societies of the world suggest a Mediterranean-like diet as the ideal dietary profile to preserve the health status, and to reduce the occurrence of the most important chronic diseases. However, despite a worldwide promotion of this nutritional model, a progressive shift to Westernised food habits has been developed in Southern European regions, and a loss of the original cultures concerning nutrition has been observed [8].

The Mediterranean-style diet is not a specific diet, but rather a collection of eating habits traditionally followed by people in the different countries bordering the Mediterranean Sea. According to the original definition of Keys as "the dietary pattern of people living in Southern Italy in the 1960s", the MD is characterised by high consumption of olive oil, as the prevalent added fat, vegetables, legumes, whole grain products, fruits, and nuts. The intake of saturated animal fats is relatively low, and moderate fish consumption (depending on the proximity to the sea) provides an adequate level of polyunsaturated fats. Finally, red wine, generally consumed during meals, is the main alcohol intake and is more prevalent respect to other alcoholic beverages. Nevertheless, it is beyond doubt that there is not a single MD; dietary habits of countries bordering the Mediterranean Sea vary considerably, and even inside the same country relevant differences in dietary pattern exist.

Therefore, the MD should be considered not just a dietary pattern, though an integrated way of living where foods represent only one of the relevant components along with culture, beliefs, tradition, and pleasure. This complexity explains why a general definition of such dietary pattern is difficult to obtain, and the methods of measurements are not easy to evaluate.

For decades, studies have targeted the evaluation of single dietary components of the MD in relation to different health outcomes. A vast amount of literature supports the evidence that an increased consumption of some food groups such as fruits and vegetables, fish, or whole-grain cereals is somewhat beneficial for health. Such studies, however, adopted the translational concept that, if a dietary pattern contains plenty of a specific food group, and this food group has been shown in turn to be associated with a reduced incidence of diseases, the resulting diet will be beneficial. It seems clear, on the other hand, that such a reductionist approach presents several conceptual and methodological limitations because food components present synergistic and antagonist interactions, and most importantly, because people eat a complex of nutrients and not just isolated food components.

Thus, research efforts in this field switched progressively to the evaluation of a score for the adherence to the Mediterranean dietary pattern, rather than to the identification of single nutrients associated with the disease. As a result, an increasing number of studies have been carried out by summing foods considered to be important for health to provide an overall measure of dietary quality, i.e. a quality diet score. A large number of indirect indices have been proposed, with the use of two different approaches [9]. One approach has been based on the composition of predefined quality indices using current nutrition recommendations from the major scientific associations. This method is defined as "theoretically defined dietary adherence method". The other approach is based on "empirical adherence to dietary patterns" and statistical analyses such as cluster analyses.

Mediterranean Diet and Cardiovascular Disease

The first evidence about the possible benefit of the MD in relation to cardiovascular disease was derived from the Seven Countries' study [1]. The reduced incidence of cardiovascular disease reported by the countries of the Mediterranean basin during this study opened a new field of investigation, both epidemiological and clinical, aimed at confirming the preliminary results.

With regard to primary prevention, the most relevant data are those derived from the EPIC-Elderly Prospective Cohort Study, a prospective multicentre study that analysed subjects from ten different European countries. Among others, Trichopoulou et al. published an important paper which analysed data from over 22,000 people in the Greek cohort [10]. In order to find a useful tool to define the degree of adherence to the MD, the authors established a score of adherence that takes into account the main dietary variables, divided into food groups. This adherence score, based on food groups typically present in the Mediterranean diet (bread, pasta, fruit, vegetables, fish, legumes, moderate red wine consumption, and olive oil), gives a positive score to people who consume more than the median of the overall population for these groups of foods, and a negative score to those who consume a higher amount of foods which are not typical of the MD. Hence, a score of 0 represents the lowest adherence to the MD, while a score of nine represents the highest adherence to the MD. Through such score it was reported that the risk of mortality was inversely related to the degree of adherence to the MD in a population of patients followed for more than 4 years. Indeed, an increase of two points in this score was significantly associated with a 33 % reduction in mortality from cardiovascular causes (RR 0.67, 95 % CI 0.47–0.94) after adjustment for all the confounding factors [10].

Recently, a large intervention study conducted in Spain confirmed the beneficial effects of MD versus the occurrence of cardiovascular diseases in primary prevention [11]. In a sample of 7747 adults at high risk of cardiovascular disease but without a manifested disease (age range: 55–80 years) who were followed for an average of 4.8 years, three different dietary interventions were tested. The participants were randomly assigned to a MD supplemented with extra-virgin olive oil, a MD supplemented with nuts, or a control diet with a low contribution from fats. At the end of the follow-up subjects who had followed the MD with either supplementation of extra-virgin olive oil or mixed nuts demonstrated a reduced risk of occurrence for cardiovascular disease. The hazard ratios were 0.70 (95 % CI, 0.54–0.92) and 0.72 (95 % CI, 0.54–0.96) respectively, versus the control group.

These data were recently confirmed by two cohort studies carried out again in Spain [12, 13]. In the first one, on a sample of 13,609 adults (mean age: 38 years) who were followed for an average of 4.9 years, the adherence to the MD was associated with a reduced incidence of cardiovascular disease. The participants were evaluated by using a frequency questionnaire and those who had followed the MD with higher adherence had a 59 % reduction in the risk of cardiovascular disease compared to those who reported a lower adherence (RR: 0.41, 95 % CI 0.18–0.95). In particular, an increase of two points in the Mediterranean dietary score was associated with a 26 % reduction in the onset of coronary artery disease (RR: 0.74, 95 % CI 0.55–0.99) [12]. In the second study, carried out on the cohort of 41,078 subjects aged between 29 and 69 years, and followed for a mean follow-up of 10.4 years, it was shown a 40 % reduction in cardiovascular events in subjects who followed more closely the Mediterranean dietary pattern (RR: 0.60, 95 % CI 0.47–0.77), compared to those who reported a lower adherence [13].

A similar conclusion was also reached by the longitudinal study HALE, including the SENECA and FINE studies, both multicentre studies from different European countries, Mediterranean and non-Mediterranean, of 2239 elderly (>70 years of age) followed for a mean follow-up of 10 years. Adherence to a healthy lifestyle, considered as the combination of four major risk factors, such as adherence to the MD, moderate alcohol consumption, smoking cessation, and a regular physical activity, determined a lower risk of mortality from coronary heart disease by 39 % (RR: 0.61, 95 % CI 0.43–0.88) and from cardiovascular disease by 29 % (RR 0.71, 95 % CI 0.58–0.88) [14].

The protective effect of the MD in relation to cardiovascular disease was also demonstrated in non-Mediterranean populations, such as in the USA. Indeed, in two large cohort studies, adherence to MD was found to significantly modify the cardiovascular risk profile [15, 16]. The first study by Mitrou et al. 2007 [15] analysed 214,284 people, between 50 and 71 years of age for a follow-up period of about 10 years. The population of patients who had a greater adherence to the MD had a 22 % reduction in cardiovascular mortality in men (RR: 0.78, 95 % CI 0.69–0.87) and 29 % in women (RR: 0.81, 95 % CI 0.68–0.97). The second study, comprising a population of 74,486 women that attended the Nurses' Health Study and evaluated for 20 years of follow-up, confirmed the protective effect of adherence to the MD. Women who reported a higher adherence to the MD had a significant protection of 29 % (RR 0.71, 95 % CI 0.62–0.82) against coronary heart disease, with a reduction in overall mortality from cardiovascular disease by approximately 40 % (RR: 0.61, 95 % CI 0.49–0.76) [16].

The evidence for a protective effect is not limited to ischemic heart disease but also extends to cerebrovascular disease. Recent studies have shown that adherence to the MD is also able to reduce the risk of ischemic stroke. In the aforementioned study of Fung et al. [16] a greater adherence to the MD reduced by 13 % (RR: 0.87, 95 % CI 0.73–1.02), the risk of experiencing an ischemic stroke in the population of women attending the Nurses' Health Study. Similarly, a case–control study conducted in a population of 250 patients with ischemic stroke compared with 500 control subjects confirmed the potential protective effect of a greater adherence to the MD in relation to this disease (−12 %) (RR: 0.88, 95 % CI 0.82–0.94) [17].

Similar results were also reported in groups of patients already suffering from cardiovascular disease, therefore in secondary prevention. One of the most important studies is the Lyon Diet Heart Study [18], a clinical trial in which 605 patients with previous myocardial infarction were divided and assigned to an intervention group who followed a MD and to a control group that followed a so-called Prudent Diet. After a median follow-up period of 27 months, the rate of coronary events and mortality in the intervention group was reduced by 73 % and 70 % respectively, thus concluding that implementation of a MD enriched with one gram of α-linolenic acid (an essential n3-fatty acid), was able to reduce quickly, markedly and for prolonged time the risk of death, non-fatal myocardial re-infarction, and other clinical end-points.

Another important study in secondary prevention was conducted on 11,323 patients with prior myocardial infarction from 172 Italian hospitals. This study, called the GISSI-Prevention, showed that the MD was able to reduce by half the risk of mortality and cardiovascular recurrences in this type of selected high-risk patients, regardless of medication and lifestyle (RR: 0.51, 95 % CI 0.44–0.59) [19]. In addition, two studies that included subjects from the same cohort of the EPIC study with a previous diagnosis of myocardial infarction, confirmed the association between adherence to the MD and survival [20, 21]. In the first study, the Greek cohort of patients with prior coronary artery disease ($n=1302$) were followed for a mean follow-up of approximately 4 years, reporting a reduction in cardiovascular mortality by 27 % (RR: 0.73, 95 % CI 0.58–0.93) [20]. In the latest study, the population included all persons from the countries of the EPIC study with a previous diagnosis of myocardial infarction ($n=2671$) followed by a median follow-up of 7 years. In this analysis, an increase of two units in the score of adherence to the MD was associated with an 18 %-reduction in mortality (RR: 0.82, 95 % CI 0.73–0.93) [21].

Recently, in order to perform a review of the literature, our group conducted three systematic reviews and meta-analyses of prospective epidemiological studies that evaluated the adherence to the MD through a numerical score and health status [22–24]. The clinical events considered in these reports were all-cause mortality, mortality and incidence of cardiovascular disease and cancer, and the incidence of neurodegenerative diseases such as Alzheimer's disease and Parkinson's disease. In a pooled analysis of the selected studies we showed that an increase of two points in the score of adherence to the MD resulted in a 9 % reduction in the incidence and/or mortality from cardiovascular disease (RR: 0.91, 95 % CI 0.87–0.95, $p<0.0001$) [22].

An update of the latter meta-analysis, conducted 2 years later, confirmed the results of the first systematic review with a significant reduction in the incidence and mortality of cardiovascular and cerebrovascular disease (RR: 0.90, 95 % CI 0.87–0.93) even including a larger population (+7 cohort studies for cardiovascular disease, +534,064 individuals analysed) [23]. Most recently, an additional update of the systematic review and meta-analysis reinforced the significant protective role (−10 %) of greater adherence to MD versus the occurrence of cardiovascular disease (RR: 0.90; 95 % CI 0.87–0.92), in an overall analysis comprising 20 cohort prospective studies (Fig. 7.1) [24].

Adherence to MD and Inflammatory Parameters

Until now, the beneficial effect of the MD against cardiovascular disease has been attributed to its influence over classical atherosclerosis risk factors, but, recently, some authors have suggested that an anti-inflammatory effect in the vascular wall may be another important mechanism to explain the link between the MD and low cardiovascular mortality. Moreover, the important role of inflammation in the pathogenesis of atherosclerosis has led to the belief that dietary preventive measures act in part by modifying related inflammatory pathways.

In 2004, Chrysohoou et al. demonstrated, in a wide population, that subjects who were in the highest tertile of the diet score had significantly lower levels of CRP, IL-6, white blood cell count and fibrinogen [25]. Subsequently, these findings have been confirmed by Fung et al., who reported a significant inverse relationship between a higher score of diet and CRP, IL-6, and E-selectin as well as some markers of endothelial dysfunction [26]. Recently, results coming from a multicentre longitudinal study in 1003 myocardial infarction survivors from several European regions supported these findings, by showing a protective effect of adherence to MD versus a pro-inflammatory status [27]. For each unit of increasing adherence to the MD score, in fact, there was a reduction of 3.1 % in the mean levels of CRP, and of 1.9 % in the mean levels of IL-6.

Likewise, a 2-year randomised trial with a Mediterranean-style diet reported that it was effective in reducing CRP and IL-6 in individuals with metabolic syndrome [28], whereas in another 3-month randomised trial, the traditional MD was more effective in reducing oxidised LDL-C levels than a low-fat diet [29]. These findings have been more recently confirmed by a 2-year randomised trial conducted by Shai et al. in a population of 322 moderately obese subjects [30]. In this study group the intervention with a MD resulted in significant weight loss and in a more favourable health status in terms of risk parameters for cardiovascular diseases such as LDL-C and ratio of total to HDL-cholesterol, being more effective than low-fat and low-carbohydrate diets.

Finally, the results of the most important intervention study in this field, the PREDIMED study, confirmed the beneficial effects of MD on inflammatory profile of patients at risk of developing cardiovascular disease [31]. In this study, a population of 516 subjects at high risk were randomised into three intervention groups, MD with supplementation of olive oil, MD with supplementation of nuts, and low-fat diet. After 1 year of treatment, the results supported the beneficial role of MD either with supplementation of virgin olive oil or nuts, on several inflammatory parameters such as tumour necrosis factor and IL-6.

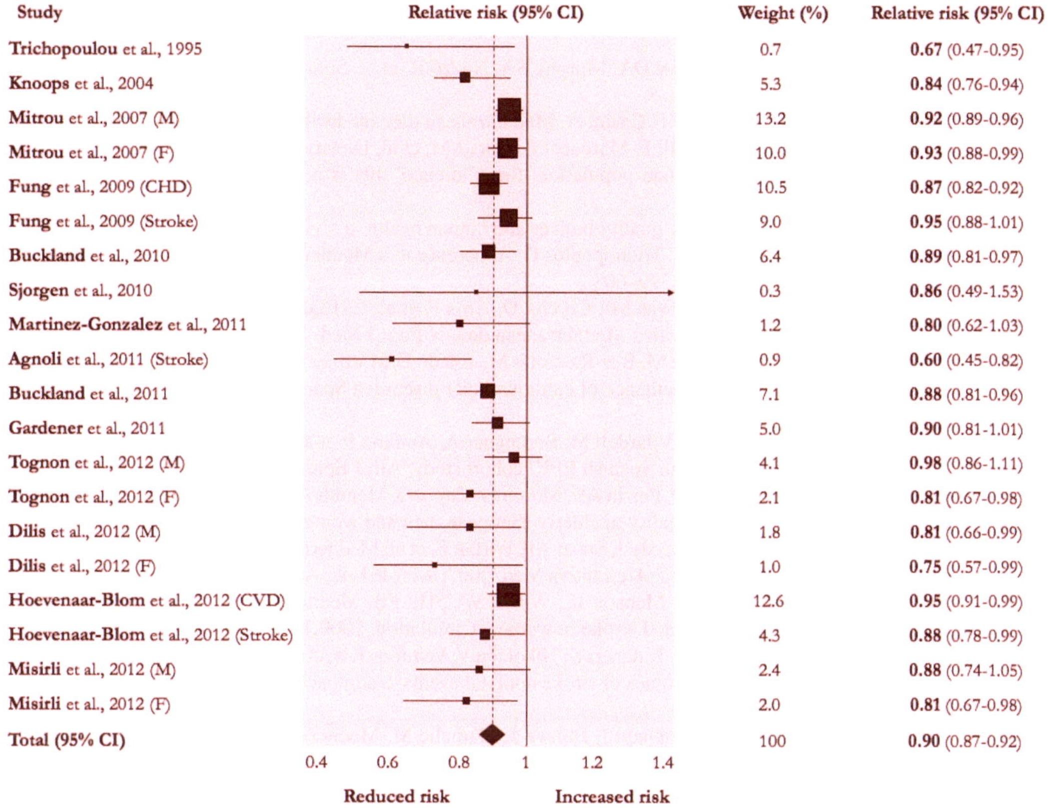

Fig. 7.1 Updated meta-analysis on greater adherence to Mediterranean diet score (two-point increase) and cardiovascular incidence and/or mortality risk

Conclusions

In conclusion, there is a vast amount of literature, to date, that demonstrates a strict relation between MD and health status in both general population and population of patients with a manifested disease. MD is able to decrease the risk of mortality and reduce the incidence of some of the most important disease states, but also is able to determine a reduction of many inflammatory parameters, possibly contributing to the decrease of this relevant risk factor of cardiovascular disease.

References

1. Keys A, Menotti A, Karvonen MJ, Aravanis C, Blackburn H, Buzina R, et al. The diet and 15-year death rate in the seven countries study. Am J Epidemiol. 1986;124:903–15.
2. Serra-Majem L, Roman B, Estruch R. Scientific evidence of interventions using the Mediterranean diet: a systematic review. Nutr Rev. 2006;64:S27–47.
3. Libby P. Inflammation in atherosclerosis. Nature. 2002;420:868–74.
4. Pearson TA, Mensah GA, Alexander RW, Anderson JL, Cannon 3rd RO, Criqui M, et al. Markers of inflammation and cardiovascular disease: application to clinical and public health practice: a statement for healthcare professionals from the centers for disease control and prevention and the American heart association. Circulation. 2003;107:499–511.

5. Ridker PM. Clinical application of C-reactive protein for cardiovascular disease detection and prevention. Circulation. 2003;107:363–9.
6. Schönbeck U, Varo N, Libby P, Morrow DA, Murphy SA, Nuzzo R, et al. Soluble CD40L and cardiovascular risk in women. Circulation. 2001;104:2266–8.
7. Sofi F, Macchi C, Abbate R, Gensini GF, Casini A. Mediterranean diet and health. Biofactors. 2013;39:335–42.
8. Sofi F, Vecchio S, Giuliani G, Martinelli F, Marcucci R, Gori AM, et al. Dietary habits lifestyle and cardiovascular risk factors in a clinically healthy Italian population: the 'Florence' diet is not Mediterranean. Eur J Clin Nutr. 2003;59:584–91.
9. Kourlaba G, Panagiotakos DB. Dietary quality indices and human health: a review. Maturitas. 2009;62:1–8.
10. Trichopoulou A, Costacou T, Bamia C, Trichopoulos D. Adherence to a Mediterranean diet and survival in a Greek population. N Engl J Med. 2003;348:2599–608.
11. Estruch R, Ros E, Salas-Salvadò J, Covas MI, Corella D, Aròs F, et al. PREDIMED study investigators. Primary prevention of cardiovascular disease with a Mediterranean diet. N Engl J Med. 2013;368:1279–90.
12. Martinez-Gonzalez MA, Garcia-Lopez M, Bes-Rastrollo M, Toledo E, Martínez-Lapiscina EH, Delgado-Rodriguez M, et al. Mediterranean diet and the incidence of cardiovascular disease: a Spanish cohort. Nutr Metab Cardiovasc Dis. 2011;21:237–44.
13. Buckland G, Gonzalez CA, Agudo A, Vilardell M, Berenguer A, Amiano P, et al. Adherence to Mediterranean diet and risk of coronary heart disease in the Spanish EPIC cohort study. Am J Epidemiol. 2009;170:1518–29.
14. Knoops KTB, de Groot L, Kromhout D, Perrin AE, Moreiras-Varela O, Menotti A, van Staveren MA. Mediterranean diet, lifestyle factors, and 10-year mortality in elderly European men and women. JAMA. 2004;292:1433–9.
15. Mitrou PN, Kipnis V, Thiebaut ACM, Reedy J, Subar AF, Wirfält E, et al. Mediterranean dietary pattern and prediction of all-cause mortality in a US population. Arch Intern Med. 2007;167:2461–8.
16. Fung T, Rexrode KM, Mantzoros CS, Manson JE, Willett WC, Hu FB. Mediterranean diet and incidence of and mortality from coronary heart disease and stroke in women. Circulation. 2009;119:1093–100.
17. Kastorini CM, Milionis HJ, Ioannidi A, Kalantzi K, Nikolaou V, Vemmos KN, et al. Adherence to the Mediterranean diet in relation to acute coronary syndromes or stroke nonfatal events: a comparative analysis of a case/case-control study. Am Heart J. 2011;162:717–24.
18. de Lorgeril M, Salen P, Martin JL, Monjaud I, Delaye J, Mamelle M. Mediterranean diet, traditional risk factors, and the rate of cardiovascular complications after myocardial infarction: final report of the Lyon Diet Heart Study. Circulation. 1999;99:779–85.
19. Barzi F, Woodward M, Marfisi RM, Tavazzi L, Valagussa F. Marchioli R; GISSI-Prevenzione Investigators. Mediterranean diet and all-causes mortality after myocardial infarction: results from the GISSI-Prevenzione trial. Eur J Clin Nutr. 2003;57:604–11.
20. Trichopoulou A, Bamia C, Trichopoulos D. Mediterranean diet and survival among patients with coronary heart disease in Greece. Arch Intern Med. 2005;165:929–35.
21. Trichopoulou A, Bamia C, Norat T, Overvad K, Schmidt EB, Tjønneland A, et al. Modified Mediterranean diet and survival after myocardial infarction: the EPIC-Elderly study. Eur J Epidemiol. 2007;22:871–81.
22. Sofi F, Cesari F, Abbate R, Gensini GF, Casini A. Adherence to Mediterranean diet and health status: a meta-analysis. BMJ. 2008;337:a1344.
23. Sofi F, Abbate R, Gensini GF, Casini A. Accruing evidence about benefits of adherence to Mediterranean diet on health: an updated systematic review with meta-analysis. Am J Clin Nutr. 2010;92:1189–96.
24. Sofi F, Macchi C, Abbate R, Gensini GF, Casini A. Mediterranean diet and health status: an updated meta-analysis and a proposal for a literature-based adherence score. Public Health Nutr. 2014;17:2769–82.
25. Chrysohoou C, Panagiotakos DB, Pitsavos C, Das UN, Stefanadis C. Adherence to the Mediterranean diet attenuates inflammation and coagulation process in healthy adults. The ATTICA study. J Am Coll Cardiol. 2004;44:152–8.
26. Fung TT, McCullough ML, Newby PK, Manson JE, Meigs JB, Rifai N, et al. Diet-quality scores and plasma concentrations of markers of inflammation and endothelial dysfunction. Am J Clin Nutr. 2005;82:163–73.
27. Panagiotakos DB, Dimakopoulou K, Katsouyanni K, Bellander T, Grau M, Keonig W, et al. Mediterranean diet and inflammatory response in myocardial infarction survivors. Int J Epidemiol. 2009;38:856–66.
28. Esposito K, Marfella R, Ciotola M, Di Palo C, Giugliano F, Giugliano G, et al. Effect of a Mediterranean-style diet on endothelial dysfunction and markers of vascular inflammation in the metabolic syndrome: a randomized trial. JAMA. 2004;292:1440–6.
29. Fito M, Guxens M, Corella D, Saez G, Estruch R, de la Torre R, et al. Effect of a traditional Mediterranean diet in lipoprotein oxidation: a randomized controlled trial. Arch Intern Med. 2007;167:1195–203.
30. Shai I, Schwarzfuchs D, Henkin Y, Shahar DR, Witkow S, Greenberg I, et al. Weight loss with a low-carbohydrate, Mediterranean, or low-fat diet. N Engl J Med. 2008;359:229–41.
31. Urpi-Sarda M, Casas R, Chiva-Blanch G, Romero-Mamani ES, Valderas-Martinez P, Salas-Salvado J, et al. The Mediterranean diet pattern and its main components are associated with lower plasma concentrations of tumor necrosis factor receptor 60 in patients at high risk of cardiovascular disease. J Nutr. 2012;142:1019–25.

Chapter 8
Wine, Polyphenols, and Cardioprotection

Brandon J. Sumpio, Alfredo C. Cordova, and Bauer E. Sumpio

Key Points

- Of all the components to the Mediterranean diet, red wine is arguably one of the most provocative and perhaps most investigated for its health benefit. Hypercholesterolemia, arterial hypertension, nicotine abuse, diabetes mellitus, and genetic predisposition are all major risk factors for cardiovascular disease (CVD).
- Epidemiological data, multiple clinical trials, animal models, in vivo and in vitro studies suggest an association between moderate and regular alcoholic beverage consumption, particularly red wine, and a lower risk for CVD.
- In this chapter, we discuss the epidemiological data correlating the beneficial effects of red wine on cardiovascular health. Also, we discuss the components of red wine that may be responsible for the cardioprotective effects, and some putative mechanisms of actions of red wine components on blood vessel and metabolic homeostasis.
- We conclude that coordinated actions of phenolic compounds and alcohol exert beneficial effects and reduce the risk of atherosclerosis. Regular and moderate consumption of red wine, perhaps 1–2 drinks a day with meals, should be encouraged. However, sound clinical judgment is needed to determine if alcohol consumption is an appropriate recommendation for each patient based on medical history and predisposition to dependency.

Keywords Red wine • Polyphenols • Cardiovascular disease • French paradox

B.J. Sumpio • B.E. Sumpio, M.D., Ph.D., F.A.C.S. (✉)
Department of Vascular Surgery, Yale University School of Medicine, 333 Cedar Street, BB 204, New Haven, CT 06510, USA
e-mail: bauer.sumpio@yale.edu; bauer.sumpio@yale.edu

A.C. Cordova, M.D.
Affinity Surgery/Care New England, Memorial Hospital of Rhode Island, Clinical Assistant Professor, Warren Alpert Medical School of Brown University, 333 School Street, Suite 213, Pawtucket, RI 02860, USA
e-mail: alfredo_cordova@brown.edu

D.F. Romagnolo, O.I. Selmin (eds.), *Mediterranean Diet*, Nutrition and Health,
DOI 10.1007/978-3-319-27969-5_8

Introduction

Of all the components to the Mediterranean diet, red wine is arguably one of the most provocative and perhaps most investigated for its health benefit. Red wine has a long history of use as an early form of medication. Ancient Egyptians were among the first to use wine in medicines, but it was the Greeks that took a more systematic approach to using wine as part of a healthy diet. Hippocrates advocated wine as a disinfectant for wounds and a medium to mix with drugs for consumption by patients. Greek physicians did not fully understand the biological compounds in wine, but still prescribed it for curing various ailments such a diarrhea and lethargy and to alleviate pain during childbirth. In these ancient times, religion played a significant role as well for promoting red wine's use as a health remedy.

Red wine's role as a cardioprotective agent has only recently been appreciated. Cardiovascular disease (CVD) has protean manifestations, and presents a grave problem for public health. Hypercholesterolemia, arterial hypertension, nicotine abuse, diabetes mellitus, and genetic predisposition are all major risk factors for CVD. Epidemiological data, multiple clinical trials, animal models, in vivo and in vitro studies suggest an association between moderate and regular alcoholic beverage consumption, particularly red wine, and a lower risk for CVD [1–4]. CVD is the most important cause of morbidity and mortality in Western industrialized nations, and accounts for more than 500,000 deaths from coronary artery disease (CAD) and 170,000 deaths from stroke every year in the USA. This represents approximately 40 % of the total annual mortality in the USA. In 2010 the estimated direct and indirect cost of CVD was $273.0 and for stroke in 2012 was $105.2 billion [5, 6]. In comparison, the estimated cost reported for all cancers in 2008 was $201.5 billion [7], and the estimated cost for new cases of HIV/AIDS in 2002 was $36.4 billion [8]. Worldwide, cardiovascular pathology accounted for over 18 million deaths in 2008, which is approximately 30 % of the total global mortality [9].

Alcohol's beneficial effects on the cardiovascular system have been well reported. In 1786, Heberden was the first to suggest alcohol's beneficial effects on the cardiovascular system; he noticed the relief of angina pectoris by "spirituous cordialis" [10, 11]. In 1819, international comparisons suggested the choice of a person's beverage as a protective factor. A century later, Cabot observed an inverse association between alcohol consumption and arteriosclerosis [12]. This was corroborated in the early twentieth century when pathologists observed an inverse alcohol-atherosclerosis association. However, it was not until 30 years ago when multinational epidemiological studies suggested the inverse relationship between alcohol and a lower incidence of CVD that generated interest [13]. In 1979, St. Legar and colleagues narrowed this association of alcohol and CVD to the consumption of red wine [4]. They based their study on data collected from 18 European and American countries in which mortality from ischemic heart disease was assessed in conjunction with different factors such as health-service, gross national product per capita, saturated and monounsaturated fat intake, and alcohol consumption. Renaud and associates demonstrated the same correlation in 1992 and introduced the concept of the "French paradox" [3]. Their study was based on the MONICA (MONItoring system for CArdiovascular disease) project, which included seven million men and women between 35 and 64 years of age from 37 European, American, and Asian populations, including the USA, Canada, UK, France, and China, among others. This was a tremendous effort of the World Health Organization in which collaborating investigators from 21 countries followed the subjects over a period of 10 years, from the mid-1980s to the mid-1990s. France had a markedly lower annual mortality from CAD when compared to other industrialized nations, despite the fact that cardiovascular risk factors such as cigarette smoking, blood pressure, body mass index, and serum cholesterol concentration were similar among these countries. Furthermore, France had a threefold higher intake of saturated fats than that of the USA and the UK [4]. French consume 2.8 times more lard and 3.8 times more butter than Americans, however, have a 2.5-fold lower death rate due to CVD [14]. These studies are thought to provide evidence supporting red wine's cardiovascular protective effects.

Grapes: From Vine to Vino

Red wine is produced by a process in which juices from the grapes are fermented for up to 2 weeks in the presence of the skin and seeds. This addition of the grape's skins and seeds gives red wine its characteristic color and aroma. More importantly, these skins add a plethora of organic compounds, which could play significant roles in cardioprotection. Pressing the grapes without the skin and then allowing it to ferment produces white wine [15]. During the fermentation process yeast is added and reacts with the sugars present in the grape juices to produce ethyl alcohol and carbon dioxide.

Influenced by oenologic techniques, the origin of the grape cultivar, and environmental factors, red wine's chemical composition has changed throughout time. Red wine is composed of more than 500 compounds of which only a few including water, ethanol, glycerol, sugar, and organic acids are present at levels greater than 100 mg/l (Table 8.1). These components are primarily responsible for the taste and mouth-feel sensation of wine. Aromatic compounds, most of which are fusel oils, fatty acid esters, and volatile acids, are present at concentrations of 0.8–1.2 g/l, fusel oils representing 50 % of this total [16]. Holding specific sensory characteristics related to its fragrance, red wine is composed of phenols, carbonyls, hydrocarbons, acetals, lactones, sulfur, and nitrogen compounds. The majority of the compounds in wine, 160 of which are esters, are present in concentrations ranging from 10^{-1} to 10^{-6} mg/l. Individually they play a small role, if any at all, in the human organoleptic perception (taste); collectively, their role might be significant [16]. Red wine contains a high concentration and a wide variety of polyphenolic substances, most of which come from the extraction derived from the skin and seeds during the fermentation process (Table 8.2). These compounds are responsible for the wine's bitterness, astringency, and color, as well as providing potent antioxidant effects. As such, they are wine's main preservative allowing for a long aging process [15].

Table 8.1 Chemical composition of wine[a]

	Dessert wines		Table wine	
Component	White	Red	White	Red
Water (by difference)	76	74	87	87
Sugars (mostly glucose and fructose)	8	10	0.05	0.05
Ethanol	14	14	10	10
Other volatiles	0.05	0.05	0.04	0.04
Extract	10.1	12.2	2.6	2.7
Glycerol	0.9	0.9	1.1	1.1
Acids	0.5	0.05	0.7	0.6
Pectins	0.25	0.25	0.3	0.3
Amino acids	0.2	0.2	0.25	0.25
Ash	0.2	0.2	0.2	0.2
Phenols[b]	0.01	0.1	0.01	0.2
Fats, terpenoids	0.01	0.02	0.01	0.02
Vitamins etc	0.01	0.01	0.01	0.01
Total	100	100	100	100

[a]Adapted from Soleas et al. [16]; Estimates of typical gross composition (% weight)

[b]Phenols constitute the major compositional difference between table and dessert red and white wines

Table 8.2 Typical wine phenolic levels

Phenol class	Source[a]	White Young[b]	White Aged[c]	Red Young[b]	Red Aged[c]
Flavonoids					
Flavanol monomers (i.e., catechin)	g	25	15	200	100
Proanthocyanidins and condensed tannins	g, d	20	25	750	1000
Flavonols (i.e., quercitin)	g, d	–	–	100	100
Anthocyanins (i.e., malvin-3-glucoside)	g	–	–	400	90
Others	g, d, e, m	–	–	50	75
Total mg/L		45	40	1500	1365
Non-flavonoids					
Cinnamates derivatives	g, d	154	130	165	60
Benzene Derivatives	g, d, e, m	10	15	60	60
Hydrolyzable tannins (from oak)	e	0	100	0	250
Stilbenes (i.e., resveratrol)	g, m	0.5	0.5	7	7
Total mg/L		164.5	245.5	232	377
Total all phenols		209.5	285.5	1732	1742

Adapted from Waterhouse [15]
[a] *g* grapes, *d* degradable product, *e* environment, cooperage, *m* microbes, yeast
[b] Young refers to new wine, less than 6 months of age, not having been aged or fermented in oak barrels
[c] Aged implies about 1 year for white, about 2 years for red and some oak barrel aging (or other oak contact)

Polyphenolic composition varies among different wines according to the type of berry used, vinification process used, type of yeast that participates in the fermentation, and whether or not there were grape solids present in the maceration process. Even when the same type of berry is involved, phenolic content may differ depending upon the type of soil, weather variations (temperature, rain, humidity), and other biologic effects (fungi, insecticides, fertilizers) [17]. Water deficit decreases the amount of flavanols and greatly increase the rate of loss during fruit ripening. Polyphenols also decrease as the fruit matures [18]. Since exposure of the grapes' skins to sunlight strongly favors high levels of some flavonoids many vineyards in Europe are oriented for southern sunlight exposure [19].

A typical commercial bottle of red wine contains approximately 1.8 g/L of total polyphenols, while a typical bottle of white wine contains only around 0.2–0.3 g/L of total polyphenols [20]. Therefore, the total amount of polyphenols found in a glass of red wine is around 200 mg in comparison to only 30 mg in a glass of white wine. Polyphenols are categorized as flavonoids and non-flavonoids. Flavonoids constitute the majority of these phenols in red wine. In typical wine making, about half of the phenolic compounds are extracted during the maceration process. The amount extracted is strongly affected by the types of seed extracting methods used and are higher with the use of extended maceration techniques. The presence of ethanol and its solvent properties facilitate the process of polyphenol extraction. The amounts of polyphenols in a wine decrease with prolonged storage due to the formation of polymers which precipitate in response to their insoluble states. This could also be attributed to some oxidation reactions [15].

Polyphenols have varying levels of antioxidant characteristics that depend on their chemical structures [21, 22] (Table 8.2). The phenol group is a strong electron donor and is readily oxidized [15]. In addition, red wine is rich in catechol containing compounds that also have antioxidant activity, albeit less than polyphenols. For instance, although the OH groups on quercitin and catechin possess similar arrangements, quercitin inhibits low density lipoprotein (LDL) oxidation to a greater extent, due to its 2–3 double bond and the 4-oxo structure in its C ring [23]. Conversely, anthocyanins and polymerized tannins are very poor antioxidants [24]. Even though tannins are the most abundant of the wine polyphenols, they are not absorbed due to their large molecular size and thus impart no health effects, except perhaps in the gut. Given their control over the processing of grape to reach a specific flavor, winemakers are ultimately the critical determinants of a wine's polyphenol content [15].

Have a Glass, It's Good for You

At present, there are numerous epidemiological studies reporting alcohol's favorable effects on cardiovascular disease and other pathologies. It has been widely suggested that regular and moderate intake of alcoholic beverages, a volume of 1.1 to 1.8 ounces of alcohol per day (1 fluid ounce = 29.6 ml), decreases the risk of CAD by at least 40 % (Fig. 8.1) [25–28]. In a prospective study, 51,529 men without preexisting cardiovascular or cancer disorders were followed for 12 years with food-frequency questionnaires. The investigators reached the conclusion that ethanol consumption at least three to four times a week is inversely associated with the occurrence of myocardial infarction [29, 30]. This relationship was present even with a limited consumption of 0.35–0.42 ounces of alcohol/day, which is equivalent to one drink [31]. In the majority of reports, one drink is defined as 0.5 ounces of alcohol, which is equivalent to approximately four ounces of wine (1/2 wine glass), 12 ounces of beer, or one ounce of spirits. It has been suggested that red wine consumption of 0.7 to 1.1 ounces of alcohol per day (5–9 ounces of red wine, ~150–250 ml), comparable to the French's intake, has protective properties.

Moderate consumption of alcohol by itself can increase plasma concentrations of high density lipoprotein (HDL) and decrease the adhesiveness of platelets (Table 8.3); both of which would

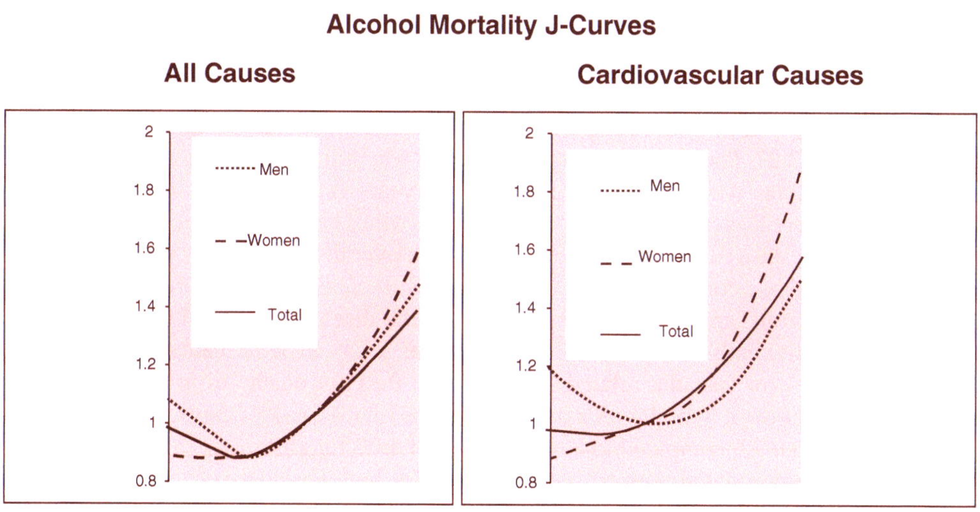

All Causes	<1 drink/month	1-2 drinks/day	3-5 drinks/day	>6 drinks/day
Men	1.1	0.9	1.1	1.5
Women	0.9	0.9	1.1	1.6
Total	1	0.9	1.1	1.4

Cardiovascular Causes	<1 drink/month	1-2 drinks/day	3-5 drinks/day	>6 drinks/day
Men	1.1	0.9	1.1	1.5
Women	0.9	0.9	1.1	1.6
Total	1	0.9	1.1	1.4

Fig. 8.1 Alcohol mortality: J-curve. Alcohol has protective effects against death from all causes, but excessive amounts of alcohol begin to have detrimental effects on overall health. A notable difference between the effects of alcohol on mortality due to cardiovascular disease compared to all causes, is that consuming 3–5 drinks per day is protective against death due to cardiovascular disease, but it has an increased relative risk of death due to other causes. One drink is defined as 0.5 ounces of alcohol, which is equivalent to approximately four ounces of wine (1/2 wine glass), 12 ounces of beer, or one ounce of spirits. Modified from Cordova et al. [48]

Table 8.3 Putative mechanisms of red wine's cardioprotective effects

Biological process	Biological effects
Antioxidant	Free radical scavenger; metal ion chelator; sparing of antioxidants (vit E and C, b-carotenoid); alteration of catalytic enzymes; modification of protein phosphorylation
Platelet aggregation modulator	Inhibition of PAF, ADP, and PDGF beta receptor; modification of phospholipase activity; inhibition of cyclo-oxygenase pathway; inhibition of thromboxane B_2 synthesis; potentiation of prostaglandin I_2
Vasorelaxation	NO release; eNOS activation; inhibition of thromboxane
Lipid regulator	Stimulation of superoxide dismutase; activation or preservation of paraoxonase activity; activation of phase II enzymes; precipitation and fecal elimination of cholesterol; inhibition of digestive lipase activity; inhibition of pancreatic lipase activity; inhibition of squalene epoxide; reduction of LDL and VLDL oxidation; enhancement of noradrenaline induced lipolysis
Inhibition of SMC proliferation and vascular hyperplasia	Cell cycle arrest; DNA strand breakage; inhibition of MMP 9; TIMP-2 overexpression; inhibition of VEGF, PDGF; inhibition of ICAM1 and VCAM1; inhibition of PI3-K and p38 MAPK; apoptosis
Sirtuin activation	Protection against cardiac hypertrophy

prevent or retard the formation of atherosclerosis and thus the risk of coronary artery disease [20]. Ethanol, present as 8–15 % of the volume of red wine, has a wide range of biological functions and can act as a fuel source, alter cholesterol composition, impair fluid balance, and alter the activity of xenobiotic metabolizing enzymes such as the p-450 cytochrome family, glutathione S-transferase superfamily, and N-acetyl-transferases [20, 32]. Meanwhile, ethanol has been demonstrated to hold a pro-oxidant effect [33, 34]. However, polyphenols, which are present in high amounts in red wine, counteract the potential pro-oxidant effect of ethanol and even confer a net antioxidant activity. In this manner, beverages which have low concentrations of phenolic compounds, such as white wine or beer, may have a pro-oxidant effect [35–37] [38].

Multiple studies have shown that red wine is the most beneficial in reducing the risks of CAD and mortality in general, when compared to other alcoholic beverages such as spirits, beer, and white wine (Fig. 8.2). The Copenhagen Heart Study, which involved 6051 men and 7234 women of 30–70 years of age who were followed for 10–12 years, reported the association between consumption of different alcoholic types of beverages (wine, beer, and spirits) and mortality. This prospective study showed the inverse correlation with overall mortality only in people consuming wine, but not in those consuming beer or spirits [38]. Increased consumption of wine decreased the risk of death from cardiovascular or cerebrovascular disease and for all causes. In comparison to abstainers, individuals who consumed 3–5 glasses a day of wine had a relative risk of 0.44 (95 % confidence) for vascular related deaths and of 0.51 for deaths from all causes. Regarding beer, the consumption of 3–5 glasses a day reduced the relative risk of cardiovascular and cerebrovascular deaths to 0.72, compared to a relative risk of 1.00 for abstainers [32]. On the other hand, spirits intake was correlated with an increased risk for both vascular-related and other causes of death. In France, alcohol intake is mainly in the form of red wine, which may explain their low incidence of CVD. However, even within France there are slight variations regarding alcoholic preferences and CAD, depending on the area. In Toulouse and the rest of the south where red wine intake is at its highest, the lowest CAD incidence is observed. In the cities in the north like Strasbourg and Lille, more spirits are consumed and there is a relatively higher incidence of this pathological process [20]. In another report, Gronbaek and associates followed 24,523 men and women of 20–98 years of age for a period of 11 years and reached the conclusion that moderate wine drinkers have a 20 % lower all-cause mortality risk than non-wine drinkers [39]. This data suggests the relative benefits of wine consumption over other alcoholic drinks.

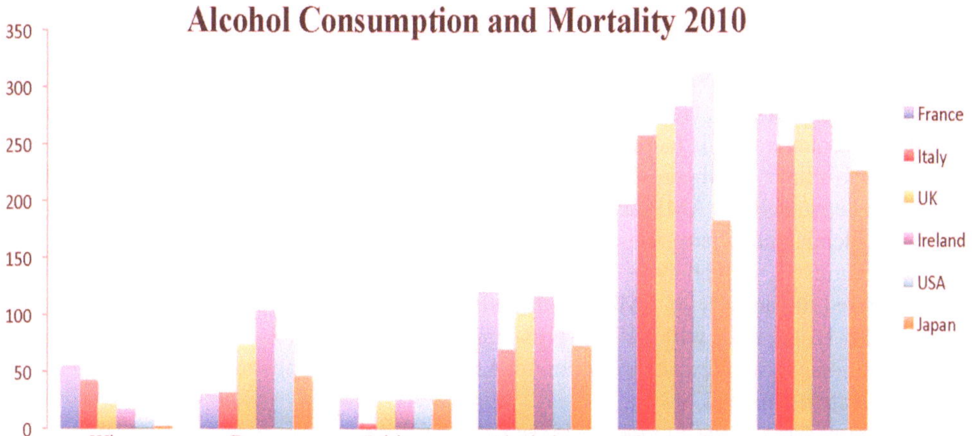

	Wine Consumption L/person/yr	Beer Consumption L/ person/yr	Spirits Consumption .1L/person/yr	Alcohol Consumption .1L/person/yr	Heart and Diabetes mortality per 100,000	Cancer Mortality per 100,000
France	54.5	30	26.2	120	197	277
Italy	42.12	31.1	4.2	69	258	249
UK	21.6	73.7	24.1	102	268	269
Ireland	16.89	103.7	25.1	116	283	272
USA	9.42	78.2	26.5	86	312	245
Japan	1.88	45.4	26.1	73	183	227

Fig. 8.2 Cardiovascular and cancer mortality and alcohol consumption. Cardiovascular disease and cancer mortality in relation to alcohol consumption by type. Note that France, while having the second highest consumption of wine in liters per person per year, has the second lowest cardiovascular disease mortality. Modified from [62–64]

Mechanisms of Action

Moderate alcohol consumption has been strongly associated with decreased cardiovascular mortality in epidemiological studies and meta-analyses. This decreased mortality has been attributed to changes in lipid profiles, decreased coagulation, increased fibrinolysis, inhibition of platelet aggregation, increased nitric oxide, and antioxidant capacities of alcoholic beverages. Most of these laboratory and animal studies, as well as intervention trials in human volunteers, have revealed many interesting mechanisms that contribute to the cardioprotective effects of alcohol, red wine, or red wine polyphenolic compounds.

The exact mechanism of red wine's effects on the cardiovascular system have not been fully elucidated, but there are many pathways in which it is thought to have a role in preventing arteriosclerosis (Table 8.3). These include increased antioxidant serum activity, increased resistance of LDL to peroxidation, [15, 24, 30, 34, 40–44] increased levels of serum HDL cholesterol, and by enhancing serum paraoxonase activation. It is apparent that alcohol by itself affects cardiovascular events by influencing the levels of lipoproteins in the blood and decreasing the adhesiveness of platelets. High levels of HDL cholesterol are associated with low risks of cardiovascular morbidity and mortality. HDL cholesterol rises with the consumption of alcohol [3, 34, 45, 46]. Epidemiological studies have shown that those who consume alcohol moderately develop a lowering of LDL cholesterol levels. High concentrations of LDL cholesterol have not been associated with a risk of coronary heart disease in men who consumed three or more drinks a day. In a controlled diet study of premenopausal women, consumption of alcohol over a three-month period was associated with an 8 % decrease in LDL cholesterol, a 10 % increase in HDL cholesterol, and no change in lipoprotein A [41]. Although alcohol increases the serum levels of HDL cholesterol, it also increases the serum level of triglycerides, which is a risk factor for cardiovascular disease. However, it may be possible that the beneficial effects of red wine via polyphenols may counteract this increase in triglycerides.

Polyphenols have also been shown to affect lipids levels. Zang et al. examined the effect of polyphenols on hepatocellular AMP-activated protein kinase (AMPK) activity and lipid levels in addition to hyperlipidemia and atherogenesis in type 1 diabetic LDL receptor-deficient mice (DMLDLR$^{-/-}$). In HepG2 hepatocytes, polyphenols, including resveratrol, apigenin, and S17834 (a synthetic polyphenol), increased the activity of AMPK with 200 times the potency of metformin. Additionally, treatment of DMLDLR$^{-/-}$ mice with S17834 prevented lipid accumulation in the liver, hyperlipidemia, and the acceleration of aortic lesion development. As a result, the polyphenols lowered lipids by activating AMPK in diabetic mice [47].

Polyphenols have been found to decrease LDL sensitivity to peroxidation as well. A study showed that subjects who consumed 375 mL/day of red wine for 2 weeks had significantly decreased lipid peroxides, thiobarbituric acid reactive substances, and conjugated dienes [42]. That antioxidant effect was associated with an increase in polyphenol plasma concentration. Moreover, alcohol free powder of red wine polyphenol extract has similar antioxidant effects on LDL as red wine [34].

The antioxidant properties of polyphenols on LDL are due to several mechanisms. Polyphenols are free radical scavengers and act as reducing agents. Additionally, polyphenols chelate transition metal ions to decrease metal free radical production. A third mechanism involves sparing vitamin E and carotenoids in LDL particles to preserve their antioxidant effects [48]. Lastly, polyphenols increase serum paraoxonase activity to promote hydrolysis of arterial cells and LDL associated lipid peroxides [33].

Alcohol has a direct effect on the status of the coagulation system. A low plasma fibrinogen level is associated with a low risk of coronary heart disease, even when LDL cholesterol concentrations are elevated. Alcohol consumption is inversely correlated with fibrinogen levels [32]. There is a positive association between moderate alcohol intake and plasma concentrations of plasminogen and endogenous tissue type plasminogen activator antigen. Moderate consumption of alcohol also enhances postprandial fibrinolytic activity, and inhibits platelet aggregation [49]. An associated decrease in thromboxane A_2 production has also been noted with consumption of alcohol. It is apparent that of the many factors that appear to account for a lower mortality in consumers of moderate alcohol, a substantial benefit might be derived from inhibited clot formation.

Polyphenols are components of wine, particularly red wine, which do not exist in spirits, and are in low concentrations in beer and malt whiskey. Polyphenols are classified as either flavonoids or non-flavonoids. The flavonoids include flavonols, which consist of quercitin and myricetin, and the flavan-3-ols that include catechin and epicatechin. The non-flavonoids include the stilbenes, hydroxycinnamates, and hydroxybenzoates [48]. All polyphenols have the basic structure of a benzene ring with multiple hydroxyl groups. It is those hydroxyl groups that are responsible for the previously mentioned powerful antioxidant properties of the compounds since they have a high affinity for binding free radical ions. That antioxidative ability has numerous physiological benefits including prevention of DNA damage, lipid peroxidation [50], inhibiting formation of harmful N-nitroso compounds [51], and alteration of oxidative enzymes. Polyphenols also indirectly have antioxidative effects by sparing the use of natural antioxidants such as urate, vitamins C and E, and β-carotene for further antioxidation.

Polyphenols putative cardioprotective mechanisms include a potent antioxidant activity, inhibition of smooth muscle cell proliferation and migration, platelet aggregation modulator, lipid modulator, and vasorelaxation (Table 8.3). They have been identified as antioxidants, antimutagens, chelators of catalytic metals, and free radical scavengers. The antioxidant effects of these phenols counter the pro-oxidant activity of alcohol [36, 37]. In a crossover study by Micallef et al. red wine consumption was found to significantly increase total plasma antioxidant status in both younger and older volunteers. These subjects either consumed 400 mL/day of red wine for 2 weeks or abstained from alcohol for 2 weeks before crossing over to the other group; blood samples were obtained both before and after red wine consumption to evaluate the antioxidant status of the blood [52]. This antioxidant effect is believed to be a result of both plasma urate levels and polyphenols [53]. Wine polyphenols decrease platelet aggregation and adhesion to endothelium, increase HDL cholesterol independent of the alcohol content of wine, and inhibit the oxidation of LDL cholesterol [37, 45, 46, 54, 55]. These compounds inhibit the cyclooxygenase and lipooxygenase of platelets and macrophages, thereby inhibiting clotting and the inflammatory mediators in a developing atheroma.

Resveratrol has been found to inhibit intracellular adhesion molecule 1 (ICAM-1) and vascular cell adhesion molecule 1 (VCAM-1) expression, which promote the adhesion of macrophages to endothelium and their entry into the intima, which then initiates the atherosclerotic plaque [56]. This is supported by another study by Sacanella et al. that showed decreased levels of CAM and several inflammatory markers in healthy women volunteering for a crossover study [57]. Moreover, our laboratory has shown that resveratrol inhibits smooth muscle cell proliferation in a dose dependent manner through induction of a block between the G1 and S phases of the cell cycle [58]. Additionally, we found that resveratrol exposure resulted in apoptosis of smooth muscle cells in vitro. This finding is significant since it is the proliferation of smooth muscle cells that contributes to atheroma formation.

Resveratrol was also found to increase in vitro platelet nitric oxide (NO) production, and thus leading to vasorelaxation. Nitric oxide production is stimulated by exposure to red wine and other red grape products, but not white wine, independent of alcohol. A study by Gresele et al noted that, in healthy volunteers, blood levels of NO increased with increased resveratrol levels [59]. They also noted in vitro that washing platelets in resveratrol 0.5 μmol/L, a concentration found to be within the range comparable to drinking 300 mL of red wine, increased their NO production [59]. Nitric oxide probably influences hemostatic mechanisms such as platelet-vessel wall (collagen) interaction, and promote vasorelaxation.

Resveratrol plays another important role as an activator of the small protein family sirtuins [59]. Sirtuins are nicotinamide adenine dinucleotide (NAD^+) dependent protein deacetylases that carry out enzymatic reactions. Research on aging has focused heavily on this group of genes, as it is believed to aid in longevity pathways. SIRT1, a human member of the sirtuin family, was shown to increase human health as well as life span [60]. When resveratrol is activated, there is an eightfold increase in SIRT1 levels, which helps it target protein substrates that fight against age-related diseases such as cancer, Alzheimer's disease, and type 2 diabetes. At the cellular level, SIRT1 controls, circadian rhythm, inflammatory pathways, insulin secretion, DNA repair and apoptosis, and mitochondrial biogenesis.

When activated, SIRT1 is a regulator of mitochondrial biogenesis, PGC-1α [61]. As humans age mitochondrial activity decreases, cause our cells to become less efficient. SIRT1 works to increase the energy output of the mitochondria. In mice studies this has been shown to increase life span by 40 %, as well as, improve running endurance. In animal studies exposed to exercise, the levels of SIRT1 activation by immunoblottting was found highest in the liver and slow-twitch red muscles.

Conclusions

There is a growing epidemic of cardiovascular disease in the Western world. The pathogenesis of cardiovascular pathology is multifactorial. Different modalities have been suggested to work together against this burden and include behavioral modification such as exercise, smoking cessation, and a healthy diet. Red wine and its "polyphenolic aid" present many beneficial characteristics against cardiovascular disease (Fig. 8.3). These are associated with their capability to lipid-peroxidize LDL, inhibit smooth muscle cell (SMC) proliferation, modulate platelet adhesiveness, enhance HDL serum levels, and produce vasorelaxation. Regular and moderate consumption of red wine, perhaps 1–2 drinks a day with meals, should be encouraged. However, sound clinical judgment should be used in

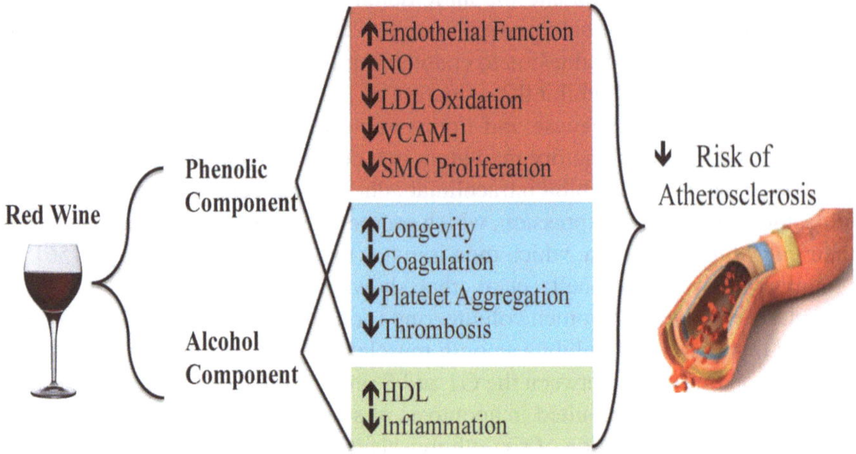

Fig. 8.3 Red wine and its beneficial effect on atherogenesis. Coordinated actions of phenolic compounds and alcohol exert beneficial effects and reduce the risk of atherosclerosis. Regular and moderate consumption of red wine, perhaps 1–2 drinks a day with meals, should be encouraged. However, sound clinical judgment is needed to determine if alcohol consumption is an appropriate recommendation for each patient based on medical history and predisposition to dependency. Abbreviations: low density lipoprotein (LDL); high density lipoprotein (HDL); smooth muscle cell (SMC); vascular cell adhesion molecule 1 (VCAM-1); nitric oxide (NO)

determining if alcohol consumption is an appropriate recommendation for each patient, taking into account factors such as contraindications with other medications and predisposition to dependency. It is also important that a distinction be made between moderate use of alcohol and its abuse. Let us keep in mind that there is a small percentage of the population that may be prone to addiction, or fails to practice moderate consumption; and therefore uncontrolled consumption may detrimental to people's health as well as present a hazard to society as a whole, via acts of violence, accidents, spousal, child, and elder abuse. Maintaining a healthy diet and lifestyle should not be a choice but a responsibility. For this reason by all means we must maintain an organized life with a healthy diet, regular exercise, and adequate sleep. Dietary and lifestyles habits proven to be beneficial by the medical community or society must be sought. In these terms, the regular consumption of red wine in a moderate fashion, 1–2 drinks a day, constitutes a solution, to some extent, to the grave public health problem of CVD.

References

1. Hennekens CH, Rosner B, Cole DS. Daily alcohol consumption and fatal coronary heart disease. Am J Epidemiol. 1978;107(3):196–200.
2. Klatsky AL, Friedman GD, Siegelaub AB. Alcohol consumption before myocardial infarction. Results from the Kaiser-Permanente epidemiologic study of myocardial infarction. Ann Intern Med. 1974;81(3):294–301.
3. Renaud S, de Lorgeril M. Wine, alcohol, platelets, and the French paradox for coronary heart disease. Lancet. 1992;339(8808):1523–6.
4. St Leger AS, Cochrane AL, Moore F. Factors associated with cardiac mortality in developed countries with particular reference to the consumption of wine. Lancet. 1979;1(8124):1017–20.
5. Ovbiagele B, Goldstein LB, Higashida RT, Howard VJ, Johnston SC, Khavjou OA, et al. Forecasting the future of stroke in the United States: a policy statement from the American Heart Association and American Stroke Association. Stroke. 2013;44(8):2361–75.
6. Heidenreich PA, Trogdon JG, Khavjou OA, Butler J, Dracup K, Ezekowitz MD, et al. Forecasting the future of cardiovascular disease in the United States: a policy statement from the American Heart Association. Circulation. 2011;123(8):933–44.

7. American Cancer Society. Cancer Facts & Figures Atlanta: American Cancer Society. 2013.
8. Hutchinson AB, Farnham PG, Dean HD, Ekwueme DU, del Rio C, Kamimoto L, et al. The economic burden of HIV in the United States in the era of highly active antiretroviral therapy: evidence of continuing racial and ethnic differences. J Acquir Immune Defic Syndr. 2006;43(4):451–7.
9. World Health Organization. [cited 2014 Jan 8]. Available from: http://www.who.int/mediacentre/factsheets/fs317/en/index.html
10. Heberden W. Some account of a disorder of the breast. Med Trans R Coll Phys (London). 1786;2:59–67.
11. Klatsky AL. Alcohol and cardiovascular diseases: a historical overview. Ann N Y Acad Sci. 2002;957:7–15.
12. Cabot RC. The relation of alcohol to arteriosclerosis. J Am Med Assoc. 1904;43:774–5.
13. Yano K, Rhoads GG, Kagan A. Coffee, alcohol and risk of coronary heart disease among Japanese men living in Hawaii. N Engl J Med. 1977;297(8):405–9.
14. Vinson JA, Teufel K, Wu N. Red wine, dealcoholized red wine, and especially grape juice, inhibit atherosclerosis in a hamster model. Atherosclerosis. 2001;156(1):67–72.
15. Waterhouse AL. Wine phenolics. Ann N Y Acad Sci. 2002;957:21–36.
16. Soleas GJ, Diamandis EP, Goldberg DM. Wine as a biological fluid: history, production, and role in disease prevention. J Clin Lab Anal. 1997;11(5):287–313.
17. Alvarez-Sala L, Slowing K, Gomez-Serranillos P, Torres F, Valderrama M, Millan J. Variabilidad del contenido de polifenoles de distintos tipos de vino y su potencial aplicaci6n al conocimiento de sus efectos biologicos. Med Clin (Barc). 2000;114:331–2.
18. Kennedy JA, Matthews MA, Waterhouse AL. Changes in grape seed polyphenols during fruit ripening. Phytochemistry. 2000;55(1):77–85.
19. Price S, Breen P, Valladao M, Watson B. Cluster sun exposure and quercetin in Pinot noir grapes and wine. Am J Enol Vitic. 1995;46:187–94.
20. Bell J, Donnovan J, Wong R, Waterhouse A, German JR, Kasim-Karacas S. (+)-catechin in human plasma after ingestion of a single serving of reconstituted red wine. Am J Clin Nutr. 2000;71:103–8.
21. Rice-Evans CA, Miller NJ, Paganga G. Structure-antioxidant activity relationships of flavonoids and phenolic acids. Free Radic Biol Med. 1996;20(7):933–56.
22. van Acker SA, van den Berg DJ, Tromp MN, Griffioen DH, van Bennekom WP, van der Vijgh WJ, et al. Structural aspects of antioxidant activity of flavonoids. Free Radic Biol Med. 1996;20(3):331–42.
23. Vinson J, Hontz B. Phenol antioxidant index: Comparative antioxidant effectiveness of red and white wines. J Agric Food Chem. 1995;43:401–3.
24. Fuhrman B, Volkova N, Suraski A, Aviram M. White wine with red wine-like properties: increased extraction of grape skin polyphenols improves the antioxidant capacity of the derived white wine. J Agric Food Chem. 2001;49(7):3164–8.
25. Boffetta P, Garfinkel L. Alcohol drinking and mortality among men enrolled in an American Cancer Society prospective study. Epidemiology. 1990;1(5):342–8.
26. Kozararevic D, McGee D, Vojvodic N, Racic Z, Dawber T, Gordon T, et al. Frequency of alcohol consumption and morbidity and mortality: The Yugoslavia Cardiovascular Disease Study. Lancet. 1980;1(8169):613–6.
27. Marmot MG, Rose G, Shipley MJ, Thomas BJ. Alcohol and mortality: a U-shaped curve. Lancet. 1981;1(8220 Pt 1):580–3.
28. Shaper AG, Wannamethee G, Walker M. Alcohol and mortality in British men: explaining the U-shaped curve. Lancet. 1988;2(8623):1267–73.
29. Mukamal KJ, Conigrave KM, Mittleman MA, Camargo Jr CA, Stampfer MJ, Willett WC, et al. Roles of drinking pattern and type of alcohol consumed in coronary heart disease in men. N Engl J Med. 2003;348(2):109–18.
30. Rimm EB, Giovannucci EL, Willett WC, Colditz GA, Ascherio A, Rosner B, et al. Prospective study of alcohol consumption and risk of coronary disease in men. Lancet. 1991;338(8765):464–8.
31. Stampfer M, Colditz G, Willet W, Speizer F, Hennekens C. A prospective study of moderate alcohol consumption and the risk of coronary disease and stroke in women. N Engl J Med. 1998;319(5):267–73.
32. Goldberg D, Hahn S, Parkes J. Beyond alcohol: beverage consumption and cardiovascular mortality. Clin Chim Acta. 1995;237:155–87.
33. Fuhrman B, Aviram M. Flavonoids protect LDL from oxidation and attenuate atherosclerosis. Curr Opin Lipidol. 2001;12(1):41–8.
34. Nigdikar SV, Williams NR, Griffin BA, Howard AN. Consumption of red wine polyphenols reduces the susceptibility of low-density lipoproteins to oxidation in vivo. Am J Clin Nutr. 1998;68(2):258–65.
35. Criqui MH, Ringel BL. Does diet or alcohol explain the French paradox? Lancet. 1994;344(8939-8940):1719–23.
36. Klatsky AL, Armstrong MA. Alcoholic beverage choice and risk of coronary artery disease mortality: do red wine drinkers fare best? Am J Cardiol. 1993;71(5):467–9.
37. Klatsky AL, Armstrong MA, Friedman GD. Relations of alcoholic beverage use to subsequent coronary artery disease hospitalization. Am J Cardiol. 1986;58(9):710–4.
38. Gronbaek M, Deis A, Sorensen TI, Becker U, Schnohr P, Jensen G. Mortality associated with moderate intakes of wine, beer, or spirits. BMJ. 1995;310(6988):1165–9.

39. Gronbaek M, Becker U, Johansen D, Gottschau A, Schnohr P, Hein HO, et al. Type of alcohol consumed and mortality from all causes, coronary heart disease, and cancer. Ann Intern Med. 2000;133(6):411–9.
40. Zou J, Huang Y, Chen Q, Wei E, Cao K, Wu JM. Effects of resveratrol on oxidative modification of human low density lipoprotein. Chin Med J. 2000;113(2):99–102.
41. Waterhouse AL, German JB, Walzem RL, Hansen RJ, Kasim-Karakas SE. Is it time for a wine trial? Am J Clin Nutr. 1998;68(2):220–1.
42. Fuhrman B, Lavy A, Aviram M. Consumption of red wine with meals reduces the susceptibility of human plasma and low-density lipoprotein to lipid peroxidation. Am J Clin Nutr. 1995;61(3):549–54.
43. Brenna OV, Pagliarini E. Multivariate analysis of antioxidant power and polyphenolic composition in red wines. J Agric Food Chem. 2001;49(10):4841–4.
44. Abu-Amsha R, Croft KD, Puddey IB, Proudfoot JM, Beilin LJ. Phenolic content of various beverages determines the extent of inhibition of human serum and low-density lipoprotein oxidation in vitro: identification and mechanism of action of some cinnamic acid derivatives from red wine. Clin Sci. 1996;91(4):449–58.
45. Araya J, Rodrigo R, Orellana M, Rivera G. Red wine raises plasma HDL and preserves long-chain polyunsaturated fatty acids in rat kidney and erythrocytes. Br J Nutr. 2001;86(2):189–95.
46. Perret B, Ruidavets JB, Vieu C, Jaspard B, Cambou JP, Terce F, et al. Alcohol consumption is associated with enrichment of high-density lipoprotein particles in polyunsaturated lipids and increased cholesterol esterification rate. Alcohol Clin Exp Res. 2002;26(8):1134–40.
47. Zang M, Xu S, Maitland-Toolan KA, Zuccollo A, Hou X, Jiang B, et al. Polyphenols stimulate AMP-activated protein kinase, lower lipids, and inhibit accelerated atherosclerosis in diabetic LDL receptor-deficient mice. Diabetes. 2006;55(8):2180–91.
48. Cordova AC, Jackson LS, Berke-Schlessel DW, Sumpio BE. The cardiovascular protective effect of red wine. J Am Coll Surg. 2005;200(3):428–39.
49. Ruf JC, Berger JL, Renaud S. Platelet rebound effect of alcohol withdrawal and wine drinking in rats. Relation to tannins and lipid peroxidation. Arterioscler Thromb Vasc Biol. 1995;15(1):140–4.
50. Pillai SP, Mitscher LA, Menon SR, Pillai CA, Shankel DM. Antimutagenic/antioxidant activity of green tea components and related compounds. J Environ Pathol Toxicol Oncol. 1999;18(3):147–58.
51. Lampe JW. Health effects of vegetables and fruit: assessing mechanisms of action in human experimental studies. Am J Clin Nutr. 1999;70(3 Suppl):475S–90.
52. Micallef M, Lexis L, Lewandowski P. Red wine consumption increases antioxidant status and decreases oxidative stress in the circulation of both young and old humans. Nutr J. 2007;6:27.
53. Modun D, Music I, Vukovic J, Brizic I, Katalinic V, Obad A, et al. The increase in human plasma antioxidant capacity after red wine consumption is due to both plasma urate and wine polyphenols. Atherosclerosis. 2008;197(1):250–6.
54. Pace-Asciak CR, Rounova O, Hahn SE, Diamandis EP, Goldberg DM. Wines and grape juices as modulators of platelet aggregation in healthy human subjects. Clin Chim Acta. 1996;246(1-2):163–82.
55. Pace-Asciak C, Hahn S, Diamandis E, Soleas G, Goldberg D. The red wine phenolics trans-resveratrol and quercitin block human platelet aggregation and eicosanoid synthesis: implications for protection against coronary heart disease. Clin Chim Acta. 1995;236:207–19.
56. Carluccio MA, Siculella L, Ancora MA, Massaro M, Scoditti E, Storelli C, et al. Olive oil and red wine antioxidant polyphenols inhibit endothelial activation: antiatherogenic properties of Mediterranean diet phytochemicals. Arterioscler Thromb Vasc Biol. 2003;23(4):622–9.
57. Sacanella E, Vazquez-Agell M, Mena MP, Antunez E, Fernandez-Sola J, Nicolas JM, et al. Down-regulation of adhesion molecules and other inflammatory biomarkers after moderate wine consumption in healthy women: a randomized trial. Am J Clin Nutr. 2007;86(5):1463–9.
58. Poussier B, Cordova AC, Becquemin JP, Sumpio BE. Resveratrol inhibits vascular smooth muscle cell proliferation and induces apoptosis. J Vasc Surg. 2005;42(6):1190–7.
59. Gresele P, Pignatelli P, Guglielmini G, Carnevale R, Mezzasoma AM, Ghiselli A, et al. Resveratrol, at concentrations attainable with moderate wine consumption, stimulates human platelet nitric oxide production. J Nutr. 2008;138(9):1602–8.
60. Baur JA, Ungvari Z, Minor RK, Le Couteur DG, de Cabo R. Are sirtuins viable targets for improving healthspan and lifespan? Nat Rev Drug Discov. 2012;11(6):443–61.
61. Menzies KJ, Singh K, Saleem A, Hood DA. Sirtuin 1-mediated effects of exercise and resveratrol on mitochondrial biogenesis. J Biol Chem. 2013;288(10):6968–79.
62. Global Market Information Database. 2002 [Jan 13, 2010]. Available from: http://www.euromonitor.com/alcoholic-drinks
63. World Health Organization. World Health Statistics 2010. 2010 [Jan 13, 2014]. Available from: http://www.who.int/whosis/whostat/2010/en/
64. Health OECD. Data 2005. Paris: organization for Economic Co-operation and. Development. 2014(January 13). Available from: http://stats.oecd.org/index.aspx?DataSetCode=HEALTH_STAT.

Chapter 9
Impact of Mediterranean Diet on Metabolic Syndrome

Golandam Khayef and Joan Sabaté

Key Points

- Due to its increasing prevalence in the past two decades and its associated health complications, metabolic syndrome (MetS) has become both a public health concern and a clinical challenge. Dietary approaches for the prevention and treatment of MetS vary, yet there is general agreement that the clinical parameters of the syndrome are greatly improved through lifestyle changes including diet.
- Existing evidence suggests a positive link between adherence to diets low in saturated fat, trans fat, cholesterol, added sugar, and sodium and high in unsaturated fats, complex unrefined carbohydrates, fruits, vegetables, and fish and improvement of metabolic abnormalities. Interestingly, these dietary features are characteristic of the traditional Mediterranean diet (MD). On the basis of the most current and available evidence including observational and intervention studies on management of MetS, adherence to the MD may be associated with improvements in various MetS parameters.
- Although most epidemiological studies recognize that the MD has preventive effects against MeS, some studies have been inconclusive possibly because of differences in methodologies, overall design of the studies, and quality of the data.
- Well-designed clinical trials are needed to investigate the cause–effect relationships between MD and onset of MetS and define the underlying mechanisms of actions of food components on pathways that contribute to the MetS.

Keywords Metabolic syndrome • Mediterranean diet • Diet • Lifestyle • Prevention • Treatment

G. Khayef, M.S., R.D.N. • J. Sabaté, M.D., Dr.P.H. (✉)
Department of Nutrition, School of Public Health, Loma Linda University,
24951 North Circle Drive, Room #1122 Nichol Hall, Loma Linda, CA 92350, USA
e-mail: gkhayef@llu.edu; jsabate@llu.edu

D.F. Romagnolo, O.I. Selmin (eds.), *Mediterranean Diet*, Nutrition and Health,
DOI 10.1007/978-3-319-27969-5_9

Introduction

Mediterranean dietary traditions have historically been linked to overall good health. Plant-based foods constitute the core of daily dietary intake of individuals who adhere to the traditional Mediterranean dietary patterns which if consumed in sufficient amounts, provide all of the essential macronutrients and micronutrients, and fiber believed to promote overall health [1]. Metabolic syndrome (MetS) or syndrome X is a collection of associated risk factors which significantly increase the risk of developing atherosclerosis and diabetes mellitus (DM) later in life. It has been suggested that individuals with MetS may benefit from aggressive lifestyle modifications through diet and physical activity, yet a uniform consensus is lacking as to which type of diet is optimal for prevention and treatment of this particular syndrome [2]. A growing body of scientific evidence has addressed the implications of the traditional Mediterranean diet (MD) and improvement of the MetS and its individual components. In this chapter, we summarize the existing scientific evidence on the impacts of the MD on MetS.

Metabolic Syndrome

Obesity, non-insulin-dependent diabetes mellitus, hypertension, and dyslipidemia, also referred to as the deadly quartet, are key characteristics of MetS. The concept of MetS was first described in 1920s by the Swedish physician, Kylin Studien, as a collection of metabolic and non-metabolic disturbances including hypertension, hyperglycemia and gout [2]. In 1947, the Marseilles physician, Jean Vague, made an important observation and drew attention to the important role that the upper body adiposity played in predisposing individuals to diabetes, atherosclerosis, and gout [2, 3]. Over the past two decades, the MeS has received increased attention from the health-care community, mainly due to a striking rise in its prevalence worldwide.

Definition and Diagnostic Criteria

Although the MeS has been in the spotlight for the past two decades, there has been considerable disagreement over the terminology, definition, and diagnosis criteria related to its diagnosis. In an effort to standardize the terminology used for MetS in the world of clinical practice, several organizations have undertaken the task of formulating simple criteria for the standardization of its diagnosis (Table 9.1) [4, 5]. The most commonly used criteria for clinical diagnosis of MetS, however, has been defined by the National Cholesterol Education Program (NCEP) Panel III (ATP III) as having at least three of the following [4, 5]:

1. Abdominal obesity (waist circumference = WC > 102 cm for men and > 88 cm for women).
2. High triglyceride (TG) levels (≥150 mg/dL).
3. Low high density lipoprotein cholesterol (HDL-C) levels (<40 mg/dL in men or <50 mg/dL in women).
4. High blood pressure (BP) (≥130/85 mmHg on at least two separate measurements).
5. High fasting glucose (≥100 mg/dL or ≥5.6 mmol/L).

In an attempt to unify the criteria for clinical diagnosis of MetS, a joint interim consensus statement was prepared and published by the International Diabetes Federation Task Force on Epidemiology and Prevention in October of 2009 [4]. The statement was the result of a joint meeting between the

Table 9.1 Criteria proposed for clinical diagnosis of metabolic syndrome

Clinical measure	WHO (1998)	EGIR	ATP III (2001)	AACE (2003)	IDF (2005)
Insulin resistance	IGT, IFG, T2DM, or lowered insulin sensitivity plus any two of the following	Plasma insulin >75th percentile plus any two of the following	None, but any three of the following five features	IGT or IFG plus any of the following based on clinical judgment	–
Body weight	Men: waist-to-hip ratio >0.90; women: waist-to-hip ratio >0.85 and/or BMI >30 kg/m^2	WC ≥94 cm in men or ≥80 cm in women	WC ≥102 cm in men or ≥88 cm in women	BMI ≥25 kg/m^2	Increased WC (population specific) plus any two of the following
Lipid	TG ≥150 mg/dL and/or HDL-C <35 mg/dL in men or <39 mg/dL in women	TG ≥150 mg/dL and/or HDL-C <39 mg/dL in men or women	TG ≥150 mg/dL HDL-C <40 mg/dL in men or <50 mg/dL in women	TG ≥150 mg/dL and HDL-C <40 mg/dL in men or <50 mg/dL in women	TG ≥150 mg/dL or on TG Rx HDL-C <40 mg/dL in men or <50 mg/dL in women or on HDL-C Rx
Blood pressure	≥140/90 mmHg	≥140/90 mmHg or on hypertension Rx	≥130/85 mmHg	≥130/85 mmHg	≥130 mmHg systolic or ≥85 mmHg diastolic or on hypertension Rx
Glucose	IGT, IFG, or T2DM	IGT or IFG (but not diabetes)	>110 mg/dL (includes diabetes)	IGT or IFG (but not diabetes)	≥100 mg/dL (includes diabetes)
Other	Microalbuminuria	–	–	Other features of insulin resistance	–

WHO World Health Organization, *EGIR* European Group for Study of Insulin Resistance, *ATP III* Adult Treatment Panel III, *AACE* American Association of Clinical Endocrinologists, *IDF* International Diabetes Foundation, *T2DM* type 2 diabetes mellitus, *IGT* impaired glucose intolerance, *IFG* impaired fasting glucose, *WC* waist circumference, *BMI* body mass index, *TG* triglycerides, *HDL-C* high density lipoprotein cholesterol. Adapted from Ref. [5]

following organizations: National Heart, Lung, and Blood Institute, the American Heart Association, World Heart Federation, International Atherosclerosis Society, and International Association for the Study of Obesity [4]. According to this new definition, MetS is defined as having at least three of the following criteria: abdominal obesity (waist circumference ≥94 cm for men and ≥80 cm for women), high blood pressure (systolic blood pressure/diastolic blood pressure ≥130/85 mmHg or antihypertensive medication), hypertriglyceridemia (≥1.7 mmol/L or fibrate medication), low HDL-cholesterolemia (<1.03 mmol/L for men or <1.29 mmol/L for women), and hyperglycemia (glycemia ≥ 5.6 mmol/L or antidiabetic medication) [4].

MeS: Prevalence and Clinical Significance

MetS is widespread among adults residing in developed countries, with a prevalence of about 20–30 %, or even higher [6]. According to reports from the National Health and Nutritional Examination Survey (NHANES), both unadjusted (27.9 ± 1.1 % to 34.1 ± 0.8 %, $P < 0.001$) and age-adjusted prevalence (29.2 ± 1.0 % to 34.2 ± 0.7 %, $P < 0.001$) of MetS among US adults showed a persistent increase from the periods 1988–1994 to 1999–2006 [7]. This increase in prevalence of MetS among US adults is a serious public health concern, given that it considerably raises the risks of developing DM and cardiovascular disease (CVD) later in life [7].

Another NHANES analysis of the prevalence and trends of MetS between 1999 and 2010 showed that while the prevalence of MetS (as it is currently defined by the ATP III) has slightly declined over time, there have been upward trends in abdominal obesity, particularly among female adults, and hyperglycemia across the entire US population compared to 1999 and 2000 [8]. This is particularly important, given that each condition related to the MeS is an independent risk factor for CVD and/or DM. However, when two or more conditions are clustered together, the MeS becomes increasingly atherogenic and diabetogenic raising the risk of stroke, diabetes-related complications including nephropathy, retinopathy, distal neuropathy, and cardiovascular morbidity and mortality [9]. In addition, MetS has been linked with other chronic diseases including fatty liver disease, some types of cancer, hypogonadism, and vascular dementia [10].

Mediterranean Diet in Prevention and Treatment of MeS

Dietary and lifestyle modification that include regular moderate to intense physical activity and reduction of central obesity remain the recommended cornerstone for the prevention and treatment of MetS [9–13]. While there is a general agreement over beneficial effects of regular physical activity and weight reduction for management of MetS, a uniform consensus is lacking as to which type of diet is optimal for this particular condition [14, 15]. Existing epidemiological evidence suggest a positive link between adherence to diets low in saturated fat, trans fat, cholesterol, added sugar, and sodium and high in unsaturated fats, complex unrefined carbohydrates, fruits, vegetables, and fish and improvement of metabolic abnormalities [10, 15]. Interestingly, these features resemble the principles of the traditional Mediterranean diet (MD) [15, 16].

Studies have documented that adherence to the MD lowers rates of morbidity, CVD, certain types of cancer, chronic inflammation, mortality, and improves overall health and quality of life [15, 16]. The term, MD, was described in 1960s and refers to dietary patterns found in olive-growing areas in the Mediterranean basin. Although there are several variations of the MD, common components include: high monounsaturated to saturated fat ratio; moderate consumption of ethanol (mainly in the form of red wine); moderate consumption of milk and dairy products (mainly in the form of cheese and yogurt); low intake of red meat and meat products; and high intake of fresh fruits and vegetables and whole grains [13–15]. One of the main characteristics of MD is the use of olive oil as the main source of fat in cooking [15–17].

Cross-Sectional Studies

Cross-sectional studies investigated the relationships between adherence to a MD and the prevalence of MetS [18–20]. The first study, known as ATTICA, was a study that randomly enrolled 1514 men and 1528 women over the age of 18 years with no history of CVD or DM from the Attica area of Greece [18]. Adherence to MD, among several other factors, was assessed by a diet score (with higher values representing a closer adherence to the MD) which incorporated the inherent characteristics of this diet. Closer adherence to the MD was associated with a 19 % lower risk of developing the MetS. Adherence to the traditional MD was also associated with a significant reduction in the concentration of inflammatory and coagulation markers [18]. The study did not find significant associations between adherence to the MD and HDL-C and TG concentrations in obese and overweight individuals but found a negative association with blood pressure [18, 21].

These first data, however, were only partially supported by the results of a second cross-sectional study which examined the intakes of cereal, fruit, legumes, vegetables, fish, nuts, monounsaturated fat to saturated fat ratio, alcohol from red wine, whole fat dairy products, and red meat among a representative sample of 578 adults (>18 years) from the Canary Islands (Spain) who were participating in the Canarian Nutrition Survey (ENCA). According to the ENCA study, once adjusted, adherence to MD showed no significant association with prevalence of the MetS. However, participants in the third tertile of the MD adherence had a 70 % lower prevalence of blood pressure criteria and 2.5 times more prevalence of the glycemic criteria with respect to the first tertile. Higher intake of red meat was associated with higher prevalence of blood pressure criteria whereas moderate alcohol intake from red wine was associated with lower prevalence of blood pressure in women and lower prevalence of HDL-C criteria in men. Fruit intake showed a protective effect on TG criteria, whereas vegetable intake showed a protective effect on insulin resistance. Whole fat dairy intake showed a protective effect on the glycemia criteria and high monounsaturated to saturated fatty acid intake had a positive impact on insulin resistance. Overall, the study concluded that the MD showed protective effects on specific components of the MetS [19].

In 2009, Babio et al. conducted a cross-sectional study in 808 elderly participants with no history of CVD, yet at high risk for developing CVD from the PREvencio´n con DIeta MEDiterra´nea (PREDIMED) study [20]. The PREDIMED was a 5-year parallel group, multicenter, controlled clinical trial that aimed to examine the effects of the MD on the primary prevention of CVD [20]. Participants in the highest quartile with the highest adherence to the MD had 47–54 % lower odds of having low HDL-C and high TG compared to those in the lowest quartile. Some components of the MD including olive oil, legumes, and red wine were associated with lower prevalence of MetS. Overall, higher adherence to the MD was significantly associated with lower odds ratio of developing MetS in a population at high risk of CVD.

Romaguera et al. assessed a cross-sectional association between adherence to a modified MD (high in foods of plant origin including vegetables, legumes, fruits, nuts, cereals, and unsaturated fatty acids), BMI, and WC in a total of 497,308 men and women (70.7 %) aged 25–70 years from 10 European countries [22]. This study was conducted in participants of the European Prospective Investigation into Center and Nutrition-Physical Activity, Nutrition, Alcohol, Cessation of Smoking, Eating Out of Home and Obesity or EPIC-PANACEA project [22]. Although there was no association between modified MD and BMI, results revealed that adherence to this type of diet, regardless of heterogeneity among regions, was strongly associated with lower abdominal obesity measured by WC in European men and women. This result was confirmed in a following cross-sectional analysis of 773 individuals aged 30–94 years (mean age of 60 years) from the Adventist Health Study 2 [23]. Results of this study suggested that a plant-based dietary pattern, similar to the modified MD, was associated with significantly lower means for all metabolic risk factors except HDL-C and a lower risk of having MetS (OR: 0.44, 95 % CI; 0.30–0.64, $P<0.001$). This relationship also persisted after adjusting for lifestyle and demographic factors.

Yahia et el. examined the association between MetS and the Mediterranean dietary patterns in a pilot study of 100 Lebanese Notre Dame University students (62 males and 38 females) aged 18–27 years. Students who had MetS had higher consumption of red meat and sweets and a lower consumption of legumes [24]. These results showed a promising trend with respect to lower consumption of animal foods and lower prevalence of MetS and its criteria.

Prospective Cohort Studies

Several prospective cohort studies have been published on the topic of adherence to MD and incidence of MetS in healthy individuals with no history of chronic diseases [25–27]. The Seguimiento University of Navarra (SUN) prospective cohort (an open-enrollment cohort) was the first study that assessed the relationship between adherence to the Mediterranean Food Pattern (MFP) and the subsequent development of MetS in 2563 Spanish university graduates (no risk factors present at baseline) for 6 years [25]. Results from the SUN cohort showed that the cumulative incidence of MetS was lower for those with the highest adherence to the MFP. In particular, participants with the highest MFP scores (highest adherence) showed an odds ratio of 0.20 (95 % CI, 0.06–0.63) in comparison to those with the lowest adherence. This difference also persisted after adjustment for age, sex, physical activity, smoking, and total energy intake [25]. Similar trends were observed by Rumawas et al. who examined the prospective association between a diet consistent with a Mediterranean-style dietary pattern and MetS traits and its incidence in 1918 nondiabetic US men and women of the Framingham Heart Study Offspring with baseline median age of 54 years followed for 7 years [26]. Results revealed that participants in the highest quintile category had a lower incidence (31.1 %) of MetS compared to those in the lowest quintile (38.5 %). Subjects with highest adherence to the diet had a 11.8 % less risk of developing MetS during the 7-year follow up period [26].

The SU.VI.MAX or Supplementation en Vitamines et Mineraux AntioXydants study was the first study that examined the association between adherence to MD and risk of MetS using three different Mediterranean diet-based scores (traditional Mediterranean diet score, MDS; an updated Mediterranean score, MED; and Mediterranean style-dietary pattern score, MSDPS) [27]. In addition, this was the first study which employed the most recent definition of MetS [4, 27]. A cohort of 3232 French MetS-free adult participants from the SU.VI.MAX study (1994–2002) was followed for 6 years. SU.VI. MAX was a randomized placebo-controlled trial that included 13,017 individuals to test the efficacy of daily supplementation with antioxidant vitamins (vitamins C, E, and β-carotene) and minerals (selenium and zinc) at nutritional doses on the incidence of cancers, ischemic heart disease, and overall mortality [28]. Results from the SU.VI.MAX cohort study showed that all MD scores were associated with reduced criteria of MetS and MetS incidence. However, the strength of the association was dependent on the score used to assess adherence to the diet. The association between MED score and lower MetS risk was stronger than that observed with the traditional MDS, suggesting a critical role of refined grains and sweetened beverages. The widely used MDS [29, 30] showed a negative association with incidence of MetS, but only WC and blood TG were negatively associated with the MDS.

A 2009 study evaluated the association between MD and incidence of MetS in 160 Iranian renal transplant patients 1 year following transplantation [31]. The incidence of MetS in renal transplant recipients is usually estimated to be ~60 % 1 year post-transplant. This high incidence is partially due to the effect of immunosuppressive medications and increased risk of weight gain, hyperlipidemia, hypertension, and glucose intolerance, which characterize the MetS. Corticosteroids may also have an important role in the incidence of post-transplant MetS. After adjustment for age and sex, results showed that participants in the highest tertile of the Mediterranean dietary pattern score had lower odds for the MetS (OR: 0.52, 95 % CI; 0.21–1.24) than those in the lowest tertile. Conversely, those patients in the highest tertile of the saturated fats and sugars dietary pattern score had greater odds of the MetS (OR: 1.29; 95 % CI; 0.54–3.06) than those in the lowest tertile [31]. These results with renal transplant patients were considered of particular significance since they extended the benefits of adherence to the MD beyond those previously observed in healthy individuals.

Intervention Trials

To date, only few intervention trials have been conducted to examine the relationships between adherence to a Mediterranean-like diet and MetS. Esposito et al. conducted a randomized single-blinded study from June 2001 to January 2004 on 180 patients with MetS at a University hospital in Italy in order to assess the effects of a Mediterranean-style diet on endothelial functions and vascular inflammatory markers [32]. The intervention group ($n=90$) was instructed to follow a Mediterranean-style diet and received advice on how to increase daily consumption of whole grains, fruits, vegetables, nuts, and olive oil. The intervention diet consisted of 50–60 % carbohydrates, 15–20 % protein, and <30 % total fat with less than 10 % coming from saturated fat and less than 300 mg cholesterol per day. Patients were encouraged to consume at least 250–300 g of fruits, 125–150 g of vegetables, 25–50 g of walnuts, 400 g of whole grains (legumes, rice, maize, and wheat) per day and to increase their intake of olive oil. The control group ($n=90$) followed a prudent diet which consisted of 50–60 % carbohydrates, 15–20 % protein, and <30 % total fat. Compared with patients consuming the control diet, patients consuming the intervention diet had significantly reduced serum concentrations of inflammatory markers as well as insulin resistance. Endothelial function score also significantly improved in the intervention group (mean [±SD] change, +1.9 [±0.6]; $P<0.001$) but remained nearly stable in the control group (+0.2 [±0.2]; $P=0.33$). At 2 years of follow-up, only 40 patients in the intervention group were still classified as having MetS, compared to 78 patients in the control group ($P<0.001$) [32].

In a 2008 PREDIMED study, 1 year effect of two behavioral interventions was compared with two high-fat, non-energy-restricted MDs, one supplemented with 1 L/week virgin olive oil (MD+VOO) and another supplemented with 30 g/day mixed nuts as 15 g walnuts, 7.5 g hazelnuts, and 7.5 g almonds (MD+nuts), with that of advice on a low-fat diet (control diet) in volunteers at high risk for CVD [33]. The study included 1224 participants who were recruited into the PREDIMED trial. All diets were ad libitum and there was no increase in physical activity for any of the intervention groups. After 1 year, the prevalence of MetS was significantly lower in the MD+nuts group (13.7 % vs. 6.7 % and 2.0 % in the MD+VOO and the control group respectively). Furthermore, logistic regression analysis confirmed that the MD+nuts was associated with lowering of MetS among those subjects who had the syndrome at baseline whereas the incident rates were not significantly different among groups (Fig. 9.1). The authors concluded that a non-energy restricted traditional MD supplemented with mixed nuts (high in fat, high in unsaturated fat, and palatable) was a useful approach in management of MetS [33]. The authors also stated that the study duration was too short to address clinical outcomes and that a longer follow-up of the entire PREDIMED cohort might provide stronger evidence on protective effects of the MD on CVD.

One possibility is that the protective effects of the MD on MetS observed in most studies may be due to the weight loss that occurs when individuals change their behaviors and incorporate a healthier eating plan. In order to examine the modifying effects of weight loss on the impact of the MD on CVD risk factors, Richard et al. assessed the efficacy of MD with and without weight loss on CVD risk factors in 26 men (aged 24–62 years) with MetS [34]. Participants consumed a North American control diet for 5 weeks followed by a 5-week MD, both under-weight-maintaining conditions. Participants then underwent a 20-week weight loss period, after which they consumed the MD for 5 weeks under-weight-stable conditions. All foods were provided to participants during the

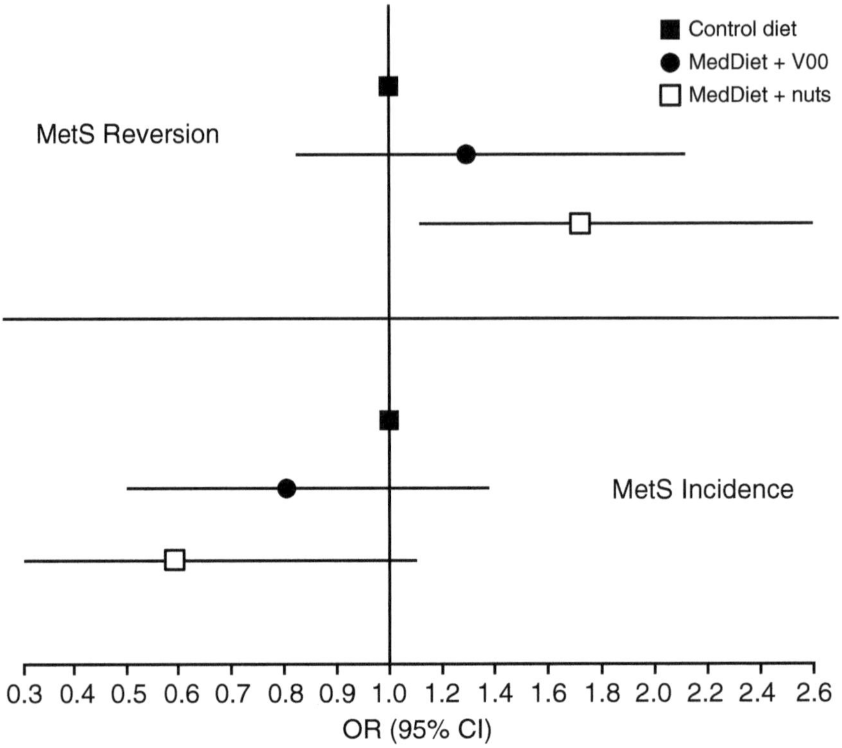

Fig. 9.1 Impact of Mediterranean diet, virgin olive oil, and nuts on MeS. Data represent odds ratio and confidence interval of 1-year reversion among participants with MetS at baseline and incidence among participants without MetS at baseline in the two MD groups in comparison with the control group [33]

weight-stable phases of the study. Results showed that in the absence of weight loss, the MD reduced total plasma cholesterol, LDL-C, and total cholesterol to HDL-C ratio compared to the control diet (all $P<0.04$). The MD in combination with weight loss resulted in reduction of systolic blood pressure, diastolic blood pressure, TG, apolipoprotein B, fasting glucose and insulin compared to the control diet (all $P<0.001$). Overall, the conclusion was that the MD in the absence of weight loss led to significant changes in plasma cholesterol concentration but had minor effects on other cardiometabolic risk factors of MetS [34].

In a 2011 study, the impact of a Mediterranean-style low-glycemic-load diet was examined in women with MetS [35]. In this 12-week, two-arm randomized clinical trial, women in the control group ($n=44$) consumed a Mediterranean-style low-glycemic-load diet and women in the intervention group ($n=45$) consumed the same diet as the control group plus a medical food containing phytosterols, soy protein, and extracts from hops and acacia. After 12 weeks, all participants showed significant decreases in WC, systolic and diastolic BP, and plasma TG in ($P<0.001$ for all) with no differences between arms. The HDL-C levels significantly decreased in week eight but returned to baseline levels by week 12 while plasma glucose concentration did not change over the course of the study. Addition of the medical food resulted in a less atherogenic lipoprotein profile and lower plasma homocysteine in the intervention arm. Both groups experienced a significant weight loss despite the fact that no caloric restriction was applied in this study. Overall, a Mediterranean-style low-glycemic-load diet effectively reduced the variables of MetS in the women of this study [15, 35].

Recently, the results of a 1-year intervention study with the MD on plasma fatty acid composition and MetS were reported in a subset of high risk participants ($n=424$, aged 55–80 years) who were randomly selected from the PREDIMED trial after completing a 1-year intervention program [6]. The detailed protocol of the PREDIMED study has been described earlier in this chapter [20, 33]. After a full year of intervention, the MD+VOO group showed a significant increase in plasma levels of palmitic and oleic acids and reduced proportions of margaric, stearic, and linoleic acids whereas MD+nuts group showed a significant rise in levels of palmitic, linoleic, and α-linolenic acids, but reduced proportions of myristic, margaric, palmitoleic, and dihomo-γ-linoleic acids. No significant weigh changes were observed in any of the study arms. Increases in the biomarkers of foods supplied to the MD groups, i.e., oleic and α-linolenic acids, were beneficially associated with the incidence, improvement, and prevalence of MetS. In conclusion, both the MD+VOO and MD+nuts diets resulted in a fatty acid composition that showed promising effects on MetS. Therefore, according to the authors of this study, a MD that is rich in fats of plant origin may be beneficial for the management of MetS without the need for concerns over potential weight gain due to the high fat content of the diet. Another recent study confirmed the beneficial effects of adherence to the MD for three months on metabolic, oxidative, and inflammatory abnormalities in 84 healthy Algerian participants (11 males and 73 females) with MetS [36]. Participants were simply advised to reduce their intake of simple carbohydrate, saturated fats, cholesterol, animal proteins, and increase intake of monounsaturated fats, olive oil, fiber, fruits, and vegetables for 3 months.

Meta-analyses

In addition to major studies reviewed so far in this chapter, several smaller clinical trials and epidemiological studies have also examined the effects of adherence to the MD on MetS and its individual components. Kastorini et al. conducted a meta-analysis of original research including epidemiological studies and randomized clinical trials until April 30, 2010 through a computer-assisted published search of PubMed, Embase, Scopus, and the Cochrane Central Register of Controlled Trials database [37]. A total of 50 original studies including 35 clinical trials, two prospective cohort studies, and 13 cross-sectional studies with 534,906 participants were included in the final analysis. Analysis of prospective and clinical studies showed that adherence to the MD was associated with reduced risk of MetS (HR = 0.96; 95 % CI, 1.24–1.16) [37]. Results of clinical studies also revealed that the MD had a protective effect on individual components of the MeS, such as WC (mean difference, 0.42 cm), HDL-C (1.17 mg/dL), TG (6.14 mg/dL), glucose (3.89 mg/dL), and systolic blood pressure (2.35 mmHg) and diastolic blood pressure (1.58 mmHg). Overall, results from clinical studies, cross-sectional studies, and prospective studies support the health benefits of the MD against MeS (Fig. 9.2).

Conclusions and Future Opportunities

Dietary approaches for the prevention and treatment of MetS vary, but there is general agreement that clinical parameters associated with the MeS can be greatly improved through lifestyle changes related to diet and physical activity. In nutritional epidemiology research, interest has shifted from the study of single nutrients to the study of food groups and more recently, to learning more about dietary patterns and how interactions between nutrients (rather than single nutrients) produce protective effects against chronic diseases and improve overall health and quality of life. In this context, the study of the Mediterranean dietary patterns in respect to MetS has received considerable interest. A substantial

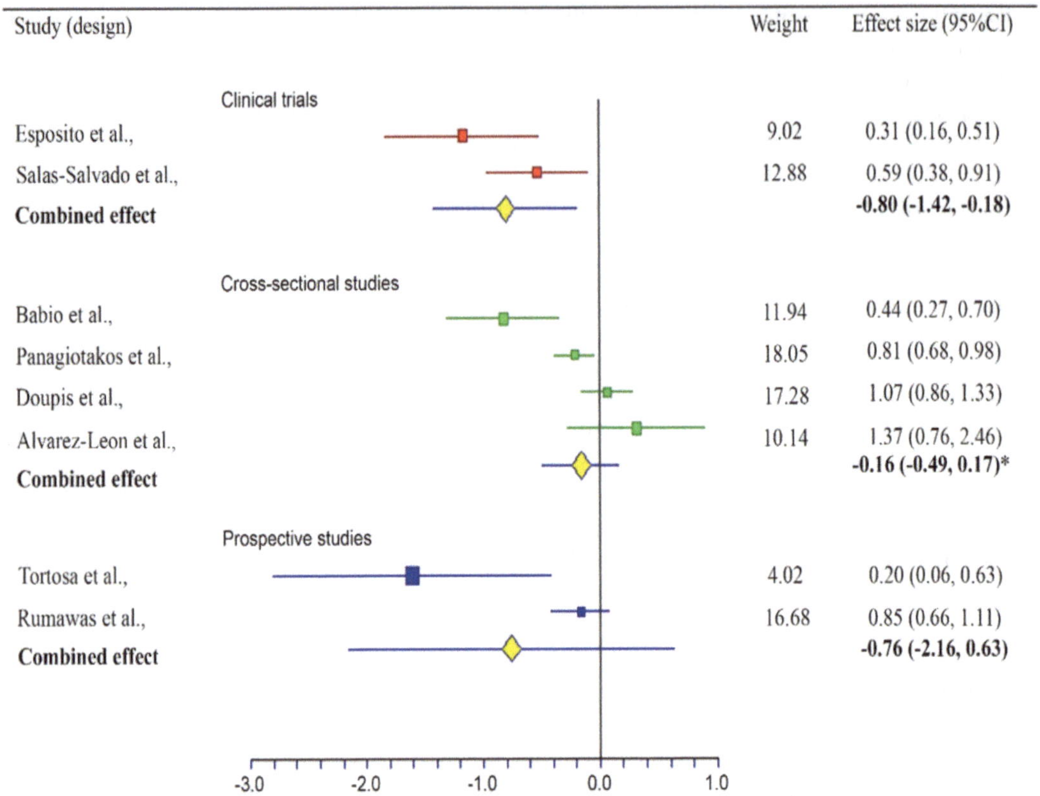

Fig. 9.2 Mediterranean diet and metabolic syndrome. Adherence to the Mediterranean diet was associated with a protective effect in two of two clinical trials, two of four cross-sectional studies, and one of two prospective studies, as compared with lower compliance with this pattern or with a control diet [37]

proportion of individuals living in the Western nations suffer from multiple metabolic abnormalities that place them at a much greater risk category for developing CVD and DM. On the basis of the most current and available evidence from observational and intervention studies, the MD may be beneficial for ameliorating conditions associated with the MeS. Although there are variations of the MD, the term essentially refers to a primarily plant-based diet that constitutes an abundance of fruits, vegetables, whole-grain cereals, nuts, and legumes; with olive oil as the primary source of fat; fish and poultry consumed in low-to-moderate amounts and relatively low consumption of red meat and dairy; and with moderate consumption of wine, normally with meals. Although the MD has been shown to contribute to weight loss in many studies, the beneficial effects of the MD on MetS seem to be independent of the weight loss.

Finally, it should be considered whether or not opportunities exist for the implementation of the MD for the prevention of MeS in Western societies. On a daily basis, the majority of people in the Western world consume large amounts of processed foods high in saturated fats, added sugar, and salt. People in Western countries spend little or no time in the kitchen cooking their meals, but more time in fast-food driving lanes picking up daily meals and restaurant franchises. Because of complex cultural and economic conditions, adherence to a Mediterranean dietary pattern remains challenging in Western societies. More studies are needed to obtain research-based evidence about the health benefits of MD against MeS and development of nutrition and lifestyle education programs for its prevention.

References

1. Willett WC, Sacks F, Trichopoulou A, Drescher G, Ferro-Luzzi A, Helsing E, et al. Mediterranean diet pyramid: a cultural model for healthy eating. Am J Clin Nutr. 1995;61(6):1402S–6.
2. Eckel RH, Grundy SM, Zimmet PZ. The metabolic Syndrome. Lancet. 2005;365:1415–28.
3. Vague J. La differenciation sexuelle, facteur determinant des formes de l'obesite. Presse Med. 1947;30:339–40.
4. Alberti KGMM, Eckel RH, Grundy SM, Zimmet PZ, Cleeman JI, Donato KA, et al. Harmonizing metabolic syndrome: A Joint interim statement of the International and Blood Institute; American Heart Association; World Heart Federation; International Diabetes Federation Task Force on Epidemiology and Prevention; National Heart, Lung, and Blood Institute; American Heart Association; World Heart Federation; International Atherosclerosis Society; and International Association for the Study of Obesity. Circulation. 2009;120:1640–45.
5. Grundy SM. Diagnosis and management of the metabolic syndrome An American Heart Association/National Heart, Lung, and Blood Institute Scientific Statement. Circulation. 2005;112:2735–52.
6. Mayneris-Perxachs J, Sala-Vila A, Chisaguano M, Castellote AI, Estruch R, Covas MI, et al. Effect of 1-year intervention with a Mediterranean diet on plasma fatty acid composition and metabolic syndrome in a population at high cardiovascular risk. PLoS ONE. 2014;9(3), e85202.
7. Mozumdar A, Liguori G. Persistent increase of prevalence of metabolic syndrome among U.S. adults: NHANES III to NHEANES 1999-2006. Diabetes Care. 2011;34:216–9.
8. Beltrán-Sánchez H, Harhay MO, Harhay MM, McElligott S. Prevalence and trends of metabolic syndrome in the adults U.S. population, 1999-2010. J Am Coll Cardiol. 2013;62(8):697–703.
9. Panagiotakos DB, Polychronopoulos E. The role of Mediterranean diet in the epidemiology of metabolic syndrome: Converting epidemiology to clinical practice. Lipids Health Dis. 2005;4:7.
10. Anagnostis P. Metabolic syndrome in the Mediterranean region: Current Status. Ind J Endocrinol Metab. 2012;16(1):72–80.
11. Cornier MA, Dabelea D, Hernandez TL, Lindstrom RC, Steig AJ, Stob NR, et al. The metabolic syndrome. Endocr Rev. 2008;29:777–822.
12. World Health Organization Study Group: Diet, Nutrition, and the Prevention of Chronic Diseases. Geneva, Switzerland: World Health Organization; Technical Report Series, 916, 2003.
13. Kontogianni MD, Panagiotakos DB. Current epidemiological and clinical evidence on the relationship between Mediterranean diet and the metabolic syndrome. Curr Nutr Food Sci. 2007;3:296–9.
14. Baxter AJ, Coyne T, McClintock C. Dietary patterns and metabolic syndrome—a review of epidemiologic evidence. Asia Pac J Clin Nutr. 2006;15:134–42.
15. Kiortsis DN, Simos YV. Mediterranean diet for the prevention and treatment of metabolic syndrome: is it worth it? Angiology. 2014;65(1):5–8.
16. Pe'rez-Lo'pez FR, Chedraui P, Haya J, Cuadros JL. Effects of the Mediterranean diet on longevity and age-related morbid conditions. Maturitas. 2009;64:67–79.
17. Minich DM, Bland JS. Dietary management of the metabolic syndrome beyond macronutrients. Nutr Rev. 2008;66(8):429–44.
18. Panagiotakos DB, Pitsavos CH, Chrysohoou C, Skoumas J, Tousoulis D, Toutouza M, et al. Impact of lifestyle habits on the prevalence of the metabolic syndrome among Greek adults from the ATTICA study. Am Heart J. 2004;147:106–12.
19. Alvarez León EE, Henríquez P, Serra-Majem L. Mediterranean diet and metabolic syndrome: A cross-sectional study in the Canary Islands. Publ Health Nutr. 2006;9:1089–98.
20. Babio N, Bullò B, Basora J, Martínez-González MA. Fernández- Ballart J, Márquez-Sandoval F, et al. Adherence to the Mediterranean diet and risk of metabolic syndrome and its components. Nutr Metab Cardiovasc Dis. 2009;19:563–70.
21. Tzima N, Pitsavos C, Panagiotakos DB, et al. Mediterranean diet and insulin sensitivity, lipid profile and blood pressure levels, in overweight and obese people; The Attica study. Lipids Health Dis. 2007;6:22.
22. Romaguera D, Norat T, Mouw T, May AM, Bamia C, Slimani N. Adherence to the Mediterranean diet is associated with lower abdominal obesity in European men and women. J Nutr. 2009;139:1728–37.
23. Rizzo NS, Sabate J, Jaceldo-Siegl K, Fraser GE. Vegetarian dietary patterns are associated with a lower risk of metabolic syndrome. Diabetes Care. 2011;34:1225–7.
24. Yahia N, Hayek G, Shahin S. Obesity, metabolic syndrome, and the Mediterranean diet in a sample of Lebanese university students. Nutr Today. 2011;46(3):138–45.
25. Tortosa A, Bes-Rastrollo M, Sanchez-Villegas A, Basterra-Gortari FJ, Nunez-Cordoba JM, Martinez-Gonzalez MA. Mediterranean diet inversely associate with the incidence of metabolic syndrome: The SUN prospective cohort. Diabetes Care. 2007;30(11):2957–9.

26. Rumawas ME, Meigs JB, Dwyer JT, McKeown NM, Jacques PF. Mediterranea-style dietary pattern, reduced risk of metabolic syndrome traits, and incidence in the Framingham offspring cohort. Am J Clin Nutr. 2009;90:1608–14.
27. Kesse-Guyot E, Ahluwalia N, Lassale C, Hercberg S, Fezeu L, Lairon D. Adherence to Mediterranean diet reduces the risk of metabolic syndrome: A 6-year prospective study. Nutr Metab Cardiovasc Dis. 2013;23:677–83.
28. Hercberg S, Galan P, Preziosi P, Bertrais S, Mennen L, Malvy D, et al. The SU.VI.MAX Study: A randomized, placebo-controlled trial of the health effects of antioxidant vitamins and minerals. Arch Intern Med. 2004;164(21):2335e42.
29. Trichopoulou A, Kouris-Blazos A, Wahlqvist ML, Gnardellis C, Lagiou P, Polychronopoulos E, et al. Diet and overall survival in elderly people. Br Med J. 1995;311(7018):1457e60.
30. Trichopoulou A, Costacou T, Bamia C, Trichopoulos D. Adherence to a Mediterranean diet and survival in a Greek population. N Engl J Med. 2003;348(26):2599e608.
31. Nafar M, Noori N, Jalali-Farahani S, Hosseinpanah F, Poorrezagholi F, Ahmadpoor P, et al. Mediterranean diets are associated with a lower incidence of metabolic syndrome one year following renal transplantation. Kidney Int. 2009;76:1199–206.
32. Esposito K, Marfella R, Ciotola M, et al. Effect of a Mediterranean-style diet on endothelial dysfunction and markers of vascular inflammation in the metabolic syndrome. A randomized trial. J Am Med Assoc. 2004;292(12):1440–6.
33. Salas-Salvado J, Fernandez-Ballart J, Ros E, Martinez-Gonzalez MA, Fito M, Estruch R, et al. Effect of a Mediterranean diet supplemented with nuts on metabolic syndrome status: One-year results from the PREDIMED randomized trial. Arch Intern Med. 2008;168(22):2449–58.
34. Richard C, Couture P, Charest A, Lamarche B. Effect of the Mediterranean diet with and without weight loss on cardiovascular risk factors in men with the metabolic syndrome. Nutr Metab Cardiovasc Dis. 2011;21:628–35.
35. Jones JL, Fernandez ML, McIntosh MS, Naim W, Calle MC. Kalynch c, et al. A Mediterranean-style low-glycemic-load diet improves variables of metabolic syndrome in women, and addition of a phytochemical-rich medical food enhances benefits on lipoprotein metabolism. J Clin Lipidol. 2011;5(3):188–96.
36. Bekkouche L, Bouchenak M, Malaisse WJ, Yahia DA. The Mediterranean diet adoption improves metabolic, oxidative, and inflammatory abnormalities in Algerian metabolic syndrome patients. Horm Metab Res. 2014;46:274–82.
37. Kastorini CM, Milionis HJ, Esposito K, Giugliano D, Goudevenos JA, Panagiotakos DB. The effect of Mediterranean diet on metabolic syndrome and its components. J Am Coll Cardiol. 2011;57:1299–313.

Chapter 10
Effects of Mediterranean Diet on the Metabolome

Jessica A. Martinez, Hector C. Keun, and Alexandros P. Siskos

Key Points

- The metabolome has been defined as the sum of all low molecular weight metabolites or chemicals present in a cell, organ, tissue, biological fluid, or organism. Metabolic profiling (metabolomics/metabonomics) experiments are typically conducted using nuclear magnetic resonance (NMR) or mass spectrometry (MS) coupled to either liquid chromatography (LC) or gas chromatography (GC).
- Metabolomics experiments can be either untargeted, i.e., metabolome wide (hypothesis generating), or targeted to characterize a specific class of metabolites or those metabolites involved in a particular biochemical pathway/mechanism, food, drug, or bioactive food component (hypothesis testing).
- Metabolomics offers substantial opportunity for nutrition researchers to understand the health effects of total diets or of individual components of diet.
- This chapter discusses the effects of foods found in the Mediterranean diet on the metabolome, with a focus on the bioactive food components found within those foods.

Keywords Mediterranean diet • Metabolomics • Metabonomics • Chronic disease • Cancer • Diabetes • Bioactive food component • Microbiome

Introduction

The metabolome has been defined as the sum of all low molecular weight metabolites or chemicals present in a cell, organ, tissue, biological fluid, or organism. It is a highly complex collection of lipids, small peptides, carbohydrates, vitamins, and other cofactors derived from both the metabolism of the host and the symbiotic microbiota, with more than 20,000 metabolites known in humans [1–3].

J.A. Martinez, Ph.D. (✉)
Department of Nutritional Sciences and The University of Arizona Cancer Center, The University of Arizona, 1501 N. Campbell Avenue, Tucson, AZ 85724, USA
e-mail: jam1@email.arizona.edu

H.C. Keun, Ph.D. • A.P. Siskos, Ph.D.
Department of Surgery and Cancer, Imperial College, South Kensington Campus, London SW7 2AZ UK
e-mail: h.keun@imperial.ac.uk; a.siskos@imperial.ac.uk

D.F. Romagnolo, O.I. Selmin (eds.), *Mediterranean Diet*, Nutrition and Health,
DOI 10.1007/978-3-319-27969-5_10

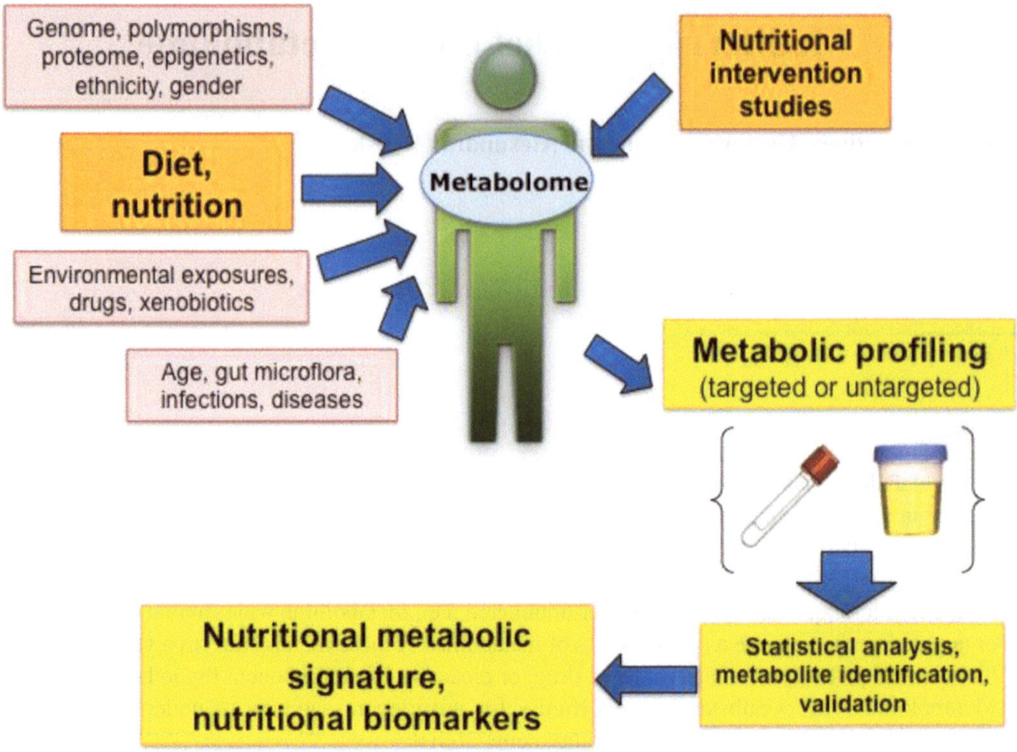

Fig. 10.1 Nutritional metabolomics. The human metabolome is the collective result of multiple interactions between dietary and lifestyle factors, as well as the products of one's genome, epigenome, transcriptome, and proteome. Metabolic profiling together with epidemiological and nutritional intervention studies can reveal the metabolic signature and metabolic effects of diet

Metabolic profiling is the study of the metabolome. Two terms, close in meaning, have been used interchangeably to describe metabolic profiling. Metabonomics was first defined by Nicholson et al. [4], whereas metabolomics was coined in 2002 by Fiehn et al. [5]. The main difference is that while metabolomics aims to characterize and quantify all the small molecules in a biological sample, metabonomics focuses on understanding the metabolic responses of living systems to pathophysiological stimuli. For consistency, the term "metabolomics" is used throughout this chapter.

An individual's metabolome reflects their exposure experience, the "exposome." It includes all dietary and lifestyle factors, as well as the products of their genome, epigenome, transcriptome, and proteome (Fig. 10.1). In this sense, the metabolome can be considered to be closer to the phenotype of one individual. The metabolome differs from other "omes" in that it represents the cumulative response of the host to a given exposure, whereas the genome and proteome represent the host's potential. Thus, metabolomics offers substantial opportunity for nutrition researchers to understand the effect of total diet or components of diet on an individual's health [6, 7]. Recently two databases that will greatly facilitate the research field of nutritional metabolomics have been established. FooDB is the world's largest and most comprehensive resource on food constituents, chemistry and biology (http://www.foodb.ca/) and is now part of the Human Metabolome Database (http://www.hmdb.ca/). In addition, Phenol-Explorer (http://www.phenol-explorer.eu/) is a comprehensive database on polyphenol content in foods, and also provides data on polyphenol metabolism and the effects of food processing and cooking. Websites like these provide a valuable repository of information that will facilitate our understanding of how exposure to diets and diet components affect an individual's metabolome.

Metabolic profiling experiments are typically conducted using either nuclear magnetic resonance (NMR) or mass spectrometry (MS) coupled to either liquid chromatography (LC) or gas chromatography (GC). The major advantage of NMR is that it is non-destructive and that no sample pretreatment is necessary. Therefore, results are highly reproducible and metabolites can be identified with high confidence. The disadvantages of NMR are its low sensitivity, poor dynamic range, and the need for relatively high volumes of samples. In MS-based metabolomics, while analysis requires destruction of the sample, there is typically a wide dynamic range, excellent sensitivity, and rich structural information. In a biological specimen during a single run, NMR-based metabolomics can typically detect up to 50 metabolites, GC-MS on the order of a couple hundred, LC-MS on the order of a few thousand depending on the MS type. Therefore, as LC-MS technology advances, it is becoming a mainstay for metabolomics experiments.

As the ability to measure more metabolites in a given experiment increases, so does the need for appropriate statistical tools to analyze the data. Typically data is first analyzed using principal components analysis (PCA), which creates a visual summary of the data. PCA facilitates the simultaneous comparison of a large number of metabolites between different study groups without a priori knowledge of the metabolite compositions. More supervised data analysis techniques include discriminant analysis based on partial least-squares regression (PLS-DA) and orthogonal partial least-squares discriminant analysis (OPLS-DA) which models structured noise separately and is thus more straightforward than PLS-DA [8, 9]. A major challenge with statistical analysis of metabolomics data is incorporating the fact that most metabolites are interconnected in a biological network. Further specific analytical challenges are beyond the scope of this chapter. However, it is important to note that the statistical approach including data preprocessing and normalization will depend on whether the experiment is an untargeted metabolome-wide analyses (hypothesis generating) or targeted, pathway-based profiling (hypothesis testing of a well-defined pathway or group of metabolites) [10]. Results from examples of both approaches to evaluate the effect of components of the Mediterranean diet on the metabolome are included in this chapter.

Despite its challenges, metabolomics offers a strategy for not only assessing intake, but also for assessing individual response to dietary exposure without the need for prior knowledge of food composition/chemistry [11, 12]. A Mediterranean-style eating pattern is rich with bioactive food components that have diverse heath-effects; metabolomics profiling offers a strategy to capture the systemic effects of those components. Given the associations with the Mediterranean style diet and various beneficial health outcomes, there is a need to strengthen the evidence base for dietary recommendations of specific foods as well as for monitoring the effects of dietary interventions. This chapter discusses the effects of foods found in the Mediterranean diet on the metabolome, biomarkers of intake discovered from metabolomics analyses, as well as the metabolome-wide effects of specific bioactive food components. The effect of diet on metabolites produced by the gut microbiome is also highlighted throughout.

Epidemiological Studies

The application of omics and specific metabolomics technologies to large population-based studies and their associated biobanks raise exciting new opportunities for the assessment of diet patterns [13]. Metabolic phenotypes represent the collective result of interactions among a variety of factors mainly nutritional, dietary, gut microbial, genetic, lifestyle, or environmental. Nutri-metabolomics, the application of metabolomics to nutritional sciences, offers the possibility to measure metabolic responses associated with the consumption of specific nutrients and foods [14, 15]. Metabolic profiles show large interindividual differences and are characteristic of an individual at a particular time in their life. Moreover, differences can be observed at the population level when comparing for example populations from different regions. While there have been no epidemiologic studies completed to date which have been designed to specifically capture the effects of the Mediterranean diet on the metabolome, many of these large cohort studies have elucidated the role of elements of the Mediterranean diet such as olive oil, fish consumption, and fiber intake.

In a recent study of 4,630 individuals from 16 sites across four countries (China, Japan, the UK, and the USA), part of the INTERMAP project (International Study of Macro/micronutrients and Blood Pressure) the diversity of human metabolic phenotype was associated with diet and blood pressure [16, 17]. Two matched 24-h urine samples were analyzed by ^{1}H NMR spectroscopy and a range of pattern recognition tools. This work showed that metabolic profiles could differentiate population centers as well as dietary habits. Importantly, the metabolites responsible for these discriminations across individuals, in particular formate, were associated with blood pressure (hypertension) across individuals, a prognostic factor for coronary disease and component of the metabolic syndrome phenotype. Moreover, distinction between Chinese subjects according to the dietary source of proteins (vegetable or animal) using untargeted profiling was achieved. Within INTERMAP, it was also determined that lower intake of total and raw vegetables and fresh fruits, identified through dietary assessment and metabolomics analysis, possibly accounted for higher blood pressure of the African Americans compared with White Americans [18]. Taken together, these studies through the INTERMAP cohort demonstrated that metabolic phenotyping of high quality epidemiological data can elucidate the mechanisms and provide novel biomarkers related to cardiovascular disease risk.

The European Prospective Investigation into Cancer and Nutrition (EPIC) study is a multicenter prospective cohort of healthy, middle-aged subjects who are followed throughout their lives in order to investigate the relationships between diet, nutritional status, lifestyle, and environmental factors and the incidence of cancer and other chronic diseases [19]. Thus far over 521,000 participants have been recruited. In a nested case–control pilot study of colon (24 cases and 23 controls) and breast (19 cases and 20 controls) cancers, authors identified plasma ^{1}H NMR metabolomics signatures as an intermediate biomarker of colon cancer risk related to low dietary fiber intake [20]. The link between dietary fiber and colorectal cancer prevention was strengthened in a cohort of 477,312 EPIC participants (HR per 10 g/day increase in fiber 0.87, 95 % CI: 0.79–0.96) [21]. Metabolomics work to identify intermediate biomarkers of risk has yet to be conducted with this large of a sample within EPIC.

Using targeted metabolomics approaches, dietary patterns have been associated with phospholipids or their constituting fatty acids in two different population studies [22, 23]. Plasma phospholipid fatty acids were correlated to fish, olive oil and margarine intake in the EPIC study [22], whereas in the Cooperative Health Research in the Region of Augsburg (KORA) study higher saturation and shorter chain length in phospholipids were associated with high dietary fiber intake [23]. Both these studies indicated that these metabolites could be used as biomarkers of exposure in epidemiological studies.

An ongoing trial called the NU-AGE project is based on the hypothesis that adherence to the Mediterranean whole diet for 1 year will reduce "inflammaging," the low grade inflammatory status that is a major characteristic of aging and plays a critical role in the pathogenesis of age-related diseases. Before and after the dietary intervention a comprehensive set of omics analyses, including metabolomics will be performed to identify the underpinning molecular mechanisms [24]. This trial is projected to complete in May 2016.

In addition to these large, prospective cohort studies, multiple clinical trials, animal studies, and cell culture experiments have investigated the effect of interventions with particular foods and components within the Mediterranean diet on the metabolome. There have also been multiple studies to investigate biomarkers of intake of particular foods. These studies are presented in the following sections organized by food group.

Olive Oil

Consumption of high levels of olive oil is probably the most recognized component of a Mediterranean style eating pattern. Olive oil extracted from the olive fruit is comprised of more than 98 % monounsaturated, polyunsaturated and saturated fatty acids mainly in the form of triacylglycerols. It is also a good source of free fatty acids (mono- and di-acylglycerols), sterols, and natural antioxidants such as polyphenols, tocopherols, terpenols, and terpenic acids. The levels of the components of olive oil, however, can vary due to region in which the olives were collected, soil, processing, and storage [25, 26]. Therefore, assessment of intake of these components is difficult when relying on traditional diet assessment tools such as food frequency questionnaires or 24-h diet recall.

Despite variability in the exact components, high olive oil diets have been consistently associated with reduced risk for diabetes, cardiovascular disease, various cancers, and other chronic diseases [27]. A series of studies conducted by Razquin et al. indicate that, while genetic factors play a role, weight loss is improved when individuals follow a Mediterranean diet supplemented with extra-virgin olive oil, compared to supplementation with nuts or the Mediterranean diet alone [28–30]. While the positive health effects of olive oil were initially attributed to the monounsaturated oleic acid, the phenolic components also probably play a role due to their antioxidant, anti-inflammatory, and antimicrobial activities.

Given that olive oil contains multiple components that result in a wide range of health effects through varying metabolic pathways, a metabolomics approach to understanding its systemic effects makes good sense. To date, limited metabolomics work has been conducted and most studies focus on bioavailability of specific, known olive oil components, hydroxytyrosol, tryosol, and oleuropein [31]. Garcia-Villalba et al. characterized phase I and phase II metabolites of olive oil in the urine of ten healthy volunteers (5 male, 5 female, ages 24–35 years). This study identified 60 phenolic metabolites in urine after olive oil consumption; in particular, metabolites derived from deacetoxy oleuropein were identified as putative biomarkers of olive oil consumption [32]. Oleuropein is a secoiridoid glycoside with several pharmacological properties, including antioxidant, cardioprotective, antiatherogenic effects, and has been commercially available as an Herbal Medicinal Product [33]. Oleuropein may also have a direct effect on the gut, as indicated in a metabolomics analysis of colorectal cancer cell culture and medium, where oleuropein aglycone (and its derivatives) as well as quercetin were identified as the main compounds in olive oil that exerted an antiproliferative effect [34]. Future work should determine whether these metabolites are associated with the protective effects of olive oil against colon cancer as well as whether they can be used as a biomarker of olive oil consumption for future dietary studies.

The beneficial effects of olive oil may also be attributed to modulation of metabolism through changes in the gut microbiota. The phenolic compounds in olive oil are not completely absorbed by the upper gastrointestinal (GI) tract and thus reach the lower GI where they are metabolized by the gut microflora and selectively stimulate the beneficial bacteria, *Lactobacillus*, and may alter cholesterol metabolism [35]. Given that variations in gut microbiota and their corresponding metabolite profiles have been demonstrated to have an effect on mammalian health [36], future metabolomics studies to evaluate the effects of olive oil in humans should also take into consideration the influence of host–microbiota interactions on metabolism.

Fish and Seafood

A Mediterranean-style eating pattern includes high fish and seafood intake, with an emphasis on those high in the ω-3 fatty acids eicosapentaenoic acid (EPA) and docosahexaenoic acid (DHA). There is an inverse relationship between fish consumption and cardiovascular disease in epidemiological studies [37], and EPA and DHA are mechanistically associated with cardioprotection [38]. The ω-3 fatty acids found in fish have been associated with reduced risk for multiple cancers, and in particular colorectal cancer [39].

While EPA and DHA are the primary fatty acids in fish, actual composition varies depending on whether the fish was wild or farmed as well as its feeding pattern [40]. An NMR-based metabolomics analysis of sea bass determined that farmed fish had roughly six times higher levels of di-unsaturated fatty acids, and much lower total polyunsaturated fatty acids, EPA and DHA. Levels of fatty acids, cholesterol, choline, trimethylamine-*N*-oxide (TMAO), glycine, fumaric acid, and malic acid also varied depending on whether the bass was wild or farmed [41]. These studies support a role for metabolomics analysis in assessing exposure to specific food components rather than deriving estimated intake using traditional dietary assessment techniques.

To our knowledge, only one study to date has investigated the effect of whole fish intake on the human metabolome. Lloyd et al. employed a metabolomics-based approach for assessing dietary exposure to smoked salmon (among other test foods). TMAO, anserine, and its metabolites 1- and 3-methylhistidine, were all increased in postprandial urine after a smoked salmon dietary challenge [42]. TMAO is an oxidation product of trimethylamine, and a common metabolite of choline (found in all meat products) produced by the gut flora [43]. The authors conclude that 1-methylhistidine could be a biomarker for fish consumption given that the parent compound, anserine, is low in other meat sources.

Perhaps because of the challenges associated with whole food metabolomics, the vast majority of metabolomics work has focused on EPA and DHA supplementation. EPA and DHA are metabolized by cyclooxygenase 2 (COX-2), which is expressed in epithelium, adipose, stroma, and collagen to produce anti-inflammatory metabolites. Conversely, COX-2 also metabolizes the ω-6 fatty acids, including arachidonic acid, to produce pro-inflammatory prostaglandins such as prostaglandin E_2 (PGE_2) [44]. Overproduction of PGE_2 is associated with multiple cancer types, inflammation-related chronic diseases and chronic pain [45–47]. In addition to COX-2, ω-6 and ω-3 fatty acids are also metabolized through two other major enzymatic pathways, lipoxygenases (LOX) and cytochrome P450 (CYP450), producing over 100 measureable metabolites and breakdown products called oxylipins. Many oxylipins have known clinical activity (protective if derived from ω-3) relating to pain, blood pressure, inflammation, cancer and cardiovascular health when studied individually [44, 48, 49]. In an effort to understand the relationship between this pathway and clinical outcomes, Dr. Bruce Hammock's group at the University of California, Davis has developed a targeted profiling method of the oxylipin metabolome in order to quantify 108 oxylipins using MS-based methods [50]. Using their methods, Schuchardt et al. demonstrated that after 12 weeks ω-3 fatty acid supplementation, both hyper- and normolipidemic men demonstrated significant increases in anti-inflammatory ω-3 derived oxylipins with a concurrent decrease in pro-inflammatory ω-6 derived oxylipins [51]. It is possible that diets high in ω-3 fatty acids, such as the Mediterranean diet, are associated with beneficial health outcomes because of the availability of ω-3 precursors for anti-inflammatory metabolites.

Because inflammation is a known tumor-promoter, there have been clinical trials using EPA as an anti-inflammatory agent in the context of cancer prevention. For example, in a randomized, double-blind, placebo-controlled trial of patients with familial adenomatous polyposis, 2 g EPA supplementation daily for 6 months had a comparable effect on reduced polyp number and size to that of the COX-2 inhibitor, celecoxib [52]. Currently, there is a randomized, double-blind, placebo-controlled, 2×2 factorial efficacy study trial, called The seAFOod Polyp Prevention Trial, actively recruiting. The primary aim of this trial is to determine whether EPA prevents colorectal adenomas, either alone or in combination with aspirin. Bioactive lipid mediators such as ω-3 PUFAs, 18R-HEPE, RvE1, and PGE-M in plasma, urine, erythrocytes, and rectal mucosa will also be measured in order to gain insight into the mechanism(s) of action of EPA and aspirin, alone and in combination, as well as to discover predictive biomarkers of EPA and/or aspirin chemoprevention efficacy [53]. Comprehensive assessment of ω-6 and ω-3 fatty acid metabolites in future studies through both targeted and untargeted approaches will continue to elucidate their relationship to cancer and other chronic diseases.

Low Red Meat

Low consumption of red meat is also considered an aspect of a Mediterranean style eating pattern. Because meat type (beef, chicken, pork, fish, etc.) is related to health outcomes, reliable and specific biomarkers of meat intake are needed as compliance markers for human trials. Of those metabolites identified thus far (e.g., creatine, creatinine, carnosine, anserine, ophidine, sulfate, and sulfite) none have proved specific or reliable enough for clinical use [54]. A metabolomics approach then may offer the opportunity to explore new biomarkers that are specific to the meat source.

There have been a few studies that aimed to assess the effect of whole meat intake on the metabolome. In a feeding study conducted by Dr. Jeremy Nicholson's group at Imperial College, U.K., discrimination between high meat, low meat, and vegetarian dietary treatments was dominated by elevated excretion of creatinine, creatine, TMAO, taurine, and 1- and 3-methylhistidine in the high meat diet and p-hydroxyphenylacetate with a vegetarian diet [55]. In a similar study, TMAO was the primary discriminating metabolite and was lower in strict lactovegetarians compared to omnivores [56]. O'Sullivan et al. identified phenylacetylglutamine as a biomarker of high vegetable intake, and *O*-acetylcarnitine as a marker of red meat intake in a double-blind, randomized, placebo-controlled dietary intervention ($N=160$) [57]. All of these studies were conducted using NMR as the metabolomics platform; it is possible that the use of more sensitive techniques could elucidate a more specific meat biomarker.

Because it is produced by the gut flora, TMAO may be a good biomarker of changes in the host gut flora and cardiovascular risk that are associated with high red meat intake. In a prospective cohort ($N=1876$), Wang et al. found a dose-dependent relationship between TMAO and risk of cardiovascular disease. In a mouse model these investigators determined that TMAO plasma levels were significantly related to atherosclerotic plaque size. TMAO was suppressed by broad spectrum antibiotics, with a concurrent decrease in macrophage foam cell formation [58]. In another smaller study with seven healthy volunteers, core metabolomes remained stable after food challenge, however metabolites produced by the gut microbiome changed considerably. Specifically, after consumption of animal protein, choline and related microbial metabolites (including TMAO) were most affected [59]. Taken together, these studies indicate that TMAO may be a useful biomarker of gut flora status and exemplify the interplay between the host and gut microbiome.

Whole Grains

Consumption of whole grains, in form of bread, pasta, and rice, is a major characteristic of the Mediterranean style eating pattern and has been associated with reduced risk for multiple cancer types, type 2 diabetes, obesity, and cardiovascular disease [60–62]. In one of the first investigations of biomarkers of whole grain intake, a crossover metabolomics study of pig urine, a whole-grain diet was characterized by betaine and hippurate excretion while creatinine excretion was associated with the non-whole-grain diet [63]. In a dietary intervention study of 77 overweight subjects, urinary hippurate was associated with fiber intake [64]. In the KORA study mentioned earlier, higher saturation and shorter chain length in phospholipids were associated with high dietary fiber intake [23]. Future work should relate metabolites associated with whole grains or fiber to dietary intake as well as health outcomes.

High Fruits and Vegetables

Epidemiological evidence suggests that diets comprised of high fruits and vegetables, such as the Mediterranean diet are associated with reduced risk for cardiovascular disease, cancer, and other chronic diseases [65]. The health effects of fruits and vegetables have been largely attributed to a wide range of phytochemicals that act as bioactive food components. According to Dr. Duke's Phytochemical and Ethnobotanical Database (www.ars-grin.gov/duke/plants.html) there are 100–300 known phytochemicals in any given plant. Many of these phytochemicals affect multiple biological pathways [66], therefore, recent efforts focused on their effects both as purified supplements and as components of whole food on the metabolome, as well as their associated health effects. In feeding studies, the metabolomic changes induced by plant polyphenols seem to be primarily derived from the microbiome [67]. In order to more effectively study these changes, a GC-MS method has been developed specifically for phenolic microbial fermentation products in urine, plasma, and fecal water [68]. Future metabolomics studies should investigate interactions between dietary polyphenols and the gut microbiome and their association with health and disease states.

In a dietary study designed to determine the effect of polyphenols on the metabolome, healthy participants (12 women, 9 men) provided first void urine samples following randomization to either their normal diet, a 2-day low-phytochemical diet, or a 2-day standard phytochemical diet [69]. Hippurate excretion was characteristic of the standardized phytochemical and normal diets while creatinine and methylhistidine excretion discriminated the low-phytochemical diet. Other discriminating ions were not identified; however, this was one of the first studies to suggest that phytochemicals in fruits and vegetables significantly change metabolomics profiles and that profiles could be used to identify biomarkers of intake.

Raspberries as well as broccoli contain high levels of polyphenols [70, 71]. Lloyd et al. showed that metabolite biomarkers in urine present after raspberry challenge were caffeoyl sulfate, ascorbate, methyl-epicatechin sulfate, 3-hydroxyhippuric acid, and naringenin glucuronide [42]. In the same study, Lloyd et al. also showed that biomarkers in urine present after broccoli challenge were ascorbate, tetronic acids, tetronic acid derivative, L-xylonate/L-lyxonate, threitol/erythritol, naringenin glucuronide, and hesperitin glucuronide [42]. The authors concluded that each of these metabolites is a putative biomarker of exposure to raspberry or broccoli intake, and that further studies should investigate the relationships between these biomarkers and health outcomes.

Citrus comprises a large proportion of the fruit consumed within a Mediterranean-style eating pattern and is associated with multiple health benefits. In a controlled feeding study conducted by the group of Jeremy Nicholson at Imperial College, proline betaine was identified as a novel short-term marker of citrus consumption using NMR-based metabolomics profiling [72]. Lloyd et al. also identified proline betaine as a marker of habitual intake as well as acute exposure in urine using a metabolomics approach [73]. In a study comparing orange juice, a proline betaine supplement, and placebo, Atkinson demonstrated that while proline betaine increased in urine with either orange juice or supplementation, it was not present in plasma [74].

Limonene is the major component in the essential oils of citrus fruits. In the context of animal models of solid tumors, limonene affects multiple pathways, and likely multiple targets within a pathway [75]. In order to identify systemic markers of limonene activity, we performed metabolomics analysis on plasma samples collected from our recently completed trial with early stage breast cancer patients [76]. Pathway-based alterations included a general increase in bile acids; a general decrease in sulfated adrenal/gonadal steroids; an increase in collagen breakdown products; changes in energy metabolism as well as changes in markers suggesting an overall decrease in inflammation. There was also a significant decrease in the cell proliferation marker cyclin D1 in breast tumor tissue. In the current metabolomics analysis, we identified 53 metabolites whose change from pre- to post-intervention was significantly correlated with the reduction in cyclin D1. Changes were primarily observed in two classes of compounds: acylcarnitines and lysoglycerophosphocholines. Our results suggest that surrogate markers of limonene effect in breast tissue are detectable in plasma [77].

Legumes

Legumes comprise numerous elements of the Mediterranean diet; examples include alfalfa, clover, lupins, green beans and peas, peanuts, soybeans, dry beans, broad beans, dry peas, chickpeas, and lentils [78]. Soybeans are of particular interest for metabolomics studies because of their high concentration of isoflavones, which have been widely studied for their health benefits [79, 80].

Solanky et al. conducted one of the first metabolomics analyses of a dietary soy intervention using NMR [81]. Healthy premenopausal women (N=5) were given a controlled diet for 1 month. After this period, 60 g soy protein, corresponding to 45 mg isoflavones, was added to the basal diet. Metabolomics profiling of plasma revealed a decrease in sugars and an increase in lactate as well as variations in isoleucine, valine, triglycerols, and choline. Two years later, the same group conducted a dietary intervention in premenopausal women with either 60 g conjugated isoflavones (in the form of soy texturized vegetable protein) or 50 g unconjugated isoflavones (miso) [82]. The authors reported subtle changes post interventions in urinary metabolic profiles associated with osmolyte fluctuation and energy metabolism. Specifically, in 24-h urine there were increased levels of TMAO, *N*-acetylglutamate, citrate, methylamine, and dimethylamine; and reduced creatine and hippurate. This was one of the first studies to demonstrate that metabolomics profiling could be used to assess novel soy biomarkers of intake.

In terms of relating metabolites to clinical outcomes, one case control study within a multiethnic cohort, used MS to assess a panel of urinary phytoestrogens in relationship to breast cancer. Although dietary soy intake was not measured, excretion of genistein and an index of total isoflavones were significantly lower among women with breast cancer, suggesting a protective effect of dietary soy and lignans [83]. Future studies should integrate changes in the "isoflavone metabolome" with changes in host innate metabolome after soy intervention in order to understand individual response to soy.

Red Wine

Light to moderate red wine consumption is associated with reduced all-cause mortality and specifically, protection against cardiovascular disease. These benefits are observed for consumption of up to two glasses of wine (~300 mL/day) for men and one glass for women [84]. The protective effects of wine may be associated with the high polyphenol content. In order to understand systemic responses to wine consumption, Grun et al. has developed a GC-TOF-MS method to profile phenolic compounds that included red wine phenols derived from the gut flora in human urine, plasma, and feces [68]. This group then used this method to examine differences in urine polyphenol profiles of men and women (N=58) after consumption of extracts from red wine and from grape juice for 4 weeks. Results documented significant increases in 19 microbial-derived polyphenol metabolites [85]. Jacobs et al developed a method using NMR to characterize the metabolome of human feces. This method was applied to a small, randomized, cross-over clinical study in which participants ($N = 39$) consumed a polyphenol-rich diet of either grape juice or ethanol-free red wine extract for 4 weeks. Interestingly, no consistent polyphenol-related changes were observed in the stool samples [86]. Vazques-Fresno et al. was the first to compare NMR metabolomics profiles in urine of men and women (N=61) after consumption of red wine, alcohol-free red wine, and gin. They found that the branched chain amino acid metabolite, 3-methyl-2-oxovalerate was higher in the wine groups indicating interaction with this metabolic pathway by both wines but not gin. Tartrate, a compound that improves polyphenol bioavailability, was higher in urine after wine intake (with or without alcohol) compared to gin. The authors concluded that tartrate could be a potential biomarker of red wine intake [87]. Boto-Ordonez conducted metabolomics profiling of urine using UPLC-MS/MS in healthy men (N=36) after dealcoholized red wine consumption. A total of 37 metabolites were identified, of these 21 phase II metabolites and 28 microbial metabolites increased significantly with dealcoholized red wine consumption [88]. While relationship to health outcomes remains to be elucidated, these studies highlighted the advantage of metabolomics approaches to elucidate systemic responses to wine, and the role of the gut microbiota in red wine polyphenol metabolism.

While many red wine phenols have biological activity, the bioactive component that has received the most attention is resveratrol [89]. Resveratrol belongs to a class of defense molecules called phytoalexins produced in response to stress such as infection or UV irradiation. It is produced naturally by 72 different plant species in addition to grapevines, particularly pines and legumes [90]. Since its presence was first reported in red wine, scientists have speculated that the cardioprotective effects of red wine (so called French paradox) may be attributed to resveratrol [91, 92]. In addition to its putative cardioprotective effects, it has also been investigated extensively for its potential health promoting properties including antioxidant, anti-neurodegenerative, anticancer, antimutagenic, chemopreventive, anti-inflammatory, and antiplatelet effects [93, 94].

Zamora-Ros et al. conducted a profiling study of urinary resveratrol metabolites in order to determine if they could be used as a biomarker of wine consumption in free-living adults. Resveratrol metabolites correlated directly with reported daily amounts of wine consumed ($R=0.895$; $P<0.001$) and even one drink per week could be detected. Wine consumers from non-wine consumers could be discriminated with 93.3 % (CI: 91.5–94.7 %) sensitivity and 92.1 % (CI: 90.2–93.7 %) specificity [95]. This study indicated that urinary levels of resveratrol metabolites could potentially be used as a biomarker to investigate the relationship between wine consumption and health benefits.

Resveratrol has demonstrated cancer chemopreventive activity in vivo in a wide variety of tumors including skin, mammary, gastrointestinal, and liver cancer models [96–102]. Resveratrol has been shown to inhibit carcinogenesis by affecting various molecular events in the initiation, promotion and progression stages [103–106]. Despite the range in anticancer activities, metabolomics studies of resveratrol in the context of cancer have been limited in number. In breast cancer cell lines MDA-MB-231 and MCF-7, resveratrol administration (5–100 μM concentration range) resulted in significantly reduced cell viability. There was a concurrent increase in the synthesis of serotonin, kynurenine, and spermidine up to 61-fold indicating that resveratrol may interact with cellular biogenic amine metabolism. Resveratrol also resulted in a pronounced increase in arachidonic acid and its metabolite 12-HETE, which may indicate oxidative stress, with a decrease in the tumor-promoting metabolite, PGE_2 [107]. Because resveratrol is known to act as a calorie restricting mimetic, Massimi et al. conducted a metabolomics analysis of the exometabolome of resveratrol-treated hepatoblastoma cell line, HepG2. The metabolite profiles indicated a metabolic switch from glucose and amino acid utilization to fat utilization for energy with resveratrol treatment [108].

Outside the cancer setting, resveratrol may also have the effect of energy restriction through interaction with metabolic pathways [109, 110]. There has been one metabolomics analysis in mice fed a high-fat diet. A combination of transcriptomics and metabolomics profiling of the mouse livers showed that a combination of resveratrol (0.2 %) and quercetin (0.2 %) (a flavonol also abundant in red wine) changed glucose/lipid metabolic profiles as well as inflammatory and cardiovascular profiles back to those mice fed control chow and more than when fed alone (both at 0.4 % diet) [111]. Future metabolomics studies should investigate the effect of both red wine and of resveratrol alone on energy restricting pathways in humans.

Coffee

While not always considered a part of the Mediterranean diet per se, there is high coffee consumption among individuals in the Mediterranean region [112]. Coffee contains multiple polyphenols that have been associated with positive health outcomes including reduced cancer risk, protection against neurodegenerative disorders, Parkinson's, and diabetes [113]. Some case–control studies suggest increased risk for cardiovascular disease; however, prospective cohort studies do not support this association and suggest a protective effect [113]. Coffee's most abundant polyphenolic constituents are chlorogenic acids (quinic acid esters of hydroxycinnamates) accounting for 6–10 % of coffee on a dry-weight basis [114]. However, roasted coffee consists of more than 800 components, including caffeine, vitamins, minerals, lipids, diterpenes, carbohydrates, as well as volatile and nonvolatile acids [115].

In order to understand which coffee components are associated with putative health outcomes, and to understand the individuals' response to coffee, several research groups have developed methods to measure coffee polyphenols and other components in blood and urine. In a targeted approach, Ito et al. quantified 15 polyphenols in the urine of 9 subjects (4 men, 5 women) using HPLC-MS after consumption of coffee and other beverages [116]; m-coumaric acid, a microbial metabolite of caffeic acid and chlorogenic acid, were identified as biomarkers of coffee consumption. Allard et al. then compared capillary electrophoresis-mass spectrometry "fingerprints" of urine samples obtained after intake of coffee, tea, or water [117]. Urine samples were collected from 13 individuals 2 h after intake of each beverage for 3 days at three separate occasions. The authors identified "fingerprint" profiles that differentiated each beverage. Further, they were able to confirm the results of Ito et al. identifying coumaric acid, caffeic acid, and chlorogenic acids as putative urinary biomarkers of coffee intake.

Using both NMR and HPLC-MS, Stalmach et al. identified 21 metabolites, primarily sulfates and glucuronides in urine and plasma of human subjects 24-h after ingestion of 200 mL instant coffee [118]. Coffee conjugates indicated colonic microflora-mediated conversion of caffeoylquinic acids to caffeic acid and dihydrocaffeic acid, and feruloylquinic acids to ferulic acid and dihydrocaffeic acid. The 0- to 24-h excretion of the parent compounds and their metabolites corresponded to 29.1 % of intake. These results suggested coffee chlorogenic acids are bioavailable to a much greater extent than other flavonoids and phenolic compounds present in coffee. The authors concluded that urinary dihydrocaffeic acid-3-*O*-sulfate and feruloylglycine would serve as very sensitive biomarkers for the consumption of relatively small amounts of coffee.

Using LC-MS, Nagy et al. were the first group to identify dimethoxycinnamic acids as potential coffee biomarkers in human plasma [119]. The same group identified a total of 34 coffee metabolites in the plasma of 9 healthy subjects (4 male, 5 female) using UPLC-MS/MS [120]. A total of 22 phenolic acid derivatives and 12 chlorogenic acid derivatives appeared in human plasma as a result of coffee consumption, metabolites mainly reduced include sulfated and methylated forms of caffeic acid, coumaric acid, caffeoylquinic acid and caffeoylquinic acid lactone. The same authors identified 19 novel circulating coffee metabolites for the first time in human plasma without enzymatic treatment; these included feruloylquinic acid lactone, sulfated and glucuronidated forms of feruloylquinic acid lactone, and sulfated forms of coumaric acid.

Altimair et al. examined the consequences of coffee consumption on human metabolism using serum from participants of the KORA study population, specifically males ($N=284$) between 55 and 79 years of age. Using a targeted lipidomics approach with LC-MS/MS and derivatization, they measured 363 metabolites. Coffee intake was positively associated with levels of cholesterol as well as two classes of sphingomyelins, one containing a hydroxy-group and the other having an additional carboxy-group. Long- and medium-chain acylcarnitines were found to decrease with increasing coffee consumption. The authors concluded that the association between hydroxylated and carboxylated sphingolipid species and coffee intake may be either related to changes in the cholesterol levels or that these molecules may act as scavengers of oxidative species, which decrease with higher coffee intake [121]. Further research is necessary to determine which of the discussed biomarkers, if any, in human plasma or urine may be associated with health outcomes related to coffee intake.

Reduced Body Size

One of the consequences of a Mediterranean versus Westernized eating pattern is reduced body size [122]. A few studies have investigated the difference between metabolite profiles of healthy obese vs lean individuals. Using NMR-based metabolomics, Kochlar et al. found that compared to obese subjects, plasma levels of choline and citrate were elevated in both male and female lean participants (BMI<21 kg/m2), whereas tyrosine, isoleucine, and glycoprotein levels were reduced. In urine, citrate was unrelated to BMI in females, whereas it was lower in lean vs obese males [123]. A growing body of evidence indicates that branched chain amino acids are increased in obese vs lean individuals and may play a role in the etiology of insulin resistance and diabetes; this evidence is reviewed by Morris et al. [124].

Although the exact mechanisms linking the metabolome to body size have yet to be determined, a growing body of evidence indicates that the composition of the gut microflora may play a role [125]. An understanding of the relationship between the metabolome and body size could inform on implementation of weight loss interventions based on Mediterranean diet and other dietary pattern approaches.

Conclusions

Metabolomics offers tremendous potential to evaluate individual responses to the Mediterranean diet in a noninvasive and dynamic way. Perhaps the most exciting long-term prospect for the application of metabolomics to nutritional science research and dietetics is the opportunity to elucidate causal mechanisms that link changes in systemic metabolism to reduced health. Biomarkers derived from these studies, if validated, can direct the optimization of nutritional interventions to prevent disease and indeed help to target those subsets of the population most likely to benefit from such interventions. The success of such investigations will depend on collaborative efforts that integrate metabolomics data from epidemiological, clinical, and preclinical studies.

References

1. Lindon JC, Holmes E, Nicholson JK. Metabonomics in pharmaceutical R&D. FEBS J. 2007;274(5):1140–51.
2. Wishart DS, Jewison T, Guo AC, Wilson M, Knox C, Liu Y, Djoumbou Y, Mandal R, Azia F, Dong E, et al. HMDB 3.0—the human metabolome database in 2013. Nucleic Acids Res. 2013;41(Database issue):D801–7.
3. Goodacre R, Vaidyanathan S, Dunn WB, Harrigan GG, Kell DB. Metabolomics by numbers: acquiring and understanding global metabolite data. Trends Biotechnol. 2004;22(5):245–52.
4. Nicholson JK, Lindon JC, Holmes E. 'Metabonomics': understanding the metabolic responses of living systems to pathophysiological stimuli via multivariate statistical analysis of biological NMR spectroscopic data. Xenobiotica. 1999;29(11):1181–9.
5. Fiehn O. Metabolomics—the link between genotypes and phenotypes. Plant Mol Biol. 2002;48(1-2):155–71.
6. Nicholson JK, Lindon JC. Systems biology: metabonomics. Nature. 2008;455(7216):1054–6.
7. Holmes E, Wilson ID, Nicholson JK. Metabolic phenotyping in health and disease. Cell. 2008;134(5):714–7.
8. Cloarec O, Dumas ME, Tryg J, Craig A, Barton RH, Lindon JC, Nicholson JK, Holmes E. Evaluation of the orthogonal projection on latent structure model limitations caused by chemical shift variability and improved visualization of biomarker changes in 1H NMR spectroscopic metabonomic studies. Anal Chem. 2005;77(2):517–26.
9. Cloarec O, Dumas ME, Craig A, Barton RH, Trygg J, Hudson J, Blancher C, Gauguier D, Lindon JC, Holmes E, et al. Statistical total correlation spectroscopy: an exploratory approach for latent biomarker identification from metabolic 1H NMR data sets. Anal Chem. 2005;77(5):1282–9.
10. Astarita G, Langridge J. An emerging role for metabolomics in nutrition science. J Nutrigenet Nutrigenomics. 2013;6(4):179–98.

11. Fave G, Beckmann ME, Draper JH, Mathers JC. Measurement of dietary exposure: a challenging problem which may be overcome thanks to metabolomics? Genes Nutr. 2009;4(2):135–41.
12. Scalbert A, Brennan L, Fiehn O, Hankemeier T, Kristal BS, van Ommen B, Pujos-Guillot E, Verheij E, Wishart D, Wopereis S. Mass-spectrometry-based metabolomics: limitations and recommendations for future progress with particular focus on nutrition research. Metabolomics. 2009;5(4):435–58.
13. Wild CP, Scalbert A, Herceg Z. Measuring the exposome: a powerful basis for evaluating environmental exposures and cancer risk. Environ Mol Mutagen. 2013;54(7):480–99.
14. Martin FP, Montoli I, Kochhar S, Rezzi S. Chemometric strategy for modeling metabolic biological space along the gastrointestinal tract and assessing microbial influences. Anal Chem. 2010;82(23):9803–11.
15. Llorach R, Garcia-Aloy M, Tulipani S, Vazquez-Fresn R, Andres-Lacueva C. Nutrimetabolomic strategies to develop new biomarkers of intake and health effects. J Agric Food Chem. 2012;60(36):8797–808.
16. Santosh C, Brennan D, McCabe C, Macrae IM, Holmes WM, Graham DI, Gallaghe L, Condon B, Hadley DM, Muir KW, et al. Potential use of oxygen as a metabolic biosensor in combination with T2*-weighted MRI to define the ischemic penumbra. J Cereb Blood Flow Metab. 2008;28(10):1742–53.
17. Yap IK, Brown IJ, Chan Q, Wijeyesekera A, Garcia-Perez I, Bictash M, Loo RL, Chadeau-Hyam M, Ebbels T, De Iorio M, et al. Metabolome-wide association study identifies multiple biomarkers that discriminate north and south Chinese populations at differing risks of cardiovascular disease: INTERMAP study. J Proteome Res. 2010;9(12):6647–54.
18. Stamler J, Brown IJ, Yap IK, Chan Q, Wijeyesekera A, Garcia-Perez I, Chadeau-Hyam M, Ebbels TM, De Iorio M, Posma J, et al. Dietary and urinary metabonomic factors possibly accounting for higher blood pressure of black compared with white Americans: results of International Collaborative Study on macro-/micronutrients and blood pressure. Hypertension. 2013;62(6):1074–80.
19. Riboli E, Kaaks R. The EPIC Project: rationale and study design. European Prospective Investigation into Cancer and Nutrition. Int J Epidemiol. 1997;26 Suppl 1:S6–14.
20. Chadeau-Hyam M, Athersuch TJ, Keun HC, De Iorio M, Ebbels TM, Jenab M, Sacerdote C, Bruce SJ, Holmes E, Vineis P. Meeting-in-the-middle using metabolic profiling—a strategy for the identification of intermediate biomarkers in cohort studies. Biomarkers. 2011;16(1):83–8.
21. Murphy N, Norat T, Ferrari P, Jenab M, Bueno-de-Mesquita B, Skeie G, Dahm CC, Overvad K, Olsen A, Tjonneland A, et al. Dietary fibre intake and risks of cancers of the colon and rectum in the European prospective investigation into cancer and nutrition (EPIC). PLoS One. 2012;7(6), e39361.
22. Saadatian-Elahi M, Slimani N, Chajes V, Jenab M, Goudable J, Biessy C, Ferrari P, Byrnes G, Autier P, Peeters PH, et al. Plasma phospholipid fatty acid profiles and their association with food intakes: results from a cross-sectional study within the European Prospective Investigation into Cancer and Nutrition. Am J Clin Nutr. 2009;89(1):331–46.
23. Altmaier E, Kastenmuller G, Romisch-Margl W, Thorand B, Weinberger KM, Illig T, Adamski J, Doring A, Suhre K. Questionnaire-based self-reported nutrition habits associate with serum metabolism as revealed by quantitative targeted metabolomics. Eur J Epidemiol. 2011;26(2):145–56.
24. Santoro A, Pini E, Scurti M, Palmas G, Berendsen A, Brzozowska A, Pietruszka B, Szczecinska A, Cano N, Meunier N, et al. Combating inflammaging through a Mediterranean whole diet approach: The NU-AGE project's conceptual framework and design. Mech Ageing Dev. 2014;136–137:3–13.
25. Dais P, Hatzakis E. Quality assessment and authentication of virgin olive oil by NMR spectroscopy: a critical review. Anal Chim Acta. 2013;765:1–27.
26. D'Imperio M, Mannina L, Capitani D, Bidet O, Enrico R, Bucarelli FM, Quaglia GB, Annalaura S. NMR and statistical study of olive oils from Lazio: A geographical, ecological and agronomic characterization. Food Chem. 2007;105:1256–67.
27. Martin-Pelaez S, Covas MI, Fito M, Kusar A, Pravst I. Health effects of olive oil polyphenols: recent advances and possibilities for the use of health claims. Mol Nutr Food Res. 2013;57(5):760–71.
28. Razquin C, Martinez JA, Martinez-Gonzalez MA, Fernandez-Crehuet J, Santos JM, Marti A. A Mediterranean diet rich in virgin olive oil may reverse the effects of the -174G/C IL6 gene variant on 3-year body weight change. Mol Nutr Food Res. 2010;54 Suppl 1:S75–82.
29. Razquin C, Martinez JA, Martinez-Gonzalez MA, Bes-Rastrollo M, Fernandez-Crehuet J, Marti A. A 3-year intervention with a Mediterranean diet modified the association between the rs9939609 gene variant in FTO and body weight changes. Int J Obes. 2010;34(2):266–72.
30. Razquin C, Martine JA, Martinez-Gonzalez MA, Salas-Salvado J, Estruch R, Marti A. A 3-year Mediterranean-style dietary intervention may modulate the association between adiponectin gene variants and body weight change. Eur J Nutr. 2010;49(5):311–9.
31. Waterman E, Lockwood B. Active components and clinical applications of olive oil. Altern Med Rev. 2007;12(4):331–42.
32. Garcia-Villalba R, Carrasco-Pancorbo A, Nevedomskaya E, Mayboroda OA, Deelder AM, Segura-Carretero A, Fernandez-Gutierrez A. Exploratory analysis of human urine by LC-ESI-TOF MS after high intake of olive oil: understanding the metabolism of polyphenols. Anal Bioanal Chem. 2010;398(1):463–75.

33. Lemonakis N, Gikas E, Halabalaki M, Skaltsounis AL. Development and validation of a combined methodology for assessing the total quality control of herbal medicinal products—application to oleuropein preparations. PLoS One. 2013;8(10), e78277.
34. Fernandez-Arroyo S, Gomez-Martinez A, Rocamora-Reverte L, Quirantes-Pine R, Segura-Carretero A, Fernandez-Gutierrez A, Ferragut JA. Application of nanoLC-ESI-TOF-MS for the metabolomic analysis of phenolic compounds from extra-virgin olive oil in treated colon-cancer cells. J Pharm Biomed Anal. 2012;63:128–34.
35. Corona G, Tzounis X, Assunta Dessi M, Deiana M, Debnam ES, Visioli F, Spencer JP. The fate of olive oil polyphenols in the gastrointestinal tract: implications of gastric and colonic microflora-dependent biotransformation. Free Radic Res. 2006;40(6):647–58.
36. Wikoff WR, Anfora AT, Liu J, Schultz PG, Lesley SA, Peters EC, Siuzdak G. Metabolomics analysis reveals large effects of gut microflora on mammalian blood metabolites. Proc Natl Acad Sci U S A. 2009;106(10):3698–703.
37. Stradling C, Hamid M, Fisher K, Taheri S, Thomas GN. A review of dietary influences on cardiovascular health: part 1: the role of dietary nutrients. Cardiovasc Hematol Disord Drug Targets. 2013;13(3):208–30.
38. Arnold C, Konkel A, Fischer R, Schunck WH. Cytochrome P450-dependent metabolism of omega-6 and omega-3 long-chain polyunsaturated fatty acids. Pharmacol Rep. 2010;62(3):536–47.
39. Chapkin RS, Seo J, McMurray DN, Lupton JR. Mechanisms by which docosahexaenoic acid and related fatty acids reduce colon cancer risk and inflammatory disorders of the intestine. Chem Phys Lipids. 2008;153(1):14–23.
40. Mannina L, Sobolev AP, Capitani D. Applications of NMR metabolomics to the study of foodstuffs: truffle, kiwifruit, lettuce, and sea bass. Electrophoresis. 2012;33(15):2290–313.
41. Mannina L, Sobolev AP, Capitani D, Iaffaldano N, Rosato MP, Ragni P, Reale A, Sorrentino E, D'Amico I, Coppola R. NMR metabolic profiling of organic and aqueous sea bass extracts: implications in the discrimination of wild and cultured sea bass. Talanta. 2008;77(1):433–44.
42. Lloyd AJ, Fave G, Beckmann M, Lin W, Tailliart K, Xie L, Mathers JC, Draper J. Use of mass spectrometry fingerprinting to identify urinary metabolites after consumption of specific foods. Am J Clin Nutr. 2011;94(4):981–91.
43. al-Waiz M, Mikov M, Mitchell SC, Smith RL. The exogenous origin of trimethylamine in the mouse. Metab Clin Exp. 1992;41(2):135–6.
44. Nakanishi M, Rosenberg DW. Multifaceted roles of PGE2 in inflammation and cancer. Semin Immunopathol. 2013;35(2):123–37.
45. Zhao Y, Agarwal VR, Mendelson CR, Simpson ER. Estrogen biosynthesis proximal to a breast tumor is stimulated by PGE2 via cyclic AMP, leading to activation of promoter II of the CYP19 (aromatase) gene. Endocrinology. 1996;137(12):5739–42.
46. Brudvik KW, Tasken K. Modulation of T cell immune functions by the prostaglandin E(2)—cAMP pathway in chronic inflammatory states. Br J Pharmacol. 2012;166(2):411–9.
47. Kawabata A. Prostaglandin E2 and pain—an update. Biol Pharm Bull. 2011;34(8):1170–3.
48. Ding XZ, Hennig R, Adrian TE. Lipoxygenase and cyclooxygenase metabolism: new insights in treatment and chemoprevention of pancreatic cancer. Mol Cancer. 2003;2:10.
49. Matsuyama M, Yoshimura R. The target of arachidonic acid pathway is a new anticancer strategy for human prostate cancer. Biologics. 2008;2(4):725–32.
50. Yang J, Schmelzer K, Georgi K, Hammock BD. Quantitative profiling method for oxylipin metabolome by liquid chromatography electrospray ionization tandem mass spectrometry. Anal Chem. 2009;81(19):8085–93.
51. Schuchardt JP, Schmidt S, Kressel G, Willenberg I, Hammock BD, Hahn A, Schebb NH. Modulation of blood oxylipin levels by long-chain omega-3 fatty acid supplementation in hyper- and normolipidemic men. Prostaglandins Leukot Essent Fat Acids. 2014;90(2–3):27–37.
52. West NJ, Clark SK, Phillips RK, Hutchinson JM, Leicester RJ, Belluzzi A, Hull MA. Eicosapentaenoic acid reduces rectal polyp number and size in familial adenomatous polyposis. Gut. 2010;59(7):918–25.
53. Hull MA, Sandell AC, Montgomery AA, Logan RF, Clifford GM, Rees CJ, Loadman PM, Whitham D. A randomized controlled trial of eicosapentaenoic acid and/or aspirin for colorectal adenoma prevention during colonoscopic surveillance in the NHS Bowel Cancer Screening Programme (The seAFOod Polyp Prevention Trial): study protocol for a randomized controlled trial. Trials. 2013;14(1):237.
54. Dragsted LO. Biomarkers of meat intake and the application of nutrigenomics. Meat Sci. 2010;84(2):301–7.
55. Stella C, Beckwith-Hall B, Cloarec O, Holmes E, Lindon JC, Powell J, van der Ouderaa F, Bingham S, Cross AJ, Nicholson JK. Susceptibility of human metabolic phenotypes to dietary modulation. J Proteome Res. 2006;5(10):2780–8.
56. Xu J, Yang S, Cai S, Dong J, Li X, Chen Z. Identification of biochemical changes in lactovegetarian urine using 1H NMR spectroscopy and pattern recognition. Anal Bioanal Chem. 2010;396(4):1451–63.
57. O'Sullivan A, Gibney MJ, Brennan L. Dietary intake patterns are reflected in metabolomic profiles: potential role in dietary assessment studies. Am J Clin Nutr. 2011;93(2):314–21.
58. Wang Z, Klipfell E, Bennett BJ, Koeth R, Levison BS, Dugar B, Feldstein AE, Britt EB, Fu X, Chung YM, et al. Gut flora metabolism of phosphatidylcholine promotes cardiovascular disease. Nature. 2011;472(7341):57–63.

59. Heinzmann SS, Merrifield CA, Rezzi S, Kochhar S, Lindon JC, Holmes E, Nicholson JK. Stability and robustness of human metabolic phenotypes in response to sequential food challenges. J Proteome Res. 2012;11(2):643–55.
60. Grosso G, Buscemi S, Galvano F, Mistretta A, Marventano S, Vela V, Drago F, Gangi S, Basile F, Biondi A. Mediterranean diet and cancer: epidemiological evidence and mechanism of selected aspects. BMC Surg. 2013;13 Suppl 2:S14.
61. Cho SS, Qi L, Fahey Jr GC, Klurfeld DM. Consumption of cereal fiber, mixtures of whole grains and bran, and whole grains and risk reduction in type 2 diabetes, obesity, and cardiovascular disease. Am J Clin Nutr. 2013;98(2):594–619.
62. Martinez-Gonzalez MA, Fernandez-Jarne E, Martinez-Losa E, Prado-Santamaria M, Brugarolas-Brufau C, Serrano-Martinez M. Role of fibre and fruit in the Mediterranean diet to protect against myocardial infarction: a case-control study in Spain. Eur J Clin Nutr. 2002;56(8):715–22.
63. Bertram HC, Bach Knudsen KE, Serena A, Malmendal A, Nielsen NC, Frette XC, Andersen HJ. NMR-based metabonomic studies reveal changes in the biochemical profile of plasma and urine from pigs fed high-fibre rye bread. Br J Nutr. 2006;95(5):955–62.
64. Rasmussen LG, Winning H, Savorani F, Ritz C, Engelsen SB, Astrup A, Larsen TM, Dragsted LO. Assessment of dietary exposure related to dietary GI and fibre intake in a nutritional metabolomic study of human urine. Genes Nutr. 2012;7(2):281–93.
65. Boeing H, Bechthold A, Bub A, Ellinger S, Haller D, Kroke A, Leschik-Bonnet E, Muller MJ, Oberritter H, Schulze M, et al. Critical review: vegetables and fruit in the prevention of chronic diseases. Eur J Nutr. 2012;51(6):637–63.
66. Manach C, Hubert J, Llorach R, Scalbert A. The complex links between dietary phytochemicals and human health deciphered by metabolomics. Mol Nutr Food Res. 2009;53(10):1303–15.
67. van Duynhoven J, Vaughan EE, Jacobs DM, Kemperman RA, van Velzen EJ, Gross G, Roger LC, Possemiers S, Smilde AK, Dore J, et al. Metabolic fate of polyphenols in the human superorganism. Proc Natl Acad Sci U S A. 2011;108 Suppl 1:4531–8.
68. Grun CH, van Dorsten FA, Jacobs DM, Le Belleguic M, van Velzen EJ, Bingham MO, Janssen HG, van Duynhoven JP. GC-MS methods for metabolic profiling of microbial fermentation products of dietary polyphenols in human and in vitro intervention studies. J Chromatogr B Anal Technol Biomed Life Sci. 2008;871(2):212–9.
69. Walsh MC, Brennan L, Pujos-Guillot E, Sebedio JL, Scalbert A, Fagan A, Higgins DG, Gibney MJ. Influence of acute phytochemical intake on human urinary metabolomic profiles. Am J Clin Nutr. 2007;86(6):1687–93.
70. Nile SH, Park SW. Edible berries: bioactive components and their effect on human health. Nutrition. 2014;30(2):134–44.
71. Sun J, Xiao Z, Lin LZ, Lester GE, Wang Q, Harnly JM, Chen P. Profiling polyphenols in five Brassica species microgreens by UHPLC-PDA-ESI/HRMS(n.). J Agric Food Chem. 2013;61(46):10960–70.
72. Heinzmann SS, Brown IJ, Chan Q, Bictash M, Dumas ME, Kochhar S, Stamler J, Holmes E, Elliott P, Nicholson JK. Metabolic profiling strategy for discovery of nutritional biomarkers: proline betaine as a marker of citrus consumption. Am J Clin Nutr. 2010;92(2):436–43.
73. Lloyd AJ, Beckmann M, Fave G, Mathers JC, Draper J. Proline betaine and its biotransformation products in fasting urine samples are potential biomarkers of habitual citrus fruit consumption. Br J Nutr. 2011;106(6):812–24.
74. Atkinson W, Downer P, Lever M, Chambers ST, George PM. Effects of orange juice and proline betaine on glycine betaine and homocysteine in healthy male subjects. Eur J Nutr. 2007;46(8):446–52.
75. Miller JA, Thompson PA, Hakim IA, Chow H-HS, Thomson CA. D-limonene: a bioactive food component in the Mediterranean diet and evidence for a potential role in breast cancer prevention. Oncol Rev. 2011;5:31–42.
76. Miller JA, Lang JE, Ley M, Nagle R, Hsu CH, Thompson PA, Cordova C, Waer A, Chow HH. Human breast tissue disposition and bioactivity of limonene in women with early-stage breast cancer. Cancer Prev Res. 2013;6(6):577–84.
77. Miller JA, Pappan K, Wulff J, Want EJ, Siskos AP, Keun HC, Hu C, Thompson PA, Lang JE, Chow HHS. Analysis of changes in the plasma metabolomic profiles of breast cancer patients after short-term limonene intervention. Cancer Prev Res. 2015;8(1):86–93.
78. Bouchenak M, Lamri-Senhadji M. Nutritional quality of legumes, and their role in cardiometabolic risk prevention: a review. J Med Food. 2013;16(3):185–98.
79. Nagaraju GP, Zafar SF, El-Rayes BF. Pleiotropic effects of genistein in metabolic, inflammatory, and malignant diseases. Nutr Rev. 2013;71(8):562–72.
80. Cassidy A. Potential risks and benefits of phytoestrogen-rich diets. Int J Vitam Nutr Res. 2003;73(2):120–6.
81. Solanky KS, Bailey NJ, Beckwith-Hall BM, Davis A, Bingham S, Holmes E, Nicholson JK, Cassidy A. Application of biofluid 1H nuclear magnetic resonance-based metabonomic techniques for the analysis of the biochemical effects of dietary isoflavones on human plasma profile. Anal Biochem. 2003;323(2):197–204.
82. Solanky KS, Bailey NJ, Beckwith-Hall BM, Bingham S, Davis A, Holmes E, Nicholson JK, Cassidy A. Biofluid 1H NMR-based metabonomic techniques in nutrition research—metabolic effects of dietary isoflavones in humans. J Nutr Biochem. 2005;16(4):236–44.

83. Goodman MT, Shvetsov YB, Wilkens LR, Franke AA, Le Marchand L, Kakazu KK, Nomura AM, Henderson BE, Kolonel LN. Urinary phytoestrogen excretion and postmenopausal breast cancer risk: the multiethnic cohort study. Cancer Prev Res (Phila). 2009;2(10):887–94.
84. Chiva-Blanch G, Arranz S, Lamuela-Raventos RM, Estruch R. Effects of wine, alcohol and polyphenols on cardiovascular disease risk factors: evidences from human studies. Alcohol Alcohol. 2013;48(3):270–7.
85. van Dorsten FA, Grun CH, van Velzen EJ, Jacobs DM, Draijer R, van Duynhoven JP. The metabolic fate of red wine and grape juice polyphenols in humans assessed by metabolomics. Mol Nutr Food Res. 2010;54(7):897–908.
86. Jacobs DM, Deltimple N, van Velzen E, van Dorsten FA, Bingham M, Vaughan EE, van Duynhoven J. (1)H NMR metabolite profiling of feces as a tool to assess the impact of nutrition on the human microbiome. NMR Biomed. 2008;21(6):615–26.
87. Vazquez-Fresno R, Llorach R, Alcaro F, Rodriguez MA, Vinaixa M, Chiva-Blanch G, Estruch R, Correig X, Andres-Lacueva C. (1)H-NMR-based metabolomic analysis of the effect of moderate wine consumption on subjects with cardiovascular risk factors. Electrophoresis. 2012;33(15):2345–54.
88. Boto-Ordonez M, Urpi-Sarda M, Queipo-Ortuno MI, Corella D, Tinahones FJ, Estruch R, Andres-Lacueva C. Microbial metabolomic fingerprinting in urine after regular dealcoholized red wine consumption in humans. J Agric Food Chem. 2013;61(38):9166–75.
89. Brown L, Kroon PA, Das DK, Das S, Tosaki A, Chan V, Singer MV, Feick P. The biological responses to resveratrol and other polyphenols from alcoholic beverages. Alcohol Clin Exp Res. 2009;33(9):1513–23.
90. Soleas GJ, Diamandis EP, Goldberg DM. Resveratrol: a molecule whose time has come? And gone? Clin Biochem. 1997;30(2):91–113.
91. Kopp P. Resveratrol, a phytoestrogen found in red wine. A possible explanation for the conundrum of the 'French paradox'? Eur J Endocrinol. 1998;138(6):619–20.
92. Catalgol B, Batirel S, Taga Y, Ozer NK. Resveratrol: French paradox revisited. Front Pharmacol. 2012;3:141.
93. Szekeres T, Fritzer-Szekeres M, Saiko P, Jager W. Resveratrol and resveratrol analogues—structure-activity relationship. Pharm Res. 2010;27(6):1042–8.
94. Kroon PA, Iyer A, Chunduri P, Chan V, Brown L. The cardiovascular nutrapharmacology of resveratrol: pharmacokinetics, molecular mechanisms and therapeutic potential. Curr Med Chem. 2010;17(23):2442–55.
95. Zamora-Ros R, Urpi-Sarda M, Lamuela-Raventos RM, Estruch R, Martinez-Gonzalez MA, Bullo M, Aros F, Cherubini A, Andres-Lacueva C. Resveratrol metabolites in urine as a biomarker of wine intake in free-living subjects: The PREDIMED Study. Free Radic Biol Med. 2009;46(12):1562–6.
96. Bhat KP, Lantvit D, Christov K, Mehta RG, Moon RC, Pezzuto JM. Estrogenic and antiestrogenic properties of resveratrol in mammary tumor models. Cancer Res. 2001;61(20):7456–63.
97. Jang M, Cai L, Udeani GO, Slowing KV, Thomas CF, Beecher CW, Fong HH, Farnsworth NR, Kinghorn AD, Mehta RG, et al. Cancer chemopreventive activity of resveratrol, a natural product derived from grapes. Science. 1997;275(5297):218–20.
98. Jang M, Pezzuto JM. Effects of resveratrol on 12-O-tetradecanoylphorbol-13-acetate-induced oxidative events and gene expression in mouse skin. Cancer Lett. 1998;134(1):81–9.
99. Li ZG, Hong T, Shimada Y, Komoto I, Kawabe A, Ding Y, Kaganoi J, Hashimoto Y, Imamura M. Suppression of N-nitrosomethylbenzylamine (NMBA)-induced esophageal tumorigenesis in F344 rats by resveratrol. Carcinogenesis. 2002;23(9):1531–6.
100. Schneider Y, Duranton B, Gosse F, Schleiffer R, Seiler N, Raul F. Resveratrol inhibits intestinal tumorigenesis and modulates host-defense-related gene expression in an animal model of human familial adenomatous polyposis. Nutr Cancer. 2001;39(1):102–7.
101. Provinciali M, Re F, Donnini A, Orlando F, Bartozzi B, Di Stasio G, Smorlesi A. Effect of resveratrol on the development of spontaneous mammary tumors in HER-2/neu transgenic mice. Int J Cancer. 2005;115(1):36–45.
102. Carbo N, Costelli P, Baccino FM, Lopez-Soriano FJ, Argiles JM. Resveratrol, a natural product present in wine, decreases tumour growth in a rat tumour model. Biochem Biophys Res Commun. 1999;254(3):739–43.
103. Delmas D, Lancon A, Colin D, Jannin B, Latruffe N. Resveratrol as a chemopreventive agent: a promising molecule for fighting cancer. Curr Drug Targets. 2006;7(4):423–42.
104. Signorelli P, Ghidoni R. Resveratrol as an anticancer nutrient: molecular basis, open questions and promises. J Nutr Biochem. 2005;16(8):449–66.
105. Aggarwal BB, Bhardwaj A, Aggarwal RS, Seeram NP, Shishodia S, Takada Y. Role of resveratrol in prevention and therapy of cancer: preclinical and clinical studies. Anticancer Res. 2004;24(5A):2783–840.
106. Athar M, Back JH, Tang X, Kim KH, Kopelovich L, Bickers DR, Kim AL. Resveratrol: a review of preclinical studies for human cancer prevention. Toxicol Appl Pharmacol. 2007;224(3):274–83.
107. Jager W, Gruber A, Giessrigl B, Krupitza G, Szekeres T, Sonntag D. Metabolomic analysis of resveratrol-induced effects in the human breast cancer cell lines MCF-7 and MDA-MB-231. OMICS. 2011;15(1-2):9–14.
108. Massimi M, Tomassini A, Sciubba F, Sobolev AP, Devirgiliis LC, Miccheli A. Effects of resveratrol on HepG2 cells as revealed by (1)H-NMR based metabolic profiling. Biochim Biophys Acta. 2012;1820(1):1–8.

109. Baur JA, Sinclair DA. Therapeutic potential of resveratrol: the in vivo evidence. Nat Rev Drug Discov. 2006;5(6):493–506.
110. Rivera L, Moron R, Zarzuelo A, Galisteo M. Long-term resveratrol administration reduces metabolic disturbances and lowers blood pressure in obese Zucker rats. Biochem Pharmacol. 2009;77(6):1053–63.
111. Zhou M, Wang S, Zhao A, Wang K, Fan Z, Yang H, Liao W, Bao S, Zhao L, Zhang Y, et al. Transcriptomic and metabonomic profiling reveal synergistic effects of quercetin and resveratrol supplementation in high fat diet fed mice. J Proteome Res. 2012;11(10):4961–71.
112. Valls-Pedret C, Lamuela-Raventos RM, Medina-Remon A, Quintana M, Corella D, Pinto X, Martinez-Gonzalez MA, Estruch R, Ros E. Polyphenol-rich foods in the Mediterranean diet are associated with better cognitive function in elderly subjects at high cardiovascular risk. J Alzheimers Dis. 2012;29(4):773–82.
113. Butt MS, Sultan MT. Coffee and its consumption: benefits and risks. Crit Rev Food Sci Nutr. 2011;51(4):363–73.
114. Crozier A, Jaganath IB, Clifford MN. Dietary phenolics: chemistry, bioavailability and effects on health. Nat Prod Rep. 2009;26(8):1001–43.
115. Spiller MA. Caffeine. Boca Raton: CRC Press; 1998.
116. Ito H, Gonthier MP, Manach C, Morand C, Mennen L, Remesy C, Scalbert A. Polyphenol levels in human urine after intake of six different polyphenol-rich beverages. Br J Nutr. 2005;94(4):500–9.
117. Allard E, Backstrom D, Danielsson R, Sjoberg PJ, Bergquist J. Comparing capillary electrophoresis-mass spectrometry fingerprints of urine samples obtained after intake of coffee, tea, or water. Anal Chem. 2008;80(23):8946–55.
118. Stalmach A, Mullen W, Barron D, Uchida K, Yokota T, Cavin C, Steiling H, Williamson G, Crozier A. Metabolite profiling of hydroxycinnamate derivatives in plasma and urine after the ingestion of coffee by humans: identification of biomarkers of coffee consumption. Drug Metab Dispos. 2009;37(8):1749–58.
119. Nagy K, Redeuil K, Williamson G, Rezzi S, Dionisi F, Longet K, Destaillats F, Renouf M. First identification of dimethoxycinnamic acids in human plasma after coffee intake by liquid chromatography-mass spectrometry. J Chromatogr A. 2011;1218(3):491–7.
120. Redeuil K, Smarrito-Menozzi C, Guy P, Rezzi S, Dionisi F, Williamson G, Nagy K, Renouf M. Identification of novel circulating coffee metabolites in human plasma by liquid chromatography-mass spectrometry. J Chromatogr A. 2011;1218(29):4678–88.
121. Altmaier E, Kastenmuller G, Romisch-Margl W, Thorand B, Weinberger KM, Adamski J, Illig T, Doring A, Suhre K. Variation in the human lipidome associated with coffee consumption as revealed by quantitative targeted metabolomics. Mol Nutr Food Res. 2009;53(11):1357–65.
122. Mendez MA, Popkin BM, Jakszyn P, Berenguer A, Tormo MJ, Sanchez MJ, Quiros JR, Pera G, Navarro C, Martinez C, et al. Adherence to a Mediterranean diet is associated with reduced 3-year incidence of obesity. J Nutr. 2006;136(11):2934–8.
123. Kochhar S, Jacobs DM, Ramadan Z, Berruex F, Fuerholz A, Fay LB. Probing gender-specific metabolism differences in humans by nuclear magnetic resonance-based metabonomics. Anal Biochem. 2006;352(2):274–81.
124. Morris C, O'Grada C, Ryan M, Roche HM, Gibney MJ, Gibney ER, Brennan L. The relationship between BMI and metabolomic profiles: a focus on amino acids. Proc Nutr Soc. 2012;71(4):634–8.
125. Shanahan F. Microbes and metabolic health. Gut. 2012;61(12):1655–6.

Part IV
Aging and Cancer Risk

Chapter 11
The Value of the Mediterranean Diet for Older Adults: Emphasis on Obesity Interventions

Kathryn N. Porter Starr and Connie W. Bales

Key Points

- The aim of this book chapter is to describe the beneficial properties of a Mediterranean diet in regard to healthy, overweight, and obese older adults, and to summarize the characteristics, prevalence, pathophysiology, impact, and controversial nature of late life obesity.
- Weight loss interventions in obese older adults show numerous health benefits ranging from improved physical function, glycemic control, total cholesterol, and hypertension.
- Furthermore, the Mediterranean diet relies heavily on healthy components such as fruits, vegetables, whole grains, unsaturated fatty acids, and lean meats and offers a regimen of nutrient dense foods that provide viable, healthy, and gradual weight loss while also reducing a number of the chronic health conditions that are so prevalent in this population.

Keywords Mediterranean diet • Weight loss intervention • Older adults • Obesity • Aging

Introduction

By 2050, older adults 65 and older are expected to comprise almost one-fifth of the entire US population, increasing from 35 million in 2000 to 72 million [1]. Additionally, the 85 and older cohort is predicted to continue to grow to 19 million by 2050. Since 1970, life expectancy has increased 11 % from 71 to 79 years; however, this increase is due in large part to the medical advancements that extend the length but not necessarily the quality of one's life [2]. Nationally, two-thirds of older adults have at least one chronic health condition, with the most prevalent being hypertension, arthritis, heart disease, diabetes, and cancer [1]. These most typical diseases account for a disproportionate portion of health care dollar expenditures [3].

It is well established that changes in body composition occur over one's life. Even if body weight remains constant, there is a shift (reduction) in the proportion of lean tissue to adipose tissue that occurs with aging. A major factor in this body composition shift is sarcopenia, a term which refers to the process of age-related skeletal muscle loss and function (strength) [4, 5]. Sarcopenia is also the major contributor to physical frailty in older adults. Moreover, as lean and fat mass are redistributed,

K.N. Porter Starr, Ph.D., R.D. • C.W. Bales, Ph.D., R.D. (✉)
Center for the Study of Aging and Human Development, Duke University Medical Center, Box 3003, Durham, NC 27710, USA
e-mail: Kathryn.starr@duke.edu; connie.bales@duke.edu

D.F. Romagnolo, O.I. Selmin (eds.), *Mediterranean Diet*, Nutrition and Health,
DOI 10.1007/978-3-319-27969-5_11

there is an increase in intra-abdominal fat and a greater loss of lean mass in peripheral tissue. Sarcopenic obesity, which refers to excessive body fat relative to skeletal muscle mass, is directly linked with impaired instrumental activities of daily living in elderly men and women [6]. Additionally, aging is associated with an increase in lipid infiltration in lean muscle mass which leads to reduced muscle strength [7] and physical function [8] as well as promoting insulin resistance [9].

Mediterranean Diet and Healthy Aging

The Mediterranean diet is identified as a healthy dietary pattern due to the high intake of plant foods, including whole grains, fruits and vegetables, legumes, and olive oil along with moderate intakes of wine, fish, and poultry, and limited amounts of saturated fats from meat and dairy products. The Mediterranean diet has been linked to healthy aging [10], longevity [11], and potentially longer leukocyte telomere length and telomerase activity [12]. Numerous observational studies have illustrated the positive impact of a Mediterranean diet pattern on chronic conditions affecting the health of older adults. These benefits include reductions in blood pressure, blood cholesterol, diabetes, inflammatory markers, coronary syndromes, cardiovascular disease, BMI, and obesity [13, 14]. In a systematic review of the literature, Tyrovolas et al. illustrated a multitude of observational studies linking reduced risk of cardiovascular disease (CVD) and some cancers in the older adult population [15]. Furthermore, intervention studies have shown improvements in lipid profiles and reduced inflammatory markers in older adults when consuming a Mediterranean diet [16, 17]. Specifically, Camargo et al. found that healthy older adults who adhered to a Mediterranean diet had lower expressions of inflammatory genes and an increased expression in anti-inflammatory genes compared to a typical high saturated fat and a high carbohydrate diet [18].

In regards to the association between the Mediterranean diet and obesity in older adults, results have been mixed. Findings from the European Prospective Investigation into Cancer Nutrition (EPIC) found no relationship between adherence to the Mediterranean diet and BMI [19]; however, Tyrovolas et al. reported that greater adherence to the Mediterranean Diet was associated with a lower risk of obesity in older adults [20]. In a study of 1553 healthy adults, older participants (>62 years) adherent to the Mediterranean diet had significantly less body fat compared to their non-adherent counterparts, but no between-group differences regarding BMI, waist circumference, or obesity were found [21]. Finally, in the PREDMIED study, older, obese adults receiving a Mediterranean diet intervention, including olive oil or walnuts, did not see an increase in weight despite their increase in fat consumption [16]. Randomized controlled trials in older adults are needed to determine the relationship between Mediterranean diets and obesity.

There are a number of foods included in the Mediterranean diet that might contribute to its marked health benefits, including dietary fiber, monounsaturated fatty acids (MUFA), antioxidants, polyphenols, magnesium; reduction in intakes of saturated and trans-fatty acids, refined grains, and processed foods is also beneficial [22]. However, it does not appear to be one particular nutrient, but rather the combination of all these nutrients that leads to the numerous health benefits associated with this dietary pattern. Table 11.1 illustrates the physiological changes associated with aging and the additional nutritional needs associated with the aging process. The high representation of fruits, vegetables, whole grains, legumes, lean protein, unsaturated fatty acid, and low-fat dairy products in the Mediterranean diet enhances its ability to meet the nutritional needs of older adults.

Definition, Prevalence and Pathophysiology of Obesity

Obesity is defined by the World Health Organization as a chronic disease that results from excess body fat accumulation that may have negative impacts on overall health and increase the risk for chronic health conditions and mortality. BMI utilizes weight and height to classify individuals as

Table 11.1 Mediterranean diet components can meet age-related changes in nutritional needs

Age-related changes	Nutritional needs	Foods/nutrients in Mediterranean diet
↓ Muscle mass	↓ Need for energy, ↑ Protein	Fatty fish, lean meats, plant-based protein
↓ Bone density	Ca and vitamin D	Low-fat dairy products*
↓ Immune function	Many nutrients	Fruits, vegetables, whole grains, unsaturated fatty acids, lean protein
↓ Gastric motility	↑ Fiber and water	Vegetables, fruit, whole grains
↓ PTH in wintertime	Vitamin D (800 IU/day all year)	Low-fat dairy products*
↓ Ca bioavailability	Ca and vitamin D (supplements)	Low-fat dairy products*
↑ Oxidative stress	Beta-carotene, vitamin C, vitamin E	Fruits, vegetables, whole grains, unsaturated fatty acids
↑ Homocysteine	Folate, vitamin B12, and vitamin B6	Fruits, vegetables, legumes, unsaturated fatty acids, lean proteins
↓ Vitamin absorption	↑ Foods with high nutrient density	Fruits, vegetables, whole grains, unsaturated fatty acids, lean protein
↑ Gastric pH	Vitamin B12, B6, folic acid, Ca, Fe, Zn	Fruits, vegetables, legumes, unsaturated fatty acids, lean protein

*Dietary supplement of calcium and vitamin D is also recommended

underweight (BMI <18.5 kg/m^2), healthy weight (BMI 18.5–24.9 kg/m^2), overweight (BMI 25–29.9 kg/m^2), and obese (≥30 kg/m^2). The obesity epidemic has not spared the older adult cohort. More than two-thirds of the older adult population is overweight, while fully one-third is obese [1]. Furthermore, the prevalence of obesity in older women has increased from 31.5 % in 2004 to 38.1 % in 2012 [23]. This prevalence increases in older populations are seen worldwide [24, 25] and likely to be a global health challenge in the decades to come [26].

Aging is associated with a reduction in energy requirements such that even with no change in calorie intake there is a gradual accumulation of body fat with age. Basal energy needs are reduced as a result of age-associated decreases in resting metabolic rates and thermic effects of food. Furthermore, energy expended from physical activity decreases with age, leading to a further reduction in total energy expenditure. As a result of the decline in total energy expenditure and stable energy intake, a positive energy balance may ensue leading to increased fat mass. Additionally, hormonal changes including reduction of growth hormone and testosterone, a decline in the body's ability to respond to thyroid hormone and leptin are associated with reduced lean muscle, increased fat mass, and decreased ability to regulate satiety [27]. Energy intake must be reduced and/or physical activity increased in order to contain gain weight. While mean energy intakes do decline somewhat with age, only 14 % of adults 65–74 and 4 % of adults 75 years of age and older meet physical activity guidelines of 150 min/week of moderate activity; thus, net energy balance remains positive and the resulting obesity is anticipated to threaten health outcomes in a growing number of older adults [1].

The Controversial Nature of Geriatric Obesity

Mortality

In young and middle aged adults, obesity has been shown to lessen life expectancy, often due to obesity-related chronic health conditions. In contrast, numerous epidemiological studies have reported an inverse relationship between mortality and BMI later in life [28–30]. In a recent meta-analysis,

Orenpoulus et al. reported that being overweight or obese was associated with lower mortality rates even in older adults with CVD [31]. Although a scientific explanation for these paradoxical findings is still lacking, one could hypothesize that being overweight may actually reduce the presence of chronic health conditions.

Potential explanations for the seemingly paradoxical increased BMI/reduced mortality relationships include selective survival; imprecisions in the measurement of obesity in older individuals; and difficulty in distinguishing intentional from unintentional weight loss. First, individuals more susceptible to obesity-related health conditions are more likely to die before attaining an old age and are not included in longitudinal survival studies; moreover, those elderly subjects who leave longer may carry factors that confer resistance to obesity-related health conditions [31, 32]. Secondly, BMI may be a poor measurement of body fat in older adults [33] Body mass index is frequently used in clinical and community settings to assess adiposity, nutritional risk, and health status [34] However, BMI is a direct calculation of height and weight such that BMI = body weight (kg)/height (m)^2, and thus does not consider the distribution of fat. BMI has been shown to be more accurate in assessing total body fatness than using body weight alone and compared to bioelectric impedance and height-weight charts, BMI provides equivalent measures [35]. But individuals with low muscle mass and/or loss of muscle mass (e.g., older adults) may have a BMI that underestimates their body fatness. As individuals age, a number of physiological changes may impact the accuracy of assessing adiposity using BMI, including spice curvature disorders (i.e., reduced height due to kyphosis of the spine) [36] and loss of muscle mass due to sarcopenia [37].

Finally, unintentional weight loss due to occult disease may contribute to the obesity paradox. In a recent longitudinal study of 3834 men, Myers et al. reported an inverse association between weight lost and mortality such that there was a 4 % increase in mortality risk per pound of weigh lost over 7 years [38]. However, more than half of the deaths in the weight loss group were associated with muscle wasting conditions and not intentional weight loss. Regardless, a positive association between weight loss and mortality was found in the weight stable participants. Similar findings were observed in a large longitudinal study of 5722 Swedish men [39]. Because it is extremely difficult to define intentionality in observational studies, controlled trials are needed to disentangle the relationships between mortality risk and overweight/obesity in elderly populations.

Morbidity: The Pros and Cons of Being Overweight vs. Obese in Elderly

Along with the possible positive correlation of BMI and mortality, other physiological aspects of being overweight might be beneficial in the later years of life. It is well known that older adults with higher body mass have greater bone mineral density and are therefore at less risk for osteoporosis-related fractures [40]. Furthermore, body fat provides extra cushion and may serve as protection in the event of a fall. Obesity may also serve as an energy reserve in the presence of serious inflammatory conditions. This may explain, at least in part, the "reverse epidemiology" of obesity, i.e., the suggestion that obese older adults with certain diseases such as end stage renal failure, heart failure, and chronic obstructive pulmonary disease have increased survival rates compared to their normal weight counterparts [41, 42].

The potential health benefits of being heavier later in life may be influenced by the extent of the adiposity. For example, being just overweight (BMI >25<30 kg/m^2) may not exert detrimental effects on morbidity and mortality in older adults [43, 44]. In contrast, as illustrated in Fig. 11.1, adiposity in obese subjects (BMI >30 kg/m^2) contributes to an array of negative health outcomes in the older population, leading to significant morbidity, disability, decreased quality of life and, in some cases, even increased rates of mortality, in addition to increased healthcare costs [45–47]. Metabolic syndrome and type 2 diabetes are most strongly associated with obesity and are on the rise in the older adult population.

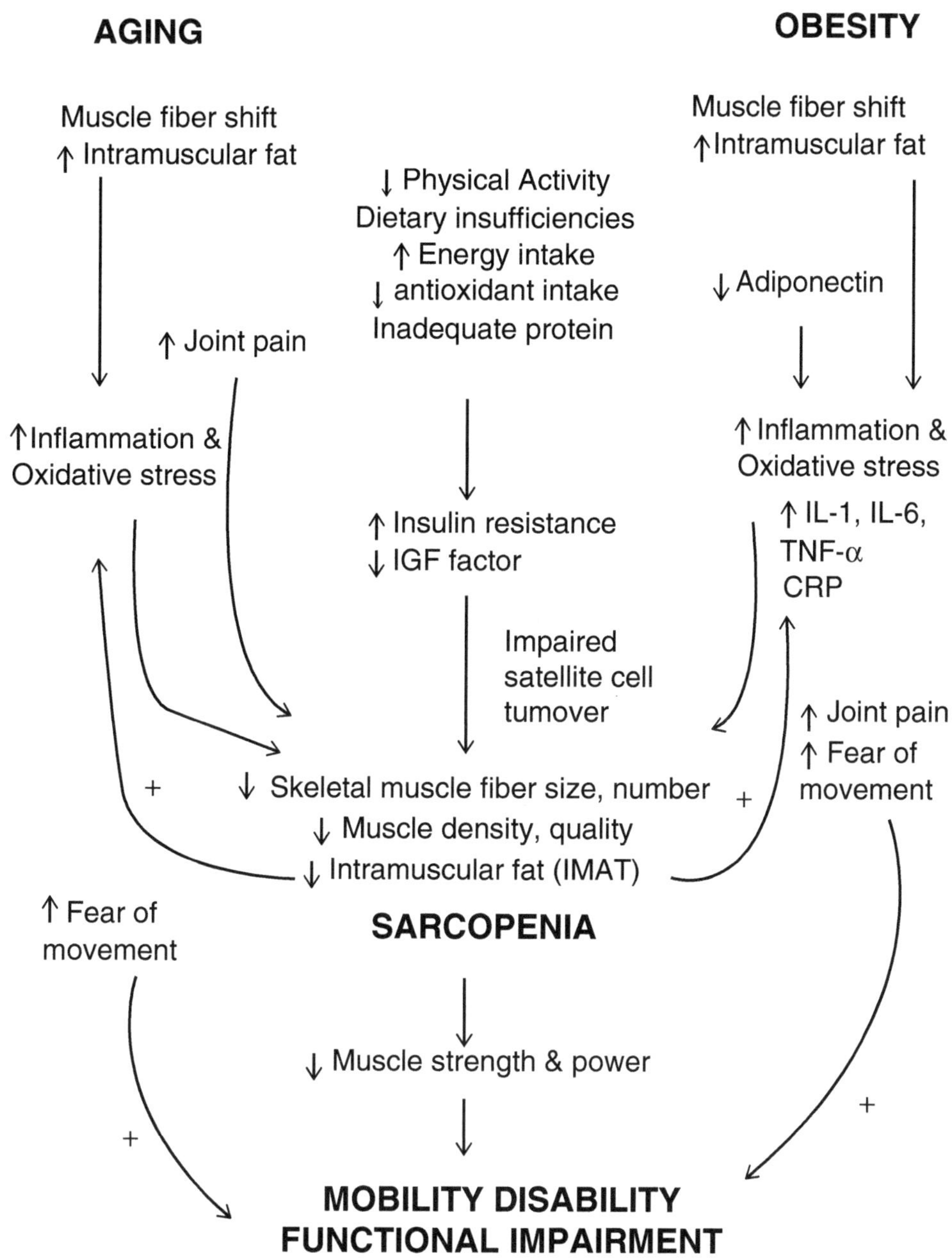

Fig. 11.1 Proposed model of the contributing factors to muscle mass insufficiency and sarcopenia in obese, older adults. *AOX* antioxidant, *IGF* insulin-like growth factor, *IMAT* intramuscular adipose tissue, *IL-1* interleukin-1, *IL-6* interleukin-6, *TNFα* tumor necrosis factor α, *CRP* C-reactive protein. The sign + denotes a positive effect on the downstream variable

Currently 33 % of adults 65 years of age and older are diabetic, and by 2050 the prevalence is expected to be 4.5 times higher [48–50]. In addition, obesity significantly impacts physical functions by worsening the age-related decline caused by sarcopenia and degenerative joint disease. These age-related changes in addition to excessive adiposity markedly increase the development of physical frailty, thereby further impairing quality of life and leading to increased nursing home admission [51, 52].

Weight Loss Interventions for Obese Older Adults

The marked increase in rate of obesity amongst older adults demands that appropriate interventions be considered. However, for reasons already mentioned, the development of weight reduction interventions for geriatric obesity has lagged behind that for children, adolescents, and younger adults. Only recently, randomized controlled weight loss intervention trials have begun to document significant improvements in cardiovascular risk factors, improved physical function, and health-related quality of life with moderate weight loss of 5–10 % [53–55]. In a recent review of the literature, intentional weight loss interventions have been shown to provide benefits in reducing chronic health conditions and nursing home placement, and improving physical function, and quality of life. Furthermore, when compared to younger adults, older adults attained greater weight loss [56]. Additionally, in a systematic review of the literature, Bales and Buhr [57] reported that intentional weight reduction in obese older adults showed improvements in osteoarthritis, physical function, CHD, and type 2 diabetes. While a recent review by Waters et al. illustrates the negative impact that weight loss has on bone mineral density and lean muscle loss, these unwanted effects could be attenuated when weight loss programs are combined with exercise [58]. Finally, as noted in our recent review [59], lifestyle interventions for obesity can improve not only physical functions, but also reduce lipid accumulation in the muscle and markers of inflammation.

Traditional Weight Loss Interventions

A number of studies have explored the effectiveness of traditional weight loss regimens in older adults. Because of the importance in considering the long-term effects of weight loss interventions in this population, we have listed in Table 11.2 only those interventional studies lasting 12 months or more. These regimens were hypocaloric but nutritionally balanced diets designed to reduce weight by 1–2 lb/week; reported mean weight losses ranged from 2.1 to 9.9 kg.

Studies of Mediterranean Diet Interventions in Older Adults

Only a few studies have examined the health impact of the Mediterranean diet in the obese, older adult population. This diet may be more optimal for obese older adults due to the anti-inflammatory and antioxidant components of MUFAs [60] and the potential muscle preserving lean protein [61]. In Table 11.2, we included three studies whose participants were on average 50 years old or older. The three studies demonstrated weight loss ranging from approximately 4–10 kg of weight loss in addition to improvements in numerous metabolic serum biomarkers. Two of the three studies used a low-carbohydrate Mediterranean diet that focused on fats high in MUFA and lean proteins including fish and poultry. In the Dietary Intervention Randomized Controlled Trial (DIRECT), Shai et al. assessed the impact of a restricted calorie Mediterranean, restricted calorie low-fat, and non-restricted low-carbohydrate diets on weight loss and blood biomarkers [62]. The calorie restricted Mediterranean diet was 35 % fat calories with 30–35 g coming from olive oil and nuts. It was rich in vegetables, and poultry and fish replaced meat and lamb. The low-fat calorie restricted diet was 30 % fat calories with 10 % of calories coming from saturated fat and no more than 300 mg/day of cholesterol. The low-carbohydrate diet was based on the Atkins diet with a recommended 120 g/day of carbohydrates. Following the 24-month intervention all groups lost weight; however, significantly greater weight loss was seen in the low-carbohydrate diet (-4.7 ± 6.5 kg) and Mediterranean diet (-4.4 ± 6.0 kg) groups

Table 11.2 Long-term weight loss interventions (≥12 months)

Weight loss intervention	Participants	Design	Weight loss	Health outcomes
Non-Mediterranean diet only and diet + exercise intervention				
Anderson et al. 2014	N = 329 Mean age = 64 BMI = 30.7 kg/m²	12 month RCT: Lifestyle intervention, control	3.5 kg (3.9 %) weight loss in lifestyle intervention arm compared to 0.8 kg (0.8 %) loss in control arm. Significant difference between arms	Significant improvements in systolic and diastolic blood pressure and blood glucose measures
Beavers et al. 2014	N = 288 Mean age = 67 Mean BMI = 32.8 kg/m²	18 month RCT: Diet + Exercise, Exercise only, control	Diet + Exercise arm lost 2.5 kg compared to 0.7 kg in exercise only arm and 0.8 kg in control arm Significant difference between Diet + Exercise vs. Exercise only and control	Significant reduction in fat mass and increase in lean mass in the Diet + Exercise arm
Crandell et al. 2006	N = 646 Mean age = 66 Mean BMI = 30.5 kg/m²	38 month RCT: Traditional Diet + Exercise, diabetes medication, or control	6.4 kg weight loss in Diet + Exercise arm	Reduced diabetes risk by 55 % in Diet + Exercise arm. Older age was associated with greater improvements
Mayer-Davis et al. 2004	N = 152 Mean age = 60 Mean BMI = 36.7 kg/m²	12 month RCT: Intensive lifestyle, reduced time lifestyle, and control	2.2 kg weight loss for intensive lifestyle arm, 0.7 kg for reduced time lifestyle, and 0.3 kg loss for control Significant difference in intensive lifestyle arm	Not reported
Messier et al. 2004	N = 316 Mean age = 69 Mean BMI = 34 kg/m²	18 month RCT: Traditional Diet only, Exercise only, Traditional Diet + Exercise, or control	4.6 kg (4.9 %) decrease in body weight in Diet only arm, 5.2 kg (5.7 %) decrease in body weight in Diet + Exercise arm, 3.5 kg (3.7 %) weight loss in the exercise only arm, and 1.1 kg (1.2 %) weight loss in the control arm. Significant reduction in Diet and Diet + Exercise arms	Significant improvements in physical function in Diet + Exercise arm. Reduced mortality risk for all intervention arms compared to control
Morey et al. 2009	N = 641 Mean age = 73 Mean BMI = 29 kg/m²	12 month RCT: Diet + Exercise, control	2.1 kg weight loss in Diet + Exercise arm, 0.9 kg weight loss in control. Significant difference compared to control	Significant improvements in physical activity, quality of life, and diet behaviors. Physical function declined less in treatment arm
Toobert et al. 2000	N = 28 Mean age = 64 Mean BMI = 32 kg/m²	24 month RCT: Diet + Exercise, control	Significant decrease in BMI in Diet + Exercise arm	Significant improvements in total and HDL cholesterol, blood pressure, and Framingham risk score

(continued)

Table 11.2 (continued)

Weight loss intervention	Participants	Design	Weight loss	Health outcomes
Villareal et al. 2008	*N*=27 Mean age=70 Mean BMI=39 kg/m²	12 month RCT: Diet+Exercise or control	9.9 kg (10 %) decrease in body weight in Diet+Exercise arm compared to a 1 % gain in the control arm. Significant difference between arms	Significant improvements in strength in Diet+Exercise arm
Villareal et al. 2011	*N*=93 Mean age=70 Mean BMI=37.2 kg/m²	12 month RCT: Diet, Exercise, Diet+Exercise, control	9.7 kg (10 %) weight loss in Diet only, 8.6 kg (9 %) in Diet+Exercise, 0.5 kg in Exercise, 0.1 kg in control Significant difference between Diet only and Diet+Exercise compared to control	Physical function and VO2 max improved in all three intervention arms, with Diet+Exercise having the greatest improvements. Strength, balance, and gait improved in the Diet+Exercise arm
Mediterranean diet only intervention				
Elhayany et al. 2010	*N*=194 Mean age=55 Mean BMI=31.4 kg/m²	12 month RCT: Low-carbohydrate Mediterranean diet, traditional Mediterranean diet, and American Diabetic Association diet	10.1 kg weight loss in low-carbohydrate Mediterranean diet, 7.8 kg in the ADA diet, and 7.4 kg in traditional weight loss diet	All groups had significant improvements. The low-carbohydrate diet had the greatest improvements in HDL, LDL, and HbA1C
Esposito et al. 2009	*N*=215 Mean age=52 Mean BMI=29.6 kg/m²	4 year RCT: Mediterranean diet, low-fat diet Physical activity recommended in each arm	6.2 kg weight loss in Mediterranean diet and 4.2 kg in low-fat diet	Mediterranean diet arm had greater improvements in glycemic control and coronary risk measures compared to the low-fat diet arm
Shai et al. 2008	*N*=322 Mean age=52 Mean BMI=30.9 kg/m²	24 month RCT: Mediterranean diet, low-fat diet, low-carbohydrate diet Physical activity recommended in each arm	4.4 kg of weight loss in the Mediterranean arm, 4.7 kg in the low-carbohydrate diet arm, and 2.9 kg in the low-fat diet arm. Significant reductions in both low-carbohydrate and Mediterranean diet compared to low-fat diet	Significant improvement in fasting plasma glucose in diabetics in Mediterranean diet compared to diabetics in other arms. Significant improvements in total and HDL cholesterol in low-carbohydrate diet compared to low-fat diet

compared to the low-fat diet group (−2.9 ± 4.2 kg). HDL-cholesterol levels increased in all three groups, with the low-carbohydrate arm having the greatest improvement in cholesterol to HDL ratio. High-sensitivity C-reactive protein decreased only in the low-carbohydrate diet and Mediterranean diet arm, while adiponectin increased and leptin decreased in all three arms. In diabetic participants, the Mediterranean diet was the only arm to show a decrease in fasting glucose and greater improvements in HOMA-IR compared to the other arms.

Esposito et al. conducted a 4-year randomized controlled trial in newly diagnosed diabetic participants to assess the impact of two calorie restricted diets, a low-carbohydrate Mediterranean diet or a low-fat diet, on the need for anti-hyperglycemic drug therapy [63]. Participants were also advised to exercise 30 min/day. Diets were restricted to 1500 kcal/day for women and 1800 kcal/day for men. Participants consuming the Mediterranean diet were instructed to consume less than 50 % of daily calories as carbohydrates and no less than 30 % of calories from fat, with 30–50 g/day of olive oil. The low-fat diet was based on the American Heart Association (AHA) guidelines and participants were instructed to consume no more than 30 % of their calories from fat with no more than 10 % of those calories coming from saturated fat. After 1 year into the trial, participants in the Mediterranean diet had lost more weight (−6.2 ± 4.2 vs. −4.2 ± 3.5 kg) and had greater reductions in BMI (−2.4 ± 1.6 vs. −1.4 ± 0.9 kg/m^2) and waist circumference (−4.8 ± 3.0 vs. −3.5 ± 2.8 cm) compared to those in the low-fat diet. However, at years 3 and 4 there was no difference in weight loss between the two groups. Participants in the Mediterranean diet were less likely to need anti-hyperglycemic drug therapy at 18 months (12 % vs. 24 %) and at 4 years (44 % vs. 70 %); and had greater reductions in fasting plasma glucose and HbA_{1C}, and improved insulin sensitivity and adiponectin levels. Finally, those in the Mediterranean diet had increases in HDL-cholesterol, and decreases in triglyceride levels and systolic blood pressure. Both groups increased their physical activity levels during the trial.

In a similar study, Elhayany et al. investigated the impact of weight loss diets on obese and older diabetic individuals [64]. This 12-month intervention included three diets, a low-carbohydrate Mediterranean diet (35 % low glycemic index (LGI) carbohydrates, 45 % fats high in MUFA, 15–20 % proteins), a traditional Mediterranean diet (50–55 % LGI carbohydrates, 30 % fats high in MUFA, 15–20 % proteins) and the American Diabetic Association (ADA) diabetic diet (50–55 % carbohydrates, 30 % fats, 20 % proteins). All diet groups were advised to exercise for 30–45 min/day at least 3 days/week. Significant weight loss was seen in all three groups with the low-carbohydrate Mediterranean diet having the greatest weight loss (−10.1 kg), followed by the ADA diet (−7.8 kg), and the traditional Mediterranean diet (−7.4 kg). The low-carbohydrate Mediterranean diet also had the greatest reduction in LDL cholesterol and was the only diet to increase HDL. Finally, HbA1c was reduced more in the low-carbohydrate Mediterranean diet (−2.0) and traditional Mediterranean diet (−1.8) than the ADA diet (−1.6).

Benefits of the Mediterranean Diet for Overweight Older Adults

As previously noted, weight reduction is mainly advocated for older adults with a BMI >30 [31, 65]. This recommendation would exclude a large percentage of overweight older adults who are at high-risk for age and weight-related conditions such as cardiovascular disease, type 2 diabetes, and hypertension. Salas-Salvado et al. assessed the impact of three non-calorie restricted diets including, Mediterranean diet with extra-virgin olive oil, Mediterranean diet with nuts, and a low-fat control diet on the development of diabetes in a high cardiovascular risk group of older adults. At the 4-year follow-up, individuals consuming the Mediterranean diet with extra-virgin olive oil had a 40 % reduction, and those consuming the Mediterranean diet with mixed nuts an 18 % reduction, in relative risk of diabetes compared to the control diet [66]. These findings illustrated some of the beneficial effects the Mediterranean diet can exert on older adults at risk for type 2 diabetes even without using a calorie-restricted diet.

Conclusions

The composition of the Mediterranean diet is well suited to support the less aggressive weight management approach advocated for older adults. Although the high intake of fat characteristic of the Mediterranean diet might be of concern when the need for weight loss is substantial, it may not be a problem when weight loss goals are modest, and managing the health problems associated with aging is a priority. In recent assessments of weight loss and macronutrient compositions, Forouhi et al. [67] concluded that their findings did not support the use of low-fat diets to prevent weight gain. Sacks et al. [68] found that reduced-calorie diets resulted in clinically meaningful weight loss regardless of which macronutrients they emphasize. However, participants consuming reduced calorie diets with a higher distribution of fat reported better adherence than those consuming a low-fat diet. Furthermore, when recommending a calorie-reduced diet for older adults it is essential for the diet to be well balanced and high in micronutrients. Since the Mediterranean diet relies heavily on fruits, vegetables, whole grains, unsaturated fatty acids, and lean meats, it offers a regimen of high nutrient density, suitable for healthy older adults and gradual weight loss while also helping to alleviate a number of chronic health conditions (i.e., type 2 diabetes) that are so prevalent in this population.

References

1. Federal Interagency Forum on Aging-Related Statistics. Older Americans 2012: key indicators of well-being. Washington, DC: U.S. Government Printing Office; 2012.
2. Kochanek KD, Arias E, Anderson RN. How did cause of death contribute to racial differences in life expectancy in the United States in 2010? Hyattsville, MD: National Center for Health Statistics; 2013.
3. Hoffman C, Rice D, Sung HY. Persons with chronic conditions. Their prevalence and costs. JAMA. 1996; 276(18):1473–9.
4. Cruz-Jentoft AJ, Baeyens JP, Bauer JM, Boirie Y, Cederholm T, Landi F, et al. Sarcopenia: European Consensus on Definition and Diagnosis: Report of the European Working Group on sarcopenia in older people. Age Ageing. 2010;39(4):412–23.
5. Rosenberg EI. Summary comments: epidemiological and methodological problems in determining nutritional status of older persons. Am J Clin Nutr. 1989;50:1231–3.
6. Baumgartner RN, Wayne SJ, Waters DL, Janssen I, Gallagher D, Morley JE. Sarcopenic obesity predicts instrumental activities of daily living disability in the elderly. Obes Res. 2004;12(12):1995–2004.
7. Visser M, Kritchevsky SB, Goodpaster BH, Newman AB, Nevitt M, Stamm E, et al. Leg muscle mass and composition in relation to lower extremity performance in men and women aged 70 to 79: the health, aging and body composition study. J Am Geriatr Soc. 2002;50(5):897–904.
8. Visser M, Goodpaster BH, Kritchevsky SB, Newman AB, Nevitt M, Rubin SM, et al. Muscle mass, muscle strength, and muscle fat infiltration as predictors of incident mobility limitations in well-functioning older persons. J Gerontol A Biol Sci Med Sci. 2005;60(3):324–33.
9. Beaufrere B, Morio B. Fat and protein redistribution with aging: metabolic considerations. Eur J Clin Nutr. 2000;54 Suppl 3:S48–53.
10. Haveman-Nies A, de Groot LPGM, Burema J, Cruz JAA, Osler M, van Staveren WA. Dietary quality and lifestyle factors in relation to 10-year mortality in older Europeans: The SENECA study. Am J Epidemiol. 2002;156(10):962–8.
11. Trichopoulou A. Traditional Mediterranean diet and longevity in the elderly: a review. Public Health Nutr. 2004;7(7):943–7.
12. Boccardi V, Esposito A, Rizzo MR, Marfella R, Barbieri M, Paolisso G. Mediterranean diet, telomere maintenance and health status among elderly. PLoS One. 2013;8(4):e62781.
13. Roman B, Carta L, Martinez-Gonzalez MA, Serra-Majem L. Effectiveness of the Mediterranean diet in the elderly. Clin Interv Aging. 2008;3(1):97–109.
14. Schroder H, Marrugat J, Vila J, Covas MI, Elosua R. Adherence to the traditional Mediterranean diet is inversely associated with body mass index and obesity in a Spanish population. J Nutr. 2004;134(12):3355–61.
15. Tyrovolas S, Panagiotakos DB. The role of Mediterranean type of diet on the development of cancer and cardiovascular disease, in the elderly: a systematic review. Maturitas. 2010;65(2):122–30.

16. Estruch R, Martinez-Gonzalez MA, Corella D, Salas-Salvado J, Ruiz-Gutierrez V, Covas MI, et al. Effects of a Mediterranean-style diet on cardiovascular risk factors: a randomized trial. Ann Intern Med. 2006;145(1):1–11.
17. Fito M, Guxens M, Corella D, Saez G, Estruch R, de la Torre R, et al. Effect of a traditional Mediterranean diet on lipoprotein oxidation: a randomized controlled trial. Arch Intern Med. 2007;167(11):1195–203.
18. Camargo A, Delgado-Lista J, Garcia-Rios A, Cruz-Teno C, Yubero-Serrano EM, Perez-Martinez P, et al. Expression of proinflammatory, proatherogenic genes is reduced by the Mediterranean diet in elderly people. Br J Nutr. 2012;108(3):500–8.
19. Trichopoulou A, Naska A, Orfanos P, Trichopoulos D. Mediterranean diet in relation to body mass index and waist-to-hip ratio: the Greek European Prospective Investigation into Cancer and Nutrition Study. Am J Clin Nutr. 2005;82(5):935–40.
20. Tyrovolas S, Bountziouka V, Papairakleous N, Zeimbekis A, Anastassiou F, Gotsis E, et al. Adherence to the Mediterranean diet is associated with lower prevalence of obesity among elderly people living in Mediterranean islands: the MEDIS study. Int J Food Sci Nutr. 2009;60(S6):137–50.
21. Patino-Alonso MC, Recio-Rodríguez JI, Belio JFM, Colominas-Garrido R, Lema-Bartolomé J, Arranz AG, et al. Factors associated with adherence to the Mediterranean diet in the adult population. J Acad Nutr Diet. 2014;114(4):583–9.
22. Schroder H. Protective mechanisms of the Mediterranean diet in obesity and type 2 diabetes. J Nutr Biochem. 2007;18(3):149–60.
23. Ogden CL, Carroll MD, Kit BK, Flegal KM. Prevalence of childhood and adult obesity in the United States, 2011–2012. JAMA. 2014;311(8):806–14.
24. Andreyeva T, Michaud PC, van Soest A. Obesity and health in Europeans aged 50 years and older. Public Health. 2007;121(7):497–509.
25. von Ruesten A, Steffen A, Floegel A, van der A D, Masala G, Tjonneland A, et al. Trend in obesity prevalence in European adult cohort populations during follow-up since 1996 and their predictions to 2015. PLoS One. 2011;6(11):e27455.
26. Kimokoti RW, Millen BE. Diet, the global obesity epidemic, and prevention. J Am Diet Assoc. 2011; 111(8):1137–40.
27. Villareal DT, Apovian CM, Kushner RF, Klein S. Obesity in older adults: technical review and position statement of the American Society for Nutrition and NAASO, The Obesity Society. Am J Clin Nutr. 2005;82(5):923–34.
28. Harris TB, Launer LJ, Madans J, Feldman JJ. Cohort study of effect of being overweight and change in weight on risk of coronary heart disease in old age. BMJ. 1997;314(7097):1791–4.
29. Losonczy KG, Harris TB, Cornoni-Huntley J, Simonsick EM, Wallace RB, Cook NR, et al. Does weight loss from middle age to old age explain the inverse weight mortality relation in old age? Am J Epidemiol. 1995; 141(4):312–21.
30. Stevens J, Cai J, Pamuk ER, Williamson DF, Thun MJ, Wood JL. The effect of age on the association between body-mass index and mortality. N Engl J Med. 1998;338(1):1–7.
31. Oreopoulos A, Kalantar-Zadeh K, Sharma AM, Fonarow GC. The obesity paradox in the elderly: potential mechanisms and clinical implications. Clin Geriatr Med. 2009;25(4):643–59. viii.
32. Inelmen EM, Sergi G, Coin A, Miotto F, Peruzza S, Enzi G. Can obesity be a risk factor in elderly people? Obes Rev. 2003;4(3):147–55.
33. Gallagher D, Ruts E, Visser M, Heshka S, Baumgartner RN, Wang J, et al. Weight stability masks sarcopenia in elderly men and women. Am J Physiol Endocrinol Metab. 2000;279(2):E366–75.
34. Kushner RF. Clinical assessment and management of adult obesity. Circulation. 2012;126(24):2870–7.
35. Jensen MD, Ryan DH, Apovian CM, Ard JD, Comuzzie AG, Donato KA, et al. 2013 AHA/ACC/TOS guideline for the management of overweight and obesity in adults: a report of the American College of Cardiology/American Heart Association Task Force on Practice Guidelines and The Obesity Society. Circulation. 2014;129(25 Suppl 2): S102–38.
36. Cohen G, Jose SM, Ahronheim JC. Body mass index: pitfalls in elderly people. J Am Geriatr Soc. 2009;57(1): 170–2.
37. Newman AB, Lee JS, Visser M, Goodpaster BH, Kritchevsky SB, Tylavsky FA, et al. Weight change and the conservation of lean mass in old age: the Health, Aging and Body Composition Study. Am J Clin Nutr. 2005;82(4):872–8. quiz 915–6.
38. Myers J, Lata K, Chowdhury S, McAuley P, Jain N, Froelicher V. The obesity paradox and weight loss. Am J Med. 2011;124(10):924–30.
39. Nilsson PM, Nilsson JA, Hedblad B, Berglund G, Lindgarde F. The enigma of increased non-cancer mortality after weight loss in healthy men who are overweight or obese. J Intern Med. 2002;252(1):70–8.
40. De Laet C, Kanis JA, Oden A, Johanson H, Johnell O, Delmas P, et al. Body mass index as a predictor of fracture risk: a meta-analysis. Osteoporos Int. 2005;16(11):1330–8.
41. Kalantar-Zadeh K, Abbott KC, Kronenberg F, Anker SD, Horwich TB, Fonarow GC. Epidemiology of dialysis patients and heart failure patients. Semin Nephrol. 2006;26(2):118–33.

42. Kalantar-Zadeh K, Horwich TB, Oreopoulos A, Kovesdy CP, Younessi H, Anker SD, et al. Risk factor paradox in wasting diseases. Curr Opin Clin Nutr Metab Care. 2007;10(4):433–42.
43. Chapman IM. Obesity paradox during aging. Interdiscip Top Gerontol. 2010;37:20–36.
44. van Uffelen JG, Berecki-Gisolf J, Brown WJ, Dobson AJ. What is a healthy body mass index for women in their seventies? Results from the Australian longitudinal study on women's health. J Gerontol A Biol Sci Med Sci. 2010;65(8):847–53.
45. Mathus-Vliegen EM. Prevalence, pathophysiology, health consequences and treatment options of obesity in the elderly: a guideline. Obes Facts. 2012;5(3):460–83.
46. Whitmer RA, Gunderson EP, Barrett-Connor E, Quesenberry Jr CP, Yaffe K. Obesity in middle age and future risk of dementia: a 27 year longitudinal population based study. BMJ. 2005;330(7504):1360.
47. Valdes AM, Andrew T, Gardner JP, Kimura M, Oelsner E, Cherkas LF, et al. Obesity, cigarette smoking, and telomere length in women. Lancet. 2005;366(9486):662–4.
48. Boyle JP, Thompson TJ, Gregg EW, Barker LE, Williamson DF. Projection of the year 2050 burden of diabetes in the US adult population: dynamic modeling of incidence, mortality, and prediabetes prevalence. Popul Health Metr. 2010;8:29.
49. Centers for Disease Control and Prevention. National diabetes fact sheet: general information and national estimates on diabetes in the United States. Atlanta, GA: U.S. Department of Health and Human Services Centers for Disease Control and Prevention; 2011.
50. Narayan KMV, Boyle JP, Geiss LS, Saaddine JB, Thompson TJ. Impact of recent increase in incidence on future diabetes burden: U.S., 2005–2050. Diabetes Care. 2006;29(9):2114–6.
51. Villareal DT, Banks M, Siener C, Sinacore DR, Klein S. Physical frailty and body composition in obese elderly men and women. Obes Res. 2004;12(6):913–20.
52. Elkins JS, Whitmer RA, Sidney S, Sorel M, Yaffe K, Johnston SC. Midlife obesity and long-term risk of nursing home admission. Obesity (Silver Spring). 2006;14(8):1472–8.
53. Purnell JQ, Kahn SE, Albers JJ, Nevin DN, Brunzell JD, Schwartz RS. Effect of weight loss with reduction of intra-abdominal fat on lipid metabolism in older men. J Clin Endocrinol Metab. 2000;85(3):977–82.
54. Villareal DT, Banks M, Sinacore DR, Siener C, Klein S. Effect of weight loss and exercise on frailty in obese older adults. Arch Intern Med. 2006;166(8):860–6.
55. Mazzali G, Di Francesco V, Zoico E, Fantin F, Zamboni G, Benati C, et al. Interrelations between fat distribution, muscle lipid content, adipocytokines, and insulin resistance: effect of moderate weight loss in older women. Am J Clin Nutr. 2006;84(5):1193–9.
56. Crandall J, Schade D, Ma Y, Fujimoto WY, Barrett-Connor E, Fowler S, et al. The influence of age on the effects of lifestyle modification and metformin in prevention of diabetes. J Gerontol A Biol Sci Med Sci. 2006;61(10):1075–81.
57. Bales CW, Buhr G. Is obesity bad for older persons? A systematic review of the pros and cons of weight reduction in later life. J Am Med Dir Assoc. 2008;9(5):302–12.
58. Waters DL, Ward AL, Villareal DT. Weight loss in obese adults 65 years and older: a review of the controversy. Exp Gerontol. 2013;48(10):1054–61.
59. Porter Starr KN, McDonald SR, Bales CW. Obesity and physical frailty in older adults: a scoping review of lifestyle intervention trials. J Am Med Dir Assoc. 2014;15(4):240–50.
60. Bullo M, Lamuela-Raventos R, Salas-Salvado J. Mediterranean diet and oxidation: nuts and olive oil as important sources of fat and antioxidants. Curr Top Med Chem. 2011;11(14):1797–810.
61. Paddon-Jones D, Leidy H. Dietary protein and muscle in older persons. Curr Opin Clin Nutr Metab Care. 2014;17(1):5–11.
62. Shai I, Schwarzfuchs D, Henkin Y, Shahar DR, Witkow S, Greenberg I, et al. Weight loss with a low-carbohydrate, Mediterranean, or low-fat diet. N Engl J Med. 2008;359(3):229–41.
63. Esposito K, Maiorino MI, Ciotola M, Di Palo C, Scognamiglio P, Gicchino M, et al. Effects of a Mediterranean-style diet on the need for antihyperglycemic drug therapy in patients with newly diagnosed type 2 diabetes: a randomized trial. Ann Intern Med. 2009;151(5):306–14.
64. Elhayany A, Lustman A, Abel R, Attal-Singer J, Vinker S. A low carbohydrate Mediterranean diet improves cardiovascular risk factors and diabetes control among overweight patients with type 2 diabetes mellitus: a 1-year prospective randomized intervention study. Diabetes Obes Metab. 2010;12(3):204–9.
65. Mathus-Vliegen EM. Obesity and the elderly. J Clin Gastroenterol. 2012;46(7):533–44.
66. Salas-Salvado J, Bullo M, Estruch R, Ros E, Covas MI, Ibarrola-Jurado N, et al. Prevention of diabetes with Mediterranean diets: a subgroup analysis of a randomized trial. Ann Intern Med. 2014;160(1):1–10.
67. Forouhi NG, Sharp SJ, Du H, van der A D, Halkjaer J, Schulze MB, et al. Dietary fat intake and subsequent weight change in adults: results from the European Prospective Investigation into Cancer and Nutrition cohorts. Am J Clin Nutr. 2009;90(6):1632–41.
68. Sacks FM, Bray GA, Carey VJ, Smith SR, Ryan DH, Anton SD, et al. Comparison of weight-loss diets with different compositions of fat, protein, and carbohydrates. N Engl J Med. 2009;360(9):859–73.

Chapter 12
Mediterranean Diet and Neurodegenerative Diseases

Ornella I. Selmin, Alberto P.G. Romagnolo, and Donato F. Romagnolo

Key Points

- Cognitive decline, dementia, Alzheimer's (AD) and Parkinson's (PD) disease are age-related conditions that affect mature adults worldwide. Risk factors include hypercholesterolemia, obesity, diabetes, and cardiovascular factors, such as hypertension, and inflammation.
- Markers of inflammation may be useful for detection and diagnosis of neurodegenerative diseases. Studies of nutrients that are essential for optimal health produced inconsistent results about prevention of cognitive diseases. In light of the global epidemic of overweight and obesity combined with longer life expectancy, more research is needed to dissect the mechanisms involved in the development of neurodegenerative diseases and potential impact of diet and bioactive food components for prevention.
- Some studies suggest that the Mediterranean diet pattern may be beneficial for preventing and/or attenuating the process of cognitive impairment. Studies on extra-virgin olive oil, the main source of saturated fat in the Mediterranean diet, suggested protective effects on markers associated with prevention of neurodegenerative diseases.
- Improving brain mitochondrial functions using Mediterranean diet, food components, and lifestyle is an important future direction in nutrition research and treatment of cognitive impairment and neurodegeneration.

Keywords Aging • Cognitive health • Mediterranean diet

O.I. Selmin, Ph.D. (✉) • D.F. Romagnolo, Ph.D., M.Sc.
Department of Nutritional Sciences, The University of Arizona, Shantz Bldg, 85721 Tucson, AZ, USA

The University of Arizona Cancer Center, The University of Arizona, Rm 3999A, 1501 N. Campbell Avenue, Tucson, AZ 85724, USA
e-mail: selmin@u.arizona.edu; donato@u.arizona.edu

A.P.G. Romagnolo
The University of Arizona Cancer Center, The University of Arizona, Rm 3999A, 1501 N. Campbell Avenue, Tucson, AZ 85724, USA
e-mail: aroma@u.arizona.edu

D.F. Romagnolo, O.I. Selmin (eds.), *Mediterranean Diet*, Nutrition and Health,
DOI 10.1007/978-3-319-27969-5_12

Introduction

Age-related diseases that affect the brain and the neuromuscular system include Alzheimer's disease (AD), Parkinson's disease (PD), and different forms of dementia that range from mild cognitive decline to vascular dementia resulting from ischemic or hemorrhagic brain lesions. AD is the most common form of cognitive decline in elderly people accounting for ~70 % of all cases of dementia [1] (Table 12.1 and Fig. 12.1). PD is the second most common neurodegenerative disorder affecting ~1 %

Table 12.1 Key facts about dementia worldwide

• #Dementia causes deterioration in memory, thinking, behavior, and ability to perform normal everyday functions. It is the major cause of debilitation and dependency among older people worldwide. As a result, it impacts family members, healthcare practitioners and society at large
• #It is not a normal part of aging, but affects primarily older people
• #Each year, 7.7 million new cases of dementia are diagnosed. About 48 million people worldwide have dementia
• #The most common form of dementia is Alzheimer's disease which accounts for ~60–70 % of all dementia cases
• #About 5–8 % of people 60 years of age or older have dementia at any given time. The total number of people worldwide with dementia is estimated to reach ~76 million in 2030 and nearly triple to ~136 million by 2050 due to the rising numbers of people living in low- and middle-income countries

Source: World Health Organization. Available at: http://www.who.int/mediacentre/factsheets/fs362/en/

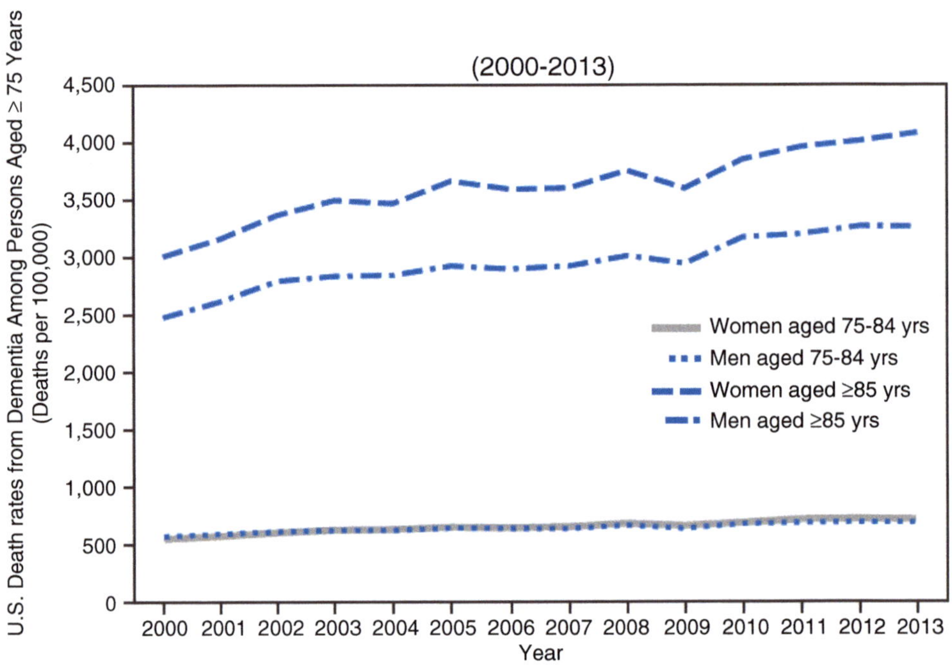

Fig. 12.1 US Death rates from dementia among persons aged ≥75 years by gender and age group, 2000–2013. Deaths from dementia include underlying and contributing causes associated with vascular dementia, unspecified dementia, or Alzheimer's disease. The figure above is a line chart showing death rates for dementia per 100,000 population increased for both men and women among persons aged 75–84 years and ≥85 years during 2000–2013. Among persons aged 75–84 years, the rate increased 21 % for men and 31 % for women. Among persons aged ≥85 years, the rate increased 32 % for men and 36 % for women. Among persons aged ≥85 years, death rates were higher for women than men throughout the period, with death rates 25 % higher among women than men in 2013 (4077.4 versus 3261.6 per 100,000 population). Source: National Vital Statistics System. Multiple cause of death data, 2000–2013. Available at http://wonder.cdc.gov/mcd-icd10.html. Reported by Ellen A. Kramarow, PhD

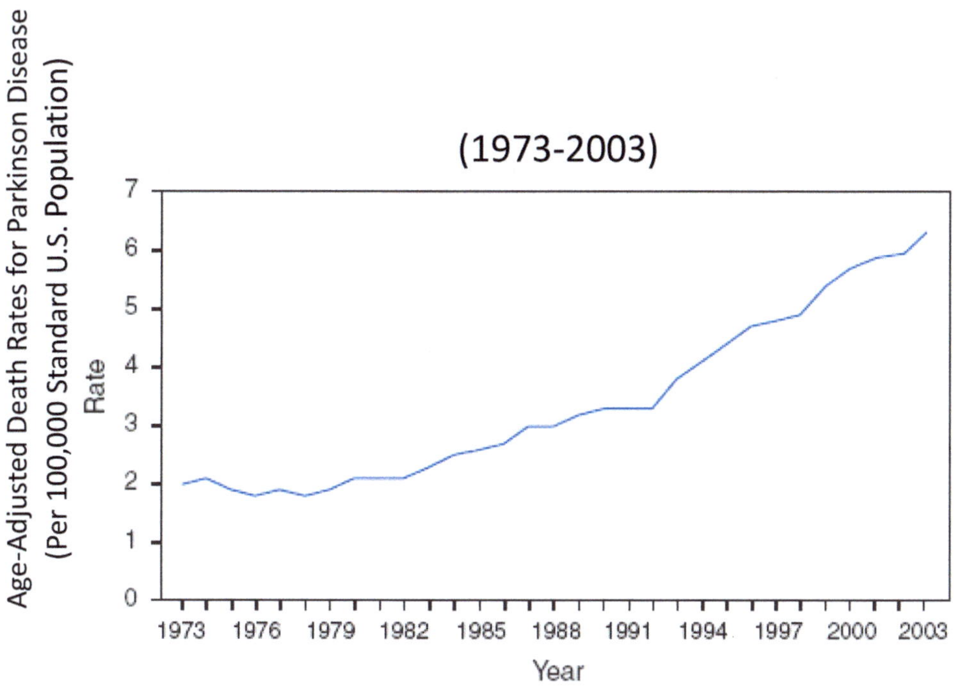

Fig. 12.2 Annual US death rates for Parkinson disease during 1973–2003. Parkinson disease became the 14th leading cause of death in the USA in 2003. This increase might be attributable to multiple factors, including an aging population, greater awareness of the disease, and improved identification of cases. Source: Hoyert DL, Heron M, Murphy SL, Kung HC. Health E-Stats. Deaths: final data for 2003. Hyattsville, MD: US Department of Health and Human Services, CDC; 2006. Available at http://www.cdc.gov/nchs/products/pubs/pubd/hestats/finaldeaths03/finaldeaths03.htm

of the population over 60 years of age in North America and Europe [2] (Fig. 12.2). Diagnosis of AD is characterized by the presence of intracellular neurofibrillary tangles of hyperphosphorylated tau; small extracellular amyloid deposits in plaques and around cerebral vessels; and of dystrophic and degenerating neurites.

Accumulation of plaques results from imbalance between amyloid deposit and clearance via autophagy. In PD patients there is a progressive degeneration of dopaminic neurons in the "*substantia grigia*" leading to difficulties in movement and progressive cognitive decline. In 2010, it was estimated that ~36 million people had some form of dementia worldwide [3], with almost 5 million new cases every year. In 2015, about 48 million people worldwide have been estimated to have dementia (Table 12.1) underscoring a ~35 % increase in only 5 years.

There are no significant worldwide geographical differences in incidence, which increases exponentially with age ranging from 1 per 1000 subjects in people between 60 and 64 years of age, to 70 per 1000 people in subjects 90 years of age or older. These data do not include people with mild cognitive disorders. Moreover, the incidence of cognitive diseases is projected to increase at a faster rate in poor countries. Epidemiological studies suggested an important role of dietary and lifestyle factors in the development of neurodegenerative disorders. Therefore, this chapter summarizes recent research evidence related to dietary and lifestyle patterns of the Mediterranean region and their usefulness for the prevention and/or amelioration of cognitive decline.

Inflammation and Aging

Inflammation plays a central role in the development of cardiovascular pathologies that in turn can predispose to cognitive decline and dementia. An increase in pro-inflammatory status in elderly persons, characterized by diminishing ability to cope with antigenic load and stressors, has been described by Franceschi et al. [4] as "inflamm-aging." These authors proposed that inflammation increases naturally with age as documented by increased levels of markers of inflammation such as interleukin-6 in elderly people. However, different factors including genetics can influence the threshold at which inflammation transitions into organ-specific disorders like AD, diabetes, atherosclerosis, etc. Successful aging, therefore, rests largely with the ability of each individual to cope with an unavoidable, lifelong exposure to environmental and inflammatory stressors, which include bacteria, viruses, oxidative stress, radicals, etc. [4]. Elevated serum levels of C-reactive protein in mature adults are linked to increased risk of AD and vascular dementia [5], supporting the hypothesis that inflammation markers may be useful to assess the development of AD and for the prevention and treatment of cognitive diseases.

Diets rich in n-6 fatty acids and unrefined sugars (e.g., Westernized diets) have been linked to inflammatory diseases such as rheumatoid arthritis, inflammatory bowel disease, and non-alcoholic fatty liver. Conversely, food components of the Mediterranean diet such as n-3 fatty acids from fish and monounsaturated fatty acids (MUFA) from olive oil have been shown to reduce or prevent inflammation [6].

Hypertension and Vascular Diseases

Research evidence suggests that hypertension in midlife is predictive of development of AD or dementia later in life [7] and that a U-shape association exist between diastolic blood pressure and risk of dementia [8], whereas lowering of blood pressure has been observed after the onset of the disease [9]. Hypercholesterolemia has also been linked to increased risk of dementia, although the findings indicated that high cholesterol levels in midlife would be a risk for AD and dementia later in life, whereas lower cholesterol levels would be characteristic of established AD and dementia [10]. One of the possible confounding factors in studies that investigated the links between cholesterol levels and cognitive health is the fact that participants may use cholesterol or lipid lowering drugs (e.g., statins) whose effects on brain functions remain largely unknown [11, 12]. In addition, genetic polymorphism may affect the interpretation of associations between nutrition parameters and risk of AD. For example, carriers of the APOE4 allele are at high risk for late onset AD and coronary heart disease. The ApoE protein regulates lipid homeostasis, and subjects who carry the APOE4 polymorphism β-oxidize more efficiently long chain n-3 fatty acids than non-carriers. This shift in oxidation efficiency may explain why consumption of fish oil rich in n-3 poly unsaturated fatty acids (PUFA) may not be beneficial to APOE4 individuals with high levels of total cholesterol [13]. Moreover, in a randomized trial that investigated the effects of dietary medium chain triglycerides in AD patients, improved cognitive scores were observed in APOE4-negative patients, but not in individuals with APOE4 mutations [14].

A recent cross-sectional study of 1889 Chinese elders (mean age: 73.5 ± 5 years) found that in participants with normal homocysteine levels there was an inverse U-shape relationship between levels of total cholesterol and cognitive scores. These results suggested that both low and high cholesterol levels were associated with lower cognitive scores. However, in participants with high homocysteine levels, no association between cholesterol and cognition was found [15]. In animal models, high levels of homocysteine increased the cortex blood-brain barrier leakage [16], and population studies have shown an increased risk of cardiovascular diseases and all-cause mortality linked to high homocysteine levels [17, 18]. Possibly, the negative effects of high levels of homocysteine may mask any positive or negative influences of cholesterol levels.

Obesity and Diabetes

Recent studies indicated that midlife obesity nearly doubled the risk of dementia later in life [19]. Conversely, opposite results were reported for older adults, where higher BMI (body mass index) was protective against AD and similar pathologies [20–24]. It is important to note, however, that BMI may not be the best indicator of risk of cognitive decline as waist to hip ratio better correlates with high risk of dementia [25].

Diabetes and glucose intolerance (pre-diabetes) are strongly associated with increased AD and vascular dementia [26–28], in particular when diabetes occurs in midlife rather than later in life [29]. Such an association may be due to brain changes induced by hyperinsulinemia, or to indirect mechanisms related to diabetes, such as hypertension, dyslipidemia, oxidative stress, and inflammation [30].

Gastrointestinal Microbiome and Brain Health

Alterations in intestinal microbiome have been implicated in diverse diseases such as diabetes, non-alcoholic liver disease, autism, and multiple sclerosis [31]. In subjects with hepatic encephalopathy, for example, cognitive decline was associated with the presence of particular species of bacteria [32]. Specifically, altered flora (higher Veillonellaceae), poor cognition, endotoxemia, and inflammation (IL-6, TNF-α, IL-2, and IL-13) were found in hepatic encephalopathy patients compared with cirrhotics patients without encephalopathy. Animal studies indicated that minor changes in the microbial composition of the gut induced by dietary regimens, caused changes in mouse brain chemistry and function [33]. Moreover, dietary changes, as well as supplementation with probiotic bacteria were able to improve learning and memory in mice [34, 35]. Longevity in people has been associated, among other factors, to microbial diversity in their intestine [36, 37], and although differences in microbiomes are reduced in elders, there is temporal stability. Changes in the microbiome observed in aging people include a reduction in bacteria that produce short-chain fatty acids, necessary for the maintenance of colonic epithelia integrity and prevention of inflammation. These changes are consistent with the concept of inflamm-aging [4], as a basis for pathologies common in later life, including dementia and AD. The fact that selected dietary patterns can reverse or modify the status of chronic inflammation in animal models and people [38, 39], provide rich opportunities for research leading to solutions to improve cognitive health and quality of life in elderly populations. A large dietary intervention study, called NU-AGE [40, 41] is currently assessing both cognitive and gut health in aged groups in relation to diet.

Parkinson's Disease

Parkinson's disease (PD) is the second most common neurodegenerative disease affecting more than one million Americans [42]. Inflammation, oxidative stress, and mitochondrial dysfunction are mechanisms contributing to its development. More specifically, it has been suggested that the main cause of PD may be the degeneration of dopaminergic neurons in the "*substantia nigra*" leading to a dopaminergic deficit in the "*corpus striatum*" and consequent progress into cognitive decline and difficulties of movement. Mitochondrial dysfunction in the "*substantia nigra*" would play a central role in development of this disorder [43]. The most common deficit in mitochondria associated with

PD is reduced activity of the mitochondrial complex I (NADH:ubiquinone oxidoreductase), which is the main site of entry of electron into the respiratory chain. This leads to accumulation of ROS, depletion of ATP, and increased death of dopaminergic neurons. Reduced brain concentration of PUFA has been suggested to play a role in the progression of PD, in light of the involvement of PUFA as substrate for the synthesis of anti-inflammatory cytokines [44]. Several epidemiological studies have reported inconsistent findings regarding possible associations of dietary components with risk of PD. These discrepancies are likely attributable to the fact most of these studies relied on questionnaires about food consumption and lifestyles, and relative small sample sizes [45]. Recently, a large study by Dong et al. [46] found a positive, albeit weak, correlation between high levels of n-6 PUFA, in particular linoleic acid, and risk of PD in never-smokers and heavy coffee drinkers. Kamel et al. [47], conversely, reported that higher levels of n-3 PUFAs were directly associated with lower risk of PD.

Alcalay et al. [48] found a positive correlation between high adherence to the Mediterranean diet and 14 % reduction in PD, both in men and women. The Mediterranean diet is characterized by a high level of MUFA (mainly in extra-virgin olive oil) and n-3 PUFA from fish and vegetables. These results were confirmed after adjusting for multiple potential confounders, and highlighted the importance of considering whole dietary patterns rather than individual food components for their influence on complex disorders such as PD.

Dietary Patterns and Cognitive Decline

Ketogenic Diet

Ketogenesis is a process taking place in the mitochondrial matrix of the liver. It occurs during fasting and carbohydrate restriction as a result of an imbalance between production of acetyl-CoA via β-oxidation of fatty acids, and its utilization to generate citrate for the Krebs cycle via condensation with oxaloacetate. As a result, acetyl-CoA molecules condense to generate the ketones acetoacetate and β-hydroxybutyrate, and under conditions of severe ketogenesis, the volatile ketone, acetone. Normally, fasting or reduced carbohydrate intake depletes the glucose available for Krebs cycle and central nervous system (CNS) activities. In the absence of glucose, the CNS is unable to utilize fatty acids because they cannot cross the blood–brain barrier; however, the brain can use ketone bodies as an alternative source of energy.

The antiepileptic effects of caloric restriction have been recognized for a long time in medical history. Usually, blood levels of ketone bodies in healthy persons remain low because the CNS efficiently utilizes ketone bodies in place of glucose, and a ketogenic diet can promote positive changes in cellular processes involving stress resistance and autophagy. It has been proposed that ketogenic diets can be a useful approach to ameliorate neurodegenerative diseases, including AD and PD, because they would contrast neuronal degeneration and mitochondrial dysfunction [49]. The mechanistic explanation may lay on the ability of the CNS to utilize sources of energy independent from glycogen breakdown. In brain of Alzheimer's patients, for example, increased availability of ketones could increase the amount of energy obtained from ATP hydrolysis and in turn increase the cytoplasmic level of acetyl-CoA which would then counteract the reduction in acetylcholine characteristic of Alzheimer's brain tissues. In addition, ketones could improve mitochondrial pathways and in turn neuronal metabolism. For example, in vitro experiments and small epidemiological studies suggested that a ketogenic diet could be beneficial to Parkinson's patients mainly because of the ability of ketone bodies to bypass defects in mitochondrial complex 1 activity [45].

The Mediterranean Diet

Some epidemiological studies documented a reduced risk of cognitive disorders associated with adherence to a Mediterranean diet. For example, lower adherence to a Mediterranean diet was associated with higher AD and mild cognitive impairment compared to healthy subjects in an Australian population [50]. Similarly, Tsivgoulis et al. [51], reported that higher adherence to a Mediterranean diet was associated with lower likelihood of incident cognitive impairment. Conversely, results of a study which included 6174 participants, aged 65+ years, from the cognitive sub-study of the Women's Health Study reported no association of the Mediterranean diet with cognitive decline [52]. These discrepancies may be due to variations in methodologies used to assess adherence; different sample size; heterogeneity of groups or populations tested; and poor reliability of food questionnaires, among other factors [53]. Earlier studies indicated that a "prudent" dietary pattern, characterized by abundance of fish, grains, fruits and vegetables may be protective against PD, when compared to a Western diet, characterized by a high content of n-6 PUFA and saturated fat [54]. In a recent review, Lourida et al. [53] analyzed 12 studies and found a positive association (in 9 out of 12), between adherence to a Mediterranean diet and slower cognitive decline including onset of AD. Gu et al. [55] measured markers of inflammation and metabolic profile and found that strict adherence to a Mediterranean diet was associated with a 34 % reduction in AD, even though markers of inflammation such as C-reactive protein, indicators of diabetes and obesity such as fasting insulin and adiponectin were either modestly reduced or unchanged. More recently, Singh et al. [56] selected five studies to investigate the relationships between adherence to the Mediterranean diet and cognitive impairment. These investigators found a 33 % reduction in onset and development of both mild cognitive impairment and AD in people strictly adhering to the Mediterranean diet. A review article by Kuczmarski et al. [57] examined 11 cross-sectional and prospective studies and concluded that there is robust scientific evidence supporting a relationship between adherence to a Mediterranean style diet and slower cognitive decline. However, standardization of assessment tools is needed to better evaluate the effectiveness of the Mediterranean diet for the prevention of AD. Differences in methodologies are likely the main reason why some studies have found no correlation between adherence to a Mediterranean diet and delayed or reduced cognitive decline [58, 59]. A few studies have utilized more rigorous and quantitative assays to establish a relation between dietary behavior and cognitive health. For example, Titova and coauthors [60] published the results of an analysis conducted in a group of ~200 healthy Swedish men and women, age 70. Adherence to a Mediterranean diet was correlated to cognitive functions and brain volumes, which were measured at age 75 by magnetic resonance imaging. Cognitive assessment was measured using the seven minute screening technique [61]. The findings suggested that low consumption of meat and meat products (one of the main suggestions of the Mediterranean diet) was positively associated to healthier cognitive aging, even though no association was found between Mediterranean score and cognitive function or brain volume. Adherence to Mediterranean and DASH (Dietary Approaches to Stop Hypertension) diets have been correlated with lower risk of incident dementia and global cognitive decline in a 6- and 11-year follow-up studies [62, 63].

Physical frailty, a major component of cognitive impairment, is considered a precursor of neurodegenerative processes, including AD [64]. Numerous studies have reported an inverse association between adherence to a Mediterranean diet and lifestyle and prevalence of frailty [65–67]. In particular, physical exercise, as an essential component of the Mediterranean pyramid, has been deemed important in promoting mobility performance in elderly populations [64]. Moreover, a balanced diet, rich in vitamins and antioxidants, and low in red meat has been considered ideal to prevent states of malnutrition often associated with frailty and cognitive impairment in aging people [68].

Single food components of the Mediterranean diet, such as fish oil and moderate wine consumption, have been linked to slower cognitive decline and reduced risk of AD [69, 70]. Also, results of various studies documented a preventive role of extra virgin olive oil (EVOO) against cognitive decline. EVOO is the main source of MUFA in the Mediterranean diet and is rich in antioxidants compounds (e.g., polyphenols). A study conducted on 447 individuals (age 55–80) at high risk of cardiovascular disease, examined urinary polyphenols as markers of food consumption and their association with cognitive scores, assessed by neuropsychologists [71]. The results of this study indicated a positive association between increased levels of urinary polyphenols and better scores in verbal memory, confirming the notion that increased intake of polyphenolic components of the Mediterranean diet may prevent or ameliorate age-related cognitive disorders.

Amyloid β-deposition in the brain precedes the onset of AD. In a mice model for amyloid-β deposition, dietary supplementation for 8 weeks with oleuropein aglycone (50 mg/kg diet), the main polyphenol present in EVOO, reduced β-amyloid levels and plaque deposits, microglia migration to the plaques for phagocytosis, and astrocyte reaction. Conversely, autophagic reaction and recovery of lysosomal activity (whose dysfunction is one of the earliest disturbances that occur in AD) were dramatically induced by oleuropein aglycone [72]. The activated autophagy would reduce plaque burden, dimensions, and compactness. The senescence accelerate mouse P8 (SAMP8) has been suggested as an excellent model of early learning and memory problems since it has cholinergic deficits, oxidative damage, alterations in membrane lipids and circadian rhythm disturbances. Brains of the SAMP8 mouse overexpress amyloid precursor protein and β-amyloid, and have increased phosphorylation of tau. These results were confirmed in an animal model of AD, the SAMP8 mice, by Morley et al. [73]. Caution should be exercised, however, in extrapolating results from animal studies to human, as differences in clinical efficacy and side effects have been observed. For examples, in studies that used rodent models to examine the neuroprotective impact of caloric restriction, adverse effects were observed in the hippocampus and brain functions [74, 75].

Lastly, Trichopoulou et al. [76] recently published results of a prospective study conducted in Greek men and women residing in Athens, using a mini-mental state examination (Table 12.2) [77] on 401 subjects 65 years of age or older. The test was administered twice over a period of 7 years and found a significant inverse association between adherence to a Mediterranean diet and both mild and substantial cognitive decline, in particular in older subjects. Of the nine dietary components included in the score system, vegetable consumption had a significant inverse association, while alcohol and high MUFA:SFA (saturated fatty acids) ratio had a weak inverse association with cognitive decline, suggesting differential effects of food components. Interestingly, this study supported the idea that adherence to a Mediterranean diet may be more beneficial in older groups when cognitive decline occurs at a faster pace.

Conclusions

A large body of data indicates that main components of the Mediterranean diet, such as EVOO, low carbohydrates, high fruits and vegetables, and regular exercise have protective effects against cognitive decline, including AD and PD. In contrast, fewer epidemiological studies do not support a positive association between adherence to a Mediterranean diet and slower progression of cognitive disorders. Factors that may impact the efficacy of the Mediterranean diet on etiology of cognitive diseases include deviations in diet composition (i.e., transition to a Westernized Mediterranean diet), and interactions with genotype (e.g., mutations and/or polymorphisms). Considering the abundance of MUFA and n-3 PUFA in the Mediterranean diet and the supporting role of ketones in regulation of brain metabolism [78], it is reasonable to speculate that adherence to a Mediterranean diet that includes fish, EVOO, and fruits and vegetables; and lifestyle that includes regular physical activity, reduction of energy intake, and intermittent fasting may offer protection against (or delay) the progression of cognitive diseases.

Table 12.2 "Mini-mental state" examination

Instructions for administration of mini-mental state examination
Orientation
–#Ask for the date. Then ask specifically for parts omitted, e.g., "Can you also tell me what season it is?" One point for each correct.
–#Ask in turn "Can you tell me the name of this hospital?" (town, county, etc.). One point for each correct.
Registration
–#Ask the patient if you may test his memory. Then say the names of three unrelated objects, clearly and slowly, about 1 s for each. After you have said all the three, ask to repeat them. This first repetition determines the score (0–3) but keep saying them until the patient can repeat all the three, up to six trials. If the patient does not eventually learn all the three, recall cannot be meaningfully tested.
Attention and calculation
–#Ask the patient to begin with 100 and count backwards by 7. Stop after five subtractions (93, 86, 79, 72, 65). Score the total number of correct answers.
–#If the patient cannot or will not perform this task, ask to spell the word "world" backwards. The score is the number of letters in correct order, e.g., dlrow = 5, dlorw = 3.
Recall
–#Ask the patient to recall the three words you previously asked to remember. Score 0–3.
Language
Naming: Show the patient a wrist watch and ask what it is. Repeat for pencil. Score 0–2.
Repetition: Ask the patient to repeat the sentence after you. Allow only one trial. Score 0 or 1.
3-Stage command: Give the patient a piece of plain blank paper and repeat the command. Score 1 point for each part correctly executed.
Reading: On a blank piece of paper print the sentence "Close your eyes," in letters large enough for the patient to see clearly. Ask to read it and do what it says. Score 1 point only if the patient actually closes his/her eyes.
Writing: Give the patient a blank piece of paper and ask to write a sentence for you. Do not dictate a sentence; it is to be written spontaneously. It must contain a subject and verb and be sensible. Correct grammar and punctuation are not necessary.
Copying: On a clean piece of paper, draw intersecting pentagons, each side about 1 in., and ask to copy it exactly as it is. All 10 angles must be present and two must intersect to score 1 point. Tremor and rotation are ignored. Estimate the patient's level of sensorium along a continuum, from alert on the left to coma on the right.

Adapted from Folstein et al. [77]

References

1. Blennow K, de Leon MJ, Zetterberg H. Alzheimer's disease. Lancet. 2006;368(9533):387–403.
2. Nussbaum RL, Ellis CE. Alzheimer's disease and Parkinson's disease. N Engl J Med. 2003;348(14):1356–64.
3. Prince M, Bryce R, Albanese E, Wimo A, Ribeiro W, Ferri CP. The global prevalence of dementia: a systematic review and meta analysis. Alzheimers Dement. 2013;9(1):63–75.e2.
4. Franceschi C, Bonafè M, Valensin S, Olivieri F, De Luca M, Ottaviani E, De Benedictis G. Inflamm-aging. An evolutionary perspective on immunosenescence. Ann N Y Acad Sci. 2000;908:244–54.
5. Gorelick PB. Role of inflammation in cognitive impairment: results of observational epidemiological studies and clinical trials. Ann N Y Acad Sci. 2010;1207:155–62.
6. Huang EY, Devkota S, Moscoso D, Chang EB, Leone VA. The role of diet in triggering human inflammatory disorders in the modern age. Microbes Infect. 2013;15(12):765–74.
7. Wysocki M, Luo X, Schmeidler J, Dahlman K, Lesser GT, Grossman H, Haroutunian V, Beeri MS. Hypertension is associated with cognitive decline in elderly people at high risk for dementia. Am J Geriatr Psychiatry. 2012;20(2):179–87.
8. Peters R, Beckett N, Fagard R, Thijs L, Wang JG, Forette F, Pereira L, Fletcher A, Bulpitt C. Increased pulse pressure linked to dementia: further results from the Hypertension in the Very Elderly Trial—HYVET. J Hypertens. 2013;31(9):1868–75.

9. Duron E, Hanon O. Vascular risk factors, cognitive decline, and dementia. Vasc Health Risk Manag. 2008;4(2):363–81.
10. Solomon A, Kåreholt I, Ngandu T, Wolozin B, Macdonald SW, Winblad B, Nissinen A, Tuomilehto J, Soininen H, Kivipelto M. Serum total cholesterol, statins and cognition in non-demented elderly. Neurobiol Aging. 2009;30(6):1006–9.
11. van Vliet P. Cholesterol and late-life cognitive decline. J Alzheimers Dis. 2012;30 Suppl 2:S147–62.
12. Simić I, Reiner Z. Adverse effects of statins—myths and reality. Curr Pharm Des. 2015;21(9):1220–6.
13. Chouinard-Watkins R, Plourde M. Fatty acid metabolism in carriers of apolipoprotein E epsilon 4 allele: is it contributing to higher risk of cognitive decline and coronary heart disease? Nutrients. 2014;6(10):4452–71.
14. Henderson ST, Vogel JL, Barr LJ, Garvin F, Jones JJ, Costantini LC. Study of the ketogenic agent AC-1202 in mild to moderate Alzheimer's disease: a randomized, double-blind, placebo-controlled, multicenter trial. Nutr Metab (Lond). 2009;6:31.
15. Cheng Y, Jin Y, Unverzagt FW, Su L, Yang L, Ma F, Hake AM, Kettler C, Chen C, Liu J, Bian J, Li P, Murrell JR, Hendrie HC, Gao S. The relationship between cholesterol and cognitive function is homocysteine-dependent. Clin Interv Aging. 2014;9:1823–9.
16. Ehrlich D, Pirchl M, Humpel C. Effects of long-term moderate ethanol and cholesterol on cognition, cholinergic neurons, inflammation, and vascular impairment in rats. Neuroscience. 2012;205:154–66.
17. Bates CJ, Mansoor MA, Pentieva KD, Hamer M, Mishra GD. Biochemical risk indices, including plasma homocysteine, that prospectively predict mortality in older British people: the National Diet and Nutrition Survey of People Aged 65 Years and Over. Br J Nutr. 2010;104(6):893–9.
18. Hackam DG, Anand SS. Emerging risk factors for atherosclerotic vascular disease: a critical review of the evidence. JAMA. 2003;290(7):932–40.
19. Loef M, Walach H. Midlife obesity and dementia: meta-analysis and adjusted forecast of dementia prevalence in the United States and China. Obesity (Silver Spring). 2013;21(1):E51–5.
20. Atti AR, Palmer K, Volpato S, Winblad B, De Ronchi D, Fratiglioni L. Late-life body mass index and dementia incidence: nine-year follow-up data from the Kungsholmen Project. J Am Geriatr Soc. 2008;56(1):111–6.
21. Chu LW, Tam S, Lee PW, Yik PY, Song Y, Cheung BM, Lam KS. Late-life body mass index and waist circumference in amnestic mild cognitive impairment and Alzheimer's disease. J Alzheimers Dis. 2009;17(1):223–32.
22. Dahl AK, Löppönen M, Isoaho R, Berg S, Kivelä SL. Overweight and obesity in old age are not associated with greater dementia risk. J Am Geriatr Soc. 2008;56(12):2261–6.
23. Fitzpatrick AL, Kuller LH, Lopez OL, Diehr P, O'Meara ES, Longstreth Jr WT, Luchsinger JA. Midlife and late-life obesity and the risk of dementia: cardiovascular health study. Arch Neurol. 2009;66(3):336–42.
24. Hughes TF, Borenstein AR, Schofield E, Wu Y, Larson EB. Association between late-life body mass index and dementia: the Kame Project. Neurology. 2009;72(20):1741–6.
25. Luchsinger JA. Type 2 diabetes and cognitive impairment: linking mechanisms. J Alzheimers Dis. 2012;30 Suppl 2:S185–98.
26. Kimm H, Lee PH, Shin YJ, Park KS, Jo J, Lee Y, Kang HC, Jee SH. Mid-life and late-life vascular risk factors and dementia in Korean men and women. Arch Gerontol Geriatr. 2011;52(3):e117–22.
27. Ohara T, Doi Y, Ninomiya T, Hirakawa Y, Hata J, Iwaki T, Kanba S, Kiyohara Y. Glucose tolerance status and risk of dementia in the community: the Hisayama study. Neurology. 2011;77(12):1126–34.
28. Wang KC, Woung LC, Tsai MT, Liu CC, Su YH, Li CY. Risk of Alzheimer's disease in relation to diabetes: a population-based cohort study. Neuroepidemiology. 2012;38(4):237–44.
29. Xu WL, von Strauss E, Qiu CX, Winblad B, Fratiglioni L. Uncontrolled diabetes increases the risk of Alzheimer's disease: a population-based cohort study. Diabetologia. 2009;52(6):1031–9.
30. Xu W, Qiu C, Winblad B, Fratiglioni L. The effect of borderline diabetes on the risk of dementia and Alzheimer's disease. Diabetes. 2007;56(1):211–6.
31. de Vos WM, de Vos EA. Role of the intestinal microbiome in health and disease: from correlation to causation. Nutr Rev. 2012;70 Suppl 1:S45–56.
32. Bajaj JS, Ridlon JM, Hylemon PB, Thacker LR, Heuman DM, Smith S, Sikaroodi M, Gillevet PM. Linkage of gut microbiome with cognition in hepatic encephalopathy. Am J Physiol Gastrointest Liver Physiol. 2012;302(1):G168–75.
33. Bercik P, Denou E, Collins J, Jackson W, Lu J, Jury J, Deng Y, Blennerhassett P, Macri J, McCoy KD, Verdu EF, Collins SM. The intestinal microbiota affect central levels of brain-derived neurotropic factor and behavior in mice. Gastroenterology. 2011;141(2):599–609. 609.e1–3.
34. Ohland CL, Kish L, Bell H, Thiesen A, Hotte N, Pankiv E, Madsen KL. Effects of Lactobacillus helveticus on murine behavior are dependent on diet and genotype and correlate with alterations in the gut microbiome. Psychoneuroendocrinology. 2013;38(9):1738–47.
35. Davari S, Talaei SA, Alaei H, Salami M. Probiotics treatment improves diabetes-induced impairment of synaptic activity and cognitive function: behavioral and electrophysiological proofs for microbiome-gut-brain axis. Neuroscience. 2013;240:287–96.

36. Claesson MJ, Cusack S, O'Sullivan O, Greene-Diniz R, de Weerd H, Flannery E, Marchesi JR, Falush D, Dinan T, Fitzgerald G, Stanton C, van Sinderen D, O'Connor M, Harnedy N, O'Connor K, Henry C, O'Mahony D, Fitzgerald AP, Shanahan F, Twomey C, Hill C, Ross RP, O'Toole PW. Composition, variability, and temporal stability of the intestinal microbiota of the elderly. Proc Natl Acad Sci U S A. 2011;108 Suppl 1:4586–91.
37. Claesson MJ, Jeffery IB, Conde S, Power SE, O'Connor EM, Cusack S, Harris HM, Coakley M, Lakshminarayanan B, O'Sullivan O, Fitzgerald GF, Deane J, O'Connor M, Harnedy N, O'Connor K, O'Mahony D, van Sinderen D, Wallace M, Brennan L, Stanton C, Marchesi JR, Fitzgerald AP, Shanahan F, Hill C, Ross RP, O'Toole PW. Gut microbiota composition correlates with diet and health in the elderly. Nature. 2012;488(7410):178–84.
38. Vom Berg J, Prokop S, Miller KR, Obst J, Kälin RE, Lopategui-Cabezas I, Wegner A, Mair F, Schipke CG, Peters O, Winter Y, Becher B, Heppner FL. Inhibition of IL-12/IL-23 signaling reduces Alzheimer's disease-like pathology and cognitive decline. Nat Med. 2012;18(12):1812–9.
39. Berer K, Mues M, Koutrolos M, Rasbi ZA, Boziki M, Johner C, Wekerle H, Krishnamoorthy G. Commensal microbiota and myelin autoantigen cooperate to trigger autoimmune demyelination. Nature. 2011;479(7374):538–41.
40. Santoro A, Pini E, Scurti M, Palmas G, Berendsen A, Brzozowska A, Pietruszka B, Szczecinska A, Cano N, Meunier N, de Groot CP, Feskens E, Fairweather-Tait S, Salvioli S, Capri M, Brigidi P, Franceschi C, NU-AGE Consortium. Combating inflammaging through a Mediterranean whole diet approach: the NU-AGE project's conceptual framework and design. Mech Ageing Dev. 2014;136–137:3–13.
41. Candela M, Biagi E, Brigidi P, O'Toole PW, De Vos WM. Maintenance of a healthy trajectory of the intestinal microbiome during aging: a dietary approach. Mech Ageing Dev. 2014;136–137:70–5.
42. Bach JP, Riedel O, Klotsche J, Spottke A, Dodel R, Wittchen HU. Impact of complications and comorbidities on treatment costs and health-related quality of life of patients with Parkinson's disease. J Neurol Sci. 2012;314(1–2):41–7.
43. Camilleri A, Vassallo N. The centrality of mitochondria in the pathogenesis and treatment of Parkinson's disease. CNS Neurosci Ther. 2014;20(7):591–602.
44. Layé S. Polyunsaturated fatty acids, neuroinflammation and well being. Prostaglandins Leukot Essent Fatty Acids. 2010;82(4–6):295–303.
45. Vanitallie TB, Nonas C, Di Rocco A, Boyar K, Hyams K, Heymsfield SB. Treatment of Parkinson disease with diet-induced hyperketonemia: a feasibility study. Neurology. 2005;64(4):728–30.
46. Dong J, Beard JD, Umbach DM, Park Y, Huang X, Blair A, Kamel F, Chen H. Dietary fat intake and risk for Parkinson's disease. Mov Disord. 2014;29(13):1623–30.
47. Kamel F, Goldman SM, Umbach DM, Chen H, Richardson G, Barber MR, Meng C, Marras C, Korell M, Kasten M, Hoppin JA, Comyns K, Chade A, Blair A, Bhudhikanok GS, Webster Ross G, William Langston J, Sandler DP, Tanner CM. Dietary fat intake, pesticide use, and Parkinson's disease. Parkinsonism Relat Disord. 2014;20(1):82–7.
48. Alcalay RN, Gu Y, Mejia-Santana H, Cote L, Marder KS, Scarmeas N. The association between Mediterranean diet adherence and Parkinson's disease. Mov Disord. 2012;27(6):771–4.
49. Paoli A, Bianco A, Damiani E, Bosco G. Ketogenic diet in neuromuscular and neurodegenerative diseases. Biomed Res Int. 2014;2014:474296.
50. Gardener S, Gu Y, Rainey-Smith SR, Keogh JB, Clifton PM, Mathieson SL, Taddei K, Mondal A, Ward VK, Scarmeas N, Barnes M, Ellis KA, Head R, Masters CL, Ames D, Macaulay SL, Rowe CC, Szoeke C, Martins RN, AIBL Research Group. Adherence to a Mediterranean diet and Alzheimer's disease risk in an Australian population. Transl Psychiatry. 2012;2:e164.
51. Tsivgoulis G, Judd S, Letter AJ, Alexandrov AV, Howard G, Nahab F, Unverzagt FW, Moy C, Howard VJ, Kissela B, Wadley VG. Adherence to a Mediterranean diet and risk of incident cognitive impairment. Neurology. 2013;80(18):1684–92.
52. Samieri C, Grodstein F, Rosner BA, Kang JH, Cook NR, Manson JE, Buring JE, Willett WC, Okereke OI. Mediterranean diet and cognitive function in older age. Epidemiology. 2013;24(4):490–9.
53. Lourida I, Soni M, Thompson-Coon J, Purandare N, Lang IA, Ukoumunne OC, Llewellyn DJ. Mediterranean diet, cognitive function, and dementia: a systematic review. Epidemiology. 2013;24(4):479–89.
54. Gao X, Chen H, Fung TT, Logroscino G, Schwarzschild MA, Hu FB, Ascherio A. Prospective study of dietary pattern and risk of Parkinson disease. Am J Clin Nutr. 2007;86(5):1486–94.
55. Gu Y, Luchsinger JA, Stern Y, Scarmeas N. Mediterranean diet, inflammatory and metabolic biomarkers, and risk of Alzheimer's disease. J Alzheimers Dis. 2010;22(2):483–92.
56. Singh B, Parsaik AK, Mielke MM, Erwin PJ, Knopman DS, Petersen RC, Roberts RO. Association of Mediterranean diet with mild cognitive impairment and Alzheimer's disease: a systematic review and meta-analysis. J Alzheimers Dis. 2014;39(2):271–82.
57. Kuczmarski MF, Allegro D, Stave E. The association of healthful diets and cognitive function: a review. J Nutr Gerontol Geriatr. 2014;33(2):69–90.
58. Féart C, Jutand MA, Larrieu S, Letenneur L, Delcourt C, Combe N, Barberger-Gateau P. Energy, macronutrient and fatty acid intake of French elderly community dwellers and association with socio-demographic characteristics: data from the Bordeaux sample of the Three-City Study. Br J Nutr. 2007;98(5):1046–57.

59. Cherbuin N, Anstey KJ. The Mediterranean diet is not related to cognitive change in a large prospective investigation: the PATH Through Life study. Am J Geriatr Psychiatry. 2012;20(7):635–9.
60. Titova OE, Sjögren P, Brooks SJ, Kullberg J, Ax E, Kilander L, Riserus U, Cederholm T, Larsson EM, Johansson L, Ahlström H, Lind L, Schiöth HB, Benedict C. Dietary intake of eicosapentaenoic and docosahexaenoic acids is linked to gray matter volume and cognitive function in elderly. Age (Dordr). 2013;35(4):1495–505.
61. Solomon PR, Hirschoff A, Kelly B, Relin M, Brush M, DeVeaux RD, Pendlebury WW. A 7 minute neurocognitive screening battery highly sensitive to Alzheimer's disease. Arch Neurol. 1998;55(3):349–55.
62. Norton MC, Dew J, Smith H, Fauth E, Piercy KW, Breitner JC, Tschanz J, Wengreen H, Welsh-Bohmer K, Cache County Investigators. Lifestyle behavior pattern is associated with different levels of risk for incident dementia and Alzheimer's disease: the Cache County study. J Am Geriatr Soc. 2012;60(3):405–12.
63. Wengreen H, Munger RG, Cutler A, Quach A, Bowles A, Corcoran C, Tschanz JT, Norton MC, Welsh-Bohmer KA. Prospective study of Dietary Approaches to Stop Hypertension- and Mediterranean-style dietary patterns and age-related cognitive change: the Cache County Study on Memory, Health and Aging. Am J Clin Nutr. 2013;98(5):1263–71.
64. Panza F, Solfrizzi V, Giannini M, Seripa D, Pilotto A, Logroscino G. Nutrition, frailty, and Alzheimer's disease. Front Aging Neurosci. 2014;6:221.
65. Talegawkar SA, Bandinelli S, Bandeen-Roche K, Chen P, Milaneschi Y, Tanaka T, Semba RD, Guralnik JM, Ferrucci L. A higher adherence to a Mediterranean-style diet is inversely associated with the development of frailty in community-dwelling elderly men and women. J Nutr. 2012;142(12):2161–6.
66. Bollwein J, Diekmann R, Kaiser MJ, Bauer JM, Uter W, Sieber CC, Volkert D. Dietary quality is related to frailty in community-dwelling older adults. J Gerontol A Biol Sci Med Sci. 2013;68(4):483–9.
67. Féart C, Pérès K, Samieri C, Letenneur L, Dartigues JF, Barberger-Gateau P. Adherence to a Mediterranean diet and onset of disability in older persons. Eur J Epidemiol. 2011;26(9):747–56.
68. Morley JE. Cognition and nutrition. Curr Opin Clin Nutr Metab Care. 2014;17(1):1–4.
69. Aberg MA, Aberg N, Brisman J, Sundberg R, Winkvist A, Torén K. Fish intake of Swedish male adolescents is a predictor of cognitive performance. Acta Paediatr. 2009;98(3):555–60.
70. Stampfer MJ, Kang JH, Chen J, Cherry R, Grodstein F. Effects of moderate alcohol consumption on cognitive function in women. N Engl J Med. 2005;352(3):245–53.
71. Valls-Pedret C, Lamuela-Raventós RM, Medina-Remón A, Quintana M, Corella D, Pintó X, Martínez-González MÁ, Estruch R, Ros E. Polyphenol-rich foods in the Mediterranean diet are associated with better cognitive function in elderly subjects at high cardiovascular risk. J Alzheimers Dis. 2012;29(4):773–82.
72. Grossi C, Rigacci S, Ambrosini S, Ed Dami T, Luccarini I, Traini C, Failli P, Berti A, Casamenti F, Stefani M. The polyphenol oleuropein aglycone protects TgCRND8 mice against Aß plaque pathology. PLoS One. 2013;8(8):e71702.
73. Morley JE, Farr SA, Kumar VB, Armbrecht HJ. The SAMP8 mouse: a model to develop therapeutic interventions for Alzheimer's disease. Curr Pharm Des. 2012;18(8):1123–30.
74. Maalouf M, Rho JM, Mattson MP. The neuroprotective properties of calorie restriction, the ketogenic diet, and ketone bodies. Brain Res Rev. 2009;59(2):293–315.
75. Balietti M, Giorgetti B, Fattoretti P, Grossi Y, Di Stefano G, Casoli T, Platano D, Solazzi M, Orlando F, Aicardi G, Bertoni-Freddari C. Ketogenic diets cause opposing changes in synaptic morphology in CA1 hippocampus and dentate gyrus of late-adult rats. Rejuvenation Res. 2008;11(3):631–40.
76. Trichopoulou A, Kyrozis A, Rossi M, Katsoulis M, Trichopoulos D, La Vecchia C, Lagiou P. Mediterranean diet and cognitive decline over time in an elderly Mediterranean population. Eur J Nutr. 2015;54(8):1311–21.
77. Folstein MF, Folstein SE, McHugh PR. "Mini-mental state". A practical method for grading the cognitive state of patients for the clinician. J Psychiatr Res. 1975;12(3):189–98.
78. Molfino A, Gioia G, Fanelli FR, Muscaritoli M. The role for dietary omega-3 fatty acids supplementation in older adults. Nutrients. 2014;6(10):4058–72.

Chapter 13
Mediterranean Diet and Breast Cancer

Cynthia A. Thomson and Nicole R. Stendell-Hollis

Key Points

- Breast cancer remains the most commonly diagnosed cancer in women. Whereas some epidemiological studies generally support the role of diet in breast cancer prevention, conflicting evidence exists, making it challenging to provide a definitive answer on these risks that can be effectively translated to clinical practice and public health recommendations.
- In evaluating the relationship between dietary patterns and breast cancer risk a rather consistent picture evolves across continents suggesting diets rich in plant foods and variety are likely associated with lower breast cancer risk as compared to diets high in animal food sources. A Mediterranean dietary pattern and diets high in vegetables, fruit, fish and soy are associated with a decreased risk for breast cancer.
- This pattern is most commonly described as a diet high in vegetables, fruit, variety of plant foods, whole grains, monounsaturated fats (olives, olive oil), lean proteins (fish, lentils, beans) as well as nuts, seeds, wine, and bioactive-rich seasoning and spices. Protective mechanisms include but are not limited to effects on breast tissue density, altered estrogen metabolism, HER-2 *neu* expression, oxidative stress, and anti-inflammatory response.
- More studies evaluating the role of the Mediterranean diet in breast cancer prevention and survival are needed before a clear recommendation can be made.

Keywords Mediterranean diet • Breast cancer • Breast density • Her2-neu • Oxidative stress • Inflammation • Estrogen • Prevention • Olive oil • Monounsaturated • Fruits and vegetables

C.A. Thomson, Ph.D., R.D.N. (✉)
Health Promotion Sciences Department, The University of Arizona,
1295 N. Martin, Campus PO Box 245209, Drachman Hall A260, Tucson, AZ 85724, USA
e-mail: cthomson@email.arizona.edu

N.R. Stendell-Hollis, Ph.D., R.D.N.
Department of Nutrition, Exercise, and Health Sciences, Central Washington University,
400 University Way, Ellensburg, WA 98926, USA
e-mail: StendellHollisN@cwu.EDU

D.F. Romagnolo, O.I. Selmin (eds.), *Mediterranean Diet*, Nutrition and Health,
DOI 10.1007/978-3-319-27969-5_13

Introduction

Breast cancer remains the most commonly diagnosed cancer in women (Fig. 13.1), accounting for 1.7 new cases annually worldwide and over 200,000 cases in the USA alone [1] (Fig. 13.2). Prognosis in terms of 5 year survival rates after a diagnosis of early stage disease are high, reaching as high as 98 % in some subgroups [2]. This improvement in survival is thought to be largely driven by expanded mammography screening as well as improved and targeted treatment options particularly for estrogen receptor positive disease [3] (Fig. 13.3).

The role of diet in cancer prevention has been a topic of research for decades, gaining substantial attention after the release of the classic Doll and Peto epidemiological study suggesting dietary practices are estimated to account for over 30 % of cancers diagnosed [4]. Over the past several decades, repeat analysis of this estimates provide fairly consistent estimates. The evidence for a relationship between diet and breast cancer prevention is among the more commonly studied and provides similar estimates for a cancer-preventive effect of higher quality diets [5–7]. In fact a 2014 analysis suggested that among postmenopausal women who demonstrate adherence to the American Cancer Society guidelines for cancer prevention there was a 22 % lower risk of breast cancer [8]. These guideline scores are driven primarily by dietary factors (energy balance, vegetables/fruit, lower fat, higher fiber/whole grains, alcohol control), but also integrate physical activity.

This chapter describes the current state of the evidence evaluating the role of diet patterns in breast cancer prevention with a focus on the Mediterranean diet. A discussion of the current epidemiological evidence and mechanisms supporting a role of the Mediterranean diet including postulated mechanisms of breast cancer protection provided by the individual components within the diet is presented.

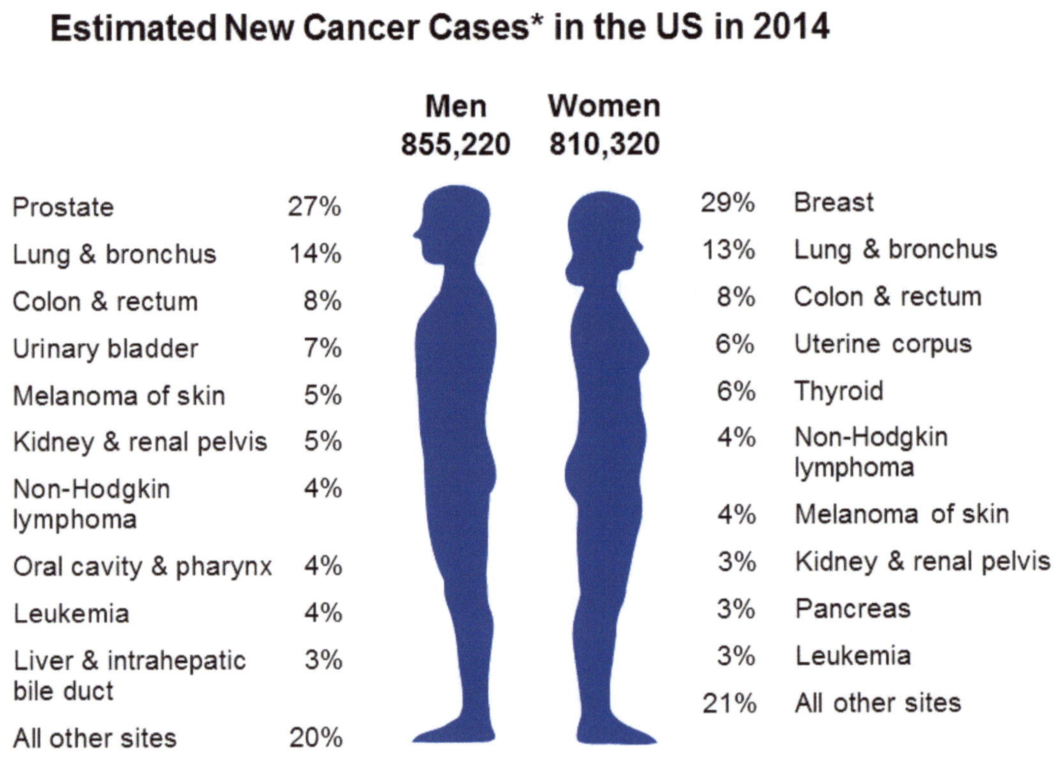

Fig. 13.1 Estimated new cancers in the USA in 2014. Breast cancer remains the most commonly diagnosed cancer in women, accounting for 1.7 new cases annually worldwide and over 200,000 cases in the USA alone

The Lifetime Probability of Developing Cancer for Women, 2008-2010*

Site	Risk
All sites†	1 in 3
Breast	1 in 8
Lung & bronchus	1 in 16
Colon & rectum	1 in 22
Uterine corpus	1 in 37
Non-Hodgkin lymphoma	1 in 52
Thyroid	1 in 62
Melanoma of the skin‡	1 in 53
Pancreas	1 in 68
Kidney & renal pelvis	1 in 83
Leukemia	1 in 86

* For those free of cancer at beginning of age interval.
† All sites exclude basal cell and squamous cell skin cancers and in situ cancers except urinary bladder.
‡ Statistic for white women.
Source: DevCan: Probability of Developing or Dying of Cancer Software, Version 6.7.0 Statistical Research and Applications Branch, National Cancer Institute, 2013.

Fig. 13.2 Risk of breast cancer in the USA. The risk of an American woman developing cancer over her lifetime is a little more than one in three

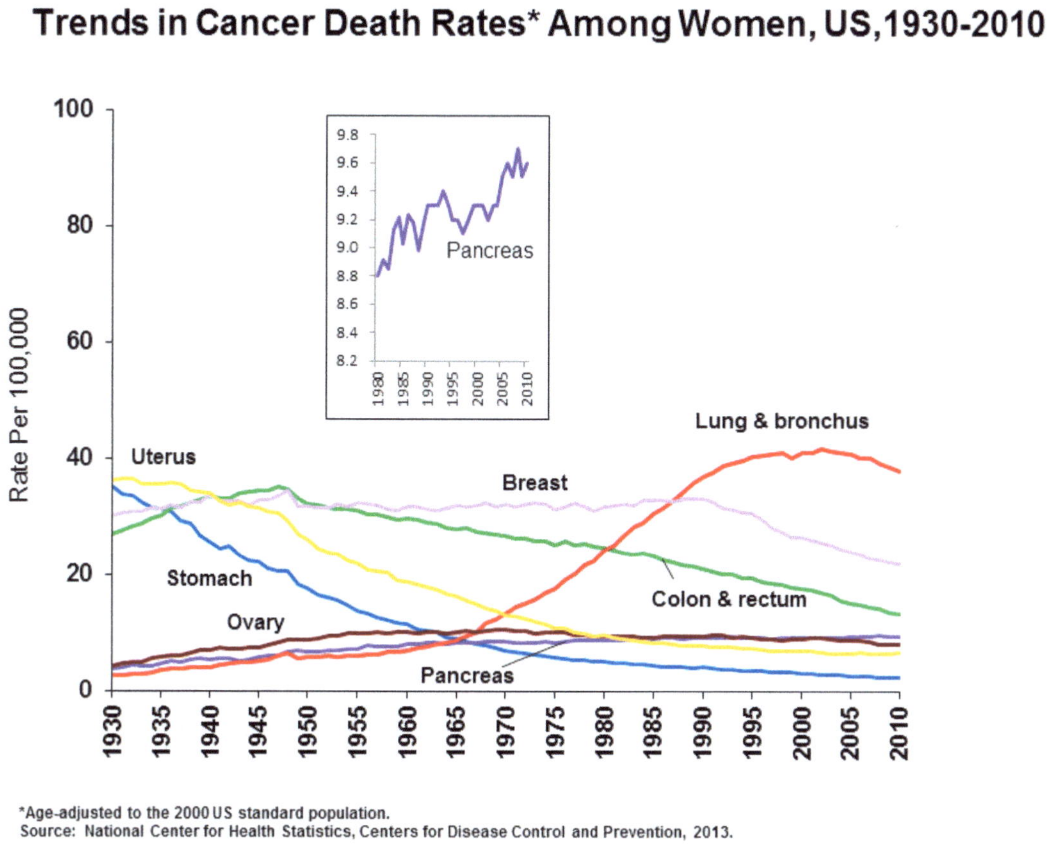

Fig. 13.3 Trends in cancer death among US women (1930–2010). Breast cancer death rates changed little between 1930 and 1990, but decreased 34 % between the peak year (1989) and 2010

State of the Evidence

Diet and Breast Cancer Risk

Epidemiological case–control and cohort studies are the mainstay of much of the evidence evaluating the relationship between diet and breast cancer risk. Only a few clinical trials have been conducted to test the hypothesis that a diet intervention reduces breast cancer incidence. Among the largest was the Women's Health Initiative Dietary Modification Trial of just over 38,000 randomized to either a low fat (<25 % energy intake) or usual diet for an average study period of 8.3 years. The results of that trial showed no significant difference in breast cancer risk between the two groups [9]; however, there was a suggestion of a 9 % lower risk in women who entered the trial within the highest quintile of dietary fat intake. Several dietary intervention trials have been conducted short term to evaluate the effect of specific food and dietary exposures on breast cancer risk factors such as mammographic density [10–12], as well as mechanism-associated risks such as inflammation [13, 14], insulin resistance [15–18], and oxidative stress [14, 19, 20]. While these studies generally support the role of diet in breast cancer prevention, conflicting evidence exists [21–23] making it challenging to provide a definitive answer on these risks that can be effectively translated to clinical practice and public health recommendations.

Methodological Issues

One interpretation of the inconsistent findings from epidemiological research has to do with the inherent limitations of self-reported dietary data and report bias [24, 25]. First and foremost any analysis of dietary patterns, including the Mediterranean diet pattern and cancer risk, requires the investigator to develop a scoring system to quantify exposure. Approaches include factor analysis, principal component analysis, and integration of preexisting scores. However, depending on the instrument applied (almost always a food frequency questionnaire, FFQ) there can be wide variability in how food items are categorized as well as the absolute number of items within a food grouping. These inherent differences will influence the final "exposure" definition and thus introduce bias in the final analysis [26].

Further, many studies have largely focused on the exposure to a single dietary component, independent of all other dietary exposures. Yet it is well known that dietary behaviors are highly correlated within individual diets both in terms of unhealthy choices (high fat, saturated fat, sodium, sugars) and healthy choices (high fiber, whole grains, vegetables, and low fat). To this end, more recent efforts to evaluate the relationship between diet and cancer risk, including breast cancer risk, have evolved to focus on dietary patterns.

Several different diet patterns have been described and been applied to the evaluation of cancer risk. At times, these dietary patterns are derived from the data (factor analysis, principle component analysis) resulting in patterns such as "Western diet," "Prudent" diet or even the "pork, processed meat, potato diet" and other times "a priori" scores are developed using previously described dietary patterns including the Healthy Eating Index score, the Alternative Healthy Eating Index score and the Mediterranean diet score.

In addition to inherent problems with defining dietary pattern scores and the known measurement error associated with dietary self-report, particularly in regard to energy under-reporting for FFQ [24, 25], other methodological concerns also plague this area of study including the possibility that in many population samples the range of intake may not be wide enough to compare biologically relevant differences in exposure or intake even at the highest levels may not be sufficient to induce the level of bioactive response to modify breast cancer risk. Further, genetic variability in nutrient and/or bioactive metabolism is not commonly evaluated and yet may play a significant role in true exposure across individuals [27].

Dietary Patterns and Breast Cancer Risk: International Perspective

In evaluating the relationship between dietary patterns and breast cancer risk a rather consistent picture evolves across continents suggesting diets rich in plant foods and variety are likely associated with lower breast cancer risk as compared to diets high in animal food sources. Yet the absolute number of studies is limited and methodological concerns including inconsistency in defining patterns of dietary exposures hinder a clear interpretation of available evidence [26]. In summarizing the evidence, the diversity in diet score pattern components is apparent, particularly across continents. Two case–control studies in Chinese women have suggested that a vegetable-soy diet as compared to a meat-sweet diet is associated with a 30 % lower risk of breast cancer [28] while a diet rich in vegetables, fruit, soy, poultry, and fish as compared to a diet high in refined grains, meat, and pickled food is associated with a 74 % lower risk for breast cancer [29]. Similar protective associations have been demonstrated in a case–control study in Japan wherein an analysis of diets from 24,218 women suggested a Prudent diet was associated with a 27 % lower risk for breast cancer [30] and an analysis of 714 women in Korea showed a 86 % lower risk in women consuming a diet rich in seafood and vegetables as compared to a diet of predominantly meat and starch [31]. One cohort study of 15,351 Germany women demonstrated a twofold higher risk for breast cancer in women reporting higher intakes of processed meat, fish, butter and other animal fats in combination with low fruit and bread intake (HR: 2.00; 95 % confidence interval 1.30–3.09), while a study in Australia of 20,967 women suggested the traditional higher fat Australian diet was associated with a 25 % greater risk for breast cancer as compared to a vegetable-rich diet. In subgroup analysis by tumor subtype, Australian women who reported higher fruit and salad intake had a 45 % lower risk for estrogen receptor positive disease and a 33 % lower risk for progesterone-receptor positive disease [32]. While many of these studies suggest "healthy" diet patterns may reduce risk as compared to "unhealthy" patterns, an analysis of three cohorts in the DIETSCAN study (the Netherlands, Italy, and Sweden) showed that risk was not lower with high vegetable intake in the Dutch or Swedish women and in fact there was evidence of a protective effect of the "pork, processed meat and potatoes" eating pattern in women residing in Italy [33]. Only one study, conducted in Germany, evaluated the relationship between diet pattern and mortality after breast. In a sample of 2522 cases, healthy as compared to unhealthy eating patterns were not significantly associated with mortality risk [34]; however the HR associated with the healthy eating pattern gave a point estimate of 0.87 while that of the unhealthy eating pattern was HR-1.34. Given the small sample size, limited numbers of deaths, and advances toward effective treatment for breast cancer, these results are not surprising.

In Italy, a country within the Mediterranean region, studies have been less consistent with one case–control study showing no association with reduced risk in women reporting intake that was vitamin and fiber-dense, and a cohort study showing a 75 % lower risk in women reporting a salad-vegetable diet pattern [35]. Of note, the case–control did demonstrate an increased risk for breast cancer in women consuming a starch-rich diet (OR: 134; 95 % confidence interval 1.10–1.65).

In the USA the Prudent versus Western dietary patterns are most frequently compared to evaluate cancer risk, including risk for breast cancer. The Prudent diet is most commonly described as rich on vegetables, fruit, salads, lean proteins, and fiber as well as low in red and processed meats, total fat, and sugars while the Western eating pattern is generally characterized but the opposite food choices. In a cohort analysis by Adebamowo et al. of 90,638 women residing in the USA, including 710 breast cancer cases, the Prudent diet pattern was not associated with a lower risk for breast cancer [36] and similar null associations were described in a cohort of 71,058 US female nurses by Fung et al. [37]. The Prudent diet was, however, associated with a 43 % lower risk for breast cancer in a study on 1901 US women [38]; in the same analysis, risk was not significantly higher in women reporting a Western dietary pattern of intake. Of note, a subgroup analysis for estrogen receptor negative disease in the Nurses' Health Study sample did show a 38 % lower risk for women reporting a Prudent dietary pattern of intake [39]. Western diet patterns were also not associated with higher risk for breast cancer in a Swedish cohort of over 61,000 women age 40–76 years, although this same analysis did demonstrate a significant 27 % higher risk for breast cancer in women who reported a "drinker" eating pattern [40], supporting other evidence suggesting that alcohol intake remains a risk factor for breast cancer [41, 42]. Importantly, the large European Prospective Investigation of Cancer (EPIC) showed a dietary intake pattern very similar to the Western pattern and concentrated in dietary fat was associated with a twofold greater risk for invasive breast cancer [43].

Two systematic reviews/meta-analyses have been conducted to evaluate the role of diet patterns and breast cancer risk. In the systematic review by Albuquerque et al. that reviewed 26 studies that met criteria for inclusion, it was concluded that the Mediterranean dietary pattern and diets high in vegetables, fruit, fish, and soy are associated with a decreased risk for breast cancer [7]. The second analysis conducted by Brennan et al. showed an 11 % lower risk for breast cancer in women who reported a Prudent/healthy eating pattern in all studies ($n=35$) and in the pooled cohort studies alone [44]. Further, a migrant study that investigated cancer rates of non-European Mediterranean individuals native to Morocco residing in France and those native to Near East and residing in Australia showed a reduced risk for breast cancer in these immigrants as compared to local-born individuals [45].

Mediterranean Diet and Breast Cancer Risk

Epidemiological Evidence

The Mediterranean diet score has received intensified interest as a dietary exposure given the relatively consistent protective association between the Mediterranean eating pattern and chronic disease risk overall [46]. This pattern is most commonly described as a diet high in vegetables, fruit, variety of plant foods, whole grains, monounsaturated fats (olives, olive oil), lean proteins (fish, lentils, beans) as well as nuts, seeds, wine, and bioactive-rich seasoning and spices. The definition is somewhat of a misnomer in that the protective diet is largely associated with dietary choices of people residing in Greece, much more so than the broader Mediterranean region. Beyond these food choices, the diet is also rich in selenium, glutathione, a balance of n-3 to n-6 fatty acids, antioxidant nutrients, fiber, as well as several chemoprotective bioactive compounds such as polyphenols, carotenoids, and allylic acid, and isothiocyanates [47]. Further, this diet provides a vegetable to meat consumption pattern wherein plant foods predominate [48]. Current estimates from epidemiological studies suggest that as much as 25 % of breast cancer could be avoided if the population were to adopt a Mediterranean eating pattern over the typical Western diet [49].

Epidemiological evidence evaluating the relationship between the Mediterranean diet pattern and breast cancer risk is limited. Of note, case–control studies are considered less analytically robust given the likelihood of dietary report bias in women asked to report their dietary habits retrospectively after a diagnosis with disease. In a case–control study by Wu et al. conducted in 2396 Asian American women age 25–74 years, the Mediterranean diet pattern was associated with a 35 % lower risk for breast cancer (OR 0.65, 95 % confidence interval: 0.44–0.95) [50] and similar results were found if the Mediterranean diet was soy free. The Four-Corners study of breast cancer also found a reduced risk for breast cancer in Hispanic as well as non-Hispanic white women in relation to adherence to a Mediterranean diet patterns (OR 0.76; 95 % confidence interval: 0.63, 0.92) [51]. Yet a case–control study from France of 1359 women that included 437 breast cancer cases showed no significant association between the Mediterranean eating pattern and risk. One study from Cyprus in 1752 women that included 935 cases between the ages of 40–70 years, was suggestive of a protective association for the Mediterranean diet at least as described by higher fruit/vegetables/fish intake (OR 0.67, 95 % confidence interval: 0.49–0.92). In the same analysis a characterization of the diet using the Martinez Gonzales score was less consistent in terms of lower (OR 0.63, 95 % confidence interval: 0.77–1.53) [52].

Prospective cohort studies show inconsistent relationships between the Mediterranean Diet and breast cancer risk, with three studies supporting a protective association, three others providing null results and one that suggested a protective association only for post-menopausal disease. In support of a protective association is a study of 65,374 French women in which the Mediterranean diet showed a 15 % lower risk for breast cancer [53], a study of 91,779 women in the USA (where a plant-based diet was associated with a 15 % lower risk for breast cancer [54] and an analysis from the EPIC cohort wherein an adapted relative Mediterranean diet score (a scoring that excludes alcohol from the Mediterranean scoring) was associated with a 6 % lower risk for breast cancer [55]. In the EPIC study the protective association was greatest in women diagnosed with estrogen receptor, progesterone receptor negative disease, a subtype that has limited treatment options and reduced overall survival as compared to estrogen receptor positive disease. The three null studies included a study from the UK of 33,731 women [56], a study of 49,258 women residing in Sweden [57] and a study from the Nurses' Health Study cohort that included 3580 breast cancer cases diagnosed over a 18 year period from 1984 to 2002 [39]. In the Greek EPIC cohort, the Mediterranean diet score was not associated with a significant reduction in risk overall, but a borderline protective association was demonstrated in post-menopausal women [58]. An interesting analysis of 80 French-Canadian families that included 89 BRCA mutation carriers who are at an elevated risk for breast cancer, the alternate Mediterranean diet was not associated with breast cancer risk, although higher Canadian Healthy Eating Index was associated with a 65 % lower risk for breast cancer in this high risk subgroup [59].

Components of the Mediterranean Diet and Breast Cancer Risk

Alcohol and Wine Constituents

There are numerous foods, nutrients, and bioactive compounds that comprise the Mediterranean diet, most of which have a large literature in relation to breast cancer risk that is beyond the scope of this chapter. However, some description of the strongest evidence is warranted in order to adequately address the complexity of evaluating the total Mediterranean diet and breast cancer risk. Among the primary dietary factors in need of discussion is alcohol. The Mediterranean diet score in its truest form recognizes a health-promoting role of alcohol, and specifically red wine, in modulating risk for chronic disease. Yet compelling evidence has shown that alcohol, even in small amounts, is associated with a higher risk for breast cancer [41, 42]. While few studies have evaluated alcohol and breast cancer risk using data of specific alcohol types (spirits, wine, beer), those that have suggested the elevated risk associated with alcohol intake did not differentiate across types of alcohol [60]. Thus, integrating alcohol into the Mediterranean diet score is problematic when assessing breast cancer risk. Of note, the one study that altered the scoring to eliminate alcohol showed a significant 6 % reduction in risk for breast cancer [55], while several other prospective studies that included alcohol in the score did not [39, 58, 59]. Interestingly, select red wine constituents have been shown to have inhibitory activity against aromatase, the enzyme responsible for increasing estrogen production [61]. A study evaluating the various flavonoid-related bioactive compounds associated with breast cancer risk suggested that flavan-3ols and flavones reduced risk by 7 and 10 %, respectively. Resveratrol was associated with a 40 % reduction in risk [62]. Of note, the protective association was related to intake of these components in grapes and other fruits. Several of these same compounds are concentrated in wine, yet wine intake was associated with a 60 % higher risk for breast cancer.

Fat/Olive Oil

Lower fat diets have been evaluated and generally suggest that lowering total fat intake, particularly in women with high fat intake, favorably modifies breast cancer risk, although evidence is not consistent. One explanation for the inconsistency in results of both clinical trials and epidemiological association studies is that evaluation of total fat may over simplify the complexity of dietary fats and related biology associated with cancer risk. For example, it is well known that saturated fats and omega-6 fatty acids in particular can induce the arachidonic acid pathway leading to elevation in pro-inflammatory cytokines known to promote carcinogenesis [63]. Yet opposing these affects are the omega-3 fatty acids that generally induce an anti-inflammatory response. This may explain why the Mediterranean diet, which is relatively high in fat but dominant in omega-3 fatty acids, is not associated with an elevated risk for breast cancer. Conversely, the evidence that omega-3 fatty acid intake is protective against breast cancer is weak [27] and for fatty fish, a source of omega-3 fatty acids, studies generally do not support a significant association [64]. One study suggested that there may be a threshold of intake of docosahexaenoic and eicosapentaenoic acids necessary to identify a protective association [65]. This implies that in the populations wherein total and variance in consumption of omega-3 fatty acids may be low there is no opportunity to effectively assess this risks. Certainly, in vitro and animal studies have supported a role for omega-3 fatty acids in attenuating tumorigenesis through not only anti-inflammatory but also antiproliferative, apoptotic, and antiangiogenic mechanisms of bioactivity [66]. A primary effect of DHA and EPA is mediation of proliferative and angiogenic factors such as vascular endothelial growth factor (VEGF), platelet-derived growth factor (PDGF), and platelet-derived endothelial cell growth factor (PDECGF). A lack of consistent association with breast cancer risk may be partially explained by the earlier diagnosis of breast as compared to other cancers. At early stages of carcinogenesis the signaling by these pro-growth, angiogenic mediators is much less pronounced and thus the suppressive effects of selected omega-3 fatty acids may be more selectively and appropriately evaluated in relation to risk of more advanced stages of disease at diagnosis. Yet the elevation of omega-3 intake in relation to stage of breast cancer diagnosis has not been evaluated in epidemiological studies.

Olive oil is a major source of dietary fat in the Mediterranean diet. Olive oil is rich in monounsaturated fat (oleic acid) and antioxidants in contrast to many other oils consumed in the human diet. Olive oil and dietary lipids in general are known to modulate cellular responses primarily through alternation of cell membrane fluidity and cell signaling [67]. Some experimental studies suggest that extra-virgin olive oil, the type most commonly consumed in the Mediterranean region, may be unique in its anticarcinogenic properties [68]. Evidence also exists to suggest that dietary fats, beyond providing a concentrated source of energy in the diet, have the capacity to modify gene expression including expression of oncogenes such as Her-2/*neu* oncogene commonly expressed in breast cancers [69–71]. In an in vitro study, breast cancer cells in culture that were exposed to oleic acid, the major fatty acid in olive oil, showed marked suppression of Her-2 oncogene [72]. Earlier epidemiological studies support the basic research and suggest that olive oil may reduce breast cancer risk [70, 71, 73, 74], although findings are not consistent [75].

Carbohydrate/Pasta

Beyond the potential protective effects of olive oil and omega-3 fatty acids in the Mediterranean diet, a few studies have evaluated the role of carbohydrates and pasta, which are food choices common to the Mediterranean region, in relation to breast cancer risk. In an analysis of two Italian case–control studies, Augustin et al. showed that higher intake of pasta was not associated with risk; however, higher bread intake was associated with a 28 % higher risk for breast cancer in this sample of 5157 women [76].

Mediterranean Diet and Mechanisms of Breast Cancer Prevention

There have been multiple studies eliciting the bioactivity of select components in the Mediterranean diet—whole foods, nutrients, and bioactive components—in relation to breast cancer risk. Reviews are also available [77, 78]. These protective mechanisms include but are not limited to effects on breast tissue density, altered estrogen metabolism, HER-2 *neu* expression, oxidative stress, and anti-inflammatory response. The current literature is described briefly below.

Breast Density

There are several mechanisms by which a Mediterranean type diet may reduce the risk for breast cancer. Among the more direct associations is early evidence suggesting that exposure to the Mediterranean diet may modulate breast density. Breast density is an accepted risk factor for breast cancer [79, 80] and considers the only well-characterized, pre-cancerous pathology inked to invasive disease. So, in addition to epidemiological studies of the relationship between diet and breast cancer risk, a few studies have also explored associations between Mediterranean diet and breast density. A study from South Germany that included a small sample of 424 women showed that adherence to the Mediterranean diet pattern was associated with reduced breast cancer risk such that for every 1 point increase in the score there was an estimated 5 % lower breast density on mammography [11]. In this same analysis, alcohol intake was associated with a 47 % higher mammographic density score. Additional support for the Mediterranean diet and breast density modulation comes from a longitudinal study in Italy wherein high breast density was significantly less prevalent in women with higher vegetable and olive oil intake; density was positively associated with wine intake [81]. In contrast, evidence from a sample of 1286 women residing in Minnesota, USA no significant associations were identified between breast density and Mediterranean diet score [82].

Modulation of Estrogen Levels

Estrogen from both exogenous hormone therapy (WHI) and endogenous sources such as adipose tissue [83] is known to promote breast cancer. Thus one interesting mechanism by which the Mediterranean diet may modify breast cancer risk is its potential to reduce free estradiol concentrations. The Mediterranean diet is rich in fiber given the plentiful integration of vegetables, fruits, whole grains, lentils, nuts, and seeds. Evidence has previously demonstrated an inverse relationship between fiber intake and estrogen [84]. In a randomized control diet conducted among 230 postmenopausal women, assignment to the Mediterranean diet was associated with a significant 40 % reduction in urinary estrogen as compared to usual dietary intake [85].

Her-2 neu Modification

As described above, there is experimental evidence that components in the Mediterranean diet, particularly extra-virgin olive oil may reduce the risk for breast cancer. Using selective breast cancer cell lines, a study demonstrated a 55 % reduction in transcriptional activity of Her-2/neu gene with exposure to oleic acid [86], with specific support that oleic acid targets the Ets protein polyomavirus enhancer activator 3 (PEA3). Alpha linolenic acid (ALA), the primary omega-3 fatty acid of the Western diet showed similar suppressive effects on Her-2 neu expression [87]. Important to breast cancer survival, the investigators have also demonstrated that specific extra-virgin olive oil polyphenols markedly increased the sensitivity of Her-2 neu positive breast cancer cells to treatment with trastuzumab [88].

Oxidative Stress

Oxidative stress and the related damage to DNA is a hallmark of cellular transformation and cancer development [89, 90]. The Mediterranean diet is rich in vegetables and fruit, including a wide variety of carotenoids. Dietary carotenoid intake and more specifically plasma concentrations of carotenoids have been demonstrated to be associated with a reduction in oxidative stress [91, 92]. In addition, dietary interventions targeting an increase in vegetables and/or fruit rich in carotenoids have been shown to reduce oxidative stress in individuals with high baseline levels [93, 94]. But even beyond the potential for the vegetables and fruits of the Mediterranean diet to favorable modulate oxidative stress, select bioactives in olive oil, including squalene, have demonstrated protective effects in relation to suppression of oxidative response in breast cancer cell lines [95]. Additionally, hydroxytyrosol, another phenol found in olive oil, was reported to reduce oxidative stress and DNA damage response is a study using both MDA-MB-231 and MCF7 breast cancer cell lines [96].

Anti-inflammatory Response

Among the more compelling mechanisms for breast cancer risk reduction in relation to intake of a diet consistent with Mediterranean habits is the role of the diet and its components in modifying the inflammatory response. The relationship between inflammation and cancer is well-documented and extend to several cancer types including breast cancer [97, 98]. As described above, the use of predominantly unsaturated fats is one reason why the Mediterranean diet has been associated with lower inflammatory response [63]. However, beyond fat sources in the diet, select herbs common to the diet have also been evaluated in relation to the anti-inflammatory response. In particular, evidence has suggested that carnosol (rosemary) demonstrates significant anti-inflammatory effects targeting NFKB [99].

Beyond experimental evidence, select epidemiological studies have also suggested that dietary patterns consistent with the Mediterranean eating pattern are associated with reduced inflammatory biomarker response. In an analysis from the Nurses' health Study, dietary patterns described as Prudent as compared to Western were associated with a significantly lower plasma concentration of C-reactive Protein (CRP); the Western diet was also positively associated with higher concentrations of E-selectin, interleukin-6, soluble ICAM, and soluble VCAM [100]. Similarly, the healthy diet pattern was associated with lower CRP in a large cohort of Japanese adult females [101]. These results are compelling and support a 2013 review on the topic, but prospective interventions to test the hypothesis that the Mediterranean diet can favorably modify inflammation are needed [102].

Practical Applications and Future Directions

The relationship between the Mediterranean diet and breast cancer risk remains inconclusive [103]. The experimental evidence that exists supports a role of select bioactives and nutrients in modifying relevant mechanisms that hold potential to modify risk in humans. Epidemiological evidence is inconsistent and limitations inherent to observational studies impede progress, to some degree, for the recommendation of the Mediterranean diet for breast cancer prevention. Randomized, controlled trials with outcomes of breast density provide early support for a potential protective association; however, trials with breast cancer endpoints are lacking. Studies evaluating the role of diet patterns, including the Mediterranean diet in breast cancer survival, are sparse and also inconclusive [104].

Despite the limitations of the current body of evidence, investigators have proposed the Mediterranean diet to reduce cancer rates in Europe [105]. Further, the more consistent inverse association of the Mediterranean diet with cardiovascular disease risk [106–108], suggests that this pattern of intake may be "Prudent" not only in regard to breast cancer risk reduction, but also in terms of overall health and perhaps even breast cancer survival given that most women diagnosed with breast cancer will not succumb to their disease, but rather face a potential increased risk or earlier age of onset of cardiovascular disease [109, 110]. Evidence from a telephone-based study of the Mediterranean diet study in adult women [111] and the PREDIMED diet study in Greece [112] certainly suggest this pattern of eating is reasonably adoptable and may be associated with improvements in several health-related measures [105, 113–115]. Recently, a secondary analysis within the PREDIMED study evaluated the effect of two interventions with Mediterranean diet vs. the advice to follow a low-fat diet (control) on breast cancer incidence. After a median follow-up of 4.8 years, investigators identified 35 confirmed incident cases of breast cancer. Observed rates (per 1000 person-years) were 1.1 for the Mediterranean diet with extra-virgin olive oil group, 1.8 for the Mediterranean diet with nuts group, and 2.9 for the control group. Investigators proposed a beneficial effect of a Mediterranean diet supplemented with extra-virgin olive oil in the primary prevention of breast cancer. They also advised these results should be confirmed in longer-term and larger studies [116].

References

1. World Health Organization. GLOBOCAN 2012: Estimated cancer incidence, mortality and prevalence worldwide in 2012. 2012. http://globocan.iarc.fr/Pages/fact_sheets_cancer.aspx. Accessed 6 Mar 2014.
2. ACS. Survival rates for breast cancer. http://www.cancer.org/cancer/breastcancer/overviewguide/breast-cancer-overview-survival-rates. Accessed 6 Mar 2014.
3. ACS. Breast cancer facts and figures. http://www.cancer.org/research/cancerfactsfigures/cancerfactsfigures/cancer-facts-figures-2013. Accessed 6 Mar 2014.
4. Peto R, Doll R, Buckley JD, Sporn MB. Can dietary beta-carotene materially reduce human cancer rates? Nature. 1981;290(5803):201–8.
5. WCRF/AICR. Food, nutrition, physical activity, and the prevention of cancer: a global perspective. 2007. http://www.dietandcancerreport.org/
6. Baena Ruiz R, Salinas Hernandez P. Diet and cancer: risk factors and epidemiological evidence. Maturitas. 2014;77(3):202–8.
7. Albuquerque RC, Baltar VT, Marchioni DM. Breast cancer and dietary patterns: a systematic review. Nutr Rev. 2014;72(1):1–17.
8. Thomson CA, McCullough ML, Wertheim BC, et al. Nutrition and physical activity cancer prevention guidelines, cancer risk, and mortality in the women's health initiative. Cancer Prev Res (Phila). 2014;7(1):42–53.
9. Prentice RL, Caan B, Chlebowski RT, et al. Low-fat dietary pattern and risk of invasive breast cancer: the Women's Health Initiative Randomized Controlled Dietary Modification Trial. JAMA. 2006;295(6):629–42.
10. Garcia-Arenzana N, Navarrete-Munoz EM, Lope V, et al. Calorie intake, olive oil consumption and mammographic density among Spanish women. Int J Cancer. 2014;134(8):1916–25.

11. Voevodina O, Billich C, Arand B, Nagel G. Association of Mediterranean diet, dietary supplements and alcohol consumption with breast density among women in South Germany: a cross-sectional study. BMC Public Health. 2013;13:203.
12. Qureshi SA, Couto E, Hilsen M, Hofvind S, Wu AH, Ursin G. Mammographic density and intake of selected nutrients and vitamins in Norwegian women. Nutr Cancer. 2011;63(7):1011–20.
13. Chajes V, Torres-Mejia G, Biessy C, et al. Omega-3 and omega-6 polyunsaturated fatty acid intakes and the risk of breast cancer in Mexican women: impact of obesity status. Cancer Epidemiol Biomarkers Prev. 2012;21(2):319–26.
14. Yeon JY, Suh YJ, Kim SW, et al. Evaluation of dietary factors in relation to the biomarkers of oxidative stress and inflammation in breast cancer risk. Nutrition. 2011;27(9):912–8.
15. Harvie M, Wright C, Pegington M, et al. The effect of intermittent energy and carbohydrate restriction v. daily energy restriction on weight loss and metabolic disease risk markers in overweight women. Br J Nutr. 2013;110(8):1534–47.
16. McCann SE, Liu S, Wang D, et al. Reduction of dietary glycaemic load modifies the expression of microRNA potentially associated with energy balance and cancer pathways in pre-menopausal women. Br J Nutr. 2012;30:1–8.
17. Tsugane S, Inoue M. Insulin resistance and cancer: epidemiological evidence. Cancer Sci. 2010;101(5):1073–9.
18. Stendell-Hollis NR, Thomson CA, Thompson PA, Bea JW, Cussler EC, Hakim IA. Green tea improves metabolic biomarkers, not weight or body composition: a pilot study in overweight breast cancer survivors. J Hum Nutr Diet. 2010;23(6):590–600.
19. Slattery ML, John EM, Torres-Mejia G, et al. Angiogenesis genes, dietary oxidative balance and breast cancer risk and progression: the Breast Cancer Health Disparities Study. Int J Cancer. 2014;134(3):629–44.
20. Bradshaw PT, Khankari NK, Teitelbaum SL, et al. Nutrient pathways and breast cancer risk: the Long Island Breast Cancer Study Project. Nutr Cancer. 2013;65(3):345–54.
21. Bertone-Johnson ER, McTiernan A, Thomson CA, et al. Vitamin D and calcium supplementation and one-year change in mammographic density in the women's health initiative calcium and vitamin D trial. Cancer Epidemiol Biomarkers Prev. 2012;21(3):462–73.
22. Martin LJ, Li Q, Melnichouk O, et al. A randomized trial of dietary intervention for breast cancer prevention. Cancer Res. 2011;71(1):123–33.
23. Wu WH, Lu SC, Wang TF, Jou HJ, Wang TA. Effects of docosahexaenoic acid supplementation on blood lipids, estrogen metabolism, and in vivo oxidative stress in postmenopausal vegetarian women. Eur J Clin Nutr. 2006;60(3):386–92.
24. Miller TM, Abdel-Maksoud MF, Crane LA, Marcus AC, Byers TE. Effects of social approval bias on self-reported fruit and vegetable consumption: a randomized controlled trial. Nutr J. 2008;7:18.
25. Hebert JR, Hurley TG, Peterson KE, et al. Social desirability trait influences on self-reported dietary measures among diverse participants in a multicenter multiple risk factor trial. J Nutr. 2008;138(1):226S–34.
26. Edefonti V, Randi G, La Vecchia C, Ferraroni M, Decarli A. Dietary patterns and breast cancer: a review with focus on methodological issues. Nutr Rev. 2009;67(6):297–314.
27. Gerber M. Omega-3 fatty acids and cancers: a systematic update review of epidemiological studies. Br J Nutr. 2012;107 Suppl 2:S228–39.
28. Cui X, Dai Q, Tseng M, Shu XO, Gao YT, Zheng W. Dietary patterns and breast cancer risk in the shanghai breast cancer study. Cancer Epidemiol Biomarkers Prev. 2007;16(7):1443–8.
29. Zhang CX, Ho SC, Cheng SZ, Chen YM, Fu JH, Lin FY. Effect of dietary fiber intake on breast cancer risk according to estrogen and progesterone receptor status. Eur J Clin Nutr. 2011;65(8):929–36.
30. Hirose K, Matsuo K, Iwata H, Tajima K. Dietary patterns and the risk of breast cancer in Japanese women. Cancer Sci. 2007;98(9):1431–8.
31. Cho YA, Kim J, Shin A, Park KS, Ro J. Dietary patterns and breast cancer risk in Korean women. Nutr Cancer. 2010;62(8):1161–9.
32. Baglietto L, Krishnan K, Severi G, et al. Dietary patterns and risk of breast cancer. Br J Cancer. 2011;104(3):524–31.
33. Mannisto S, Dixon LB, Balder HF, et al. Dietary patterns and breast cancer risk: results from three cohort studies in the DIETSCAN project. Cancer Causes Control. 2005;16(6):725–33.
34. Vrieling A, Buck K, Seibold P, et al. Dietary patterns and survival in German postmenopausal breast cancer survivors. Br J Cancer. 2013;108(1):188–92.
35. Sant M, Allemani C, Sieri S, et al. Salad vegetables dietary pattern protects against HER-2-positive breast cancer: a prospective Italian study. Int J Cancer. 2007;121(4):911–4.
36. Adebamowo CA, Hu FB, Cho E, Spiegelman D, Holmes MD, Willett WC. Dietary patterns and the risk of breast cancer. Ann Epidemiol. 2005;15(10):789–95.
37. Fung TT, Hu FB, Holmes MD, et al. Dietary patterns and the risk of postmenopausal breast cancer. Int J Cancer. 2005;116(1):116–21.

38. Kwan ML, Weltzien E, Kushi LH, Castillo A, Slattery ML, Caan BJ. Dietary patterns and breast cancer recurrence and survival among women with early-stage breast cancer. J Clin Oncol. 2009;27(6):919–26.
39. Fung TT, Hu FB, McCullough ML, Newby PK, Willett WC, Holmes MD. Diet quality is associated with the risk of estrogen receptor-negative breast cancer in postmenopausal women. J Nutr. 2006;136(2):466–72.
40. Terry P, Suzuki R, Hu FB, Wolk A. A prospective study of major dietary patterns and the risk of breast cancer. Cancer Epidemiol Biomarkers Prev. 2001;10(12):1281–5.
41. Schutze M, Boeing H, Pischon T, et al. Alcohol attributable burden of incidence of cancer in eight European countries based on results from prospective cohort study. BMJ. 2011;342:d1584.
42. Cabanes A, Pastor-Barriuso R, Garcia-Lopez M, et al. Alcohol, tobacco, and mammographic density: a population-based study. Breast Cancer Res Treat. 2011;129(1):135–47.
43. Schulz M, Hoffmann K, Weikert C, Nothlings U, Schulze MB, Boeing H. Identification of a dietary pattern characterized by high-fat food choices associated with increased risk of breast cancer: the European Prospective Investigation into Cancer and Nutrition (EPIC)-Potsdam Study. Br J Nutr. 2008;100(5):942–6.
44. Brennan SF, Cantwell MM, Cardwell CR, Velentzis LS, Woodside JV. Dietary patterns and breast cancer risk: a systematic review and meta-analysis. Am J Clin Nutr. 2010;91(5):1294–302.
45. Khlat M. Cancer in Mediterranean migrants—based on studies in France and Australia. Cancer Causes Control. 1995;6(6):525–31.
46. Panagiotakos DB, Pitsavos C, et al. Adherence to the Mediterranean food pattern predicts the prevalence of hypertension, hypercholesterolemia, diabetes and obesity among healthy adults; the accuracy of the MedDietScore. Prev Med. 2007;44(4):335–40.
47. Simopoulos AP. The traditional diet of Greece and cancer. Eur J Cancer Prev. 2004;13(3):219–30.
48. Kapiszewska M. A vegetable to meat consumption ratio as a relevant factor determining cancer preventive diet. The Mediterranean versus other European countries. Forum Nutr. 2006;59:130–53.
49. Trichopoulou A, Lagiou P, Kuper H, Trichopoulos D. Cancer and Mediterranean dietary traditions. Cancer Epidemiol Biomarkers Prev. 2000;9(9):869–73.
50. Wu AH, Yu MC, Tseng CC, Stanczyk FZ, Pike MC. Dietary patterns and breast cancer risk in Asian American women. Am J Clin Nutr. 2009;89(4):1145–54.
51. Murtaugh MA, Sweeney C, Giuliano AR, et al. Diet patterns and breast cancer risk in Hispanic and non-Hispanic white women: the Four-Corners Breast Cancer Study. Am J Clin Nutr. 2008;87(4):978–84.
52. Demetriou CA, Hadjisavvas A, Loizidou MA, et al. The Mediterranean dietary pattern and breast cancer risk in Greek-Cypriot women: a case-control study. BMC Cancer. 2012;12:113.
53. Cottet V, Touvier M, Fournier A, et al. Postmenopausal breast cancer risk and dietary patterns in the E3N-EPIC prospective cohort study. Am J Epidemiol. 2009;170(10):1257–67.
54. Link LB, Canchola AJ, Bernstein L, et al. Dietary patterns and breast cancer risk in the California Teachers Study cohort. Am J Clin Nutr. 2013;98(6):1524–32.
55. Buckland G, Travier N, Cottet V, et al. Adherence to the Mediterranean diet and risk of breast cancer in the European prospective investigation into cancer and nutrition cohort study. Int J Cancer. 2013;132(12):2918–27.
56. Cade JE, Taylor EF, Burley VJ, Greenwood DC. Does the Mediterranean dietary pattern or the Healthy Diet Index influence the risk of breast cancer in a large British cohort of women? Eur J Clin Nutr. 2011;65(8):920–8.
57. Couto E, Sandin S, Lof M, Ursin G, Adami HO, Weiderpass E. Mediterranean dietary pattern and risk of breast cancer. PLoS One. 2013;8(2):e55374.
58. Trichopoulou A, Bamia C, Lagiou P, Trichopoulos D. Conformity to traditional Mediterranean diet and breast cancer risk in the Greek EPIC (European Prospective Investigation into Cancer and Nutrition) cohort. Am J Clin Nutr. 2010;92(3):620–5.
59. Nkondjock A, Ghadirian P. Diet quality and BRCA-associated breast cancer risk. Breast Cancer Res Treat. 2007;103(3):361–9.
60. Chen WY, Rosner B, Hankinson SE, Colditz GA, Willett WC. Moderate alcohol consumption during adult life, drinking patterns, and breast cancer risk. JAMA. 2011;306(17):1884–90.
61. Shufelt C, Merz CN, Yang Y, et al. Red versus white wine as a nutritional aromatase inhibitor in premenopausal women: a pilot study. J Womens Health (Larchmt). 2012;21(3):281–4.
62. La Vecchia C, Bosetti C. Diet and cancer risk in Mediterranean countries: open issues. Public Health Nutr. 2006;9(8A):1077–82.
63. Kang JX, Weylandt KH. Modulation of inflammatory cytokines by omega-3 fatty acids. Subcell Biochem. 2008;49:133–43.
64. Engeset D, Alsaker E, Lund E, et al. Fish consumption and breast cancer risk. The European Prospective Investigation into Cancer and Nutrition (EPIC). Int J Cancer. 2006;119(1):175–82.
65. Kim J, Lim SY, Shin A, et al. Fatty fish and fish omega-3 fatty acid intakes decrease the breast cancer risk: a case-control study. BMC Cancer. 2009;9:216.
66. Spencer L, Mann C, Metcalfe M, et al. The effect of omega-3 FAs on tumour angiogenesis and their therapeutic potential. Eur J Cancer. 2009;45(12):2077–86.

67. Escrich E, Solanas M, Moral R. Olive oil and other dietary lipids in breast cancer. Cancer Treat Res. 2014;159:289–309.
68. Escrich E, Solanas M, Moral R, Escrich R. Modulatory effects and molecular mechanisms of olive oil and other dietary lipids in breast cancer. Curr Pharm Des. 2011;17(8):813–30.
69. Menendez JA, Vellon L, Colomer R, Lupu R. Oleic acid, the main monounsaturated fatty acid of olive oil, suppresses Her-2/neu (erbB-2) expression and synergistically enhances the growth inhibitory effects of trastuzumab (Herceptin) in breast cancer cells with Her-2/neu oncogene amplification. Ann Oncol. 2005;16(3):359–71.
70. Colomer R, Lupu R, Papadimitropoulou A, et al. Giacomo Castelvetro's salads. Anti-HER2 oncogene nutraceuticals since the 17th century? Clin Transl Oncol. 2008;10(1):30–4.
71. Colomer R, Menendez JA. Mediterranean diet, olive oil and cancer. Clin Transl Oncol. 2006;8(1):15–21.
72. Wahle KW, Rotondo D, Heys SD. Polyunsaturated fatty acids and gene expression in mammalian systems. Proc Nutr Soc. 2003;62(2):349–60.
73. Martin-Moreno JM, Willett WC, Gorgojo L, et al. Dietary fat, olive oil intake and breast cancer risk. Int J Cancer. 1994;58(6):774–80.
74. Trichopoulou A, Katsouyanni K, Stuver S, et al. Consumption of olive oil and specific food groups in relation to breast cancer risk in Greece. J Natl Cancer Inst. 1995;87(2):110–6.
75. Buckland G, Travier N, Agudo A, et al. Olive oil intake and breast cancer risk in the Mediterranean countries of the European Prospective Investigation into Cancer and Nutrition study. Int J Cancer. 2012;131(10):2465–9.
76. Augustin LS, Malerba S, Lugo A, et al. Associations of bread and pasta with the risk of cancer of the breast and colorectum. Ann Oncol. 2013;24(12):3094–9.
77. Escrich E, Moral R, Solanas M. Olive oil, an essential component of the Mediterranean diet, and breast cancer. Public Health Nutr. 2011;14(12A):2323–32.
78. Escrich E, Moral R, Grau L, Costa I, Solanas M. Molecular mechanisms of the effects of olive oil and other dietary lipids on cancer. Mol Nutr Food Res. 2007;51(10):1279–92.
79. Sandberg ME, Li J, Hall P, et al. Change of mammographic density predicts the risk of contralateral breast cancer—a case-control study. Breast Cancer Res. 2013;15(4):R57.
80. McCormack VA, dos Santos Silva I. Breast density and parenchymal patterns as markers of breast cancer risk: a meta-analysis. Cancer Epidemiol Biomarkers Prev. 2006;15(6):1159–69.
81. Masala G, Ambrogetti D, Assedi M, Giorgi D, Del Turco MR, Palli D. Dietary and lifestyle determinants of mammographic breast density. A longitudinal study in a Mediterranean population. Int J Cancer. 2006;118(7):1782–9.
82. Tseng M, Sellers TA, Vierkant RA, Kushi LH, Vachon CM. Mediterranean diet and breast density in the Minnesota Breast Cancer Family Study. Nutr Cancer. 2008;60(6):703–9.
83. Wang KH, Kao AP, Lin TC, Chang CC, Kuo TC. Promotion of epithelial-mesenchymal transition and tumor growth by 17beta-estradiol in an ER(+)/HER2(+) cell line derived from human breast epithelial stem cells. Biotechnol Appl Biochem. 2012;59(3):262–7.
84. Thomson CA, Rock CL, Giuliano AR, et al. Longitudinal changes in body weight and body composition among women previously treated for breast cancer consuming a high-vegetable, fruit and fiber, low-fat diet. Eur J Nutr. 2005;44(1):18–25.
85. Carruba G, Granata OM, Pala V, et al. A traditional Mediterranean diet decreases endogenous estrogens in healthy postmenopausal women. Nutr Cancer. 2006;56(2):253–9.
86. Menendez JA, Papadimitropoulou A, Vellon L, Lupu R. A genomic explanation connecting "Mediterranean diet", olive oil and cancer: oleic acid, the main monounsaturated fatty acid of olive oil, induces formation of inhibitory "PEA3 transcription factor-PEA3 DNA binding site" complexes at the Her-2/neu (erbB-2) oncogene promoter in breast, ovarian and stomach cancer cells. Eur J Cancer. 2006;42(15):2425–32.
87. Menendez JA, Vazquez-Martin A, Ropero S, Colomer R, Lupu R. HER2 (erbB-2)-targeted effects of the omega-3 polyunsaturated fatty acid, alpha-linolenic acid (ALA; 18:3n-3), in breast cancer cells: the "fat features" of the "Mediterranean diet" as an "anti-HER2 cocktail". Clin Transl Oncol. 2006;8(11):812–20.
88. Menendez JA, Vazquez-Martin A, Colomer R, et al. Olive oil's bitter principle reverses acquired autoresistance to trastuzumab (Herceptin) in HER2-overexpressing breast cancer cells. BMC Cancer. 2007;7:80.
89. Klaunig JE, Kamendulis LM. The role of oxidative stress in carcinogenesis. Annu Rev Pharmacol Toxicol. 2004;44:239–67.
90. Klaunig JE, Kamendulis LM, Hocevar BA. Oxidative stress and oxidative damage in carcinogenesis. Toxicol Pathol. 2010;38(1):96–109.
91. Thomson CA, Stendell-Hollis NR, Rock CL, Cussler EC, Flatt SW, Pierce JP. Plasma and dietary carotenoids are associated with reduced oxidative stress in women previously treated for breast cancer. Cancer Epidemiol Biomarkers Prev. 2007;16(10):2008–15.
92. Rao AV, Rao LG. Carotenoids and human health. Pharmacol Res. 2007;55(3):207–16.
93. Folchetti LD, Monfort-Pires M, de Barros CR, Martini LA, Ferreira SR. Association of fruits and vegetables consumption and related-vitamins with inflammatory and oxidative stress markers in prediabetic individuals. Diabetol Metab Syndr. 2014;6(1):22.

94. Rendo-Urteaga T, Puchau B, Chueca M, et al. Total antioxidant capacity and oxidative stress after a 10-week dietary intervention program in obese children. Eur J Pediatr. 2014;173(5):609–16.
95. Warleta F, Campos M, Allouche Y, et al. Squalene protects against oxidative DNA damage in MCF10A human mammary epithelial cells but not in MCF7 and MDA-MB-231 human breast cancer cells. Food Chem Toxicol. 2010;48(4):1092–100.
96. Warleta F, Quesada CS, Campos M, Allouche Y, Beltran G, Gaforio JJ. Hydroxytyrosol protects against oxidative DNA damage in human breast cells. Nutrients. 2011;3(10):839–57.
97. Colotta F, Allavena P, Sica A, Garlanda C, Mantovani A. Cancer-related inflammation, the seventh hallmark of cancer: links to genetic instability. Carcinogenesis. 2009;30(7):1073–81.
98. Mantovani A. Molecular pathways linking inflammation and cancer. Curr Mol Med. 2010;10(4):369–73.
99. Johnson JJ. Carnosol: a promising anti-cancer and anti-inflammatory agent. Cancer Lett. 2011;305(1):1–7.
100. Lopez-Garcia E, Schulze MB, Fung TT, et al. Major dietary patterns are related to plasma concentrations of markers of inflammation and endothelial dysfunction. Am J Clin Nutr. 2004;80(4):1029–35.
101. Nanri A, Yoshida D, Yamaji T, Mizoue T, Takayanagi R, Kono S. Dietary patterns and C-reactive protein in Japanese men and women. Am J Clin Nutr. 2008;87(5):1488–96.
102. Barbaresko J, Koch M, Schulze MB, Nothlings U. Dietary pattern analysis and biomarkers of low-grade inflammation: a systematic literature review. Nutr Rev. 2013;71(8):511–27.
103. Pauwels EK. The protective effect of the Mediterranean diet: focus on cancer and cardiovascular risk. Med Princ Pract. 2011;20(2):103–11.
104. Thomson CA, Thompson PA. Dietary patterns, risk and prognosis of breast cancer. Future Oncol. 2009;5(8):1257–69.
105. Giacosa A, Barale R, Bavaresco L, et al. Cancer prevention in Europe: the Mediterranean diet as a protective choice. Eur J Cancer Prev. 2013;22(1):90–5.
106. Reedy J, Krebs-Smith SM, Miller PE, et al. Higher diet quality is associated with decreased risk of all-cause, cardiovascular disease, and cancer mortality among older adults. J Nutr. 2014;144(6):881–9.
107. Yang J, Farioli A, Korre M, Kales SN. Modified Mediterranean diet score and cardiovascular risk in a North American working population. PLoS One. 2014;9(2):e87539.
108. Martinez-Gonzalez MA, Bes-Rastrollo M. Dietary patterns, Mediterranean diet, and cardiovascular disease. Curr Opin Lipidol. 2014;25(1):20–6.
109. Obi N, Gornyk D, Heinz J, et al. Determinants of newly diagnosed comorbidities among breast cancer survivors. J Cancer Surviv. 2014;8(3):384–93.
110. Haque R, Prout M, Geiger AM, et al. Comorbidities and cardiovascular disease risk in older breast cancer survivors. Am J Manag Care. 2014;20(1):86–92.
111. Djuric Z, Vanloon G, Radakovich K, Dilaura NM, Heilbrun LK, Sen A. Design of a Mediterranean exchange list diet implemented by telephone counseling. J Am Diet Assoc. 2008;108(12):2059–65.
112. Estruch R, Ros E, Salas-Salvado J, et al. Primary prevention of cardiovascular disease with a Mediterranean diet. N Engl J Med. 2013;368(14):1279–90.
113. Rees K, Hartley L, Flowers N, et al. 'Mediterranean' dietary pattern for the primary prevention of cardiovascular disease. Cochrane Database Syst Rev. 2013;8, CD009825.
114. Lourida I, Soni M, Thompson-Coon J, et al. Mediterranean diet, cognitive function, and dementia: a systematic review. Epidemiology. 2013;24(4):479–89.
115. Chedraui P, Perez-Lopez FR. Nutrition and health during mid-life: searching for solutions and meeting challenges for the aging population. Climacteric. 2013;16 Suppl 1:85–95.
116. Toledo E, Salas-Salvadó J, Donat-Vargas C, Buil-Cosiales P, Estruch R, Ros E, Corella D, Fitó M, Hu FB, Arós F, Gómez-Gracia E, Romaguera D, Ortega-Calvo M, Serra-Majem L, Pintó X, Schröder H, Basora J, Sorlí JV, Bulló M, Serra-Mir M, Martínez-González MA. Mediterranean diet and invasive breast cancer risk among women at high cardiovascular risk in the PREDIMED trial: a randomized clinical trial. JAMA Intern Med. 2015;14:1–9.

Chapter 14
Mediterranean Diet, Inflammatory Bowel Diseases, and Colon Cancer

Micah G. Donovan, Ornella I. Selmin, Tom C. Doetschman, and Donato F. Romagnolo

Key Points

- Mortality rates from colorectal cancers (CRC) have been declining due to advances in screening and diagnostic technology. However, they remain the third most common cancer diagnosis and fourth leading cause of cancer-related mortality worldwide.
- Inflammatory bowel disease (IBD) has been linked to an increased risk of CRC. In general, adherence to the Mediterranean dietary pattern is associated with a decreased risk of IBD and CRC. Specific components of the Mediterranean diet include lower intakes of red meat, refined sugars, and processed foods; higher intakes of fish, fruits, vegetables, whole grains, and overall dietary fiber; and increased omega-3/omega-6 ratios.
- Other hallmarks of the Mediterranean diet are the substantial consumption of extra virgin olive oil, which makes up most of daily fat intake, and moderate red wine consumption.
- The combination of Mediterranean foods and habits rather than single foods or bioactive food components is likely responsible for the beneficial impact of the Mediterranean diet on the gut microbiota and maintenance of intestinal health.

Keywords Mediterranean diet • Inflammatory bowel disease • Colorectal cancer • Microbiota • Intestinal health

Introduction

Although mortality rates from colorectal cancers (CRC) have been declining due to advances in screening and diagnostic technology [1], they remain the third most common cancer diagnosis and fourth leading cause of cancer-related mortality worldwide [2]. The initiation and development of

M.G. Donovan • O.I. Selmin, Ph.D. • D.F. Romagnolo, Ph.D., M.Sc. (✉)
Department of Nutritional Sciences, The University of Arizona, Shantz Bldg, Tucson, AZ 85721-0038, USA
e-mail: mdono123@email.arizona.edu; selmin@u.arizona.edu; donato@u.arizona.edu

T.C. Doetschman, Ph.D.
Department of Molecular and Cellular Medicine, College of Medicine, The University of Arizona, Rm 321, Tucson, AZ, USA
e-mail: tdoetsch@u.arizona.edu

D.F. Romagnolo, O.I. Selmin (eds.), *Mediterranean Diet*, Nutrition and Health,
DOI 10.1007/978-3-319-27969-5_14

colon cancer is multifactorial and influenced by a variety of genetic and modifiable risk factors [3]. Depending on dietary pattern, diet can be associated with increased or reduced risk of inflammation and CRC [4, 5]. Historically, high-fat diets have been associated with an increased risk of CRC [6]. Interestingly, the relatively high-fat intakes (28–40 %) in Mediterranean populations with traditional lower risk of CRC suggest that types of fat, rather than total fat, consumed and overall dietary exposures should be considered when assessing intestinal chronic diseases [7–10].

The Mediterranean diet is the result of a combination of ancient dietary patterns and religious, economic, and cultural practices of the many countries surrounding the Mediterranean Sea [8, 10, 11]. In general, adherence to the Mediterranean dietary pattern is associated with a decreased risk of CRC, whereas the Western diet is associated with increased risk [12–14]. Interestingly, current statistics from the World Health Organization indicate that the prevalence of CRC in Northern Mediterranean countries (e.g., Italy, France, Spain) is trending toward those of other developed Western countries in Europe (e.g., U.K., Germany), North America (e.g., USA, Canada), and Oceania (Australia, New Zealand), whereas countries along the Southern Mediterranean coast (e.g., Morocco, Algeria, Libya) have a lower risk similar to that of Asian countries (e.g., China, India) [15] (Fig. 14.1). The adoption of typical Western diets and lifestyle may be at the basis of the increased prevalence of chronic diseases, including CRC, observed in some Mediterranean countries.

Diet can influence the risk of CRC by altering expression of genes involved in intestinal inflammation, gut microbiome [12, 13, 16–19], and metabolism of xenobiotics [20]. In general, it takes ~15–20 years for a microadenoma of the colon to develop into metastatic colorectal tumor [21] (Fig. 14.2). Therefore, diet may play an important role in prevention or slowing the progression of CRC. The Western-style dietary pattern is characterized by the overconsumption of red and processed

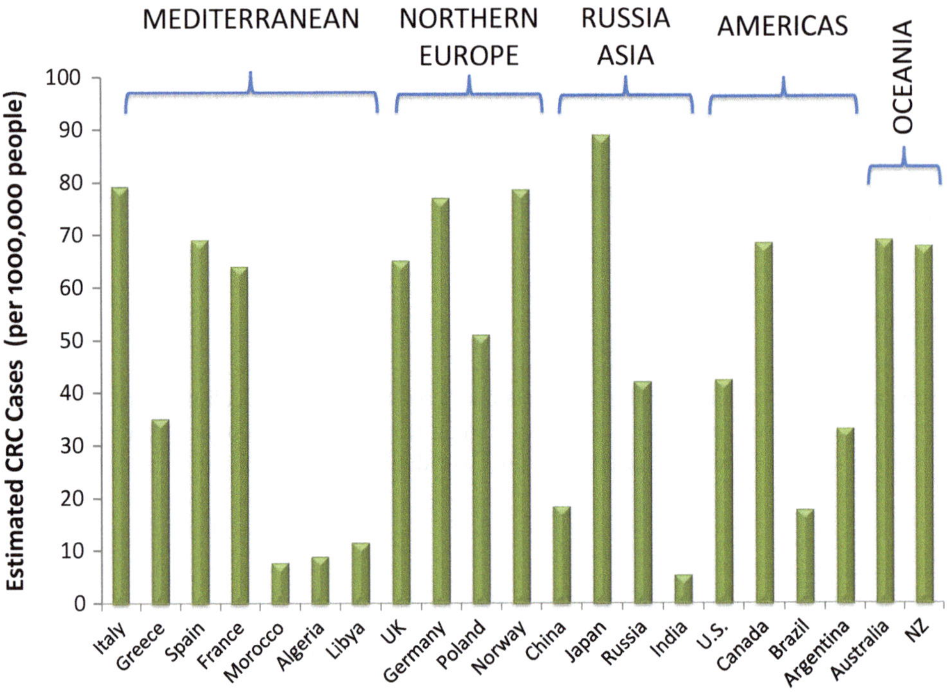

Fig. 14.1 Estimated colorectal cancer incidence by country per 100,000 inhabitants in 2014. Results represent pooled data for men and women [15]

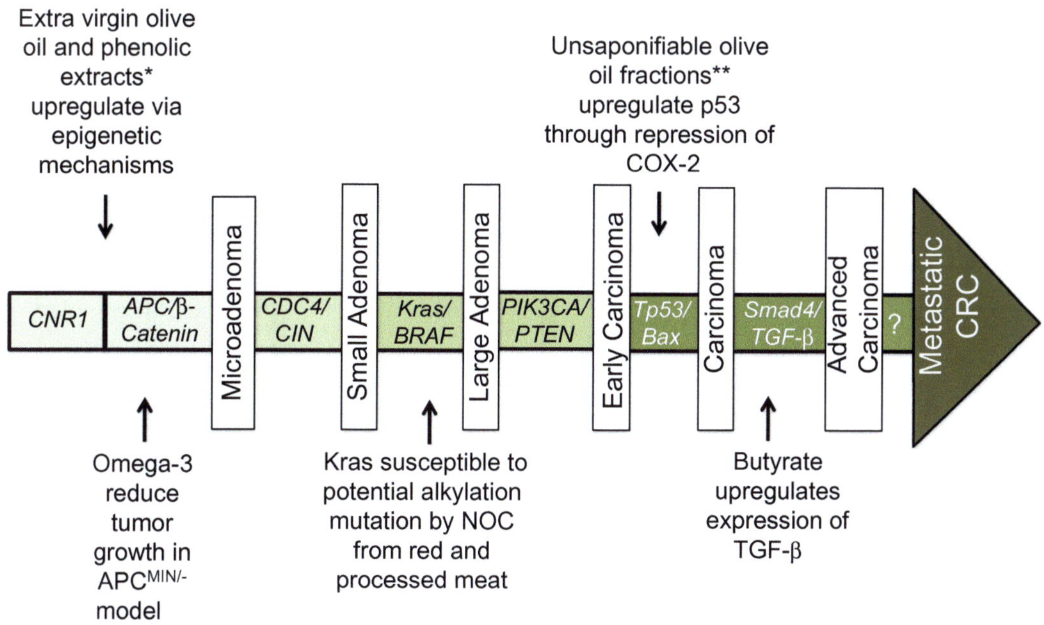

Fig. 14.2 The sequence of known genetic mutations that accumulate and manifest as metastatic colorectal cancer, and the dietary influences that may act upon them. *Asterisk*, tyrosol and hydroxytyrosol; *double asterisk,* squalene, sterols, β-sitosterol, triterpenic dialcohols, aliphatic alcohols, metilsterols, and α-tocopherol; *NOC N*-nitrosocompounds [21]

meats, high-fat foods, and refined sugars; an insufficient intake of fruits, vegetables, and dietary fiber; and a lower ratio of omega-3 to omega-6 fatty acids [22, 23]. Conversely, the Mediterranean diet is associated with lower intakes of red meat, refined sugars, and processed foods; higher intakes of fish, fruits, vegetables, whole grains, and overall dietary fiber; and increased omega-3/omega-6 ratios [8, 10, 11, 24]. Other hallmarks of the Mediterranean diet are the higher consumption of extra virgin olive oil, which makes up most of daily fat intake, and moderate red wine consumption [10]. In this chapter, we discuss the health implications of adopting Mediterranean and Western diets, and the impact of specific dietary components commonly present in these diets on inflammation and CRC risk. Because of limited space, we will focus our discussion on the effects of selected foods, specifically olive oil, omega-3 and -6 fatty acids, and fiber. Finally, we will briefly discuss the effects of red wine polyphenols and red meat consumption on systemic and colon-specific inflammation and CRC risk.

Inflammation

The adoption of a Mediterranean diet and lifestyle has been suggested as means to reduce inflammation [25]. The prevalence of IBD in Mediterranean countries, such as Italy, Greece, Lebanon, and Turkey, is lower compared to that of other developed countries such as the UK, USA, Canada, and New Zealand (Fig. 14.3) [26]. In this section, we summarized in vitro, animal and human studies that have evaluated the impact of Mediterranean food components and diets on biochemical processes associated with colonic inflammation.

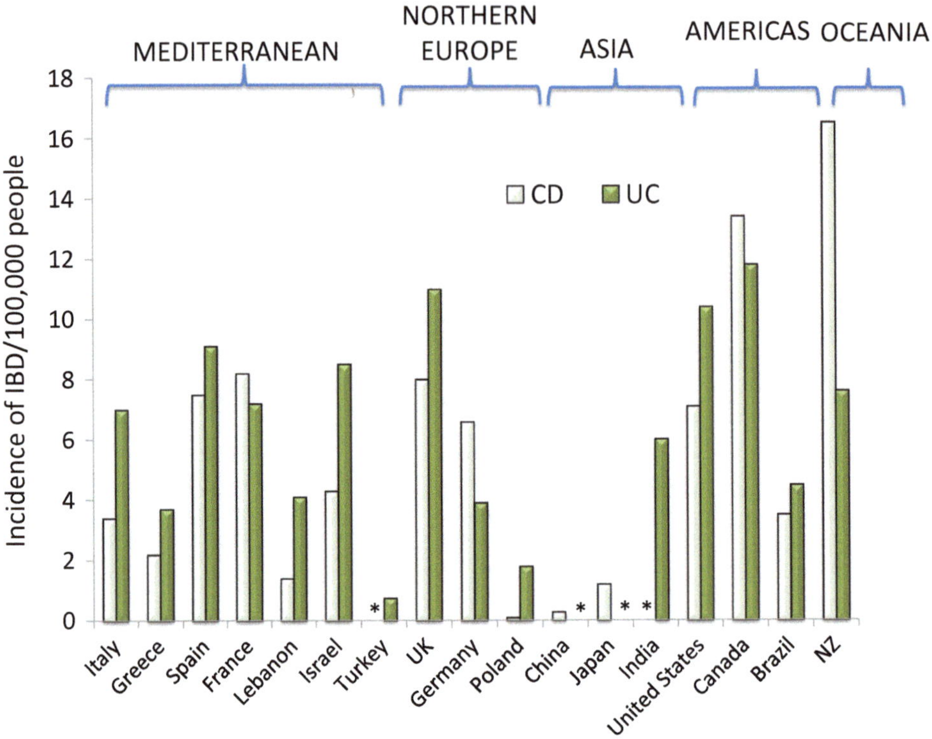

Fig. 14.3 Annual incidence of inflammatory bowel diseases (Crohn's disease, and ulcerative colitis), per 100,000 inhabitants from various time points, by country. *Asterisk,* no data available [26]

Olive Oil

In Vitro Studies

Olive oil comprises various fatty acids, of which oleic acid (18:1) accounts for about 70 % of the fat content; phenolic compounds such as tyrosol, hydroxytyrosol, catechin, epicatechin, epigallocatechin gallate, oleuropein, quercetin, and rutin; and traces of squalene, lignans, tocopherols, sterols (i.e., β-sitosterol), and alcohols [27, 28]. In vitro studies attributed the anti-inflammatory properties of olive oil to repression of cyclooxygenase-2 (COX-2) expression by phenolic compounds rather than oleic acid alone. For example, whole olive oil, but not oleic acid, downregulated COX-2 expression in HT-29 and Caco 2 human colon cancer cell lines [29]. Other investigations documented that hydroxytyrosol (50 and 100 μM) downregulated COX-2 expression and prostaglandin E2 (PGE2) synthesis, in vitro in isolated human monocytes [30]. Similarly, treatment with hydroxytyrosol (1 and 10 μM) decreased the expression of phorbol-myristate acetate (PMA)-induced matrix metallopeptidase 9 (MMP-9), PGE2, and COX-2 in both peripheral blood mononuclear cells and U937 human monocytes. Additionally, 10 μM hydroxytyrosol reduced in U937 monocytes expression of nuclear factor kappa-light-chain-enhancer of activated B cells (NF-κB), PKCα, and PKCβ1, which are upstream regulators of COX-2 and MMP-9 genes [31]. In murine macrophages cultured in vitro, tyrosol decreased in a concentration-dependent manner (from 50 to 250 μM) PMA-induced arachidonic acid release, superoxide formation, COX-2 expression, and PGE2 and leukotriene B4 (LTB_4)

synthesis [32]. Finally, an in vitro study with RAW 264.7 macrophages indicated that polyphenols of olive oil and wine and ß-sitosterol of olive oil led to the modulation of the effects of oxidized low-density lipoprotein (oxLDL) on oxidative stress and PGE2 synthesis [33].

Animal Studies

Extra virgin olive oil (EVOO)-enriched diet (5 %) administered to 6-week-old male Sprague-Dawley rats with dextran sulfate sodium (DSS)-induced colitis (a model of ulcerative colitis) improved disease activity indexes, assessed by the presence of rectal bleeding, weight loss, and stool consistency; improved colonic histology scores; and decreased expression of COX-2, inducible nitric oxide synthase (iNOS), and signal transducer and activator of transcription 3 (STAT3) in colonic mucosa tissue [34]. Similarly, an EVOO-enriched diet (10 %), fed to 6-week-old mice with DSS-induced colitis, attenuated disease activity index scores and histological signs of damage. These diets supplemented with hydroxytyrosol (40 mg/kg of diet) showed improved results over EVOO alone. Additionally, EVOO and EVOO supplemented with hydroxytyrosol decreased levels of TNFα and IL-10, and expression of COX-2 and iNOS in colonic tissue compared to control mice [35]. The unsaponifiable fraction of extra virgin olive oil also displayed efficacy in attenuating inflammation associated with ulcerative colitis. For example, EVOO-enriched diet (10 %) and unsaponifiable fractions attenuated inflammatory processes in a DSS-induced colitis mouse model. This was reflected by improved disease activity indexes and histological damage scores, and reduced expression of MCP-1, TNFα, COX-2, and iNOS in colonic mucosal tissue [36].

Clinical Studies

Clinical trials have investigated the anti-inflammatory effects of olive oil. In Spanish coronary heart disease patients, mean 68 years of age (SD=7 years), daily doses of 50 ml of unprocessed extra virgin olive oil over two 3-week periods, improved serum levels of IL-6 and c-reactive protein (CRP), compared to control subjects given refined olive oil [37]. Another trial assessed the effects of extra virgin olive oil consumption on HDL anti-inflammatory activity in both young and elderly, men and women, aged 20–30 years and 65–85 years, respectively. Subjects in the intervention group consumed 25 ml of olive oil per day for 12 weeks. Olive oil consumption increased the anti-inflammatory activity of HDL, which was reflected in the decreased expression of intracellular adhesion molecule-1 [38]. These data suggested that olive oil, in particular extra virgin olive oil, may be useful for the prevention of inflammatory responses [39].

Omega-3 Fatty Acids

In Vitro Studies

A mixture of fish oil containing approximately 50 % eicosapentaenoic acid (EPA) and docosahexaenoic acid (DHA) was reported to downregulate COX-2 expression in HT-29 and Caco-2 human colon cancer cells (4 h post-treatment) [29]. Another study reported that in vitro treatment of macrophages (extracted from wild-type mice) with DHA (50 μM) and EPA (25 and 50 μM) decreased COX-2, TNFα, and iNOS expression. These effects were not seen in macrophages extracted from knockout *Nrf2* mice. These findings indicated that Nrf2-dependent signaling may play a critical role in the anti-inflammatory activities of EPA and DHA [40]. Increasing Nrf2 activity has been suggested as a strategy to attenuate inflammatory processes [41].

Animal Studies

Omega-3 polyunsaturated fatty acids (PUFA) have been shown to attenuate DSS-induced colitis in animal models of IBD. For example, male Sprague-Dawley weanling rats fed diets with 2:1 ratio of linoleic acid (LA, omega-6) to α-linolenic acid (ALA, omega-3) had significantly improved disease activity index scores, as determined by body weight, stool consistency, and presence of fecal occult blood or gross rectal bleeding; and increased levels of TNFα, IL-1β, MPO, and alkaline phosphatase activity in the colonic mucosa, compared to rats fed diets with lower ratios of LA to ALA [42]. Similarly, in 6-week-old male C57BL/6 mice, an omega-3 enriched diet (2:1 LA:ALA) significantly attenuated DSS-induced increases in TNFα, keratinocyte-derived chemokine, and IL-17 mRNA expression in colonic tissue compared to control mice fed diets with higher ratios of LA:ALA [43]. Furthermore, in male Wistar rats with trinitrobenzene sulfonic acid-induced colitis, the administration of diets enriched with omega-3 (10 %) improved histological index scores, lowered colonic alkaline phosphatase and gamma-glutamyltranspeptidase activities, and lowered mucosal levels of PGE2 and LTB_4 compared to control diets [44].

Clinical Studies

Eicosanoids produced from the metabolism of omega-6 PUFA, such as PGE2, are considered "pro-inflammatory," whereas eicosanoids formed from omega-3 PUFA are considered "anti-inflammatory." Omega-3 and omega-6 PUFAs are substrates for the same metabolic enzymes and higher intake of omega-3 has been shown to reduce omega-6 eicosanoid precursors in phospholipids of human plasma [45].

A clinical trial examined the effects of omega-3 supplementation in overweight males with BMI >25 kg/m^2 and 25–65 years of age. Results suggested that supplementation with omega-3 (57.5 mg EPA and 32.5 mg DHA, from krill) for 4 weeks decreased blood levels of IL-1β, IL-6, and TNFα, and increased blood levels of adiponectin [46]. These results were confirmed by another study that investigated the effect of daily supplementation with 4 g fish oil capsule (0.8 g EPA and 1.6 g DHA) in a Mexican population with multiple sclerosis, 18–55 years of age, and currently undergoing interferon therapy. After 1-year intervention, subjects supplemented with fish oil had significantly lower levels of serum TNFα, IL-1β, IL-6, and NO metabolites, compared to control subjects dosed with excipient of fish oil capsules [47]. These results indicated that dietary omega-3 fatty acids can lower pro-inflammatory cytokines and markers of systemic inflammation.

A prospective study in the UK using 7-day food diaries from 25,639 subjects aged 45–74 years reported a decreased risk (odds ratio = 0.43) of ulcerative colitis in association with DHA intake, and borderline significant decreased risk with EPA (OR = 0.53) and total omega-3 intake (OR = 0.56) [48]. Clinical studies in patients with active ulcerative colitis taking prednisone found that 4-month supplementation with fish oil (3.24 g EPA; and 2.16 g DHA) decreased rectal LTB_4 levels; improved acute and total histology index scores; and decreased the average needed dose of prednisone compared to placebo supplementation with isocaloric amounts of vegetable oil [49]. In addition, supplementation with fish oil (EPA 3.2 g, DHA 2.4 g) for 6 months significantly reduced natural killer cell cytotoxicity and serum IL-2 in ulcerative colitis patients [50]. Overall, these clinical studies supported a protective effect of EPA and DHA against development of IBDs.

Fiber

Animal Studies

Several studies have been conducted in animal models to investigate the role of fiber and prebiotics on gut inflammation. In the HLA-B27 transgenic rat model of Crohn's disease, 13 weeks administration of a high fiber diet (5 % psyllium seed by weight) decreased nitric oxide, LTB_4, and TNFα levels in colonic tissue [51]. Similarly, in the HLA-B27 rat model, 7 weeks placement on high fiber intake in the form of a 1:1 mixture of long-chain inulin and short-chain inulin (found in wheat, onion, banana, garlic, and leek among other sources) at 5 g/kg body weight/day decreased IL-1β and increased TGF-β levels in cecal tissue [52, 53]. In addition, dietary lactulose, a semi-synthetic disaccharide of galactose and fructose, solubilized in drinking water (2.5 %) and administered for 2 weeks, reduced TNFα and leukotriene levels in colon tissue of female Wistar rats with trinitrobenzenesulfonic acid (TNBS)-induced colitis [54]. Decreased levels of cecal TNFα and leukotrienes were observed in male Wistar rats with DSS-induced colitis and given oral lactulose (1000 mg/kg) twice daily for 6 days [55]. Finally, dietary supplementation with butyrate (0.5 %) increased TGF-β concentration; decreased IL-10 concentrations; and decreased memory T lymphocytes and dendritic cells in Peyer's patches in the intestinal mucosa of DSS-induced colitis mice compared to controls diets [56].

Clinical Studies

A systematic cross-sectional analysis investigated the effects of dietary fiber on serum cytokine levels of 88 cancer-free subjects (men and women, aged 35–65 years) from the Italian cohort of the EPIC studies. Dietary fiber intake, assessed with dietary questionnaires during enrollment, was inversely associated with IL-1β, IL-4, IL-5, IL-6, IL-13, and TNF-α levels in the blood [57]. A clinical trial with ulcerative colitis patients examined the effects of dietary fiber intake in the form of 20–30 g of germinated barley foodstuff on endoscopic index parameters such as erythema, edema, friability, granularity, and erosion. Clinical activity scores included the number of episodes of diarrhea, the presence of nocturnal diarrhea, the degree of visible blood in the stools, the presence of fecal incontinence, the degree of abdominal pain or cramping, general well-being, the degree of abdominal tenderness, and the need for antidiarrheal drugs. Significantly decreased endoscopic index and clinical activity index parameters were observed in patients receiving fiber supplementation, compared to patients receiving control diets [58]. Overall, these studies suggested dietary fiber may attenuate symptoms associated with systemic and gastrointestinal inflammation.

Red Wine Polyphenols

Animal Studies

Preclinical evidence has emerged indicating red wine polyphenols may reduce gut inflammation. In the peptidoglycan-polysaccharide (PG-PS) rat model of Crohn's disease, 100 mg/kg of oral resveratrol, administered 27 days after PG-PS injection, significantly decreased expression of IL-1β, IL-6, TNFα, and TGFβ in the cecum, compared to control animals receiving vehicle [59]. Similarly, daily intake of a resveratrol-enriched diet (3 mg/kg body weight) decreased expression of prostaglandin E synthase-1, COX-2, and iNOS transcripts; decreased levels of TNFα and IL-1β; and increased IL-10 in colonic tissue of mice with DSS-induced colitis [60]. Resveratrol administered at 10 mg/kg diet per day lowered levels of PGE2, COX-2, and NF-κB in colonic mucosa of male Wistar rats with TNBS-induced colitis [61].

Clinical Studies

The efficacy of resveratrol as an anti-inflammatory agent was investigated in a 6-week double-blinded randomized controlled trial. Oral ingestion of 500 mg/day of resveratrol decreased plasma TNFα and hs-CRP, and reduced NF-κB nuclear activity in peripheral blood mononuclear cells of ulcerative colitis patients [62].

Mixed Diet

Clinical Studies

To investigate the effects of the Mediterranean diet on inflammation, Schwingshackl and Hoffman conducted a meta-analysis of 17 randomized controlled trials, ranging from 12 weeks to 48 months, in participants at least 19 years old [4]. The studies included in the meta-analysis had to satisfy two or more of the following criteria of adherence to the Mediterranean diet: high monounsaturated/saturated fat ratio; low to moderate red wine consumption; high consumption of legumes; high consumption of grains and cereals; high consumption of fruits and vegetables; low consumption of meat and meat products, increased consumption of fish; and moderate consumption of milk and dairy products. Inflammation was assessed by pooling study-specific weighted mean differences for levels of circulating adiponectin, IL-6, hs-CRP, and intracellular adhesion molecule 1. The Mediterranean diet was associated with increased adiponectin (weighted mean difference (WMD) = 1.69 μg/ml, $I^2 = 78$ %) and decreased hs-CRP (WMD: −0.98 mg/l, $I^2 = 91$ %), IL-6 (weighted mean difference: −0.42, $I^2 = 81$ %), and intracellular adhesion molecule-1 (WMD: −23.73 ng/ml, $I^2 = 34$ %). Overall, these data suggested adherence to the Mediterranean diet decreased the levels of biomarkers associated with systemic inflammation.

Observational studies in healthy 70-year-old men and women from the 1936 Lothian birth cohort documented the adoption of Mediterranean diet patterns, defined by greater consumption of vegetables, fish, poultry, pasta, rice, water, tomato-based-sauces, oil and vinegar dressing, and beans over the lifetime, was associated with reduced levels of fibrinogen, a biomarker of systemic inflammation [63]. Another study reported reduced IL-6, TNFα, and homocysteine levels with moderate to high compliance with Mediterranean diet patterns, calculated using the MedDietScore over a 10-year period, in men and women aged 18–89 years in the Athenian province of Attica. This study also found decreased CRP and fibrinogen levels with high Mediterranean diet compliance [64].

A crossover trial compared the effects of the Mediterranean diet to those of a high saturated fat (SFA-rich) or low-fat-high-carbohydrate diet (LFHC) on the postprandial inflammatory state of elderly men and women from Córdoba Spain (mean age 67.1 years). The Mediterranean and SFA-rich diets provided the same total percentage of calories from fat (38 %) but the types of fat were different: for the Mediterranean diet, 24 % of calories were from MUFA (virgin olive oil), <10 % from SFA, and 4 % from PUFA of which 0.4 % was ALA; the high SFA diet had 12 % of calories from MUFA, 22 % from SFA, and 4 % from PUFA with 0.4 % ALA. At the end of a 3-week intervention trial, subjects on the Mediterranean diet had decreased fasting and postprandial expression of the p65 subunit of NFκB compared to the SFA-rich diet, and decreased postprandial expression of p65 and TNFα compared to subjects on the LFHC diet [65].

One study examined the effects of a Mediterranean diet over a period of 2 years on markers of inflammation in men and women with metabolic syndrome (mean age 43 years), and who were outpatients of the Division of Metabolic Diseases at the Second University of Naples, in Italy. The kcal breakdown for the Mediterranean diet group was carbohydrates 50–60 %, fat <30 % (less than 10 % saturated), protein 15–20 %, with less than 300 mg of cholesterol per day and advice to consume 250–300 g of fruits, 125–150 g of vegetables, 25–50 g of walnuts, and 400 g of whole grains per day. An additional suggestion was to increase olive oil consumption. Control subjects had similar basal diet but were only given general advice about healthy eating. At the end of the 2-year intervention, subjects following the Mediterranean diet had higher levels of HDL and lower levels of serum IL-6, IL-7, IL-18, and hs-CRP compared to controls [66].

A study performed with Crohn's disease patients ($n=8$) investigated the anti-inflammatory potential of an experimental Mediterranean diet comprising salmon, organic avocados, kumara, a variety of sweet potato, gluten-free bread, New Zealand EVOO, green tea, and honey and fish oil capsules. After 6 weeks of adherence to the Mediterranean diet, serum measures of CRP and the presence of micronuclei in the cytoplasm of bi-nucleated lymphocyte cells (a validated method for determining DNA damage in peripheral blood lymphocytes cells) were reduced albeit not to a significant degree. However, using a transcriptomics approach, investigators found that experimental diets modified the expression of 3551 genes, of which 1902 genes were upregulated and 1649 downregulated [67]. Characterization of these proteomic changes may provide new clues about the impact of a Mediterranean diet on biochemical pathways associated with Crohn's disease.

Colorectal Cancer

Cumulative evidence from preclinical and clinical studies suggests that inflammatory responses may predispose to the development of CRC [68]. The colonic epithelium is lined with small invaginations known as crypts, which expand the epithelial surface area and contribute to the functionality of the colon. Terminally differentiated epithelial cells align the top portion of the crypt and mediate the secretory and absorptive properties of the colonic mucosa. These cell populations are short-lived and, after undergoing apoptosis, slough off into the intestinal lumen every few days (3–5 days in humans and 2–3 in mice) [69]. Renewal of this cell population is mediated by pluripotent stem cells found at the base of the crypts, which upon asymmetric division give rise to transit amplifying (TA) cells that migrate up the crypt wall and further differentiate into the functional epithelial cells at the mouth of the crypt [70]. Maintenance of a healthy colonic mucosa is therefore dependent on precise homeostatic regulation of the balance between apoptosis of differentiated epithelial cells and proliferation and differentiation of stem and TA cells.

Sporadic CRC differ from hereditary tumors in that, rather than being the result of heritable mutations in the germ line, they are due to long-term and sequential aggregation of aberrations in various oncogenic and tumor suppressive pathways [71] (Fig. 14.2). The initiation of CRC is associated with loss of APC functions resulting in the formation of precancerous microadenomas [16]. Progression from microadenomas to large adenomas is associated with downregulation of the tumor suppressive CDC4/CIN and upregulation of the oncogenic KRAS/BRAF pathways. Finally, progression from large benign adenomas to malignant tumors is the result of downregulation of the TP53/BAX and SMAD4/TGFβ pathways and upregulation of the PIK3CA/PTEN pathway. The transition from microadenoma to advanced carcinoma occurs over a period of ~15–20 years whereas advancement from carcinomas to metastatic tumors takes only 2–3 years. The relatively slow development throughout the benign stages of this process begs the question whether windows of opportunity exist for early CRC prevention through dietary strategies that include bioactive components and foods that are characteristic of the Mediterranean dietary pattern.

Olive Oil

In Vitro and Animal Studies

In vitro studies attributed antiproliferative and proapoptotic activity of olive oil extracts to modulation of the cellular oxidative state. For example, hydroxytyrosol (50, 100, and 200 μM) selectively decreased (within 24–48 h post-treatment) antioxidant defense capacity of colon cancer DLD1 cells, leading to apoptosis and reduced cell proliferation. These effects were not seen in normal colonic epithelial 1807 cells [72]. In the same study, the treatment of DLD1 cells with hydroxytyrosol, selected as a prototype of phenolic compounds present in olive oil extracts, increased cellular reactive oxygen species (ROS) and stimulated the phosphoinositide 3-kinase/Akt pathway leading to repression of FOXO3a and its downstream (antioxidant) target genes [72]. Studies in HT-29 human colon cancer cells investigated the effects of the unsaponifiable fraction of olive oil, which consists of squalene, triterpenic or aliphatic alcohols, sterols, tocopherols, and other compounds. The unsaponifiable fraction (250–500 μg/ml) decreased proliferation (within 48 h post-treatment) and increased apoptosis (~24 h with 500 μg/ml). The latter changes were associated with upregulation of p53 (500 μg/ml, 48 h) and PPARγ (250 and 500 μg/ml, 2 h); downregulation of COX-2 (500 μg/ml, 48 h); and accumulation of IKBα, an inhibitor of pro-inflammatory NFκB [73].

The type 1 cannabinoid receptor (CB1) is a tumor suppressor gene that is part of the endocannabinoid system, with antiproliferative and proapoptotic effects on CRC cells [74]. Loss of CB1 has been shown to facilitate the growth of colonic adenomas in the *APCMin/+* mouse model of familial adenomatous polyposis (FAP) [75]. In vitro studies with Caco-2 human colon cancer cells showed that both whole EVOO and the phenolic extracts oleuropein, and hydroxytyrosol upregulated *CNR1* and CB1 expression; these changes were paralleled by decreased methylation on the *CNR1* promoter. In the same study, female Sprague-Dawley rats receiving dietary extra virgin olive oil for 10 days had increased expression of CB1 mRNA and protein in colonic tissue [76]. These cumulative data suggest that epigenetic silencing of the *CNR1* gene may be a predisposing event leading to loss of APC expression and CRC development, but this process may be preventable or counteracted by compounds present in extra virgin olive oil.

Omega-3 Fatty Acids

Animal Studies

A review of studies that cataloged the risk factors associated with colonic tumorigenesis suggested that omega-3 fatty acids may protect against chemically induced tumor incidence and multiplicity, compared to omega-6, which tend to enhance tumor growth [77]. For example, the administration of a fish-oil-enriched diet (18 % by weight) over a period of 36 weeks had protective effects against 1,2-dimethylhydrazine-induced preneoplastic lesion and adenoma development in Wistar male rats, compared to animals administered soybean oil (rich in omega-6) as a control [78]. Supporting evidence that omega-6 fatty acids may promote colon carcinogenesis was also provided by results of studies in which male Donryu rats fed a LA-enriched diet (5 % by weight) had significantly enhanced growth of chemically induced colonic tumors compared to rats fed a diet enriched with an isocaloric amount of SFA [79]. The tumor enhancing effects of omega-6 fatty acids may be due to increased levels of omega-6 metabolites, specifically PGE2 which has been shown to be elevated in the colonic mucosa of patients during initiation of CRC and in advanced tumors [80, 81]. Thus, Mediterranean diets enriched in omega-3 fatty acids may exert colon cancer protective effects by increasing the production of antitumorigenic 3-series eicosanoids, e.g., PGE 3 while reducing the formation of omega-6 eicosanoid precursors [82].

Studies conducted in an *APC* knockout mouse model (*Apc*$^{\Delta 716}$) showed that administration of a DHA-enriched diet (3 %) for 7 weeks reduced the number of colonic polyps formed in female mice, whereas DHA-fed males showed no significant decrease in the polyp number [83]. Similar studies conducted in mouse strains with mutated *APC* (*APCMin/+*), a mouse model of FAP, corroborated the gender-specific protection of omega-3 supplementation, which reduced the number of precancerous polyps in female mice (but not in male mice) administered a diet with various concentrations (0.4, 1.25, or 2.5 %) of fish oil blend containing 54.4 % EPA and 30.3 % DHA [84]. On the other hand, studies conducted in *APCMin*$^{/+}$ male mice found that feeding an EPA-enriched diet (31 g/kg) caused a 50 % reduction in tumor multiplicity [85]. Similarly, *APCMin*$^{/+}$ male mice fed a 2.5 or 5 % EPA-enriched diet had a decreased total number and size of intestinal polyps compared to animals fed a control diet [86]. Clearly, more studies are needed to clarify whether or not dose and timing of exposure exert gender-specific effects on the development of CRC associated with loss of APC function.

Clinical Studies

A clinical study investigated the effects of DHA supplementation in three Japanese FAP patients, aged 31–59 who had undergone total or subtotal colectomy [87]. Subjects were supplied with capsules containing 90 mg of DHA and instructed to begin taking 6 capsules/day, gradually increasing to 24 capsules/day during the first 2 months and then maintaining this dosage over a 2-year period. At the end of the trial, there was no significant decrease in the number of polyps in any of the patients. However, 12 months after the conclusion of the trial one subject had developed endometrial cancer; another developed colon cancer after 24 months; and the third patient developed lung cancer after 12 months. Given the small number of patients it is difficult to assess the significance of these results. On the other hand, they raise the question about possible harmful effects of overdosing with fish oils. Conversely, a shorter, however significantly larger ($n=58$), trial was performed in FAP patients under the age of 18 (recruited from the Polyposis Registry, St Mark's Hospital, London), who had previously undergone surgical colectomy with ileorectal anastomosis. Subjects were divided into two groups and supplied with EPA capsules (500 mg) or placebo capsules (capric and caprylic acid medium chain triglycerides), and instructed to take them twice daily (total daily = 1000 mg), with food, for 6 months. Both groups had similar numbers of polyps at baseline. However, after the 6-month intervention period the number of polyps measured in the same area analyzed at baseline had decreased by ~13.0 % in the EPA group. Conversely, during the same time, an increase (~10 %) was observed in the number of polyps for the placebo group [88]. Clearly, larger clinical intervention studies are needed to assess the impact of age, gender, timing, and dose of exposure to omega-3 PUFA on colon cancer development.

Fiber

Human Studies

The human digestive tract does not secrete enzymes that catalyze the breakdown of dietary fiber, which accelerates transit of digests through the large intestine and reduces its exposure to potential carcinogens (i.e., secondary bile acids) [89]. Observational studies of fiber intake and CRC incidence in men and women, aged 25–70 years who enrolled in the EPIC study, suggested that doubling fiber intake in subjects with low-fiber intake could reduce CRC risk by ~40 % [90]. A clinical trial conducted in the USA with men and women 55–74 years of age compared food intakes of patients with confirmed distal colon adenoma with those of healthy controlled subjects and found that higher fiber intake was associated with a decreased risk of developing adenomas [91]. Subjects in the highest quintile of dietary fiber intake had a 27 % lower risk of adenoma than those in the lowest quintile. The effect was strongest for fiber from grains and cereals, and fruits. In keeping with these findings, a case-control study in Italian men and women reported a positive association between risk of CRC and higher glycemic index [92]. Low intake of fiber amplified the adverse consequences of high glycemic load. High fiber intake has also been associated with improved insulin resistance resulting in reduced levels of IGF-1, a well-characterized promoter of cell proliferation, and antiapoptotic factor [93].

In the large intestine, undigested fiber is fermented by gut bacteria, which generate short-chain fatty acids, namely butyrate, acetate, and propionate [94]. In studies performed in the RKO human colon cancer cell line, butyrate (40–100 mM) inhibited proliferation, suppressed cell migration (10–50 mM), and induced apoptosis (10–50 mM, after 4 h) [95]. A study that compared metabolite production from in vitro colonic fermentation of dietary fiber from two European diets (Mediterranean vs. Scandinavian) concluded the dietary fiber of the Mediterranean diet (mostly from cereals, fruits, and vegetables) supported a higher production of acetate and butyrate compared to that of the Scandinavian dietary fiber mostly from cereals [96]. These results clearly highlighted that source and composition of dietary fiber influences metabolite production during colonic fermentation.

Red Meat

Human Studies

Red meat has been shown to support the production of genotoxic *N*-nitroso compounds (NOC) in the intestine. The formation of NOC-specific DNA adduct, *O*(6)-carboxymethyl guanine (*O*(6)CMG), was significantly higher in patients on a high red meat diet (420 g red meat/day for 15 days) compared with subjects on a vegetarian (30 g fiber as nonstarch polysaccharides) or high red meat (420 g) + fiber (30 g) diets [97]. The intestinal exposure to NOC compounds is likely limited in subjects that adhere to a Mediterranean diet. For example, a dietary analysis of men and women aged 29–69 within the Spanish cohort of the EPIC study assessed the intake and food sources of nitrites and *N*-nitrosodimethylamine, and overall NOC exposure. Results suggested that intake of potential NOC generating compounds was lower in the cohort adopting a Mediterranean diet [98]. NOC induce mutations by causing deamination of DNA bases leading to DNA polymerase errors, mismatch errors, or the formation of abasic sites [99]. Mutations observed in K-ras, specifically G>A transitions at codon 12 or 13, are characteristic of alkylating reactions induced by NOC [100].

Mixed Diet

Recently, Agnoli et al. [12] performed a secondary analysis from the EPIC study of CRC risk in an Italian cohort of men and women (42,275 participants) with no cancer history. Based on dietary questionnaires, adherence to a Mediterranean diet was assessed using the Italian Mediterranean Index, in which participants were scored favorably based on high intakes of pasta, raw tomatoes, leafy vegetables, onion, garlic, salad, and fruits and vegetables; and low intakes of soft drinks, butter, red meat, and potatoes. Results suggested that adherence to the Mediterranean diet was inversely related (HR: 0.50; 95 % CI: 0.35–0.71) to the risk of CRC irrespective of gender. The protective effects were seen mainly for distal colon and rectal cancer but not for proximal colon cancer. In a similar study, Bamia et al. [13] examined the effect of Mediterranean diet adherence on the incidence and mortality of CRC in a cohort of men and women aged 25–70 years from various European countries including France, Italy, Norway, and Spain, among others. Adherence was calculated by cataloging data from dietary questionnaires using two 10-unit scales, the Modified Mediterranean Diet Score (MMDS) and the Centre-Specific MMDS, which regarded favorably subjects with high consumption of Mediterranean foods (vegetables, legumes, fruits/nuts, fish/seafood, and cereals) and low consumption of red and processed meats and dairy. Adherence to the Mediterranean diet was associated with an 8–11 % decrease in CRC risk. Interestingly, a 2-unit increment in either Mediterranean scale was associated with a 3–4 % reduction in CRC risk. Overall, results of these human studies confirmed the notion that adherence to a Mediterranean diet may reduce CRC risk.

Gut Microbia, Inflammation, and Colon Cancer

Butyrate Paradox

It is widely known that dietary intake influences the microbial environment and metabolism in the gut [101]. Microbia of the phylum *Firmicutes* are the major producers of the short-chain fatty acid (SCFA) butyrate from fermentation of dietary fiber. They preferentially colonize the mucosal layer which maximizes bioavailability of butyrate [102]. Conversely, non-butyrate-producing *Bacteroidetes* and *Proteobacteria* phyla are significant constituents of the colonic luminal area [103]. The production of butyrate is often associated with *Bacteroidetes* and *Actinobacteria* [104].

It should be noted that in normal rat colon epithelium physiological levels of butyrate (<10–15 mM) stimulate cell growth, whereas at higher concentrations (>15–20 mM) it inhibits the growth of cultured colon cells [105]. This apparent paradox may be explained given that butyrate provides ~80 % of the energy used by the colonic mucosa [106]. Consequently, at normal concentrations it would stimulate growth whereas, at higher levels, it would inhibit growth to maintain homeostasis [107]. Resolution of this paradox may lie in whether or not colon epithelial cells are subject to the Warburg effect (high glucose environment for aerobic glycolysis instead of oxidative metabolism). When HCT116 human colon tumor cells were cultured under Warburg effect conditions (high glucose), butyrate inhibited cell growth whereas under healthy colon conditions (no Warburg effect, low glucose) cell growth was stimulated.

The dependency on the Warburg effect may result from the epigenetic states of histones. In the normal colon environment where butyrate is a source of oxidative energy, butyrate is converted to acetyl-CoA, which not only feeds carbons into the tricarboxylic acid cycle but also induces histone acetyltransferase activity. In the colon tumor environment where the tricarboxylic acid cycle is inhibited, butyrate, as an oxidative energy source, is inhibited from producing acetyl-CoA. Under these conditions, butyrate accumulates, acetyl-CoA is reduced, and histone deacetylase (HDAC) activity is inhibited, which is known to hamper the growth of many tumor types. Consequently, depending upon the metabolic state of the colonic epithelial cell, butyrate can differentially affect growth as well as the epigenetic state of the cell [108].

To add more complexity to the paradoxical effects of butyrate, a recent study suggested that butyrate may play a role in the protection or induction of colon cancer depending upon the genetic signature of the tumor. Mouse studies that used the *APCMin*$^{/+}$ or DSS-based models showed that butyrate inhibited inflammation, tumor cell growth, and polyp formation. The *APC* gene is mutated in over 80 % of human colon cancer and has a chromosomal instability (CIN) genetic signature (Fig. 14.2) [109].

Another genetic signature of colon cancer is microsatellite instability (MSI). Mismatch repair deficiency leads to MSI, which results in mutations that cause colon cancer as well as other types of malignancies. MSI is found in approximately 15 % of all colon cancers [110]. An analysis of a mouse model that combines the CIN and MSI genetic signatures, *APCMin*$^{/+}$*MSH2*$^{-/-}$ (*MSH2* is the most frequently mutated mismatch repair gene in human MSI colon cancers), revealed that butyrate levels normally found in the distal colon stimulated, rather than inhibited, the proliferation of colon mucosal epithelial cells compared to wild-type control mice. Higher butyrate concentrations did not stimulate growth [111]. Altogether, these results suggest that butyrate may affect tumor cell growth depending upon the genetic signature of the tumor. Normal levels of butyrate may inhibit growth in tumors with CIN signatures, but stimulate growth in tumors with MSI signatures. From this it is clear that butyrate levels are important in determining colon cancer risk. Its production is determined by a combination of diet, of which the Mediterranean diet high in fiber can play a significant role, and profile of the gut microbiota.

Inflammation

Several strains of gut bacteria enhance T regulatory (Treg) cell development, which protects against inflammation. Butyrate, produced by several *Clostridia* species, stimulates Treg-cell development through epigenetic modification of the FoxP3 transcription factor gene, which is responsible for Treg-cell development [112]. In addition, the G protein coupled receptor for niacin also binds butyrate, which can induce the anti-inflammatory cytokine IL18. Removal of the receptor from colonic dendritic and macrophage cells prevents IL18 induction by butyrate [113]. Similarly, *Bacteriodes fragilis* can also stimulate Treg-cell development. When polysaccharide A (PSA), a product of *B. fragilis*, binds to the innate immune receptor TLR2 on Treg cells, it induces further Treg-cell production, thereby inhibiting intestinal inflammation. Removal of PSA from *B. fragilis* eliminates this response [114].

On the other hand, there are strains of bacteria that stimulate inflammation. Some species within the family *Clostridiacea* are segmented filamentous bacteria, which enhance the production of IL17-producing T cells (Th17), and shift the homeostatic balance towards inflammation [115]. Also, *Fusobacterium nucleatum* expresses the virulence factor FadA that adheres to intestinal epithelium, thereby subjecting gut epithelium to penetration by other gut bacteria resulting in an increased inflammatory environment [116].

Roles for chronic infection in IBD and colon cancer development have been identified in a rodent model deficient for recombinase-activating gene-2 (RAG2$^{-/-}$). RAG2-deficient mice are devoid of B and T cells, and *Helicobacter hepaticus* induces inflammation and colon cancer mediated by TNFα-induced iNOS, which induces nitrosative stress. Conversely, the treatment of RAG2-deficient mice with IL10 reduces TNFα and iNOS expression and reduces cancer [117]. These results highlighted the role of interactions between *Helicobacter hepaticus*-induced inflammation and induction of colon cancer.

It has been demonstrated that the combination of nitrosative and oxidative stress can generate mutagenic DNA adducts (etheno-dC) of the type found in Crohn's and ulcerative colitis patients [118]. Some bacteria such as *Enterococcus faecalis* produce extracellular superoxide, possibly through oxygen reduction by dimethyl-mena-quinone that is membrane bound. The amounts produced have been shown to be sufficient to induce DNA damage in colon epithelial cells [119]. Bacterial products such as toxins and carcinogens can also cause DNA damage in gut epithelial cells.

For example, *E. coli* of the group B2 produces a toxin called polyketide-peptide, or colibactin, which has DNA crosslinking activity leading to double strand breaks (DSB). It has been shown in a mouse colon loop model that infection with colibactin-producing *E. coli* induces DSB [120]. Also, mice treated with the carcinogen azoxymethane had a much higher tumor multiplicity if they were infected with colibactin-producing *E. coli* compared with an isogenic strain lacking the colibactin gene [121]. Finally, some *Bacteroides* species produce fecapentaenes, ether-like polyunsaturated lipids. These compounds that are thought to induce DNA damage through DNA alkylation and/or oxidative DNA damage through formation of 8-oxo-dG adducts [122].

In conjunction with the heterocyclic amines that are produced in fried meats, such as the procarcinogen quinolone IQ, *Eubacterium* can metabolize IQ into the carcinogenic quinolone HOIQ [123]. The mutagenic effects of IQ have been tested in rodent models. Colon cells from animals treated with IQ had greater DNA damage than untreated animals, and co-treatment with a glucosinolate contained in cruciferous vegetables known to have chemoprotective effects against carcinogens reduced the DNA damage [124].

One study investigating the effects of moderate red wine consumption (272 ml/day for 20 days) in healthy men volunteers identified positive changes in the gut microflora. Specifically, the number of *Enterococcus*, *Bacteroidetes*, *Bifidobacterium*, and *Prevotella* was increased and accompanied by a decrease in the *Clostridium* species. Also, systolic and diastolic blood pressures, triglycerides, total cholesterol, HDL cholesterols, and CRP levels decreased significantly [125]. Bacteria from the *Clostridium* genera are generally considered a deleterious species, with some exceptions, and are associated with obesity, aging, cancer, and neurodegeneration; in addition many are known to possess the 7α-dehydroxylase enzyme responsible for secondary BA formation [126]. Fruit intake has also been associated with positive changes in gut microbia including increases in *Bifidobacteria* and *Lactobacilli* [104]. These examples highlight the fact that foods commonly present in the Mediterranean diet (i.e., wine, fruits) may positively impact health through modifications of the gut microflora potentiating the growth of probiotic bacteria (e.g., *Bifidobacteria*).

Probiotic bacterial species have been shown to play a beneficial role by downregulating the expression of various pro-inflammatory genes [127]. For example, the growth of beneficial *Bifidobacteria* is associated with decreased CRP, indicating a repressive effect on systemic inflammation [126]. The gut microbia also influence systemic inflammation by maintaining gut-barrier integrity. Overgrowth of certain species such as *Proteobacteria* (named after the Greek god Proteus = many shapes) may result in increased gut permeability, which can lead to systemic exposure to bacterial lipopolysaccharide, which induces inflammatory cytokine responses [128, 129].

Summary and Conclusions

In summary, the risk of developing IBD and CRC is highly dependent on a combination of dietary, genetic, and epigenetic factors. The Mediterranean dietary pattern is associated with a lower risk of IBD and CRC, whereas the Western diet is associated with higher risk of these diseases. The health promoting effects of a Mediterranean diet are likely not attributable to variations in total fat intake given the relatively high consumption of dietary fats seen in both Mediterranean and Western regions. The potential anti-inflammatory and anticancer effects of the Mediterranean diet are likely linked to increased consumption of monounsaturated fatty acids and polyphenolic compounds from olive oil, omega-3 fatty acids from fish, dietary fiber, moderate consumption of red wine, and lower intakes of red meat. We propose that the combination of Mediterranean foods, rather than specific

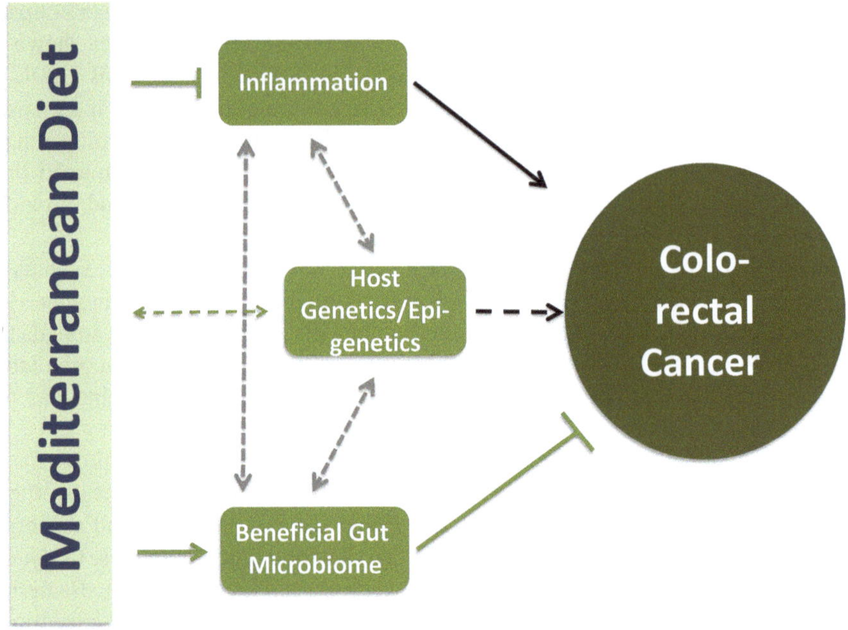

Fig. 14.4 Summary of influences of the Mediterranean diet on colorectal cancer. Mediterranean foods are proposed to protect against colorectal inflammation while favoring the expansion of a beneficial gut microbiome. The host genetic and epigenetic background interacts with food components and influences the establishment of the gut microbiome and susceptibility to colorectal inflammation. Overall, adherence to a Mediterranean diet is expected to reduce the risk of colorectal cancer. *Solid lines* suggest directs effects. *Dashed lines* indicate interactions

ones or bioactive compounds found in Mediterranean diet, impacts the gut microbiome and contributes to the maintenance of intestinal health and the prevention of inflammation and cancer of the colon (Fig. 14.4).

References

1. Quintero E, Hassan C, Senore C, Saito Y. Progress and challenges in colorectal cancer screening. Gastroenterol Res Pract. 2012;2012:846985.
2. Ferlay J, Soerjomataram I, Dikshit R, Eser S, Mathers C, Rebelo M, et al. Cancer incidence and mortality worldwide: sources, methods and major patterns in GLOBOCAN 2012. Int J Cancer. 2015;136(5):E359–86.
3. Quadrilatero J, Hoffman-Goetz L. Physical activity and colon cancer. A systematic review of potential mechanisms. J Sports Med Phys Fitness. 2003;43(2):121–38.
4. Schwingshackl L, Hoffmann G. Adherence to Mediterranean diet and risk of cancer: a systematic review and meta-analysis of observational studies. Int J Cancer. 2014;135(8):1884–97.
5. Gingras D, Béliveau R. Colorectal cancer prevention through dietary and lifestyle modifications. Cancer Microenviron. 2011;4(2):133–9.
6. Reddy BS. Dietary fat and colon cancer: animal model studies. Lipids. 1992;27(10):807–13.
7. Slattery ML, Potter JD, Duncan DM, Berry TD. Dietary fats and colon cancer: assessment of risk associated with specific fatty acids. Int J Cancer. 1997;73(5):670–7.
8. Willett WC, Sacks F, Trichopoulou A, Drescher G, Ferro-Luzzi A, Helsing E, et al. Mediterranean diet pyramid: a cultural model for healthy eating. Am J Clin Nutr. 1995;61(6 Suppl):1402S–6.
9. Austin GL, Ogden LG, Hill JO. Trends in carbohydrate, fat, and protein intakes and association with energy intake in normal-weight, overweight, and obese individuals: 1971–2006. Am J Clin Nutr. 2011;93(4):836–43.

10. Simopoulos AP. The traditional diet of Greece and cancer. Eur J Cancer Prev. 2004;13(3):219–30.
11. Trichopoulou A, Lagiou P. Healthy traditional Mediterranean diet: an expression of culture, history, and lifestyle. Nutr Rev. 1997;55(11 Pt 1):383–9.
12. Agnoli C, Grioni S, Sieri S, Palli D, Masala G, Sacerdote C, et al. Italian Mediterranean Index and risk of colorectal cancer in the Italian section of the EPIC cohort. Int J Cancer. 2013;132(6):1404–11.
13. Bamia C, Lagiou P, Buckland G, Grioni S, Agnoli C, Taylor AJ, et al. Mediterranean diet and colorectal cancer risk: results from a European cohort. Eur J Epidemiol. 2013;28(4):317–28.
14. Yusof AS, Isa ZM, Shah SA. Dietary patterns and risk of colorectal cancer: a systematic review of cohort studies (2000–2011). Asian Pac J Cancer Prev. 2012;13(9):4713–7.
15. WHO. Cancer country profiles 2014. Geneva: World Health Organization; 2014.
16. Berrino F, Muti P. Mediterranean diet and cancer. Eur J Clin Nutr. 1989;43 Suppl 2:49–55.
17. Okabayashi K, Ashrafian H, Hasegawa H, Yoo JH, Patel VM, Harling L, et al. Body mass index category as a risk factor for colorectal adenomas: a systematic review and meta-analysis. Am J Gastroenterol. 2012;107(8):1175–85.
18. Moghaddam AA, Woodward M, Huxley R. Obesity and risk of colorectal cancer: a meta-analysis of 31 studies with 70,000 events. Cancer Epidemiol Biomarkers Prev. 2007;16(12):2533–47.
19. Hullar MA, Fu BC. Diet, the gut microbiome, and epigenetics. Cancer J. 2014;20(3):170–5.
20. Modan B. Role of diet in cancer etiology. Cancer. 1977;40(4 Suppl):1887–91.
21. Jones S, Chen WD, Parmigiani G, Diehl F, Beerenwinkel N, Antal T, et al. Comparative lesion sequencing provides insights into tumor evolution. Proc Natl Acad Sci U S A. 2008;105(11):4283–8.
22. Kasdagly M, Radhakrishnan S, Reddivari L, Veeramachaneni DN, Vanamala J. Colon carcinogenesis: influence of Western diet-induced obesity and targeting stem cells using dietary bioactive compounds. Nutrition. 2014;30(11–12):1242–56.
23. Simopoulos AP. Evolutionary aspects of diet: the omega-6/omega-3 ratio and the brain. Mol Neurobiol. 2011;44(2):203–15.
24. Dernini S, Berry EM. Mediterranean diet: from a healthy diet to a sustainable dietary pattern. Front Nutr. 2015;2:15.
25. Ahluwalia N, Andreeva VA, Kesse-Guyot E, Hercberg S. Dietary patterns, inflammation and the metabolic syndrome. Diabetes Metab. 2013;39(2):99–110.
26. Talley NJ, Abreu MT, Achkar JP, Bernstein CN, Dubinsky MC, Hanauer SB, et al. An evidence-based systematic review on medical therapies for inflammatory bowel disease. Am J Gastroenterol. 2011;106 Suppl 1:S2–25.
27. Gosetti F, Bolfi B, Manfredi M, Calabrese G, Marengo E. Determination of eight polyphenols and pantothenic acid in extra-virgin olive oil samples by a simple, fast, high-throughput and sensitive ultra high performance liquid chromatography with tandem mass spectrometry method. J Sep Sci. 2015. doi:10.1002/jssc.201500452.
28. Allouche Y, Jiménez A, Gaforio JJ, Uceda M, Beltrán G. How heating affects extra virgin olive oil quality indexes and chemical composition. J Agric Food Chem. 2007;55(23):9646–54.
29. Llor X, Pons E, Roca A, Alvarez M, Mañé J, Fernández-Bañares F, et al. The effects of fish oil, olive oil, oleic acid and linoleic acid on colorectal neoplastic processes. Clin Nutr. 2003;22(1):71–9.
30. Rosignoli P, Fuccelli R, Fabiani R, Servili M, Morozzi G. Effect of olive oil phenols on the production of inflammatory mediators in freshly isolated human monocytes. J Nutr Biochem. 2013;24(8):1513–9.
31. Scoditti E, Nestola A, Massaro M, Calabriso N, Storelli C, De Caterina R, et al. Hydroxytyrosol suppresses MMP-9 and COX-2 activity and expression in activated human monocytes via PKCα and PKCβ1 inhibition. Atherosclerosis. 2014;232(1):17–24.
32. Moreno JJ. Effect of olive oil minor components on oxidative stress and arachidonic acid mobilization and metabolism by macrophages RAW 264.7. Free Radic Biol Med. 2003;35(9):1073–81.
33. Vivancos M, Moreno JJ. Effect of resveratrol, tyrosol and beta-sitosterol on oxidised low-density lipoprotein-stimulated oxidative stress, arachidonic acid release and prostaglandin E2 synthesis by RAW 264.7 macrophages. Br J Nutr. 2008;99(6):1199–207.
34. Takashima T, Sakata Y, Iwakiri R, Shiraishi R, Oda Y, Inoue N, et al. Feeding with olive oil attenuates inflammation in dextran sulfate sodium-induced colitis in rat. J Nutr Biochem. 2014;25(2):186–92.
35. Sánchez-Fidalgo S, Sánchez de Ibargüen L, Cárdeno A, Alarcón de la Lastra C. Influence of extra virgin olive oil diet enriched with hydroxytyrosol in a chronic DSS colitis model. Eur J Nutr. 2012;51(4):497–506.
36. Sánchez-Fidalgo S, Cárdeno A, Sánchez-Hidalgo M, Aparicio-Soto M, Villegas I, Rosillo MA, et al. Dietary unsaponifiable fraction from extra virgin olive oil supplementation attenuates acute ulcerative colitis in mice. Eur J Pharm Sci. 2013;48(3):572–81.
37. Fitó M, Cladellas M, de la Torre R, Martí J, Muñoz D, Schröder H, Alcántara M, et al. Anti-inflammatory effect of virgin olive oil in stable coronary disease patients: a randomized, crossover, controlled trial. Eur J Clin Nutr. 2008;62(4):570–4.
38. Loued S, Berrougui H, Componova P, Ikhlef S, Helal O, Khalil A. Extra-virgin olive oil consumption reduces the age-related decrease in HDL and paraoxonase 1 anti-inflammatory activities. Br J Nutr. 2013;110(7):1272–84.

39. Kwan HY, Chao X, Su T, Fu X, Tse AK, Fong WF, et al. The anti-cancer and anti-obesity effects of Mediterranean diet. Crit Rev Food Sci Nutr. 2015 Apr 1:0.
40. Wang H, Khor TO, Saw CL, Lin W, Wu T, Huang Y, et al. Role of Nrf2 in suppressing LPS-induced inflammation in mouse peritoneal macrophages by polyunsaturated fatty acids docosahexaenoic acid and eicosapentaenoic acid. Mol Pharm. 2010;7(6):2185–93.
41. Pall ML, Levine S. Nrf2, a master regulator of detoxification and also antioxidant, anti-inflammatory and other cytoprotective mechanisms, is raised by health promoting factors. Sheng Li Xue Bao. 2015;67(1):1–18.
42. Tyagi A, Kumar U, Reddy S, Santosh VS, Mohammed SB, Ehtesham NZ, et al. Attenuation of colonic inflammation by partial replacement of dietary linoleic acid with α-linolenic acid in a rat model of inflammatory bowel disease. Br J Nutr. 2012;108(9):1612–22.
43. Huang CH, Hou YC, Yeh CL, Yeh SL. A soybean and fish oil mixture with different n-6/n-3 PUFA ratios modulates the inflammatory reaction in mice with dextran sulfate sodium-induced acute colitis. Clin Nutr. 2015;34(5):1018–24.
44. Nieto N, Fernandez MI, Torres MI, Ríos A, Suarez MD, Gil A. Dietary monounsaturated n-3 and n-6 long-chain polyunsaturated fatty acids affect cellular antioxidant defense system in rats with experimental ulcerative colitis induced by trinitrobenzene sulfonic acid. Dig Dis Sci. 1998;43(12):2676–87.
45. Lands WE, Libelt B, Morris A, Kramer NC, Prewitt TE, Bowen P, et al. Maintenance of lower proportions of (n-6) eicosanoid precursors in phospholipids of human plasma in response to added dietary (n-3) fatty acids. Biochim Biophys Acta. 1992;1180(2):147–62.
46. Paoli A, Moro T, Bosco G, Bianco A, Grimaldi KA, Camporesi E, et al. Effects of n-3 polyunsaturated fatty acids (ω-3) supplementation on some cardiovascular risk factors with a ketogenic Mediterranean diet. Mar Drugs. 2015;13(2):996–1009.
47. Ramirez-Ramirez V, Macias-Islas MA, Ortiz GG, Pacheco-Moises F, Torres-Sanchez ED, Sorto-Gomez TE, et al. Efficacy of fish oil on serum of TNF α, IL-1 β, and IL-6 oxidative stress markers in multiple sclerosis treated with interferon beta-1b. Oxid Med Cell Longev. 2013;2013:709493.
48. John S, Luben R, Shrestha SS, Welch A, Khaw KT, Hart AR. Dietary n-3 polyunsaturated fatty acids and the aetiology of ulcerative colitis: a UK prospective cohort study. Eur J Gastroenterol Hepatol. 2010;22(5):602–6.
49. Stenson WF, Cort D, Rodgers J, Burakoff R, DeSchryver-Kecskemeti K, Gramlich TL, Beeken W. Dietary supplementation with fish oil in ulcerative colitis. Ann Intern Med. 1992;116(8):609–14.
50. Almallah YZ, El-Tahir A, Heys SD, Richardson S, Eremin O. Distal procto-colitis and n-3 polyunsaturated fatty acids: the mechanism(s) of natural cytotoxicity inhibition. Eur J Clin Invest. 2000;30(1):58–65.
51. Rodríguez-Cabezas ME, Gálvez J, Camuesco D, Lorente MD, Concha A, Martinez-Augustin O, et al. Intestinal anti-inflammatory activity of dietary fiber (Plantago ovata seeds) in HLA-B27 transgenic rats. Clin Nutr. 2003;22(5):463–71.
52. Hoentjen F, Welling GW, Harmsen HJ, Zhang X, Snart J, Tannock GW, et al. Reduction of colitis by prebiotics in HLA-B27 transgenic rats is associated with microflora changes and immunomodulation. Inflamm Bowel Dis. 2005;11(11):977–85.
53. Roberfroid MB. Introducing inulin-type fructans. Br J Nutr. 2005;93 Suppl 1:S13–25. Review.
54. Camuesco D, Peran L, Comalada M, Nieto A, Di Stasi LC, Rodriguez-Cabezas ME, et al. Preventative effects of lactulose in the trinitrobenzenesulphonic acid model of rat colitis. Inflamm Bowel Dis. 2005;11(3):265–71.
55. Rumi G, Tsubouchi R, Okayama M, Kato S, Mózsik G, Takeuchi K. Protective effect of lactulose on dextran sulfate sodium-induced colonic inflammation in rats. Dig Dis Sci. 2004;49(9):1466–72.
56. Vieira EL, Leonel AJ, Sad AP, Beltrão NR, Costa TF, Ferreira TM, et al. Oral administration of sodium butyrate attenuates inflammation and mucosal lesion in experimental acute ulcerative colitis. J Nutr Biochem. 2012;23(5):430–6.
57. Chuang SC, Vermeulen R, Sharabiani MT, Sacerdote C, Fatemeh SH, Berrino F, et al. The intake of grain fibers modulates cytokine levels in blood. Biomarkers. 2011;16(6):504–10.
58. Kanauchi O, Suga T, Tochihara M, Hibi T, Naganuma M, Homma T, et al. Treatment of ulcerative colitis by feeding with germinated barley foodstuff: first report of a multicenter open control trial. J Gastroenterol. 2002;37 Suppl 14:67–72.
59. Rahal K, Schmiedlin-Ren P, Adler J, Dhanani M, Sultani V, Rittershaus AC, et al. Resveratrol has antiinflammatory and antifibrotic effects in the peptidoglycan-polysaccharide rat model of Crohn's disease. Inflamm Bowel Dis. 2012;18(4):613–23.
60. Sánchez-Fidalgo S, Cárdeno A, Villegas I, Talero E, de la Lastra CA. Dietary supplementation of resveratrol attenuates chronic colonic inflammation in mice. Eur J Pharmacol. 2010;633(1–3):78–84.
61. Martín AR, Villegas I, Sánchez-Hidalgo M, de la Lastra CA. The effects of resveratrol, a phytoalexin derived from red wines, on chronic inflammation induced in an experimentally induced colitis model. Br J Pharmacol. 2006;147(8):873–85.
62. Samsami-Kor M, Daryani NE, Asl PR, Hekmatdoost A. Anti-inflammatory effects of resveratrol in patients with ulcerative colitis: a randomized, double-blind. Placebo-controlled pilot study. Arch Med Res. 2015;46(4):280–5.

63. Corley J, Kyle JA, Starr JM, McNeill G, Deary IJ. Dietary factors and biomarkers of systemic inflammation in older people: the Lothian Birth Cohort 1936. Br J Nutr. 2015;7:1–11.
64. Koloverou E, Panagiotakos DB, Pitsavos C, Chrysohoou C, Georgousopoulou EN, Grekas A, et al., ATTICA Study Group. Adherence to Mediterranean diet and 10-year incidence (2002–2012) of diabetes: correlations with inflammatory and oxidative stress biomarkers in the ATTICA cohort study. Diabetes Metab Res Rev. 2015. doi:10.1002/dmrr.2672.
65. Camargo A, Delgado-Lista J, Garcia-Rios A, Cruz-Teno C, Yubero-Serrano EM, Perez-Martinez P, et al. Expression of proinflammatory, proatherogenic genes is reduced by the Mediterranean diet in elderly people. Br J Nutr. 2012;108(3):500–8.
66. Esposito K, Marfella R, Ciotola M, Di Palo C, Giugliano F, Giugliano G, et al. Effect of a Mediterranean-style diet on endothelial dysfunction and markers of vascular inflammation in the metabolic syndrome: a randomized trial. JAMA. 2004;292(12):1440–6.
67. Marlow G, Ellett S, Ferguson IR, Zhu S, Karunasinghe N, Jesuthasan AC, et al. Transcriptomics to study the effect of a Mediterranean-inspired diet on inflammation in Crohn's disease patients. Hum Genomics. 2013;7:24.
68. Janakiram NB, Rao CV. The role of inflammation in colon cancer. Adv Exp Med Biol. 2014;816:25–52.
69. van der Wath RC, Gardiner BS, Burgess AW, Smith DW. Cell organisation in the colonic crypt: a theoretical comparison of the pedigree and niche concepts. PLoS One. 2013;8(9):e73204.
70. Tan CW, Hirokawa Y, Gardiner BS, Smith DW, Burgess AW. Colon cryptogenesis: asymmetric budding. PLoS One. 2013;8(10):e78519.
71. Mundade R, Imperiale TF, Prabhu L, Loehrer PJ, Lu T. Genetic pathways, prevention, and treatment of sporadic colorectal cancer. Oncoscience. 2014;1(6):400–6.
72. Sun L, Luo C, Liu J. Hydroxytyrosol induces apoptosis in human colon cancer cells through ROS generation. Food Funct. 2014;5(8):1909–14.
73. Cárdeno A, Sánchez-Hidalgo M, Cortes-Delgado A, Alarcón de la Lastra C. Mechanisms involved in the antiproliferative and proapoptotic effects of unsaponifiable fraction of extra virgin olive oil on HT-29 cancer cells. Nutr Cancer. 2013;65(6):908–18.
74. Izzo AA, Camilleri M. Cannabinoids in intestinal inflammation and cancer. Pharmacol Res. 2009;60(2):117–25.
75. Wang D, Wang H, Ning W, Backlund MG, Dey SK, DuBois RN. Loss of cannabinoid receptor 1 accelerates intestinal tumor growth. Cancer Res. 2008;68(15):6468–76.
76. Di Francesco A, Falconi A, Di Germanio C, Micioni Di Bonaventura MV, Costa A, Caramuta S, et al. Extravirgin olive oil up-regulates CB1 tumor suppressor gene in human colon cancer cells and in rat colon via epigenetic mechanisms. J Nutr Biochem. 2015;26(3):250–8.
77. Cave Jr WT. Dietary n-3 (omega-3) polyunsaturated fatty acid effects on animal tumorigenesis. FASEB J. 1991;5(8):2160–6.
78. Moreira AP, Sabarense CM, Dias CM, Lunz W, Natali AJ, Glória MB, et al. Fish oil ingestion reduces the number of aberrant crypt foci and adenoma in 1,2-dimethylhydrazine-induced colon cancer in rats. Braz J Med Biol Res. 2009;42(12):1167–72.
79. Sakaguchi M, Hiramatsu Y, Takada H, Yamamura M, Hioki K, Saito K, et al. Effect of dietary unsaturated and saturated fats on azoxymethane-induced colon carcinogenesis in rats. Cancer Res. 1984;44(4):1472–7.
80. Kulkarni N, Zang E, Kelloff G, Reddy BS. Effect of the chemopreventive agents piroxicam and D, L-alpha-difluoromethylornithine on intermediate biomarkers of colon carcinogenesis. Carcinogenesis. 1992;13(6):995–1000.
81. Rigas B, Goldman IS, Levine L. Altered eicosanoid levels in human colon cancer. J Lab Clin Med. 1993;122(5):518–23.
82. Cockbain AJ, Toogood GJ, Hull MA. Omega-3 polyunsaturated fatty acids for the treatment and prevention of colorectal cancer. Gut. 2012;61(1):135–49.
83. Oshima M, Takahashi M, Oshima H, Tsutsumi M, Yazawa K, Sugimura T, et al. Effects of docosahexaenoic acid (DHA) on intestinal polyp development in Apc delta 716 knockout mice. Carcinogenesis. 1995;16(11):2605–7.
84. Paulsen JE, Elvsaas IK, Steffensen IL, Alexander J. A fish oil derived concentrate enriched in eicosapentaenoic and docosahexaenoic acid as ethyl ester suppresses the formation and growth of intestinal polyps in the Min mouse. Carcinogenesis. 1997;18(10):1905–10.
85. Petrik MB, McEntee MF, Johnson BT, Obukowicz MG, Whelan J. Highly unsaturated (n-3) fatty acids, but not alpha-linolenic, conjugated linoleic or gamma-linolenic acids, reduce tumorigenesis in Apc(Min/+) mice. J Nutr. 2000;130(10):2434–43.
86. Fini L, Piazzi G, Ceccarelli C, Daoud Y, Belluzzi A, Munarini A, et al. Highly purified eicosapentaenoic acid as free fatty acids strongly suppresses polyps in Apc(Min/+) mice. Clin Cancer Res. 2010;16(23):5703–11.
87. Akedo I, Ishikawa H, Nakamura T, Kimura K, Takeyama I, Suzuki T, et al. Three cases with familial adenomatous polyposis diagnosed as having malignant lesions in the course of a long-term trial using docosahexanoic acid (DHA)-concentrated fish oil capsules. Jpn J Clin Oncol. 1998;28(12):762–5.
88. West NJ, Clark SK, Phillips RK, Hutchinson JM, Leicester RJ, Belluzzi A, et al. Eicosapentaenoic acid reduces rectal polyp number and size in familial adenomatous polyposis. Gut. 2010;59(7):918–25.

89. Williams MT, Hord NG. The role of dietary factors in cancer prevention: beyond fruits and vegetables. Nutr Clin Pract. 2005;20(4):451–9.
90. Bingham SA, Day NE, Luben R, Ferrari P, Slimani N, Norat T, et al. Dietary fibre in food and protection against colorectal cancer in the European Prospective Investigation into Cancer and Nutrition (EPIC): an observational study. Lancet. 2003;361(9368):1496–501.
91. Peters U, Sinha R, Chatterjee N, Subar AF, Ziegler RG, Kulldorff M, et al. Dietary fibre and colorectal adenoma in a colorectal cancer early detection programme. Lancet. 2003;361(9368):1491–5.
92. Franceschi S, Dal Maso L, Augustin L, Negri E, Parpinel M, Boyle P, et al. Dietary glycemic load and colorectal cancer risk. Ann Oncol. 2001;12(2):173–8.
93. Yu H, Rohan T. Role of the insulin-like growth factor family in cancer development and progression. J Natl Cancer Inst. 2000;92(18):1472–89.
94. Pryde SE, Duncan SH, Hold GL, Stewart CS, Flint HJ. The microbiology of butyrate formation in the human colon. FEMS Microbiol Lett. 2002;217(2):133–9.
95. Zuo L, Lu M, Zhou Q, Wei W, Wang Y. Butyrate suppresses proliferation and migration of RKO colon cancer cells though regulating endocan expression by MAPK signaling pathway. Food Chem Toxicol. 2013. doi:10.1016/j.fct.2013.10.028. pii: S0278-6915(13)00703-5.
96. Tabernero M, Venema K, Maathuis AJ, Saura-Calixto FD. Metabolite production during in vitro colonic fermentation of dietary fiber: analysis and comparison of two European diets. J Agric Food Chem. 2011;59(16):8968–75.
97. Lewin MH, Bailey N, Bandaletova T, Bowman R, Cross AJ, Pollock J, et al. Red meat enhances the colonic formation of the DNA adduct O6-carboxymethyl guanine: implications for colorectal cancer risk. Cancer Res. 2006;66(3):1859–65.
98. Jakszyn P, Agudo A, Berenguer A, Ibáñez R, Amiano P, Pera G, et al. Intake and food sources of nitrites and N-nitrosodimethylamine in Spain. Public Health Nutr. 2006;9(6):785–91.
99. Pessêgo M, Rosa da Costa AM, Moreira JA. Importance of phenols structure on their activity as antinitrosating agents: a kinetic study. J Pharm Bioallied Sci. 2011;3(1):128–34.
100. Bingham SA, Pignatelli B, Pollock JR, Ellul A, Malaveille C, Gross G, et al. Does increased endogenous formation of N-nitroso compounds in the human colon explain the association between red meat and colon cancer? Carcinogenesis. 1996;17(3):515–23.
101. Sears CL, Garrett WS. Microbes, microbiota, and colon cancer. Cell Host Microbe. 2014;15(3):317–28.
102. Louis P, Flint HJ. Diversity, metabolism and microbial ecology of butyrate-producing bacteria from the human large intestine. FEMS Microbiol Lett. 2009;294(1):1–8.
103. Van den Abbeele P, Belzer C, Goossens M, Kleerebezem M, De Vos WM, Thas O, et al. Butyrate-producing Clostridium cluster XIVa species specifically colonize mucins in an in vitro gut model. ISME J. 2013;7(5):949–61.
104. Lopez-Legarrea P, Fuller NR, Zulet MA, Martinez JA, Caterson ID. The influence of Mediterranean, carbohydrate and high protein diets on gut microbiota composition in the treatment of obesity and associated inflammatory state. Asia Pac J Clin Nutr. 2014;23(3):360–8.
105. Lupton JR. Butyrate and colonic cytokinetics: differences between in vitro and in vivo studies. Eur J Cancer Prev. 1995;4(5):373–8.
106. Roediger WE. Utilization of nutrients by isolated epithelial cells of the rat colon. Gastroenterology. 1982;83(2):424–9.
107. Lupton JR. Microbial degradation products influence colon cancer risk: the butyrate controversy. J Nutr. 2004;134(2):479–82.
108. Donohoe DR, Collins LB, Wali A, Bigler R, Sun W, Bultman SJ. The Warburg effect dictates the mechanism of butyrate-mediated histone acetylation and cell proliferation. Mol Cell. 2012;48(4):612–26.
109. Pino MS, Chung DC. The chromosomal instability pathway in colon cancer. Gastroenterology. 2010;138(6):2059–72. doi:10.1053/j.gastro.2009.12.065.
110. Boland CR, Goel A. Microsatellite instability in colorectal cancer. Gastroenterology. 2010;138(6):2073–87.e3.
111. Belcheva A, Irrazabal T, Robertson SJ, Streutker C, Maughan H, Rubino S, et al. Gut microbial metabolism drives transformation of MSH2-deficient colon epithelial cells. Cell. 2014;158(2):288–99.
112. Arpaia N, Campbell C, Fan X, Dikiy S, van der Veeken J, deRoos P, et al. Metabolites produced by commensal bacteria promote peripheral regulatory T-cell generation. Nature. 2013;504(7480):451–5.
113. Singh N, Gurav A, Sivaprakasam S, Brady E, Padia R, Shi H, et al. Activation of Gpr109a, receptor for niacin and the commensal metabolite butyrate, suppresses colonic inflammation and carcinogenesis. Immunity. 2014;40(1):128–39.
114. Round JL, Lee SM, Li J, Tran G, Jabri B, Chatila TA, et al. The Toll-like receptor 2 pathway establishes colonization by a commensal of the human microbiota. Science. 2011;332(6032):974–7.
115. Gaboriau-Routhiau V, Rakotobe S, Lécuyer E, Mulder I, Lan A, Bridonneau C, et al. The key role of segmented filamentous bacteria in the coordinated maturation of gut helper T cell responses. Immunity. 2009;31(4):677–89.

116. Xu M, Yamada M, Li M, Liu H, Chen SG, Han YW. FadA from Fusobacterium nucleatum utilizes both secreted and nonsecreted forms for functional oligomerization for attachment and invasion of host cells. J Biol Chem. 2007;282(34):25000–9.
117. Erdman SE, Rao VP, Poutahidis T, Rogers AB, Taylor CL, Jackson EA, et al. Nitric oxide and TNF-alpha trigger colonic inflammation and carcinogenesis in Helicobacter hepaticus-infected, Rag2-deficient mice. Proc Natl Acad Sci U S A. 2009;106(4):1027–32.
118. Nair J, Gansauge F, Beger H, Dolara P, Winde G, Bartsch H. Increased etheno-DNA adducts in affected tissues of patients suffering from Crohn's disease, ulcerative colitis, and chronic pancreatitis. Antioxid Redox Signal. 2006;8(5–6):1003–10.
119. Wang X, Huycke MM. Extracellular superoxide production by Enterococcus faecalis promotes chromosomal instability in mammalian cells. Gastroenterology. 2007;132(2):551–61. Epub 2006 Nov 29.
120. Cuevas-Ramos G, Petit CR, Marcq I, Boury M, Oswald E, Nougayrède JP. Escherichia coli induces DNA damage in vivo and triggers genomic instability in mammalian cells. Proc Natl Acad Sci U S A. 2010;107(25):11537–42.
121. Arthur JC, Perez-Chanona E, Mühlbauer M, Tomkovich S, Uronis JM, Fan TJ, et al. Intestinal inflammation targets cancer-inducing activity of the microbiota. Science. 2012;338(6103):120–3.
122. Huycke MM, Gaskins HR. Commensal bacteria, redox stress, and colorectal cancer: mechanisms and models. Exp Biol Med (Maywood). 2004;229(7):586–97.
123. Carman RJ, Van Tassell RL, Kingston DG, Bashir M, Wilkins TD. Conversion of IQ, a dietary pyrolysis carcinogen to a direct-acting mutagen by normal intestinal bacteria of humans. Mutat Res. 1988;206(3):335–42.
124. Kassie F, Rabot S, Kundi M, Chabicovsky M, Qin HM, Knasmüller S. Intestinal microflora plays a crucial role in the genotoxicity of the cooked food mutagen 2-amino-3-methylimidazo [4,5-f]quinoline. Carcinogenesis. 2001;22(10):1721–5.
125. Queipo-Ortuño MI, Boto-Ordóñez M, Murri M, Gomez-Zumaquero JM, Clemente-Postigo M, et al. Influence of red wine polyphenols and ethanol on the gut microbiota ecology and biochemical biomarkers. Am J Clin Nutr. 2012;95(6):1323–34.
126. Bialonska D, Ramnani P, Kasimsetty SG, Muntha KR, Gibson GR, Ferreira D. The influence of pomegranate by-product and punicalagins on selected groups of human intestinal microbiota. Int J Food Microbiol. 2010;140(2-3):175–82.
127. Plaza-Diaz J, Gomez-Llorente C, Fontana L, Gil A. Modulation of immunity and inflammatory gene expression in the gut, in inflammatory diseases of the gut and in the liver by probiotics. World J Gastroenterol. 2014;20(42):15632–49.
128. Cani PD, Bibiloni R, Knauf C, Waget A, Neyrinck AM, Delzenne NM, et al. Changes in gut microbiota control metabolic endotoxemia-induced inflammation in high-fat diet-induced obesity and diabetes in mice. Diabetes. 2008;57(6):1470–81.
129. Cani PD, Delzenne NM. Interplay between obesity and associated metabolic disorders: new insights into the gut microbiota. Curr Opin Pharmacol. 2009;9(6):737–43.

Chapter 15
Epigenetics of Mediterranean Diet: Altering Disease Risk

Sharon A. Ross

Key Points

- A Mediterranean diet (MD) pattern is characterized by consumption of olive oil, plant foods, fish, seafood, and low-fat dairy foods, a moderate intake of wine and low consumption of red meat and processed meat products. Such a dietary pattern has been thought to counter conditions/diseases such as metabolic syndrome, atherosclerosis, cancer, diabetes, obesity, pulmonary diseases, and cognition disorders.
- The potential disease preventing activities of an MD pattern have been attributed to a number of dietary factors, including monounsaturated fatty acids, vitamins and phytochemicals. However, the underlying mechanisms remain unknown, but may be linked to epigenetics, which has emerged as a significant link between genes and the environment.
- With a great degree of complexity and flexibility, epigenetic mechanisms exert a profound influence on the regulation of how genetic information is transcribed and translated into proteins that ultimately affect health and disease.
- Dietary components have been shown to influence epigenetic mechanisms, altering gene expression and potentially modifying disease risk. Understanding how dietary factors and dietary patterns participate in modifying gene expression through epigenetics is a complex task given the range of food choices, the diversity of nutrient intakes, the individual differences in genetic backgrounds and intestinal environments where food is metabolized, as well as the numerous enzymes, protein complexes, and factors that participate in epigenetics, among other challenges.
- Recent advances concerning the relationship between dietary factors of an MD pattern and epigenetic mechanisms, and their influence on health and disease are briefly discussed. Insights from current studies may assist with future avenues of research, and ultimately intervention strategies for prevention of chronic diseases.

Keywords Dietary pattern • Olive oil • Epigenetics • Histone • DNA methylation • Cancer

S.A. Ross, Ph.D., M.P.H. (✉)
Nutritional Science Research Group, Division of Cancer Prevention, Department of Health and Human Services, National Cancer Institute, National Institutes of Health, 9609 Medical Center Drive, 5E578 MSC 9788, Bethesda, MD 20892, USA
e-mail: rosss@mail.nih.gov

D.F. Romagnolo, O.I. Selmin (eds.), *Mediterranean Diet*, Nutrition and Health,
DOI 10.1007/978-3-319-27969-5_15

Abbreviations

5hmc	5-methylhydroxycytosine
Aβ	Amyloid-β
CB_1	Type 1 cannabinoid receptor
CIN2+	Cervical intraepithelial neoplasia 2+
CLOCK	Clock circadian regulator gene
CpGs	Cytosine phosphate guanine dinucleotides
DHA	Docosahexaenoic acid
DMR	Differentially methylated region
ELOVL5	Elongase 5
EVOO	Extra-virgin olive oil
FADS2	Fatty acid desaturase-2 gene
H3K9	Histone 3 acetylation on lysine 9
HDACs	Histone deacetylases
HT	Hydroxytyrosol
IGF2	Insulin-like growth factor II
LIs	Long interspersed nucleotide element
lncRNA	Long noncoding RNA
MUFA	Monounsaturated fatty acid
OLE	Oleuropein aglycone
OO	Olive oil
OPE	Olive oil phenolic extract
PBMCs	Peripheral blood mononuclear cells
PUFA	Polyunsaturated fatty acid
SFA	Saturated fatty acid
TET	Ten-eleven translocation family of proteins
Tg	Double transgenic TgCRND8 mice (overexpressing the Swedish and Indiana mutations in the human amyloid precursor protein)
βOHB	Ketone body β-hydroxybutyrate

Introduction

Although there are many definitions of a MD pattern, it typically consists of a dietary intake high in olive oil, vegetables and fruits, plant proteins, whole grains, fish, low-fat dairy foods, moderate red wine intake, and low red meat consumption [1]. Adherence to such a dietary pattern has been associated with health promotion and disease prevention, including prevention of cardiovascular disease and various cancers [2, 3]. Clinical trial data also support a role for consumption of an MD pattern in the prevention of cardiovascular disease in individuals at high risk [4]. These beneficial activities have been attributed to a number of dietary constituents—potentially acting in combination—such as monounsaturated fatty acids (MUFAs), vitamins, and various phytochemicals [5]. It is interesting to note that olive oil itself contains several bioactive constituents (Table 15.1), including phenolic components and fatty acids, which may elicit important biological functions [6, 7]. The underlying biological mechanisms for the beneficial effects of consuming a MD are thought to involve inflammatory, antioxidant, insulin signaling and other biological processes [2]. Importantly, these processes may be influenced by genetic and epigenetic variation in genes/gene promoter regions of these processes. For example, consumption of a MD pattern was associated with a reduced risk of stroke for carriers

Table 15.1 Major bioactive constituents and representative activities found in extra-virgin olive oil.

Dietary constituent	Biological effects	Reference
Oleic acid (C18:1)	Reduce mortality, cardiovascular mortality, cardiovascular events, and stroke	[53]
Other fatty acids: palmitic acid (C16:0), linoleic acid (C18:2), stearic acid (C18:0), α-linolenic acid (C18:3)	Nutritional (i.e., energy, essential fatty acids) and sensory quality	[62]
Phenolic alcohols (i.e., hydroxytyrosol and tyrosol), phenolic acids, lignans, flavonoids, secoiridoids (oleuropein, oleocanthal)	Reduce inflammation, cancer	[63]
Oleanolic acid, maslinic acid, uvaol, erythrodiol	Reduce oxidative stress, inflammation, cancer, cardiovascular disease	[64]

of a variant of the transcription factor 7-like 2 (TCF7L2) gene, a component of the Wnt signaling pathway [2]. The significance of understanding the molecular etiology of disease in order to advance and "fine-tune" prevention and treatment options has placed the focus on genetic variation; however utilizing "omic" approaches should provide additional clues, including an understanding of epigenomic regulation of disease. Notably, epigenetic mechanisms influence the regulation of genes, thereby affecting health and disease. Epigenetics has emerged as a significant link between genes and the environment and may help to assess individual variation in response to environmental factors. Dietary components have been shown to influence epigenetic mechanisms, altering gene expression and potentially modifying disease risk. Because the whole MD has not been studied with regard to epigenetic modulation, this review will focus on the effects of parts of the MD with an emphasis on olive oil and its constituents and their effects on epigenetics in clinical and preclinical studies.

Epigenetics in Health and Disease

A recent definition for epigenetics is "molecular factors and processes around DNA that regulate genome activity independent of DNA sequence and are mitotically stable" [8]. Another current definition is "the reversible regulation of gene expression, occurring independently of DNA sequence, mediated principally through changes in DNA methylation and chromatin structure" [9]. Together, these definitions capture the important elements of the use of the term epigenetics—heritable, gene regulatory and reversible—for the purpose of this review. The most studied epigenetic mechanisms include DNA methylation of cytosine bases in cytosine phosphate guanine dinucleotides (CpGs); posttranslational modifications of histone tail domains—including methylation, acetylation, ubiquitination, and phosphorylation; regulation through noncoding RNAs; and chromatin remodeling and higher order chromatin structural alterations [10].

DNA methylation involves the transfer of a methyl group to the 5′ position of the cytosine pyrimidine ring of a CpG sequence, which is catalyzed by DNA methyltransferases (DNMTs) [11]. DNA methylation is a stable epigenetic mechanism, but is also thought to influence transcriptional flexibility in the mammalian genome [12]. Promoter DNA methylation disrupts the binding of transcription factors and attracts methyl-binding proteins that initiate chromatin compaction and gene silencing [11]. DNA methylation of gene promoters for processes such as cell differentiation or imprinting may be determined early, but likely persist throughout life, while other DNA methylation marks appear to be more plastic especially during vulnerable periods, such as rapid growth [13, 14]. Genes that retain epigenetic plasticity or flexibility may respond to environmental exposure, including dietary patterns and factors.

Altered epigenetic regulation by DNA methylation of specific genes may be a causal factor in a number of chronic diseases [15, 16]. For example, aberrant DNA methylation influences molecular processes that control critical cellular mechanisms that are altered in prostate and other cancers [17]. Region specific hypomethylation and hypermethylation of CpG islands have both been observed in human cancers. Hypomethylation usually influences repeated DNA sequences, whereas hypermethylation involves CpG islands in promoter/regulatory regions; such loss and/or gain of methylation in specific regions can contribute to carcinogenesis [18].

A nucleosome consists of 146 base pairs of DNA wrapped around an octamer of histone proteins (two molecules each of H2A, H2B, H3, and H4) [19]. In addition to their importance for packaging DNA inside the nucleus, histone proteins also influence the regulation of gene expression. Posttranslational modifications of the N-terminal tails of the histone proteins include acetylation, methylation, phosphorylation, sumoylation, and ubiquitylation; together these modifications are believed to represent a complex "histone code" that modulates gene expression and other chromatin functions [20]. Histone modifications influence the availability of the transcriptional machinery to the DNA. Some modifications persuade chromatin to condense forming heterochromatin in which the DNA and histone proteins are tightly packed. Heterochromatin blocks the access of transcription factors and other proteins/cofactors involved in gene expression and is associated with repressed transcription. An open chromatin conformation (termed "euchromatin") allows the transcriptional machinery to target DNA and drive transcription [21]. Different histone modifications have different roles in gene expression and function. For example, the addition of an acetyl group may be associated with gene activation (e.g., acetylation of histone 3 at lysines 9 and 14), whereas methylation of histone 3 at lysines 9 and 27 is associated with decreased gene expression [22]. Similar to DNA methylation, histone modifications are dynamic and regulated by a host of enzymes and cofactors, including histone acetyltransferases (HATs) and histone deacetylases (HDACs), which add and remove acetyl groups, respectively.

Although DNA methylation and histone modifications are often studied separately, it is now known that these two mechanisms interact in numerous ways for normal chromatin function. For example, histone lysine methylation may help to target DNA methylation during development [23]. Noncoding RNAs also participate as epigenetic regulators of gene expression and have been shown to influence histone posttranslational modifications [24]. For example, H19 lncRNA, a long noncoding RNA which interacts with MBD1, has been shown to regulate H3K9 methylation of several genes important in the control of embryonic growth [24]. Through interactions with MBD1, H19 lncRNA maintains the repressive chromatin mark on target genes. In addition, RNA undergoes posttranscriptional modifications that influence gene expression. For example, the N^6-methyl-adenosine (m^6A) mRNA/lncRNA modification has been linked to epigenetic regulation of gene expression, comparable to DNA methylation and histone modification and studies suggest that the m^6A modification may influence health and disease [25].

Furthermore, novel epigenetic mechanisms or marks continue to be elucidated. A mechanism for active DNA demethylation was recently discovered which involves oxidation of 5-methylcytosine to 5-methylhydroxycytosine (5hmc) by the ten-eleven translocation (TET) family of proteins [26]. In addition to 5hmc, formylcytosine and carboxylcytosine are also generated by oxidation of methylcytosine through TET enzymes. As a result, full DNA demethylation can occur, but each of these oxidation products are also thought to act as epigenetic signaling molecules [27]. It is also noteworthy that 5hmc levels have been observed to be altered in cancer and other disorders and that dysfunction and/or mutations in TET genes have been characterized in various cancers [27]. In addition to DNA methylation, histone posttranslational modifications, and noncoding RNA, gene expression is also influenced by the positioning and occupancy of nucleosomes at promoter regions [28]. To add to all this complexity, nucleosome remodeling complexes are involved in nucleosome positioning to regulate access to DNA.

Diet and Epigenetics in Health and Disease

Epigenetic mechanisms, because they are reversible, may allow rapid adaptation to dietary exposures. In fact, dietary factors have been shown to influence epigenetic mechanisms, altering gene expression and potentially modifying disease risk. The one-carbon metabolism pathway requires vitamins B_6, B_{12}, folate, betaine, and choline as well as the amino acids methionine, cysteine, serine, and glycine for proper functioning. Because one-carbon metabolism is important for the availability of *S*-adenosylmethionine, the universal methyl donor for DNA, histone and other macromolecular methylation reactions, alterations in B-vitamin status influence these epigenetic mechanisms [29]. An interesting finding from a cohort of healthy women undergoing reduction mammoplasty exemplifies the significance of nutrient concentrations [30]. These investigators found that lower breast folate concentrations were associated with hypermethylation of the tumor suppressor gene *p16INK4a* and lower P16 expression, suggesting that one-carbon metabolism may influence epigenetic variation, and perhaps, breast cancer risk. Other dietary factors also influence DNA methylation, but through other pathways and mechanisms. For example, the polyphenol epigallocatechin-3-gallate found in green tea and the isoflavone genistein found in soy have shown demethylation activity in cancer cell lines [31]. Dietary factors can also influence histone modification. Several dietary components such as curcumin and sulforaphane and diet-derived components (i.e., butyrate) display weak histone deacetylase inhibition, which is associated with upregulation of tumor suppressor genes and anticancer activity [32].

The relationship of nutrition in early life to health outcomes later in life, for which there is increasing evidence, has received much recent attention [33, 34]. DNA methylation, histone modifications and other epigenetic mechanisms are thought to be involved in conveying this developmental programming of disease. During the very early phases of normal embryonic development, DNA methylation is erased and then extensively reprogrammed. It can be envisioned, therefore, that undernutrition or overnutrition early in life can affect DNA methylation significantly during this vulnerable period. It is interesting to note here that differences in DNA methylation have been identified at the insulin-like growth factor II (*IGF2*) locus, a key factor in human growth and development which is maternally imprinted, between individuals exposed to the Dutch Hunger Winter famine compared to their unexposed siblings [35]. Because certain epigenetic marks may be more flexible and because they are important regulators of gene expression, epigenetic processes likely affect disease susceptibility throughout the lifespan. Although DNA methylation changes may be a natural outcome of aging, methylation changes in specific regions have been associated with decreased organ function, memory, bone density and other age-related health conditions [36, 37]. The future of studying epigenetics in aging may provide an understanding of preventing, perhaps through lifestyle change, such age-related health problems.

How Do Dietary Factors and Changes in Cellular Metabolism Trigger Epigenetic Modifications?

Understanding how dietary factors and dietary patterns participate in modifying gene expression through epigenetics is complex. Dietary factors might influence a global change in DNA methylation affecting multiple genes or influence DNA methylation of a specific gene or region. The mechanisms and cellular pathways that are involved in triggering these global or specific epigenetic changes have not been fully elucidated. A working hypothesis on how the cellular environment influences

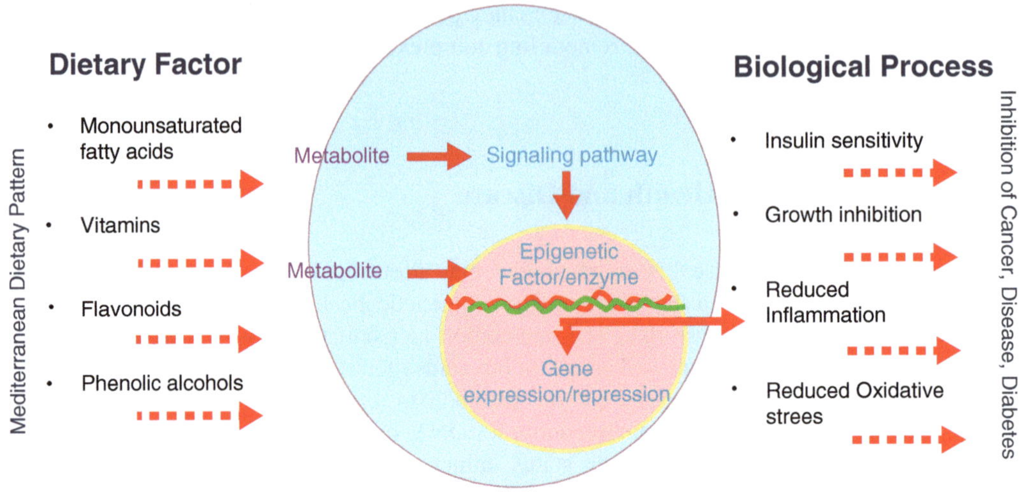

Fig. 15.1 A model for the mechanism of action of a Mediterranean dietary pattern in health promotion and disease prevention. Dietary patterns/factors and changes in cellular metabolism trigger epigenetic modifications to influence biological pathways that ultimately alter health and disease. Epigenetic factors (i.e., dietary factor or resulting metabolite) may act through either a direct or an indirect mechanism. A factor may act directly by altering activity of an epigenetic enzyme or by altering the availability of substrate involved in an epigenetic process. An indirect acting factor is one that first influences cellular signaling pathways that then alter gene regulatory proteins involved in epigenetics

epigenetic changes has been recently outlined [38]. For example, an epigenetic factor (i.e., dietary factor or resulting metabolite) may act through either a direct or an indirect mechanism. A factor may act directly by altering activity of an epigenetic enzyme or by altering the availability of substrate involved in an epigenetic process (such as methyl or one carbon availability) (Fig. 15.1). An indirect acting factor is one that first influences cellular signaling pathways that then alter gene regulatory proteins involved in epigenetics (i.e., methyl binding protein). Examples of dietary factors that act either directly or indirectly have been documented but exact mechanisms are still being characterized. As an example of a direct effect by a dietary epigenetic influence, a recent study found that caloric restriction prevented the age-related increase in HDAC2 concentration in the mouse hippocampus [39]. It may also be that caloric restriction acts indirectly to modify HDAC expression and activity through signaling molecules such as the ketone body β-hydroxybutyrate (βOHB) [40]. In this regard, βOHB might act as an endogenous metabolic intermediary of caloric restriction by influencing signaling pathways to inhibit HDACs.

There are many metabolic intermediaries that affect gene expression via chromatin modifications, including acetyl-CoA and reduced levels of NAD^+ [41]. These intermediaries may be key links between variations in the cellular environment and the epigenetic changes associated with health and disease. Dietary pattern and dietary factors are known to alter these metabolic intermediaries and other cellular metabolites, and may also alter the epigenetic regulation of gene expression through such mechanisms. Furthermore, it has been suggested that responses to environmental cues are likely driven by changes in the levels, locations, and combinations of transcription factors which act within the three dimensional epigenetic landscape that results from the spatial organization of the genome [42]. Thus, a more complete understanding of how dietary patterns influence epigenetics and biological response should involve the interrelationships between DNA and histone modification patterns and genome function, in the context of spatial organization of chromatin, including long-range chromatin interactions.

Dietary Pattern and Epigenetics

Some have speculated that compared to isolated dietary factors, the study of dietary patterns may have greater power for determining an effect of diet on DNA methylation [43]. Although a Mediterranean dietary pattern has not been examined in this regard, one study reported that a dietary pattern characterized by a high intake of vegetables and fruits was associated with a lower prevalence of global leukocyte DNA hypomethylation [43]. DNA hypomethylation of certain regions (intergenic and intronic regions of the DNA, mostly repeat sequences and transposable elements) may be associated with an increased risk of several cancers due to chromosomal instability and increased mutation events. Thus, these findings could suggest a diet high in fruits and vegetables may prevent cancer by diminishing hypomethylation of these susceptible regions. However, this study reported no association between a Western dietary pattern (characterized by high intake of meats, grains, dairy, oils, and potatoes) and global leukocyte DNA methylation. Another study found that in a cohort of women at risk for developing cervical intraepithelial neoplasia 2+ (CIN2+), those who consumed a "healthy" dietary pattern (comprised of foods such as seafood, beans, whole grains, fruits, vegetables, low fat dairy, chicken and turkey) compared to those consuming an "unhealthy" diet (including such foods as high sugar beverages, starchy foods, margarine, butter, refined grains, desserts and sweets, fatty meat, sausages and bacon) were more likely to have higher DNA methylation in the long interspersed nucleotide element (LIs) of peripheral blood mononuclear cells [44]. They also found that human papilloma virus associated risk of developing CIN2+ may be reduced with a healthy dietary pattern and that LI methylation pattern may be a biomarker of dietary effectiveness. These studies show that "healthier" diets encourage DNA methylation in regions that are normally DNA hypermethylated and silenced.

Dietary Factors of a Mediterranean Dietary Pattern Influence Epigenetics

As mentioned above, individual dietary constituents of the Mediterranean dietary pattern have been shown to modulate epigenetics in several research contexts and model systems. The epigenetic activities of dietary phytochemicals, including plant polyphenols that are considered as part of a Mediterranean dietary pattern, have been reviewed extensively, especially as they relate to cancer prevention activities [45–47]. In this regard, Hardy and Tollefsbol [48] recently coined the term "epigenetic diet" which refers to the consumption of certain foods, including the plant foods soy, grapes, cruciferous vegetables, and green tea which have individually been shown to affect epigenetic mechanisms and are associated with either a decrease in the incidence of cancer or increase in longevity. As an example, resveratrol found in grapes and red wine, has been shown to prevent BRCA-1 promoter hypermethylation and transcriptional repression induced by the aromatic hydrocarbon receptor-ligand 2,3,7,8 tetrachlorodibenzo-*p*-dioxin in breast cancer cells [49]. In addition, fish oil or their predominant fatty acids eicosapentaenoic acid (EPA) and docosahexaenoic acid (DHA), also considered as part of a Mediterranean dietary pattern, have been studied for their involvement in epigenetic regulation [50]. Much of the research, however, involves dietary supplementation of omega-3 fatty acids during the prenatal period and measuring consequent effects in offspring. For example, an intervention trial conducted in Mexican pregnant women supplemented daily with 400 mg of DHA or a placebo from gestation week 18–22 to parturition assessed DNA methylation states of the imprinted gene locus *IGF2/H19* differentially methylated region (DMR), specifically DNA methylation at *IGF2* promoter 3 (*IGF2* P3), *IGF2* DMR, and *H19* DMR from cord blood mononuclear cells [51]. This imprinted gene region was studied because of its involvement in growth and development. The investigators found that DHA supplementation was associated with an increase of *IGF2* DMR methylation in cord blood of infants of overweight mothers and a significant hypomethylation of *H19 DMR* in infants of normal-weight mothers. In addition, DHA supplementation stimulated an increase of *IGF2* P3 methylation in preterm infants. These results suggest that prenatal DHA supplementation may affect reprogramming of *IGF2/H19* DNA methylation of infants at birth, putatively protecting fetal growth and development in the offspring of overweight mothers. Although any long-term effect, especially on fat distribution and metabolic regulation, needs to be ascertained, the findings suggest that epigenetic mechanisms might be appropriate targets for modulation of fetal programming of certain human diseases.

Olive Oil and Its Bioactive Constituents Influence Epigenetic Mechanisms

Olive oil represents the typical lipid source of the Mediterranean diet [52]. The beneficial effects of olive oil consumption on reducing cardiovascular disease risk has been supported by several studies, and this activity is thought to be attributed to high amounts of MUFAs and phenolic compounds in olive oil [53]. Antioxidant activity, inflammatory protective potential and effects on blood lipid concentrations have been cited as mechanisms of the protective effects of olive oil consumption [54]. In addition, recent studies have examined olive oil and its fatty acid and/or phenolic constituents with regard to epigenetic modulation in various biological pathways, conditions, and disease states. Representative studies that include cancer, Alzheimer's disease, circadian rhythm pathways, insulin resistance and adipogenesis, as well as polyunsaturated fatty acid (PUFA) metabolism using different study designs (human clinical and observational, animal and cell culture) are described below. The findings suggest that olive oil as a protective factor of the Mediterranean dietary pattern may work through epigenetic modulation of important genes that influence chronic disease.

The effects of dietary extra-virgin olive oil (EVOO) and its phenolic compounds on the endocannabinoid system gene expression via epigenetic regulation in human colon cancer cells (Caco-2) have been recently reported [52]. Specifically, the tumor suppressor gene *CNR1*, which encodes the type 1 cannabinoid receptor (CB_1) and displays antiproliferative effects in colorectal cancer cells, was investigated. It is known that *CNR1* gene expression is reduced in Caco-2 human colon cancer cells compared to normal colon mucosa cells and this reduced gene expression is associated with DNA methylation of the *CNR1* promoter region. Treatment of Caco-2 cells with extra-virgin olive oil (EVOO at 100 ppm), olive oil phenolic extract (OPE, 50 μM) or the olive oil polyphenol hydroxytyrosol (HT, 50 μM) for 24 h was associated with decreased *CNR1* promoter methylation and increased CB_1 mRNA and protein expression. Furthermore, both OPE and HT decreased Caco-2 cell proliferation at the same doses used to induce CB_1 expression. Interestingly, treatment of cells with an EVOO extract devoid of phenolics did not result in any changes in *CNR1* methylation and mRNA levels, suggesting that the phenolic fraction of EVOO provides the beneficial effect. These results suggest that consumption of olive oil may contribute to the reduction of colorectal cancer risk in those consuming a Mediterranean dietary pattern.

Resistance to trastuzumab, a monoclonal antibody that interferes with the oncogene HER2/neu receptor, is a challenge in HER2-overexpressing metastatic breast cancer that must be alleviated [55]. Polyphenols from EVOO have been shown to modulate the activity of HER2 and other receptor tyrosine kinases in an anticancer fashion. Using the HER2 amplified JIMT-1 breast cancer cell line, investigators found that complex polyphenols found in EVOO (i.e., secoiridoids, a family of complex polyphenols found in olive oil) influenced epigenetic regulation of chromatin structure which was associated with inhibition of mitosis and promotion of G2/M cell cycle arrest, through the G2/M checkpoint-related stress sensor growth arrest and DNA damage-45 (GADD45) kinase [55]. The nuclei of JIMT-1 cells treated with secoiridoid-rich EVOO phenolic extracts (but not all EVOO phenolic extracts tested), was strongly immunoreactive when stained with the specific antibody against anti-AcH3/K18 (histone H3 acetylation at lysine 18) demonstrating that treatment with secoiridoid-rich EVOO phenolic extracts induced histone hyperacetylation in cell cycle arrested JIMT-1 cells. Thus, a molecular link between treatment of complex polyphenols found in EVOO and posttranslational modification of histones, which can lead to epigenetic regulation of chromatin structure and changes in cell physiology in response to cellular stress, suggests a possible novel strategy to alleviate resistance of HER2-positive breast carcinomas.

Dietary supplementation of oleuropein aglycone (OLE), a secoiridoid abundant in extra-virgin olive oil, has been found to improve learning and memory, decrease de novo amyloid-β (Aβ) peptide Aβ42 deposition, stimulate preformed Aβ42 plaque disassembly, and increase autophagy in the double transgenic TgCRND8 mice (overexpressing the Swedish and Indiana mutations in the human amyloid precursor protein) (Tg) mice, a model of Alzheimer's disease that mimics Aβ deposition in the brain [56] (Also please see Chap. 12). In a more recent study, these investigators examined whether OLE supplementation reduced the toxic pE3-Aβ peptide deposits in the brain of Tg mice at different ages corresponding to early, intermediate, and late stage of Aβ deposition [57]. Because evidence suggests that epigenetic modifications are involved in learning and memory [58], Luccarini et al. [57], also measured histone acetylation in the oldest animals to determine if epigenetic alterations participated in the beneficial responses observed from OLE supplementation. Tg mice fed an AIN-76A diet supplemented with OLE (50 mg/kg of diet) for 8-weeks displayed reduced deposition of the toxic pE3-Aβ. Moreover, OLE fed animals were found to have greater neuronal autophagy (which is associated with reduction and disaggregation of Aβ42 plaque deposits) even in mice at advanced or late stage pathology. Using immunohistochemistry and Western blot analysis, the levels of H3K9 and of histone 4 acetylation on lysine 5 (H4K5) were found to be higher in the brain of OLE-fed Tg mice than in untreated mice. This finding matches a decrease of histone deacetylase 2 expression with a significant improvement of synaptic function. Aberrant epigenetic posttranslational modification of proteins is an emerging factor in the pathogenesis of neurologic diseases and treatment with OLE administration might be a new approach to prevent and treat Alzheimer's disease.

Disturbances in circadian rhythm pathways may be associated with being overweight and developing metabolic syndrome and other chronic conditions. One study examined the relationship between MUFAs and PUFA intake with clock circadian regulator gene (*CLOCK*) methylation at baseline in normal-weight, overweight, and obese women who were following a 16-week weight reduction program to modify metabolic syndrome outcomes [59]. DNA methylation levels at different CpG sites of *CLOCK*, *BMAL1*, and *PER2* genes—genes involved in circadian rhythms—were analyzed by Sequenom's MassARRAY in white blood cells obtained before the intervention. Baseline nutrient intake was determined by 24-h dietary recalls of food intake, inclusive of weekends and weekdays, and the intakes of the predominant saturated fatty acids, MUFA, and PUFA were calculated from Spanish food-composition tables. In this Mediterranean cohort, characterized by a high intake of olive oil and MUFA, the methylation levels of *CLOCK* CpGs 1 and 8 were negatively associated with MUFA intake ($P<0.05$), while the association was positive with PUFA ($P<0.05$). These results suggest that fatty acid composition of the diet could influence the methylation pattern of and putative expression of genes involved in circadian rhythm regulation. Investigators also found an association between weight loss and the baseline methylation levels of *CLOCK* CpG 1, *PER2* CpG 2–3, and *PER2* CpG 25, suggesting that these epigenetic marks might be useful as biomarkers of weight loss.

Evidence suggests that the type and the amount of dietary fat consumed influences metabolic pathways in chronic disease, including obesity, metabolic syndrome, type 2 diabetes, cardiovascular disease, and cancer. The influence of diet on DNA methylation of genes in these metabolic pathways has not been studied in a genome-wide fashion until recently. In this example, investigators explored the effects of the ratio of PUFA to saturated fatty acids (SFA), the ratio of MUFA to SFA, and the ratio of MUFA + PUFA to SFA on genome-wide DNA methylation patterns in a cohort of normal-weight and obese children from Greece [60]. The methylation profile of genomic DNA isolated and purified from the peripheral whole blood from 69 Greek preadolescents was measured using HumanMethylation27

BeadChip (Illumina, San Diego, CA, USA), which examines 27,578 CpG dinucleotides covering 14,495 genes. Dietary intake for two consecutive weekdays and one weekend day was assessed using a 24-h recall technique at morning interviews with the children at their school site. Overall, the investigators found a number of CpG sites and regions that were significantly associated with the quality of fat intake, but few sites that were significantly associated with the quantity of fat intake. Among the findings for the MUFA/SFA relationship to DNA methylation was one CpG site associated with aldehyde dehydrogenase 3 family, member A2 (*ALDH3A2*), and a CpG site associated with sema domain, immunoglobulin domain, short basic domain, secreted, (semaphorin) 3G (*SEMA3G*), genes involved in insulin resistance and adipogenesis, respectively. There was some overlap between the significant CpG sites found for the different fatty acid ratios, but little overlap between all fatty acid ratios. This may signify, for example, how MUFA and PUFA affect DNA methylation in different ways. PUFA and MUFA were also found to affect the methylation of some genes in an identical way, as was the example for the site associated with *NCOA1*, a member of the p160 SRC family that interact with nuclear hormone receptors and other transcription factors to facilitate the assembly of transcriptional protein complexes for chromatin remodeling and activation of gene expression, which was more significant for (MUFA + PUFA)/SFA than for PUFA/SFA or MUFA/SFA. One study limitation is that DNA methylation can vary by blood cell type, and therefore the methylation changes associated with the variables investigated in this study may represent an alteration in blood cell composition, rather than a change in methylation; furthermore, methylation patterns observed in blood may not always reflect the pattern in other tissues. Regardless, these results suggest that specific changes in DNA methylation may have an important role in the mechanisms involved in the physiological responses to different types of dietary fat. Using controlled, randomized designs, future studies might reveal additional influences of dietary fat quality on DNA methylation and perhaps investigate further the downstream effects of this process, such as mRNA and protein expression.

Investigators recently assessed whether fatty acid supplementation induced differential changes in the DNA methylation of genes involved in long-chain n-3 PUFA biosynthesis [61]. To do so, they supplemented renal patients (male and female) with 4 g daily of either n-3 PUFAs or olive oil (OO) for 8 weeks and measured the DNA promoter methylation status of genes involved in PUFA biosynthesis from peripheral blood mononuclear cells (PBMCs). Compared to baseline, both OO and n-3 PUFA supplementation induced significant changes in the level of methylation of individual CpG loci in specific genes involved in PUFA metabolism in PBMCs, which appeared to be differential by gender. For example, supplementation with OO increased the level of methylation compared to baseline at CpG-806 in the fatty acid desaturase (Fads)-2 gene (FADS2) by 13 % and at CpG-775 by 24.0 % in males. In females, supplementation with OO increased methylation at in FADS2 gene at CpGs −1119 (6.3 %), −1101 (14.6 %), −871 (13.1 %), −869 (16.5 %), −855 (13.3 %), −817 (17.5 %), −806 (13.9 %), and CpG −775 (8.9 %) compared to baseline. In males, there was no significant effect of supplementation with OO on the methylation of CpG loci in elongase 5 (ELOVL5). In females, however, supplementation with OO decreased methylation in ELOVL5 at CpG −686 (3.1 %), but increased methylation of CpG −269 (7.6 %) and CpG −259 (4.6 %) compared to baseline. Although the mRNA expression of FADS2 was reduced significantly in all dietary groups, ELOVL5 expression was reduced in females who received the OO supplement and in males who received with the OO or n-3 PUFA supplement compared to baseline. Although these results do not support a tight one-to-one relationship between the level of promoter CpG methylation and mRNA expression of the corresponding transcript, they suggest that increased intakes of n-3 PUFA or olive oil may reduce PUFA biosynthesis via changes in the epigenetic regulation of FADS2 and ELOVL5 that affect gene transcription. The results may assist in understanding the mechanisms for the health benefits associated with higher consumption of fish oil or olive oil and that with supplementation of specific fatty acids it may be possible to target individual CpG loci. This has implications for understanding the effect of fatty acids on PUFA metabolism and cell function.

The above discussion outlines emerging findings that support the idea that extra-virgin olive oil, its fatty acids (e.g., MUFAs) and phenolic composition (e.g., secoiridoid-rich EVOO phenolic extracts, oleuropein aglycone, hydroxytyrosol) can modify epigenetic mechanisms, including specific DNA promoter methylation and global histone acetylation, that influence a host of biological process (e.g., endocannabinoid system, receptor tyrosine kinases, learning and memory, circadian rhythm regulation, insulin resistance and adipogenesis, long-chain polyunsaturated fatty acid biosynthesis) in health and disease. However, there is a need for more rigorous studies that assess directly the effect epigenetic modifications induced by a Mediterranean dietary pattern, or its components in combination, have on gene expression and functional biological pathways in health and disease.

Conclusions

Understanding the biological mechanisms by which specific dietary patterns contribute to health and disease may assist with intervention strategies and help to "fine-tune" dietary recommendations. Epigenetic regulation of genes by specific dietary patterns or bioactive food components is potentially an important mechanism in metabolic control and in disease risk, but there is a substantial need for studies that demonstrate a direct effect of epigenetic changes on transcription, metabolism and other biological functions and phenotypic outcome. Furthermore, the ability to characterize and understand the factors that affect individual variation in response to specific dietary patterns is also needed. The application of emerging high throughput analytical technologies in combination with established research approaches will enhance our ability to define individual differences in health, responses to dietary pattern, and the development of disease. Such emerging technologies include "omic-based" approaches such as nutrigenetics, transcriptomics, epigenomics, proteomics, and metabolomics. Because the underlying genetic sequence may influence epigenetic marks and processes, studies in humans need to differentiate epigenetic marks that are indeed due to intake of specific dietary patterns from those that are due to other environmental factors. The majority of the studies addressing the use of dietary factors of a Mediterranean dietary pattern have been conducted in vitro, often without considering the actual bioavailability and metabolic processing of the constituent in humans. The absorption of some of these dietary factors, especially polyphenols, is known to be low in human subjects, and the absorbed fractions are usually metabolized and rapidly excreted. Additionally, the effects of dietary plant compounds have often been assessed in vitro or in animal models using single compounds added at supra-physiological concentrations. Thus, models that examine dietary patterns or factors in combination at doses that are physiologically relevant rather than single dietary compounds at non-physiological concentrations are needed.

Additional research needs to include the ability to better discriminate a "healthy" epigenetic profile or epigenome from those related to specific conditions or diseases. Studies that elucidate when and where to look, and/or that assess the temporal and spatial considerations of epigenetic regulation are emerging, i.e., examination of epigenomes of adult stem cells. Furthermore, studies are needed to examine epigenomic profiles of sorted-cell populations within a tissue versus a mixed cell population. The timing of consumption of a particular dietary pattern may be important in the development and maintenance of epigenetic marks and processes. For example, it is known that maternal dietary intake during pregnancy and lactation may influence persistent changes in epigenetic regulation by DNA methylation and histone modification of genes in the tissues of offspring. Intake of specific dietary patterns in adults may stimulate altered epigenetic regulation of specific genes, although this may be transient and reversible. In this regard, investigations to understand the biological mechanisms leading to dysregulation of normal epigenetic patterns in aging, including consequences of epigenetic drift in aging are needed. Thus, epigenetics may be a possible mechanism connecting diet to gene and cell function during vulnerable periods of the life span. Epigenetic biomarkers also may be useful as biomarkers of prevention, early disease, or nutritional status, as well as function as potential molecular targets that are modulated by dietary interventions. Furthermore, the relationship between bacteria–host gene interactions, including the influence of the bacterial epigenome which may offer additional regulatory capacity, requires investigation.

Although this review focused on the effects of parts of the Mediterranean diet with an emphasis on olive oil and its bioactive constituents and their effects on epigenetics in clinical and preclinical studies, there is a need to evaluate the role of the Mediterranean dietary pattern as a whole on epigenetic regulation as well as in an epigenome-wide fashion. Understanding the influence of specific dietary patterns on the epigenome is likely to be important in elucidating dietary choices for health promotion and strategies to intervene for disease prevention.

Acknowledgements The author gratefully acknowledges Larae McCarty for assistance with figure design and Paulina Knight for assistance with systematic literature searches.

References

1. Bach-Faig A, Berry EM, Lairon D, Reguant J, Trichopoulou A, Dernini S, Medina FX, Battino M, Belahsen R, Miranda G, Serra-Majem L. Mediterranean Diet Foundation Expert Group. Mediterranean diet pyramid today. Science and cultural updates. Public Health Nutr. 2001;14:2274–84.
2. Corella D, Ordovás JM. How does the Mediterranean diet promote cardiovascular health? Current progress toward molecular mechanisms: gene-diet interactions at the genomic, transcriptomic, and epigenomic levels provide novel insights into new mechanisms. Bioessays. 2014;36:526–37.
3. Schwingshackl L, Hoffmann G. Adherence to Mediterranean diet and risk of cancer: a systematic review and meta-analysis of observational studies. Int J Cancer. 2014;135:1884–97.
4. Estruch R, Ros E, Salas-Salvadó J, Covas MI, Corella D, Arós F, Gómez-Gracia E, Ruiz-Gutiérrez V, Fiol M, Lapetra J, Lamuela-Raventos RM, Serra-Majem L, Pintó X, Basora J, Muñoz MA, Sorlí JV, Martínez JA, Martínez-González MA. PREDIMED Study Investigators. Primary prevention of cardiovascular disease with a Mediterranean diet. N Engl J Med. 2013;368:1279–90.
5. Simopoulos AP. The Mediterranean diets: what is so special about the diet of Greece? The scientific evidence. J Nutr. 2001;131 Suppl 11:S3065S–73.
6. Sánchez de Medina V, Riachy ME, Priego-Capote F, Luque de Castro MD. Composition of fatty acids in virgin olive oils from cross breeding segregating populations by gas chromatography separation-flame ionization detection. J Sci Food Agric. 2014. doi:10.1002/jsfa.7030.
7. Pérez AG, León L, Pascual M, Romero-Segura C, Sánchez-Ortiz A, de la Rosa R, et al. Variability of virgin olive oil phenolic compounds in a segregating progeny from a single cross in Olea europaea L. and sensory and nutritional quality implications. PLoS One. 2014;9(3):e92898.
8. Skinner Laboratory Epigenetics Background Definition [Internet]. Washington State University. 2015 [cited 2015 Jan 24]. Available from: http://skinner.wsu.edu/toxnews/epigeneticdefinition.html
9. Jaenisch R, Bird A. Epigenetic regulation of gene expression: how the genome integrates intrinsic and environmental signals. Nat Genet. 2003;33(Suppl):245–54.
10. Ross SA. Diet and epigenetics. In: Milner JA, Romagnolo DF, editors. Nutrition and health: bioactive compounds and cancer. New York: Springer Science+Business Media, LCC; 2010. p. 101–23.
11. Klose RJ, Bird AP. Genomic DNA methylation: the mark and its mediators. Trends Biochem Sci. 2006;31:89–97.
12. Jirtle RL, Skinner MK. Environmental epigenomics and disease susceptibility. Nat Rev Genet. 2007;8:253–62.
13. Goldberg AD, Allis CD, Bernstein E. Epigenetics: a landscape takes shape. Cell. 2007;128:635–8.
14. Szyf M. The dynamic epigenome and its implications in toxicology. Toxicol Sci. 2007;100:7–23.
15. Burdge GC, Lillycrop KA, Jackson AA. Nutrition in early life, and risk of cancer and metabolic disease: alternative endings in an epigenetic tale? Br J Nutr. 2009;101:619–30.
16. Burdge GC, Lillycrop KA. Nutrition, epigenetics, and developmental plasticity: implications for understanding human disease. Annu Rev Nutr. 2010;30:315–39.
17. Ngollo M, Dagdemir A, Karsli-Ceppioglu S, Judes G, Pajon A, Penault-Llorca F, et al. Epigenetic modifications in prostate cancer. Epigenomics. 2014;6:415–26.
18. Watanabe Y, Maekawa M. Methylation of DNA in cancer. Adv Clin Chem. 2010;52:145–67.

19. Luger K, Mäder AW, Richmond RK, Sargent DF, Richmond TJ. Crystal structure of the nucleosome core particle at 2.8 A resolution. Nature. 1997;389:251–60.
20. Rothbart SB, Strahl BD. Interpreting the language of histone and DNA modifications. Biochim Biophys Acta. 2014;1839:627–43.
21. Grewal SI, Jia S. Heterochromatin revisited. Nat Rev Genet. 2007;8:35–46.
22. Smith S, Mill J. Epigenetics and chronic diseases: an overview. In: Roach HI, Bronner F, Oreffo ROC, editors. Epigenetic aspects of chronic diseases. London: Springer; 2011. p. 1–20.
23. Rose NR, Klose RJ. Understanding the relationship between DNA methylation and histone lysine methylation. Biochim Biophys Acta. 2014;1839:1362–72.
24. Joh RI, Palmieri CM, Hill IT, Motamedi M. Regulation of histone methylation by noncoding RNAs. Biochim Biophys Acta. 2014;1839:1385–94.
25. Liu N, Pan T. RNA epigenetics. Transl Res. 2015;165:28–35.
26. Wu SC, Zhang Y. Active DNA demethylation: many roads lead to Rome. Nat Rev Mol Cell Biol. 2010;11:607–20.
27. Delatte B, Deplus R, Fuks F. Playing TETris with DNA modifications. EMBO J. 2014;33:1198–211.
28. Hesson LB, Sloane MA, Wong JW, Nunez AC, Srivastava S, Ng B, et al. Altered promoter nucleosome positioning is an early event in gene silencing. Epigenetics. 2014;9:1422–30.
29. Niculescu MD, Zeisel SH. Diet, methyl donors and DNA methylation: interactions between dietary folate, methionine and choline. J Nutr. 2002;132 Suppl 8:S2333–5.
30. Llanos AA, Dumitrescu RG, Brasky TM, Liu Z, Mason JB, Marian C, et al. Relationships among folate, alcohol consumption, gene variants in one-carbon metabolism and p16 INK4a methylation and expression in healthy breast tissues. Carcinogenesis. 2015;36:60–7.
31. Li Y, Tollefsbol TO. Impact on DNA methylation in cancer prevention and therapy by bioactive dietary components. Curr Med Chem. 2010;17:2141–51.
32. Pham TX, Lee J. Dietary regulation of histone acetylases and deacetylases for the prevention of metabolic diseases. Nutrients. 2012;4:1868–86.
33. Tammen SA, Friso S, Choi SW. Epigenetics: the link between nature and nurture. Mol Aspects Med. 2013;34:753–64.
34. Langley-Evans SC. Nutrition in early life and the programming of adult disease: a review. J Hum Nutr Diet. 2015;28 Suppl 1:S1–14.
35. Heijmans BT, Tobi EW, Stein AD, Putter H, Blauw GJ, Susser ES, et al. Persistent epigenetic differences associated with prenatal exposure to famine in humans. Proc Natl Acad Sci U S A. 2008;105:17046–9.
36. Lepeule J, Baccarelli A, Motta V, Cantone L, Litonjua AA, Sparrow D, et al. Gene promoter methylation is associated with lung function in the elderly: The Normative Aging Study. Epigenetics. 2012;7:261–9.
37. Liu L, van Groen T, Kadish I, Li Y, Wang D, James SR, et al. Insufficient DNA methylation affects healthy aging and promotes age-related health problems. Clin Epigenetics. 2011;2:349–60.
38. Kanherkar RR, Bhatia-Dey N, Csoka AB. Epigenetics across the human lifespan. Front Cell Dev Biol. 2014;2:49.
39. Chouliaras L, van den Hove DL, Kenis G, Draanen M, Hof PR, van Os J, et al. Histone deacetylase 2 in the mouse hippocampus: attenuation of age-related increase by caloric restriction. Curr Alzheimer Res. 2013;10:868–76.
40. Newman JC, Verdin E. Ketone bodies as signaling metabolites. Trends Endocrinol Metab. 2014;25:42–52.
41. Katada S, Imhof A, Sassone-Corsi P. Connecting threads: epigenetics and metabolism. Cell. 2012;148:24–8.
42. O'Sullivan JM, Doynova MD, Antony J, Pichlmuller F, Horsfield JA. Insights from space: potential role of diet in the spatial organization of chromosomes. Nutrients. 2014;6:5724–39.
43. Zhang FF, Morabia A, Carroll J, Gonzalez K, Fulda K, Kaur M, et al. Dietary patterns are associated with levels of global genomic DNA methylation in a cancer-free population. J Nutr. 2011;141:1165–71.
44. Piyathilake CJ, Badiga S, Kabagambe EK, Azuero A, Alvarez RD, Johanning GL, et al. A dietary pattern associated with LINE-1 methylation alters the risk of developing cervical intraepithelial neoplasia. Cancer Prev Res (Phila). 2012;5:385–92.
45. Vanden Berghe W. Epigenetic impact of dietary polyphenols in cancer chemoprevention: lifelong remodeling of our epigenomes. Pharmacol Res. 2012;65:565–76.
46. Link A, Balaguer F, Goel A. Cancer chemoprevention by dietary polyphenols: promising role for epigenetics. Biochem Pharmacol. 2010;80:1771–92.
47. Thakur VS, Deb G, Babcook MA, Gupta S. Plant phytochemicals as epigenetic modulators: role in cancer chemoprevention. AAPS J. 2014;16:151–63.
48. Hardy TM, Tollefsbol TO. Epigenetic diet: impact on the epigenome and cancer. Epigenomics. 2011;3:503–18.
49. Papoutsis AJ, Lamore SD, Wondrak GT, Selmin OI, Romagnolo DF. Resveratrol prevents epigenetic silencing of BRCA-1 by the aromatic hydrocarbon receptor in human breast cancer cells. J Nutr. 2010;140:1607–14.
50. Burdge GC, Lillycrop KA. Fatty acids and epigenetics. Curr Opin Clin Nutr Metab Care. 2014;17:156–61.
51. Lee HS, Barraza-Villarreal A, Biessy C, Duarte-Salles T, Sly PD, Ramakrishnan U, et al. Dietary supplementation with polyunsaturated fatty acid during pregnancy modulates DNA methylation at IGF2/H19 imprinted genes and growth of infants. Physiol Genomics. 2014;46:851–7.

52. Di Francesco A, Falconi A, Di Germanio C, Micioni Di Bonaventura MV, Costa A, Caramuta S, et al. Extravirgin olive oil up-regulates CB_1 tumor suppressor gene in human colon cancer cells and in rat colon via epigenetic mechanisms. J Nutr Biochem. 2014. doi:10.1016/j.jnutbio.2014.10.013. pii: S0955-2863(14)00241-1.
53. Schwingshackl L, Hoffmann G. Monounsaturated fatty acids, olive oil and health status: a systematic review and meta-analysis of cohort studies. Lipids Health Dis. 2014;13:154.
54. Widmer RJ, Flammer AJ, Lerman LO, Lerman A. The Mediterranean diet, its components, and cardiovascular disease. Am J Med. 2014. doi:10.1016/j.amjmed.2014.10.014. pii: S0002-9343(14)00913-9.
55. Oliveras-Ferraros C, Fernández-Arroyo S, Vazquez-Martin A, Lozano-Sánchez J, Cufí S, Joven J, et al. Crude phenolic extracts from extra virgin olive oil circumvent de novo breast cancer resistance to HER1/HER2-targeting drugs by inducing GADD45-sensed cellular stress, G2/M arrest and hyperacetylation of Histone H3. Int J Oncol. 2011;38:1533–47.
56. Grossi C, Rigacci S, Ambrosini S, Ed Dami T, Luccarini I, Traini C, et al. The polyphenol oleuropein aglycone protects TgCRND8 mice against Aβ plaque pathology. PLoS One. 2013;8(8):e71702.
57. Luccarini I, Grossi C, Rigacci S, Coppi E, Pugliese AM, Pantano D, et al. Oleuropein aglycone protects against pyroglutamylated-3 amyloid-β toxicity: biochemical, epigenetic and functional correlates. Neurobiol Aging. 2014. doi:10.1016/j.neurobiolaging.2014.08.029. pii: S0197-4580(14)00591-0.
58. Graff J, Rei D, Guan JS, Wang WY, Seo J, Hennig KM, et al. An epigenetic blockade of cognitive functions in the neuro-degenerating brain. Nature. 2012;483:222–6.
59. Milagro FI, Gómez-Abellán P, Campión J, Martínez JA, Ordovás JM, Garaulet M. CLOCK, PER2 and BMAL1 DNA methylation: association with obesity and metabolic syndrome characteristics and monounsaturated fat intake. Chronobiol Int. 2012;29:1180–94.
60. Voisin S, Almén MS, Moschonis G, Chrousos GP, Manios Y, Schiöth HB. Dietary fat quality impacts genome-wide DNA methylation patterns in a cross-sectional study of Greek preadolescents. Eur J Hum Genet. 2014. doi:10.1038/ejhg.2014.139.
61. Hoile SP, Clarke-Harris R, Huang RC, Calder PC, Mori TA, Beilin LJ, et al. Supplementation with N-3 long-chain polyunsaturated fatty acids or olive oil in men and women with renal disease induces differential changes in the DNA methylation of FADS2 and ELOVL5 in peripheral blood mononuclear cells. PLoS One. 2014;9(10):e109896.
62. Reboredo-Rodríguez P, González-Barreiro C, Cancho-Grande B, Simal-Gándara J. Quality of extra virgin olive oils produced in an emerging olive growing area in north-western Spain. Food Chem. 2014;164:418–26.
63. Cárdeno A, Sánchez-Hidalgo M, Alarcón-de-la-Lastra C. An up-date of olive oil phenols in inflammation and cancer: molecular mechanisms and clinical implications. Curr Med Chem. 2013;20:4758–76.
64. Sánchez-Quesada C, López-Biedma A, Warleta F, Campos M, Beltrán G, Gaforio JJ. Bioactive properties of the main triterpenes found in olives, virgin olive oil, and leaves of Olea europaea. J Agric Food Chem. 2013;61:12173–82.

Part V
Building a Mediterranean-Like Pyramid

Chapter 16
Physical Activity and the Mediterranean Diet

Melanie D. Hingle, Deepika R. Laddu, and Scott B. Going

Key Points

- The health benefits of physical activity (PA) are undisputed. Regular PA can mitigate or reverse risk factors common to chronic diseases including impaired glucose metabolism, dyslipidemia, and low-grade inflammation.
- Population-based studies have shown reductions on the order of 30 % or more for incident chronic disease in active individuals compared to their inactive peers. PA has been associated with increased diet quality and with a Mediterranean-style eating pattern in both men and women.
- Research suggests that the Mediterranean diet's impact on health may reflect overall lifestyle rather than diet per se, and raises the possibility that PA is a major contributor of the observed health benefits. Herein, we discuss how PA might contribute to the observed benefits of the Mediterranean lifestyle. This includes optimal frequency, intensity, type and time of PA needed for disease prevention, current PA recommendations, and the role of lifestyle PA and sedentary behaviors in chronic disease risk.
- Similar to the Mediterranean diet, PA works through multiple pathways to reduce disease risk. We conclude with examples of potentially overlapping metabolic pathways and effects shared by diet and PA, including lipoprotein and lipid metabolism, anti-thrombotic and anti-arrhythmic effects, and insulin sensitivity.

Keywords Physical activity • Chronic disease prevention • Mediterranean lifestyle • Physical activity recommendations • Physical activity dose

---

M.D. Hingle, Ph.D., M.Ph., R.D. (✉) • S.B. Going, Ph.D.
Department of Nutritional Sciences, The University of Arizona,
1177 E. 4th Street, Shantz Bldg, Room 309, Tucson, AZ 85721-0038, USA
e-mail: hinglem@u.arizona.edu; going@email.arizona.edu

D.R. Laddu, Ph.D.
Stanford Prevention Research Center, Stanford University School of Medicine,
1070 Arastradero Road, 1c052, Palo Alto, CA 94304-1334, USA
e-mail: dladdu@gmail.com

D.F. Romagnolo, O.I. Selmin (eds.), *Mediterranean Diet*, Nutrition and Health,
DOI 10.1007/978-3-319-27969-5_16

Introduction

The health benefits of the Mediterranean diet are well established. Defined by the collective eating habits of the region as described by Keys and colleagues in the 1950s [1–3], this dietary pattern is characterized by low intake of meat and meat products, moderate fruit and wine consumption, moderate to high intakes of fish, poultry, cereals, legumes, vegetables, nuts, garlic, herbs, and high olive oil consumption. Numerous systematic reviews and meta-analyses since the seminal 1970 Keys journal supplement have confirmed the protective effects of the Mediterranean diet on cardiovascular disease [4], metabolic syndrome [5], and overall mortality [6, 7]. Research also suggests that adherence to the Mediterranean diet confers protection against obesity [8], an important risk factor for numerous chronic diseases, and that this effect is partially or wholly mediated by the diet's relatively low energy and high nutrient densities [9–11].

Given the higher fat content of the Mediterranean diet (30–40 % of total energy) relative to diets consumed by populations in Northern Europe and North America [12], this outcome may be viewed as paradoxical. However, the Mediterranean pattern is distinct from other diets in its composition, low in saturated fatty acids (7–8 % of total calories) and high in monounsaturated fatty acids (>20 % of total calories) primarily as olive oil [13]. Increasing evidence suggests it is the fatty acid composition of the diet, and not quantity of fat per se, which can delay or prevent the onset of obesity and related co-morbid conditions [14]. Interestingly, different rates of oxidation have been observed between MUFA and SFA [15]. This suggests differences in energy balance and body weight in experimental [16] and observational studies evaluating the effects of dietary composition on weight outcomes [17] may be a result of differential fatty acid metabolism.

The health promoting effects of the Mediterranean diet, i.e. reduced disease risk and body weight, are thought to be mediated in part by a unique blend of dietary lipids, polyphenols, fibers, and alcohol [18], which together, exert multiple and related physiological effects on lipid fractions, blood pressure, insulin and glucose metabolism, inflammatory processes, and cardiovascular function. Similar effects may result from the action of another important and often overlooked aspect of the Mediterranean lifestyle, physical activity, the focus of this chapter.

Defining Physical Activity

Movement requires muscle contraction, which in turn requires energy expenditure, and energy expenditure balanced with energy intake is essential to health. Although the terms PA and exercise are often used interchangeably, exercise differs slightly from PA in concept. PA has been defined as any bodily movement produced by skeletal muscle contraction resulting in energy expenditure [19]. PA is further qualified by its intensity, described as lifestyle, light, moderate, or vigorous, although there is no consensus on the exact definition of these various intensity levels [20]. Exercise has been defined as planned, structured and repetitive bodily movement done to improve or maintain physical fitness (e.g., cardio-respiratory endurance, skeletal muscle strength and endurance, power, speed, flexibility, balance, and body composition) [19]. Both physical activity and exercise obviously require muscle contraction and thus contribute to energy expenditure and disease prevention. Interestingly, public health guidelines almost always use the term physical activity whereas guidelines for specific disease states frequently use exercise, in part because sedentary individuals may find it easier to begin a physical activity program, whereas a specific exercise prescription may be more effective for specific disease states and to target specific components of fitness.

Health Benefits of Physical Activity

The health benefits of physical activity (PA) are undisputed, and the overall effect of PA on health can be quite powerful [21]. Regular PA can mitigate or reverse risk factors common to chronic diseases [22, 23], including hypertension, impaired glucose metabolism, dyslipidemia, and low grade inflammation. Population-based studies have shown reductions on the order of 30 % or more for incident chronic disease in active individuals compared to their inactive peers [24–29]. Regular PA also improves functional outcomes, such as muscle strength and endurance and aerobic capacity, which are not improved by dietary modifications. Obesity, an important risk factor for chronic disease, is at least partially ameliorated by the increased energy expenditure associated with PA, depending on accompanying alterations in diet and energy intake, while lean mass can be increased or at least maintained. Even without significant weight loss, chronic disease risk factors can be improved with PA [30]. Secondarily, PA has been associated with increased diet quality [31] and importantly to this discussion, with a Mediterranean-style eating pattern in both men and women [32, 33]. Similar findings suggest that the Mediterranean diet's impact on health may reflect overall lifestyle rather than diet per se, and raises the possibility that PA is a major contributor of the observed health benefits.

Optimal Frequency, Intensity, Type and Time of Physical Activity

There is still much to be learned about the optimal dose of physical activity. The risk reduction at higher levels of activity, whether the activity is higher in frequency, intensity or duration, remains to be better defined. Questions remain regarding the minimal amount of exercise needed for health maintenance and whether there is a different threshold of activity necessary to prevent heart disease versus diabetes versus cancer. The anticipated benefits and risks are related to several characteristics of the activity, including the total and rate of energy expenditure, the frequency and duration of activity, and the nature of the activity that is undertaken. Research has shown a dose–response relationship between PA or exercise and health outcomes [21, 34]. Moderate to high levels of PA and physical fitness are associated with greater life expectancy [35, 36] compared to low levels. Also, chronic disease risk factors are more prevalent in adolescents and adults with lower fitness [37], suggesting that regular activity can affect long-term health starting at a younger age. Although a higher dose of PA produces greater benefits, research has clearly shown that people with lower fitness can achieve greater health benefits with a given increase in PA [35, 38, 39]. In fact, the curvilinear dose–response relationship is such that the greatest gains are achieved by increasing activity from low to moderate levels, suggesting that opportunities to significantly impact health through PA extend beyond traditional, structured exercise programs to "lifestyle" PA.

Physical Activity Recommendations

Many countries and organizations have published PA recommendations [20]. Initial recommendations were based on an exercise prescription model that had a central focus on higher-intensity and shorter-duration activity with the goal of improving cardio-respiratory fitness [40, 41]. While controlled exercise studies have been critical to defining the cardiovascular responses to specific PA prescriptions, they lack long-term data and do not provide any guidance on the amount and intensity of beneficial lifestyle activity, which is typically more amenable to study within the context of long-term epidemiology studies. In the 1990s, the American College of Sports Medicine, the U.S. Centers for Disease Control and Prevention (CDC), and the American Heart Association published statements acknowledging the importance of lifestyle physical activity for the reduction of disease risk [34, 42]. As a result, the focus of public health PA guidelines has gradually shifted to a lower-intensity, longer duration lifestyle physical activity model with the goal of reducing chronic disease [43, 44].

Lifestyle PA and Reducing Time Spent in Sedentary Behaviors

Lifestyle PA includes activities such as climbing stairs, walking, shoveling, gardening, sweeping, carrying loads and similar activities performed throughout the day that contribute to energy expenditure. Lifestyle PA may encompass occupational activity and can span the range of intensities, although it is generally regarded as being of a low to moderate intensity. The potential contribution of low intensity activity (e.g., standing versus sitting) to daily energy expenditure is now better appreciated and there is a growing literature on local, cellular adaptations to muscle contraction that contribute to lowering disease risk [45, 46]. There is also an extensive body of research that shows activities of daily living add significantly to total energy expenditure, contributing in important ways to obesity prevention and other aspects of disease prevention and physical and mental health [21]. Sedentary behavior has been identified as a primary risk factor for developing CVD, CHD, as well as some cancers [24, 35, 47–49]. Several longitudinal studies have shown a significant association between TV viewing and CVD mortality [50], and prolonged sitting (>4 h per day) compared to less sitting has been associated with an increased likelihood of incident CVD in postmenopausal women [51]. Interestingly, recent studies suggest that excessive sedentary behavior, even among active individuals meeting the physical activity recommendations, may increase risk of all-cause and CVD mortality [24], and that sedentary time might displace light activity [52]. Although additional work is needed to confirm these data, findings suggest that even small amounts of physical activity (e.g., standing versus sitting at work) may reduce CHD/CVD risk in unfit individuals or individuals participating in low levels of structured physical activity [24, 49, 51], and even active individuals benefit from so-called lifestyle activity.

The Role of PA in the Mediterranean Lifestyle

The Mediterranean lifestyle historically required regular PA in daily tasks [53] rather than planned exercise, which surely contributed significantly to daily energy expenditure. As Willett has suggested [53], part of the health benefits of the Mediterranean diet may be due to other aspects of Mediterranean lifestyle including PA. However, their independent contributions to health are difficult to tease apart since PA is often not controlled in studies of diet, and both diet and PA are difficult to measure accurately. It is also important to note that the introduction of the Mediterranean diet into other regions of the world may not necessarily have the same benefits as other lifestyle-related factors may be different. These limitations notwithstanding, there is an extensive literature on health benefits of PA [21] and even without direct comparisons, there is considerable work demonstrating that regular PA has strong benefits in many of the same ways as a healthy diet including the Mediterranean diet. Below we provide examples of potential overlapping mechanisms of effect shared by diet and PA on the major risk factors for chronic disease, namely lipoprotein and lipid metabolism, anti-thrombotic and anti-arrhythmic effects, and insulin sensitivity.

Plasma Lipids and Lipoproteins

The beneficial effects of physical activity on plasma lipids and lipoprotein profiles have been systematically investigated [54], and include significant reductions in serum triglycerides (TG) and low-density lipoproteins (LDL) (around 2.5 % on average), with modest (non-significant) increases in HDL concentrations. Intensity may also affect the extent to which exercise impacts blood lipids and lipoproteins. A meta-analysis of 22 randomized controlled trials of aerobic exercise trials in older adults (806 exercisers, 621 controls; ages 50 and older) suggested improvements in total cholesterol (TC) (1.1 %), HDL-C (5.6 %), LDL-C (2.5 %), and the ratio of TC to HDL-C (7.1 %), but not TG [55] with moderate intensity (55–90 % of maximum heart rate) aerobic activity; increased HDL-C and decreased ratio of TC/HDL-C were the only fractions that remained statistically significant after a sensitivity analysis to identify publication bias ($p<0.05$), suggesting that aerobic exercise might specifically target the HDL-C. Subgroup analyses suggested changes in lipids and lipoproteins were associated with changes in body weight (decreased LDL-C associated with weight reduction), BMI (decreased LDL-C and TG associated with BMI reduction) and fitness assessed by V_{02max} (defined as maximum oxygen consumption in mL/kg/min) (decreased LDL-C, TC/HDL-C, and TG associated with increased V_{02max}). However, these data focus on PA of moderate to vigorous intensities, whereas the majority of adults do not engage in intense PA regularly.

In a meta-analysis of 25 studies investigating the effects of walking (a light to moderate intensity aerobic activity) on lipids and lipoproteins in adults (692 walkers, 484 controls) suggested that regular walking (defined as 5 times per week for at least 40 min) resulted in statistically significant walking-induced reductions in LDL-C and TC/HDL-C of 5 % and 6 %, respectively. Cardiorespiratory fitness also increased significantly in the walking group (15 % over control condition). No significant changes were observed for TC, HDL-C, or TG, although changes were observed in the expected directions. Kelley and colleagues also examined body composition in this study, noting that the observed changes in lipid fractions occurred independently of body composition (which did not change significantly in either walking or control groups) [56].

Arrhythmia and Thrombosis

The benefits of regular PA include (acute) cardio-protective effects during the transition from rest to exercise, as well as (chronic) adaptations that protect against cardio-metabolic disease [57, 58] although the risks and benefits are dose and intensity-related and certainly modified by disease. Numerous studies have shown a positive association between low to moderate-intensity exercise and an overall reduction in cardiovascular disease risk and related co-morbidities in healthy individuals, as well as those with established CHD [59–64]. In contrast, individuals with pre-existing cardiovascular disease or habitually sedentary individuals who perform unaccustomed strenuous exercise are at increased risk of primary cardiac arrest during vigorous exercise [65, 66]. The precise mechanism by which vigorous exercise provokes cardiac events is not well established. Several studies have suggested possible "triggering" events that may cumulatively promote a consequential event in susceptible individuals [67, 68]. Normal responses to strenuous exercise includes increased heart rate and blood pressure, possibly resulting in increased arterial wall stress and increased coronary artery spasms in diseased arterial segments [58, 67]; this exercise-induced flexing of atherosclerotic coronary arteries [58, 69] may disrupt existing plaques, leading to thrombotic occlusion and ultimately, thrombosis. Simultaneous modifications in vascular thrombotic pathways (involving activation of coagulation and fibrinolysis) in response to catecholamines released during intense PA may have additional detrimental effects. It is important to note that circulating catecholamine levels (and therefore platelet activation) are more closely related to the relative and not absolute intensity of the PA session.

In contrast to strenuous exercise, moderate exercise desensitizes platelets and enhances plasmin formation and fibrinolytic activity without increasing activation of blood coagulation markers. Studies have shown that moderate exercise (60 % of maximal heart rate for 40 min) suppressed shear-induced platelet aggregation primarily by reducing catecholamine levels and a2-adrenergic receptor performance [64, 70]. Exercise training also enhances release of nitric oxide (NO), a potential antithrombotic compound, from platelets and endothelium [64]. Given the results from cross-sectional and longitudinal studies it seems likely regular physical activity reduces thrombolytic development and enhances blood clot degradation by increasing plasmin formation and subsequently accelerating the rate of blood fibrinolysis. These factors combined contribute to an overall reduction in reduced peripheral vascular resistance and enhanced systemic blood flow [59]. The training status of the individual is likely to influence the effect on the thrombotic modifications in coagulation, fibrinolysis and platelet activity. Importantly, three months of detraining reversed favorable adaptations [59, 71].

Effect of Physical Activity on Insulin and Glucose Metabolism

The protective effects of PA and aerobic fitness against derangements in whole body glucose metabolism and insulin regulation are well established by numerous cross-sectional [72–76] and prospective [73, 75, 77] studies. The independent benefits of physical activity remain uncertain as they likely depend on initial metabolic status, changes in body composition, and the dose and intensity of the activity.

The overall effect of insulin on glucose transport is characterized in terms of insulin sensitivity and responsiveness [78]. In skeletal muscle, significant increases in glucose transport occur during repeated muscle contractions, although the effects are short-lived (2–4 h) [79, 80]. In contrast, post-exercise benefits of insulin on glucose transport [80, 81] are characterized by an increase in proteins that activate glucose transport, as well as additional mechanism that lie downstream of the insulin signaling pathway [78].

During and after exercise, the increased insulin sensitivity is mediated, in part, by enhanced expression of glucose transport proteins (GLUT 4 or SLC2A4) [82, 83], and a subsequent increase in insulin-stimulated GLUT 4 translocation to the cell surface [84]. This post-exercise increase in insulin sensitivity requires the presence of a serum protein such as AMP-activated protein kinase (AMPK), which is stimulated in response to exercise induced increases in AMP/ATP [81]. Numerous studies have shown that AMPK plays an essential role in regulating both cellular and molecular pathways that contribute to metabolic benefits elicited with exercise. Muscle AMPK activity is increased during exercise, and some studies suggest a feed-forward regulatory control of GLUT-4 translocation [83, 85–87] may explain the association between exercise and increased insulin sensitivity.

Repeated bouts of exercise have been shown to promote cumulative adaptations in muscle phenotype [88] by mechanisms that include the up-regulation of transcription and expression of co-activators that stimulate mitochondrial biogenesis [81]. These increases in mitochondrial content improve oxidative capacity and confer greater resistance to muscle fatigue [89]. Exercise-induced increases in AMPK also influence molecular changes in mitochondrial morphology, function and efficiency [81, 88, 89]. Exercise is believed to modify many steps in increased mitochondrial biogenesis, responses that are enhanced with regular exercise [88].

Summary

Like diet, PA works through multiple pathways to reduce disease risk. Increasing evidence suggests the protective effects of exercise on cardiovascular disease are intensity- and dose-dependent. Observed metabolic adaptations in response to increasing PA (e.g., improved insulin sensitivity, glucose homeostasis, changes in lipid fractions and lipid oxidation) also underscore the importance of PA as an optimal strategy for the prevention of type 2 diabetes and associated complications [78, 90] continuous activity must be maintained in order for favorable modifications (anti-thrombotic and angiogenic) to confer lasting benefits [58]. Daily moderate PA (equivalent of brisk walking for 30–60 min) appears to be a safe and effective dose for minimizing risk of cardiovascular disease. Given that the benefits of exercise are greatest in the least active [91–95], even modest increases in minutes spent walking and the resulting energy expenditure for this and similar types of physical activities will contribute significantly to risk reduction. Importantly, PA appears to exert a protective effect on health that is independent of diet and concomitant changes in body weight change.

References

1. Keys A, Menotti A, Karvonen MJ, Aravanis C, Blackburn H, Buzina R, et al. The diet and 15-year death rate in the seven countries study. Am J Epidemiol. 1986;124(6):903–15.
2. Kromhout D, Keys A, Aravanis C, Buzina R, Fidanza F, Giampaoli S, et al. Food consumption patterns in the 1960s in seven countries. Am J Clin Nutr. 1989;49(5):889–94.
3. Keys A, Aravanis C, Blackburn H, Buzina R, Djordjevic BS, Dontas AS, et al. Coronary heart disease in seven countries. A summary. Circ J. 1970;41:1186–95.
4. Lairon D. Intervention studies on Mediterranean diet and cardiovascular risk. Mol Nutr Food Res. 2007;51(10):1209–14.
5. Esposito K, Ciotola M, Giugliano D. Mediterranean diet and the metabolic syndrome. Mol Nutr Food Res. 2007;51(10):1268–74.
6. Mitrou PN, Kipnis V, Thiebaut AC, Reedy J, Subar AF, Wirfalt E, et al. Mediterranean dietary pattern and prediction of all-cause mortality in a US population: results from the NIH-AARP Diet and Health Study. Arch Intern Med. 2007;167(22):2461–8.
7. Trichopoulou A, Costacou T, Bamia C, Trichopoulos D. Adherence to a Mediterranean diet and survival in a Greek population. N Engl J Med. 2003;348(26):2599–608.
8. Schroder H. Protective mechanisms of the Mediterranean diet in obesity and type 2 diabetes. J Nutr Biochem. 2007;18(3):149–60.
9. Howarth NC, Saltzman E, Roberts SB. Dietary fiber and weight regulation. Nutr Rev. 2001;59(5):129–39.
10. Slavin JL. Dietary fiber and body weight. Nutrition. 2005;21(3):411–8.
11. Walker KZ, O'Dea K. Is a low fat diet the optimal way to cut energy intake over the long-term in overweight people? Nutr Metab Cardiovasc Dis. 2001;11(4):244–8.
12. Keys A. Mediterranean diet and public health: personal reflections. Am J Clin Nutr. 1995;61(6 Suppl):1321S–3.
13. Mackenbach JP. The Mediterranean diet story illustrates that "why" questions are as important as "how" questions in disease explanation. J Clin Epidemiol. 2007;60(2):105–9.
14. Storlien LH, Baur LA, Kriketos AD, Pan DA, Cooney GJ, Jenkins AB, et al. Dietary fats and insulin action. Diabetologia. 1996;39(6):621–31.
15. DeLany JP, Windhauser MM, Champagne CM, Bray GA. Differential oxidation of individual dietary fatty acids in humans. Am J Clin Nutr. 2000;72(4):905–11.
16. Piers LS, Walker KZ, Stoney RM, Soares MJ, O'Dea K. Substitution of saturated with monounsaturated fat in a 4-week diet affects body weight and composition of overweight and obese men. Br J Nutr. 2003;90(3):717–27.
17. Moussavi N, Gavino V, Receveur O. Could the quality of dietary fat, and not just its quantity, be related to risk of obesity? Obesity (Silver Spring). 2008;16(1):7–15.
18. de Lorgeril M, Salen P. The Mediterranean diet: rationale and evidence for its benefit. Curr Atheroscler Rep. 2008;10(6):518–22.
19. Caspersen CJ, Powell KE, Christenson GM. Physical activity, exercise, and physical fitness: definitions and distinctions for health-related research. Public Health Rep. 1985;100(2):126–31.
20. Rahl R. Physical activity and health guidelines: recommendations for various ages, fitness levels, and conditions from 57 authoritative sources. Champaign, IL: Human Kinetics; 2010.
21. Physical Activity Guidelines for Americans. U.S. Dept. of Health and Human Services (2008). Available from: http://health.gov/paguidelines/guidelines/chapter1.aspx
22. Garber CE, Blissmer B, Deschenes MR, Franklin BA, Lamonte MJ, Lee IM, et al. American College of Sports Medicine position stand. Quantity and quality of exercise for developing and maintaining cardiorespiratory,

musculoskeletal, and neuromotor fitness in apparently healthy adults: guidance for prescribing exercise. Med Sci Sports Exerc. 2011;43(7):1334–59.
23. USDHHS. Physical activity and health: surgeon general's report. Atlanta, GA: USDHHS, Centers for Disease Control and Prevention; 1996.
24. Shiroma EJ, Lee IM. Physical activity and cardiovascular health: lessons learned from epidemiological studies across age, gender, and race/ethnicity. Circulation. 2010;122(7):743–52.
25. Smith TC, Wingard DL, Smith B, Kritz-Silverstein D, Barrett-Connor E. Walking decreased risk of cardiovascular disease mortality in older adults with diabetes. J Clin Epidemiol. 2007;60(3):309–17.
26. Stamatakis E, Hamer M, Lawlor DA. Physical activity, mortality, and cardiovascular disease: is domestic physical activity beneficial? The Scottish Health Survey—1995, 1998, and 2003. Am J Epidemiol. 2009;169(10):1191–200.
27. van Dam RM, Li T, Spiegelman D, Franco OH, Hu FB. Combined impact of lifestyle factors on mortality: prospective cohort study in US women. Br Med J (Clin Res Ed). 2008;337:a1440.
28. Mora S, Cook N, Buring JE, Ridker PM, Lee IM. Physical activity and reduced risk of cardiovascular events: potential mediating mechanisms. Circulation. 2007;116(19):2110–8.
29. Nocon M, Hiemann T, Muller-Riemenschneider F, Thalau F, Roll S, Willich SN. Association of physical activity with all-cause and cardiovascular mortality: a systematic review and meta-analysis. Eur J Cardiovasc Prev Rehabil. 2008;15(3):239–46.
30. Ross R, Janiszewski PM. Is weight loss the optimal target for obesity-related cardiovascular disease risk reduction? Can J Cardiol. 2008;24(Suppl D):25D–31.
31. Samieri C, Sun Q, Townsend MK, Chiuve SE, Okereke OI, Willett WC, et al. The association between dietary patterns at midlife and health in aging: an observational study. Ann Intern Med. 2013;159(9):584–91.
32. Grosso G, Marventano S, Giorgianni G, Raciti T, Galvano F, Mistretta A. Mediterranean diet adherence rates in Sicily, southern Italy. Public Health Nutr. 2013;14:1–9.
33. Sanchez-Villegas A, Martinez JA, De Irala J, Martinez-Gonzalez MA. Determinants of the adherence to an "a priori" defined Mediterranean dietary pattern. Eur J Nutr. 2002;41(6):249–57.
34. Pate R, Pratt M, Blair S, et al. Physical activity and public health: a recommendation from the Centers for Disease Control and Prevention and the American College of Sports Medicine. JAMA. 1995;273(5):402–7.
35. Franco OH, de Laet C, Peeters A, Jonker J, Mackenbach J, Nusselder W. Effects of physical activity on life expectancy with cardiovascular disease. Arch Intern Med. 2005;165(20):2355–60.
36. Paffenbarger RS, Hyde RT, Wing AL, Hsieh C. Physical activity, all-cause mortality, and longevity of college alumni. N Engl J Med. 1986;314:605–13.
37. Carnethon MR, Gulati M, Greenland P. Prevalence and cardiovascular disease correlates of low cardiorespiratory fitness in adolescents and adults. JAMA. 2005;294(23):2981–8.
38. Blair SN, Kohl III HW, Barlow CE, Paffenbarger RS, Gibbons LW, Macera CE. Changes in physical fitness and all-cause mortality: a prospective study of healthy and unhealthy men. J Am Med Assoc. 1995;273:1093–8.
39. Blair SN, Kohl III HW, Paffenbarger Jr RS, Clark DG, Cooper KH, Gibbons LW. Physical fitness and all-cause mortality. A prospective study of healthy men and women. J Am Med Assoc. 1989;262(17):2395–401.
40. ACSM. The recommended quantity and quality of exercise for developing and maintaining fitness in healthy adults. Med Sci Sports Exerc. 1978;10:vii–x.
41. ACSM. Position stand: the recommended quantity and quality of exercise for developing and maintaining cardiorespiratory and muscular fitness in healthy adults. Med Sci Sports Exerc. 1990;22:265–74.
42. CDC. Workshop of physical activity and public health. Sports Med Bull. 1994;28(4):7.
43. CDC. (1996) Physical activity and health: a report of the Surgeon General: U.S. Department of Health and Human Services, Centers for Disease Control and Prevention, National Center for Chronic Disease Prevention and Health Promotion.
44. Haskell WL. J.B. Wolffe Memorial Lecture. Health consequences of physical activity: understanding and challenges regarding dose-response. Med Sci Sports Exerc. 1994;26(6):649–60.
45. Novak CM, Levine JA. Central neural and endocrine mechanisms of non-exercise activity thermogenesis and their potential impact on obesity. J Neuroendocrinol. 2007;19(12):923–40.
46. Thorp AA, Owen N, Neuhaus M, Dunstan DW. Sedentary behaviors and subsequent health outcomes in adults a systematic review of longitudinal studies, 1996–2011. Am J Prev Med. 2011;41(2):207–15.
47. Ford ES, Ajani UA, Mokdad AH. The metabolic syndrome and concentrations of C-reactive protein among U.S. youth. Diabetes Care [Comparative Study Research Support, US Gov't, PHS]. 2005;28(4):878–81.
48. Nunan D, Mahtani KR, Roberts N, Heneghan C. Physical activity for the prevention and treatment of major chronic disease: an overview of systematic reviews. Syst Rev. 2013;2:56.
49. Lee IM, Sesso HD, Paffenbarger Jr RS. Physical activity and coronary heart disease risk in men: does the duration of exercise episodes predict risk? Circulation. 2000;102(9):981–6.
50. Wijndaele K, Brage S, Besson H, Khaw KT, Sharp SJ, Luben R, et al. Television viewing and incident cardiovascular disease: prospective associations and mediation analysis in the EPIC Norfolk Study. PLoS One. 2011;6(5), e20058.

51. Manson JE, Greenland P, LaCroix AZ, Stefanick ML, Mouton CP, Oberman A, et al. Walking compared with vigorous exercise for the prevention of cardiovascular events in women. N Engl J Med. 2002;347(10):716–25.
52. Mansoubi M, Pearson N, Clemes S, Biddle SJ. The relationship between sedentary behaviour and physical activity in adults: a systematic review. Prev Med. 2014;69:28–35.
53. Willett WC. The Mediterranean diet: science and practice. Public Health Nutr. 2006;9(1A):105–10.
54. Kelley GA, Kelley KS, Roberts S, Haskell W. Comparison of aerobic exercise, diet or both on lipids and lipoproteins in adults: a meta-analysis of randomized controlled trials. Clin Nutr. 2012;31(2):156–67.
55. Kelley GA, Kelley KS, Tran ZV. Exercise, lipids, and lipoproteins in older adults: a meta-analysis. Prev Cardiol. 2005;8(4):206–14.
56. Kelley GA, Kelley KS, Tran ZV. Walking, lipids, and lipoproteins: a meta-analysis of randomized controlled trials. Prev Med. 2004;38(5):651–61.
57. Thompson PD, Buchner D, Pina IL, Balady GJ, Williams MA, Marcus BH, et al. Exercise and physical activity in the prevention and treatment of atherosclerotic cardiovascular disease: a statement from the Council on Clinical Cardiology (Subcommittee on Exercise, Rehabilitation, and Prevention) and the Council on Nutrition, Physical Activity, and Metabolism (Subcommittee on Physical Activity). Circulation. 2003;107(24):3109–16.
58. Thompson PD, Franklin BA, Balady GJ, Blair SN, Corrado D, Estes 3rd NA, et al. Exercise and acute cardiovascular events placing the risks into perspective: a scientific statement from the American Heart Association Council on Nutrition, Physical Activity, and Metabolism and the Council on Clinical Cardiology. Circulation. 2007; 115(17):2358–68.
59. Ignarro LJ, Balestrieri ML, Napoli C. Nutrition, physical activity, and cardiovascular disease: an update. Cardiovasc Res. 2007;73(2):326–40.
60. Kavanagh T, Mertens DJ, Hamm LF, Beyene J, Kennedy J, Corey P, et al. Peak oxygen intake and cardiac mortality in women referred for cardiac rehabilitation. J Am Coll Cardiol. 2003;42(12):2139–43.
61. Mark DB, Lauer MS. Exercise capacity: the prognostic variable that doesn't get enough respect. Circulation. 2003;108(13):1534–6.
62. Myers J, Prakash M, Froelicher V, Do D, Partington S, Atwood JE. Exercise capacity and mortality among men referred for exercise testing. N Engl J Med. 2002;346(11):793–801.
63. Smart N, Marwick TH. Exercise training for patients with heart failure: a systematic review of factors that improve mortality and morbidity. Am J Med. 2004;116(10):693–706.
64. Wang JS. Exercise prescription and thrombogenesis. J Biomed Sci. 2006;13(6):753–61.
65. Thijssen DH, Maiorana AJ, O'Driscoll G, Cable NT, Hopman MT, Green DJ. Impact of inactivity and exercise on the vasculature in humans. Eur J Appl Physiol. 2010;108(5):845–75.
66. Thomson CA, Giuliano A, Rock CL, Ritenbaugh CK, Flatt SW, Faerber S, et al. Measuring dietary change in a diet intervention trial: comparing food frequency questionnaire and dietary recalls. Am J Epidemiol. 2003;157(8):754–62.
67. Gordon JB, Ganz P, Nabel EG, Fish RD, Zebede J, Mudge GH, et al. Atherosclerosis influences the vasomotor response of epicardial coronary arteries to exercise. J Clin Invest. 1989;83(6):1946–52.
68. Thompson PD. The cardiovascular risks of exercise. In: Thompson PD, editor. Exercise and sports cardiology. New York, NY: McGraw-Hill; 2001.
69. Black A, Black MM, Gensini G. Exertion and acute coronary artery injury. Angiology. 1975;26(11):759–83.
70. Wang JS, Liao CH. Moderate-intensity exercise suppresses platelet activation and polymorphonuclear leukocyte interaction with surface-adherent platelets under shear flow in men. Thromb Haemost. 2004;91(3):587–94.
71. Schmidt R, Fazekas F, Hayn M, Schmidt H, Kapeller P, Roob G, et al. Risk factors for microangiopathy-related cerebral damage in the Austrian stroke prevention study. J Neurol Sci. 1997;152(1):15–21.
72. Carroll S, Cooke CB, Butterly RJ. Metabolic clustering, physical activity and fitness in nonsmoking, middle-aged men. Med Sci Sports Exerc. 2000;32(12):2079–86.
73. Ekelund U, Brage S, Franks PW, Hennings S, Emms S, Wareham NJ. Physical activity energy expenditure predicts progression toward the metabolic syndrome independently of aerobic fitness in middle-aged healthy Caucasians: the Medical Research Council Ely Study. Diabetes Care. 2005;28(5):1195–200.
74. Franks PW, Ekelund U, Brage S, Wong MY, Wareham NJ. Does the association of habitual physical activity with the metabolic syndrome differ by level of cardiorespiratory fitness? Diabetes Care. 2004;27(5):1187–93.
75. Laaksonen DE, Lakka HM, Lynch J, Lakka TA, Niskanen L, Rauramaa R, et al. Cardiorespiratory fitness and vigorous leisure-time physical activity modify the association of small size at birth with the metabolic syndrome. Diabetes Care. 2003;26(7):2156–64.
76. Rennie KL, McCarthy N, Yazdgerdi S, Marmot M, Brunner E. Association of the metabolic syndrome with both vigorous and moderate physical activity. Int J Epidemiol. 2003;32(4):600–6.
77. Laaksonen DE, Lakka HM, Salonen JT, Niskanen LK, Rauramaa R, Lakka TA. Low levels of leisure-time physical activity and cardiorespiratory fitness predict development of the metabolic syndrome. Diabetes Care. 2002;25:1612–8.
78. Holloszy JO. Exercise-induced increase in muscle insulin sensitivity. J Appl Physiol (1985). 2005;99(1):338–43.

79. Richter EA. Glucose utilization. In: Rowell LB, Shepherd JT, editors. Handbook of physiology. Section 12. New York: Oxford University Press; 1996.
80. Wojtaszewski JF, Hansen BF, Gade KB, Markuns JF, Goodyear LJ, et al. Insulin signaling and insulin sensitivity after exercise in human skeletal muscle. Diabetes. 2000;49(3):325–31.
81. Healy GN, Wijndaele K, Dunstan DW, Shaw JE, Salmon J, Zimmet PZ, et al. Objectively measured sedentary time, physical activity, and metabolic risk: the Australian Diabetes, Obesity and Lifestyle Study (AusDiab). Diabetes Care. 2008;31(2):369–71.
82. Balkau B, Mhamdi L, Oppert JM, Nolan J, Golay A, Porcellati F, et al. Physical activity and insulin sensitivity: the RISC study. Diabetes. 2008;57(10):2613–8.
83. O'Gorman DJ, Karlsson HK, McQuaid S, Yousif O, Rahman Y, Gasparro D, et al. Exercise training increases insulin-stimulated glucose disposal and GLUT4 (SLC2A4) protein content in patients with type 2 diabetes. Diabetologia. 2006;49(12):2983–92.
84. Hansen PA, Nolte LA, Chen MM, Holloszy JO. Increased GLUT-4 translocation mediates enhanced insulin sensitivity of muscle glucose transport after exercise. J Appl Physiol (1985). 1998;85(4):1218–22.
85. Larance M, Ramm G, Stockli J, van Dam EM, Winata S, Wasinger V, et al. Characterization of the role of the Rab GTPase-activating protein AS160 in insulin-regulated GLUT4 trafficking. J Biol Chem. 2005;280(45): 37803–13.
86. Miinea CP, Sano H, Kane S, Sano E, Fukuda M, Peranen J, et al. AS160, the Akt substrate regulating GLUT4 translocation, has a functional Rab GTPase-activating protein domain. Biochem J. 2005;391(Pt 1):87–93.
87. Zeigerer A, McBrayer MK, McGraw TE. Insulin stimulation of GLUT4 exocytosis, but not its inhibition of endocytosis, is dependent on RabGAP AS160. Mol Biol Cell. 2004;15(10):4406–15.
88. Joseph AM, Pilegaard H, Litvintsev A, Leick L, Hood DA. Control of gene expression and mitochondrial biogenesis in the muscular adaptation to endurance exercise. Essays Biochem. 2006;42:13–29.
89. Sriwijitkamol A, Coletta DK, Wajcberg E, Balbontin GB, Reyna SM, Barrientes J, et al. Effect of acute exercise on AMPK signaling in skeletal muscle of subjects with type 2 diabetes: a time-course and dose-response study. Diabetes. 2007;56(3):836–48.
90. Sriwijitkamol A, Ivy JL, Christ-Roberts C, DeFronzo RA, Mandarino LJ, Musi N. LKB1-AMPK signaling in muscle from obese insulin-resistant Zucker rats and effects of training. Am J Physiol Endocrinol Metab. 2006;290:E925–32.
91. Blair SN, LaMonte MJ, Nichaman MZ. The evolution of physical activity recommendations: how much is enough? Am J Clin Nutr. 2004;79(5):913S–20.
92. Davis CL, Pollock NK, Waller JL, Allison JD, Dennis BA, Bassali R, et al. Exercise dose and diabetes risk in overweight and obese children: a randomized controlled trial. JAMA. 2012;308(11):1103–12.
93. Hu FB, Stampfer MJ, Solomon CG, Liu S, Willett WC, Speizer FE, et al. The impact of diabetes mellitus on mortality from all causes and coronary heart disease in women: 20 years of follow-up. Arch Intern Med. 2001;161(14):1717–23.
94. Hu G, Lindstrom J, Valle TT, Eriksson JG, Jousilahti P, Silventoinen K, et al. Physical activity, body mass index, and risk of type 2 diabetes in patients with normal or impaired glucose regulation. Arch Intern Med. 2004;164(8):892–6.
95. Rana JS, Li TY, Manson JE, Hu FB. Adiposity compared with physical inactivity and risk of type 2 diabetes in women. Diabetes Care. 2007;30(1):53–8.
96. Shai I, Schwarzfuchs D, Henkin Y, Shahar DR, Witkow S, Greenberg I, Golan R, Fraser D, Bolotin A, Vardi H, Tangi-Rozental O, Zuk-Ramot R, Sarusi B, Brickner D, Schwartz Z, Sheiner E, Marko R, Katorza E, Thiery J, Fiedler GM, Blüher M, Stumvoll M, Stampfer MJ; Dietary Intervention Randomized Controlled Trial (DIRECT) Group. Collaborators: Weitzman S, Goldbourt U, Leitersdorf E. Weight loss with a low-carbohydrate, Mediterranean, or low-fat diet. N Engl J Med. 2008;359:229–41.
97. Rock CL, Flatt SW, Sherwood NE, Karanja N, Pakiz B, Thomson CA. Effect of a free prepared meal and incentivized weight loss program on weight loss and weight loss maintenance in obese and overweight women: a randomized controlled trial. JAMA. 2010;304:1803–10.
98. Truby H, Baic S, de Looy A, Fox KR, Livingstone MB, Logan CM, Macdonald IA, Morgan LM, Taylor MA, Millward DJ. Randomised controlled trial of four commercial weight loss programmes in the UK: initial findings from the BBC "diet trials". BMJ. 2006;332(7553):1309–14.
99. Tate DF, Wing RR, Winett RA. Using Internet technology to deliver a behavioral weight loss program. JAMA. 2001;295:1172–7.
100. Laddu D, Dow C, Hingle M, Thomson C, Going S. A review of evidence-based strategies to treat obesity in adults. Nutr Clin Pract. 2011;26(5):512–25.

Chapter 17
Biodiversity, Conviviality, and Herbs in the Mediterranean *Genius Loci*

Maria R. Dalla Francesca

Key Points

- The first objective of this chapter is to discuss the link between the need for conservation and improvement of biodiversity to protect and promote in modern era two of the key components of the Mediterranean pyramid: biodiversity and conviviality.
- Biodiversity is a characteristic of a place, intimately related to the *Genius Loci*, the spirit of the place, as it was defined by the ancient Romans. The bonds between people and the place they live in contribute to the heritage and social capital of the communities involved. This heritage influence human and dietary behavior, and extends beyond regional boundaries as people and ideas migrate to different regions of the world. In the traditional Mediterranean concept of lifestyle, conviviality, i.e., eating a meal together, goes far beyond the needs of satisfying nutrition requirements.
- Sharing meals represent a moment for socialization, which is central to celebrating the culture, environment, and biodiversity of many civilizations including those that have populated for centuries the Mediterranean basin. The second objective of this chapter is to present examples of herbs that contribute to the biodiversity and are at base of the traditional Mediterranean diet pyramid with information about their origin and use in meals, and water and herbal infusions.

Keywords Mediterranean lifestyle • Biodiversity • Conviviality • Environment • Herbs

Introduction

In the 1980s, food advocates [1, 2] launched their call for the protection of regional cultures to contrast trends towards globalization of foods choices and lifestyles. The impetus behind these "slow-food" initiatives was the idea that the introduction of food solutions void of links with the local customs and regional agriculture would be disruptive of the socioeconomic elements that

The content of the chapter was revised and edited by Drs. Donato F. Romagnolo and Ornella I. Selmin, Department of Nutritional Sciences, The University of Arizona Cancer Center, Tucson, AZ, USA.

M.R.D. Francesca, B.S. (✉)
Fattoria Didattica Altaura, Via Correr 1291, loc. Altaura, 35040 Casale di Scodosia, Padova, Italy
e-mail: dfmaria@libero.it

D.F. Romagnolo, O.I. Selmin (eds.), *Mediterranean Diet*, Nutrition and Health,
DOI 10.1007/978-3-319-27969-5_17

contributed for centuries to the evolution and prosperity of regional communities. The transition from traditional agriculture practices to a modern, more intensive, production has led in recent history to global changes in food supply challenging the use and sustainability of natural resources. One objective of modern agriculture has been to more efficiently produce food for an ever growing world population. Unfortunately, this has been paralleled by an increase in food insecurity not only in undeveloped countries but also in Western societies. More urban communities have distanced themselves from traditional agricultural practices, which as the etymology of the word suggests, derives from the Greek term "*agro*" = field and Latin "*cultura*" = taking care of. Not surprisingly, during the last three decades we have witnessed an increase in efforts that promote a more sustainable and regional agriculture, attentive to the preservation of the environment and production of foods to meet the nutrition needs of local communities [3, 4]. Modern "foraging" is perhaps the metaphor that best encourages the adoption of a more eco-friendly pattern of subsistence and better use of natural resources [5–8].

Didactic programs strive to develop farm-to-table initiatives that reduce the "distance" between agricultural production and food preparation and consumption, a phenomenon that has also been referred to as "Zero Km" food. During the last three decades these "organic" approaches have found support through a myriad of initiatives that promote marketing and consumption of locally produced foods and traditional heritage. These include regional farmer-run markets; farm-to-table events; educational garden and kitchen programs; and youth agricultural education training.

The interdependency between food agriculture and culture has been recognized throughout Mediterranean history (Fig. 17.1a, b). Examples of artistic accounts of Mediterranean foods for culture are the paintings of the seventeenth century painter Bartolomeo Bimbi. Entrusted by the Grand Duke of Tuscany, Italy Cosimo III dei Medici, painter Bimbi produced paintings representing biblical foods such as pomegranate and figs, along with pears, grapes, plums, farm animals and birds in traditional landscape settings. Another example is that of the sixteenth century Italian painter Giuseppe Arcimboldo who created human images made of various fruits, vegetables, and fish. Examples of other famous artists who recognized in their work the role of agricultural landscapes, grapes and wine include Tiziano, Picasso, Rubens, Morandi, Tiepolo, and Poussin among many others. Clearly, these examples highlight the interrelationships between agriculture, foods, and communities.

Biodiversity

Biodiversity encompasses the totality of the forms of life that compose an ecosystem and the variations within [9]. Thus, biodiversity is unique to every ecological niche and intimately related to the *Genius Loci*, or "the spirit of the place," which in ancient Roman tradition was the protective spirit of a place. It was the spiritual part of the land that originated from the peculiarity of colors (e.g., the lush green of well irrigated areas compared to the sandy-brown color found characteristic of drought regions); geography (e.g., mountain ridges compared to flat agricultural plains or coastal areas); lifestyle (e.g., intense urban settings vs moderate or laidback agricultural areas); and flavors (e.g., types and freshness of local foods and meals available to communities). The dietary vocation of the Mediterranean genius loci is therefore the result of interactions between all form of life (plants and animals) and communities that have inhabited this region for millennia. The *Genius Loci* is the cumulative inspiration deriving from images, scents, flavors, views, etc. that accompanies individuals and populations even after they physically distance themselves to recreate their original customs. The conservation of the Mediterranean *Genius Loci* should therefore be considered an important societal task among inhabitants of the Mediterranean countries in order to preserve food heritages associated with healthy eating.

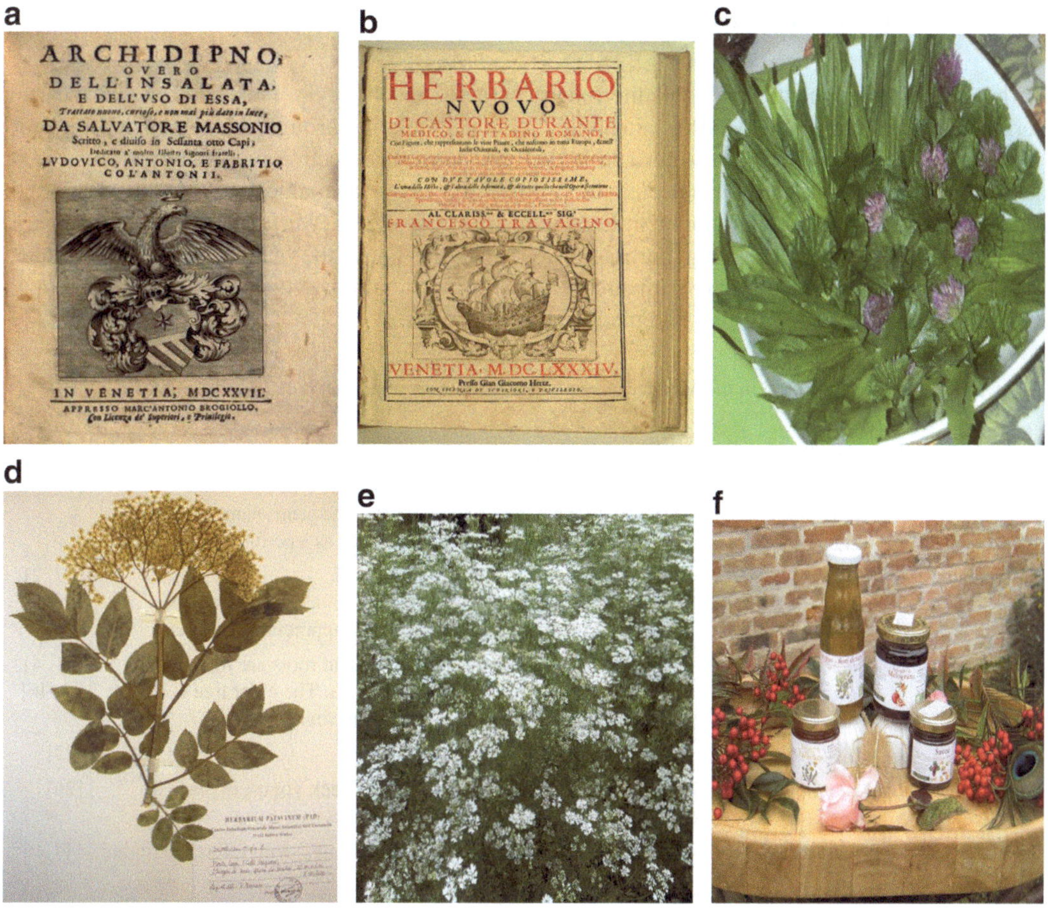

Fig. 17.1 Traditional herbs of the Mediterranean region. (**a** and **b**) Examples of seventeenth century publication about culinary use of herbs and their classification; (**c**) Green salad with common "Malva" flowers (*in purple*) (*Malva sylvestris L.*) and other green leaves; (**d**) Branch of elder tree (Sambucus nigra L.); (**e**) Coriander plants; (**f**) Fig leaf syrup, elder flower, and pomegranate syrup are examples of foods prepared using fruits and herbs that are indigenous to the Mediterranean region

Conviviality

The Mediterranean diet, declared a world heritage by UNESCO in November 2012, is an important component of a lifestyle that promotes well-being and an eco-friendly environment. In the traditional Mediterranean culture, a component of socialization is conviviality, i.e., eating a meal together not just to satisfy nutrition needs, but also to celebrate the culture, environment, and biodiversity of communities that have populated for centuries the Mediterranean basin [9–11]. Proposing, offering, and sharing of foods have been, and remain still today, very effective ways to communicate with people, while stimulating curiosity for new customs and better ways to prepare foods. In modern times, eating meals together is still a popular venue (e.g., lunch meetings, conference and town gatherings) for building and expanding a network of collective knowledge; developing new opportunities for commerce; and celebrating traditional practices that would otherwise be lost. The Mediterranean pyramid with its inclusion of conviviality is an inspirational model than can be adopted beyond the boundaries of the Mediterranean region. It provides ideas for healthy living; creates connections between people and their environment; and provides stimuli for cultural exchange.

Vernal Mediterranean Herbs

Herbs are key components of the Mediterranean pyramid and lifestyle. For centuries, home grown herbs have been part of the Mediterranean medicine and cuisine through their inclusion into food recipes or for the preparation of water and herbal infusions. This section will highlight some of the culinary and medicinal use of selected herbs that are easily available and/or cultivable in the Mediterranean region, but may not be utilized in today's way of life. We focus specifically on vernal (Latin "vernalis" = related to Spring) herbs as this season is the time of the year that in the Mediterranean region offers the richest herbal biodiversity. Table 17.1 summarizes selected herbs used in the Mediterranean region for culinary and medicinal applications.

Table 17.1 Selected herbs used in the Mediterranean region for culinary and medicinal applications

Common name	Botanical name	Properties and use	Reference
Lavender	*Lavandula angustifolia Mill.*	Flowers are used to flavor water drinks Derives its name from Latin *lavanda*. The genus name derives from the fact that it used to be added as a perfume to bath water	[17]
Lemon balm	*Melissa officinalis L.*	Flowers are used to flavor water drinks Takes its name from the Greek *melitta/melissa*, "honey bee", likely because it is a plant greatly appreciated by bees	[17, 21, 31, 33]
Elder tree	*Sambucus nigra L.*	Flowers, buds, berries, bark, leaves, and roots are for various culinary and medicinal applications. The elder tree is a plant present throughout the Mediterranean region	[21, 41, 42, 46]
Juda's tree	*Cercis siliquastrum L.*	Flowers are used in brine with capers	[23]
Borage	*Borago officinalis L.*	Flowers are used to flavor Tzatziki Greek yogurt in place of cucumber and to prepare rice dishes	[26]
Coriander	*Coriandrum sativum L.*	Derived from the Greek *koris*, "stink bug," with reference to the smelling of the plant's leaves	[47]
Common nettle	*Urtica dioica. L.*	The name is derived from the Latin *urere*, "to burn," while *dioica* derives from the Greek "two houses", indicating that male and female flowers are segregated in different plants. Leaves are used to dress cream made with ricotta cheese and with strawberry leaves. Also, used against arthritis, rheumatism, eczema, and asthma	[22]
Fig	*Ficus carica L.*	From Latin *ficus*, "fig," and *carica*, which means originating from Caria, an ancient region of Asia Minor. Figs can be consumed fresh, dried, or in jams. The leaf syrup can be used with cheese, or in herbal medicine against cough and throat aches. The "milky" latex sap that pours out from the fig is medicinal for skin diseases but can cause allergic reactions	[17, 32, 44, 48–50]
Celery	*Apium graveolens L.*	*Apium* derives from the Greek *apion*. The Latin word *graveolens* means "very scented". Celery leafs and stalks can be used to prepare soups with potatoes, lavender flowers, peas and little daisy flowers	[18, 51]
Garlic	*Garlic. Allium sativum L.*	From Latin *allium*, "garlic", which derives from a word used by the Celts. The suffix *all* in Celtic means "hot", "that burns." Commonly used in the kitchen for pasta dishes with other herbs (e.g., Laurel), and for medicinal applications	[17, 30]
Laurel	*Laurus nobilis L.*	The word is related to the Latin term *laus*, "praise", while *nobilis* means "noble". For the ancient Romans the laurel wreath, called *laurus* or *laurĕa*, symbolized victory, culture, knowledge, and power. Laurel berries are used to prepare liqueurs. It also features digestive and expectorating properties	[18, 32]

(continued)

Table 17.1 (continued)

Common name	Botanical name	Properties and use	Reference
Bermuda grass	*Cynodon dactylon* (*L.*) *Pers.*	The word *cynodon* derives from Greek *kyon*, "dog", and *odous*, "tooth". *Daktylon* is Greek for "finger", because the inflorescence is composed of five parts like the fingers of an open hand	[20, 52]
Strawberry	*Fragaria vesca L.*	*Fragaria* was used by the Roman writer Pliny the Elder (Como, 23 A.D.–Stabia, 25th August 79 A.D.) in *Naturalis Historia*, to indicate the plant. It could be derived from the Sanskrit *ghra* or the Latin *fragrans*, both referring to the fresh scent of fruits. *Vesca* derives from the Latin *vescus*, "soft" due to the softness of the fruit. Strawberry leaves are used in the kitchen to prepare herbal teas and pastries, and in herbal medicine to alleviate iron deficiencies	[17, 23]
Common hop	*Humulus lupulus L.*	Derived from Latin *humus*, "earth", with reference to the species' habitat, and *lupulus*, "small wolf", referring to the wild appearance of the plant. Used to make herbal teas	[17, 22]
Goat's beard	*Aruncus dioicus* (*W.F.*)	The term *aruncus*, derives from the Greek *aryngos*, "goat's beard", refers to its white buds which resemble the beard of a goat. Can be used to make herbal teas	[17, 22]
Butcher's broom	*Ruscus aculeatus L.*	The name *ruscus* relates to the Greek *rhynchos* meaning "beak, rostrum", *aculeatus* means "pointed"; both terms refer to the thorny branches of the plant. The young shoots can be eaten as asparagus	[17, 34, 51]
Wild asparagus	*Asparagus acutifolius L.*	The name derives from the Persian *asparag*, "bud", while *acutifolius* is a Latin term meaning "having pointed leaves". Used extensively in dishes of Mediterranean countries. A slightly bitter, diuretic, acts as painkiller against rheumatic pains	[17, 34]

Traditional Culinary Herbs, Dishes, Drinks, and Infusions

Selected herbs were selected to represent as much as possible culinary traditions of various Mediterranean countries. Because of space limitation not all relevant literature could be cited. For additional details on plant classifications, regional plants, and ecosystems we refer the reader to a number of selected publications [12–16].

Lamb's Lettuce (*Valerianella locusta* (*L.*))

This herb belongs to the genus *Valeriana*, which derives from the Latin word "*valere*" or to be strong, for its many medicinal properties [17]. The term *locusta* refers to the grasshopper that feeds on these plants. Both the common name of the species, "lamb's lettuce", and the scientific one *Valerianella*, in which the suffix *-ella* transforms *Valeriana* into its a diminutive, likely refer to the unassuming, "humble" appearance of the plant. Widely available commercially, it grows spontaneously in Mediterranean countries and is cultivated organically. There are three kinds of *Valerianella* plant with different size leaves. The cultivars available commercially have the largest leaves, while those growing spontaneously are the smallest. The smaller the leaves, the more intense are the color of the leaves and their flavor. Valerianella is used for the seasoning of egg-based dishes and vegetable soups, and it has cleansing properties [18–20].

Dandelion (Taraxacum *officinale, L., Weber ex F.H.Wigg*)

The word *Taraxacum* probably derives from the Perso-Arabic "*talkh chakok*" meaning "bitter grass", or alternatively from the Greek "*tarasso*" which means "to agitate", and therefore "the herb that can heal agitated bodies" [21]. The term "*officinale*" indicates a medicinal use, from the Latin "*officina*" meaning "laboratory". Its brined flower buds taste surprisingly similar to capers and the syrup made from the flowers is indistinguishable from dandelion honey. Its raw leaves enrich salads and can be a great cooked vegetable when sautéed with garlic. From its toasted roots, a good coffee substitute can be obtained. It has cleansing and detoxifying properties and is rich in vitamin C [20, 22].

Malva (*Malva syilvestris L.*)

The name Malva originates from the Greek word *malakhe*, meaning "emollient, benevolent", with reference to the plant's properties, while the term *sylvestris* indicates a plant growing in an uncultivated land (*from the Latin sylva*, meaning "forest"). Various parts of the plant (buds, leaves, and purple flowers) can be mixed together to prepare rice dishes and vegetable soups (Fig. 17.1c). Battering and frying of the flowers and mixing of buds in salty water are excellent to prepare tasty dishes. This plant features emollient, laxative, and anti-inflammatory properties [17, 20, 22].

Goat's Beard (*Tragopogon porrifolius L. and Tragopogon pratensis L.*)

The scientific name derives from the Greek *tragos*, "male goat" and *pogon*, "beard" with reference to its hairy seeds resembling a goat's beard. *Porrifolius* means "having the leaves of a leek" which are narrow and long, while *pratensis* means "growing in meadows", clearly connected to the species' habitat. Dried roots can be milled into flour and used to prepare breads and sweet dishes, whereas the sprouts can be used in combination with various vegetables and egg-based dishes [17, 22–24].

Borage (*Borago officinalis L.*)

The name probably derives from Latin *borra*, rough wool fabric, due to the rough feel of the plant. The blue flowers possess a cucumber-like flavor and are used fresh in vegetable salads. They possess anti-inflammatory and purifying properties. The leaves instead are dried and are served fried, or are used to prepare various handmade pasta, rice dishes, or cooked like greens [17, 22–27].

Burdock (*Arctium lappa L.*)

Derived from the Greek *arctos*, indicating the bear, *arctium* perhaps refers to the prickly appearance of the plant, while *lappa* may come from the Greek *labein*, "to hang to", because its fruits stick to clothes and for this reason are often used in children games. After boiling, stalks and roots can be served as a side dish. Various parts of the plant are also used in cosmetics or as a natural remedy against dermatitis [17, 22, 28, 29].

Peppermint (*Mentha x piperita L.*)

The genus name comes from the Greek *Míntha*, a Naiad or water nymph. *Piperita* means "with the scent of pepper" because of the strong smell and sting of this plant. Pepper in Latin is *piper*. Mint, which was nicknamed *edyosmos* ("aromatic"), was used in ancient Greece in burial rituals, along with rosemary and myrtle, to mask the odor of the decomposing body. Because of its strong scent, various parts of the plant were used as antiseptic to prepare drinking water or even as a defense against various parasites. Mint twig remains have also been found in an Egyptian tomb [17, 30–32]. This herb can be used in a variety of salads or with fresh fruits.

Judas' Tree (*Cercis siliquastrum L.*)

Derived from the Greek *kerkis*, "small boat" or "spool," and from the Latin *siliqua*, "pod", both referring to the shape of the fruit, which is similar to a small boat. The carob is called *siliqua*, and *siliquastrum* is a pejorative term indicating false carob. The tree is very common in Palestine [17, 33–35]. The flowers are edible.

Pea (*Pisum sativum L.*)

The word *pisum* is Latin for pea, while *sativum* means "edible". Raw peas are consumed regularly in Middle East countries facing the Mediterranean Sea such as Lebanon. Historic accounts document that even the Doge (Chief in command of the Venetian Republic) ate rice and peas-based dishes (*risi e bisi*) on Ascension Day (June 2nd) and on April 25th, St. Mark's day, Patron Saint of Venice. The same rice and peas dishes were consumed to celebrate the arrival of Spring [24, 25, 30, 36–40].

Primrose (*Primula vulgaris Huds*)

The genus name *Primula* is a variant of *primus* meaning "first" in Latin and indicates the precociousness of its blooming at the end of winter, beginning of spring. It is used in soups and baking of sweets [17, 23].

Chickweed (*Stellaria media, L. Vill.*)

The Latin genus name refers to its star-shaped flowers, while the term *media* means "of average size." This plant grows throughout cold winters until spring suggesting it possesses unique features of freezing tolerance. Its leaves are extremely delicate like those of vegetables grown in a greenhouse. On the other hand, once picked, it degrades much more quickly than many other vegetables [17, 20]. It is used to make salads and water infusions.

Garden Sorrel (*Rumex acetosa L.*)

The name comes from the Latin *rumex*, meaning "beam" or "spear", referring to its pointed leaves. The term *acetosa* means "acidic", with reference to the taste of the leaves, which are used in vegetables soups or mixed with fried eggs, or for thirst quenching. It has diuretic, refreshing, and anti-inflammatory properties. It can be used to prepare salads with extra virgin olive oil and salt. Due to its inherent acidity, this herb can be used in place of vinegar to prepare salads [17, 20, 35].

Sorrel (*Oxalis acetosella L.*)

It derives its name from the Greek *oxys*, "sharp", "stinging", and *hals*, "salt", due to the presence of oxalic acid, while *acetosella* is a diminutive of *acetosa*, indicating the plant acidic taste and its small size.

The leaves are used to prepare water infusions, and sweet and fruit dishes that possess detoxifying benefits. In kitchen demonstrations, the juice of oxalis can be used for pH litmus tests in place of other acidic solutions (e.g., lemon juice) along with the juice of a purple cabbage (*Brassica oleracea* L. cultivar *capitata*). The oxalis juice will turn the color of the cabbage juice from purple to pink. Then, the addition of the common oat's grass blades (*Avena sativa* L.) in place of sodium bicarbonate (a base) would turn the pink color into green [17, 18, 20, 22–24, 40].

The Elder Tree (*Sambucus nigra L.*)

The elder tree (*Sambucus nigra L.*) is also called "gypsies grapes" due to its similarity to small grape bunches (Fig. 17.1d). The Latin term, *sambucus* originates from the Greek *sambukè* [21], which is a musical instrument [41, 42]. This tree was considered sacred by the Greeks, who called it *actéa*, from Sanskrit *açnati* = nourishment. Its flowers are used to make syrups for the treatment of cough and flu symptoms; its black, glossy berries are also used to prepare excellent syrups, wines, and delicious jams. Neuralgia-soothing herbal tea can be made from its buds while the leaves can be used for dermatological applications. Also, a syrup can be made from its berries to treat airway inflammation. The bark of the elder tree has been shown to alleviate glaucoma symptoms whereas the roots exert anti-gout effects. The marrow, mixed with honey and flour, is used to soothe the pain of dislocations [17, 43].

Coriander (*Coriandrum sativum L.*)

The leaves of coriander are used throughout the Mediterranean region to prepare vegetable soups, seasoning of salad and meat dishes; and are served in combination with soft bread and ricotta cheese (Fig. 17.1e). The seeds are used to flavor many dishes and to prepare alcoholic drinks. In the sixteenth century during the Carnival festivities coriander seeds were sugar glazed, and it is for this reason that the name remained in the Italian vocabulary indicating multicolored sweets, *coriandoli*. The coriander was among the herbs offered by Egyptian kings in temples, and seeds have been found in Tutankhamun's tomb [17, 30].

Fennel (*Foeniculum vulgare Mill.*)

Foeniculum is Latin for "small hay" [33], with reference to the hay-resembling smell. The Greek name for fennel is *marathon* [21]. The name of the town Marathon, linked to the memory of the famous battle in which the Athenians defeated the Persians in 490 B.C., derives indeed from the fact that a lot of fennel grows in the area. The Roman writer Pliny the Elder, recommended fennel as a sexual stimulant. In the Medieval Ages, the crafty Venetians used to give their wine buyers some fennel to eat so as to confuse their palates; a cunning method to make them unable to distinguish a lower quality wine from the high quality one they were paying for. In Venetian regional dialect the verb "*infinocchiare*", is used to suggest "to fennel", meaning "to swindle". Fennel leaves and seeds are used extensively in Mediterranean countries to flavor salads, egg and meats dishes, and pastries.

Grapevine (*Vitis vinifera L.*)

The word *vitis* is Latin for *vitis* which derives from the Indo-European word *viere* meaning "to curve", "to weave". In Cattabiani's *Florario*, the grapevine is listed among the cosmic trees due to the fact that, since Sumerian time, wine was related to youth and eternal life, so the vine was the plant of life and immortality. Stuffed vine leave recipes with rice and cheese are used extensively in some Mediterranean countries including Lebanon and Greece among others [32, 44, 45].

Cherry Tree (*Prunus avium L.*)

The term *avium* in Latin means "of birds". This is due to the fact that birds often eat cherries [33]. Cherry blossoms are used to prepare desserts of "panna cotta", a pudding made with milk, honey, corn starch, and topped with dandelion flowers or fig leaves syrup.

Various Flowers and Leaves Can Be Used to Prepare Desserts

For example, ice creams can be flavored with elder flowers, mint or lemon balm leaves; biscuits with lavender flowers or lemon balm leaves; chocolate with lavender flowers or mint leaves; and gastronomy accompaniment crunchy bite-size desserts made with hazelnuts, honey, and dried rose petals; and syrups can be prepared using fig leafs, elder flower, and pomegranate (Fig. 17.1f).

Damask Rose (*Rosa x damascene Herrm*)

The Latin word *damascena*, means "coming from Damascus," a town in Syria. This species is spread throughout the Middle East and Europe. It has very strongly scented petals that are edible and can be used also in herbal teas.

Conclusions

Food biodiversity and conviviality represent important aspects of the Mediterranean pyramid. Herbs are at the base of the traditional Mediterranean diet, and agricultural and medicinal practices. These qualitative and lifestyle elements have contributed for centuries to the health and socioeconomic well-being, and culture of residents of Mediterranean countries [53]. They may offer a platform for improving the way of life in other communities and countries. To this end, more didactic and farm-to-table programs are needed to restore and preserve the richness of regional agriculture and cuisines that promote the production of traditional foods and ingredients for socioeconomic sustainability and healthy living.

Acknowledgements The author wishes to thank Mauro Bregolin and Karly J. Ahrens for assistance with translation; Luca Tosetto for botanical information; Jenny Gkiougki for help with editing, proofing, and Greek etymology; Serafina Contin for sharing her herbal experience; and Maria Gennusa for culinary assistance.

References

1. Petrini C. Slow food: the case for taste. New York: Columbia University Press; 2003.
2. The Slow Food Dictionary to Regional Italian Cooking. Slow Food Editore, 2011.
3. Howard A. I diritti della Terra. Bra: Slow Food Editore; 2005. p. 25–40.
4. Fukuoka M. La fattoria biologica. Roma: Edizioni Mediterranee; 2001.
5. Mabey R. Food for free. New York: Collins; 2012.

6. Irwing M. The Forager handbook. London: Ebury Press; 2009.
7. Bird F. The Forager's kitchen. London: CICO Books; 2013.
8. Lewis-Stempel J. Foraging, the essential guide to free wild food. Tadworth: Right Way; 2012.
9. Levin SA. Encyclopedia of biodiversity. New York: Academic; 2007.
10. Gepts PL, Famula TR, Bettinger RL. Biodiversity in agriculture. Cambridge: Cambridge University Press; 2012.
11. Shiva V. Tomorrow's biodiversity. London: Thames & Hudson Ltd; 2000.
12. Viggiani P. Erbe spontanee e infestanti: tecniche di riconoscimento-dicotiledoni. Bologna: Edizioni Agricole; 1998.
13. Todaro A, Brentan M, Marcucci R, Villani M, Biasiolo M, Tornadore N. Libro Rosso dei Colli Euganei. Este: Parco Regionale dei Colli Euganei; 2002.
14. Pignatti S. La flora d'Italia. Bologna: Edagricole; 1982.
15. The Plant list (2013). Version1.1. Available at http://www.theplantlist.org/. Accessed 16 Dec 2014.
16. Pauli G. Blue economy, 10 anni, 100 innovazioni, 100 milioni di posti di lavoro. Milano: Edizioni Ambiente; 2010.
17. Forum Acta Plantarum, from 2007 on - Forum for the sharing of Italian spontaneous flora information. Available at http://www.actaplantarum.org/floraitaliae/. Accessed 16 Dec 2014.
18. Azzolini B. Insalate curative e aromatiche. Trento: G. B. Monauni Editore; 1976.
19. Scudelotti C, Stoppele M, Toffaletti L. Erbe, erbette e dolci frutti di campi e boschi. San Giovanni Lupatoto: Mulino Don Chisciotte, Arsenale Editore; 2012.
20. Vaglio M. Erbe delle valli alpine, alla scoperta di 260 piante commestibili. Scarmagno: Priuli e Verlucca; 2014.
21. Carlo Schenkl, Francesco Ambrosoli, Vocabolario Greco-Italiano edizione XIII, Torino, 1894.
22. Luciano R, Gatti C, Colombo ML. Erbe spontanee commestibili. Boves: Araba Fenice; 2008.
23. Gamacchio RC. Riconoscimento e uso delle piante selvatiche. Colognola ai Colli: Demetra; 1995.
24. Massonio S. *Archidipno, overo dell'insalata, e dell'uso di essa.* appresso Marc'Antonio Brogiollo, in Venetia 1627.
25. Rizzo G. Catechismo agricolo ad uso dei contadini. Padova: Società Cooperativa Tipografica; 2003.
26. Valavanis A, Depollas Y. La cucina greca. Athina: Fotorama; 1999.
27. Fidi A. Erbe e piante medicinali. Torino: Edizioni Polaris; 1993.
28. Mabey R. Elogio delle erbacce. Milano: Saggi Ponte alle Grazie; 2011.
29. F. Coccolo, F. Vuono, Guida pratica al pronto soccorso naturale, Riza, 2007.
30. Manniche L. An ancient Egyptian herbal. London: British Museum Publications Limited; 1989.
31. Spolaore L. Tisane delle erbe officinali. Urbana: F.lli Corradin Editore; 2007.
32. Cattabiani A. Florario. Milano: Mondadori Eds; 1997.
33. Durando C. Lexicon Latina-Italicum. Torino: Tipografia e Libreria Salesiana; 1913.
34. Mazzetti A. La flora dei Colli Euganei. Padova: Editoriale Programma; 1987.
35. Castore Durante, Herbario nuovo, presso Gio. Giacomo Hertz, in Venetia 1667.
36. Da Mosto R. Il Veneto in cucina. Firenze: Giunti Martello; 1985.
37. Tamari, La cucina veneta, MP Edizioni, 2001.
38. Toffaletti L, Brunoro G. Il quaderno delle ricette di Padova. San Giovanni Lupatoto: Ecolibri; 2009.
39. Maffioli G. Cucina padovana. Padova: Franco Muzzio Editore; 2002.
40. Jones M. Fiori selvatici. Lainate: Vallardi I. G.; 1995.
41. Psilakis N. Herbs in coking. Greece: Karmanor; 2003.
42. Scolari P. Tenere erbe e dolci frutti dei campi. Sommacampagna: La casa verde; 1989.
43. Ferrari V, Ghezzi D. Le siepi in campagna. Bologna: Edagricole; 1999.
44. Cattabiani A. Erbario. Milano: Rusconi Libri; 1994.
45. Sebesta G. Il lavoro dell'uomo nel ciclo dei Mesi di Torre Aquila. Trento: Provincia Autonoma di Trento; 1996.
46. Routh S. Note di cucina di Leonardo da Vinci. Roma: Finestre Voland; 2005.
47. Forti C. Parte Quinta, La coltivazione degli ortaggi. In: Alpe V, Zecchini M, Soave M, Voglin P, editors. Nuova Enciclopedia Agraria Italiana. Torino: Società Tipografica Torinese; 1929.
48. von Peschke HP, Feldmann W. La cucina del Rinascimento. Milano: Guido Tommasi Editore; 2002.
49. Impelluso L. La natura e i suoi simboli. Milano: Electa; 2003.
50. Brosse J. Mitologia degli alberi. Milano: Bur; 2006.
51. Da Broi F. Il prato è servito-le erbe spontanee in cucina. Cison di Valmarino: Francesco Da Broi Edizioni Multimediali; 2005.
52. Rovesti P, Boni U, Patri G, Bartolomelli A. Scoprire riconoscere usare le erbe. Milano: Fabbri Editori; 1978.
53. Durando C. Lexicon Latino-Italicum. Torino: Tipografia salesiana; 1913.

Chapter 18
Food-Based Approaches for Achieving Nutritional Adequacy with the Mediterranean, DASH, and USDA Food Patterns

Michelle A. Briggs, Jennifer A. Fleming, and Penny M. Kris-Etherton

Key Points

- Inadequacies and overconsumption of various foods/nutrients in the average American diet impact the development of chronic diseases such as heart disease, diabetes, and cancer. In this chapter, we compare and contrast several healthy eating patterns including the Dietary Approaches to Stop Hypertension dietary pattern (DASH), the US Department of Agriculture food pattern (USDAFP), and the Mediterranean dietary pattern (MDP).
- Review of the evidence demonstrates that healthy eating patterns decrease the risk of chronic diseases. We also examine the nutrients of concern in the average American diet (calcium, fiber, potassium, and vitamin D as well as magnesium), their role in chronic disease, and how different healthful eating patterns can prevent nutrient inadequacies.
- Finally, we discuss how emphasizing individual foods and food groups that are recommended in the MDP, the USDAFP, and the DASH dietary pattern can be used to achieve nutrient adequacy and prevent chronic diseases.

Keywords Mediterranean dietary pattern • DASH dietary pattern • USDA food pattern • Fruit and vegetable consumption • n-3 fatty acids • Chronic disease prevention • Average American/Western diet • Achieving nutrient adequacy

Introduction

Good nutrition practices are central to all lifestyle recommendations that promote health. We have a good understanding of the nutrients necessary to achieve nutritional adequacy and prevent nutrient deficiency diseases. In addition, we understand the role that nutrients, foods, and dietary patterns play

M.A. Briggs, Ph.D., M.S. (✉)
Department of Biology, Lycoming College, 700 College Place, Williamsport, PA 17701, USA
e-mail: briggs@lycoming.edu

J.A. Fleming, M.S., R.D. • P.M. Kris-Etherton, Ph.D., R.D.
Department of Nutritional Sciences, The Pennsylvania State University,
110 Chandlee Lab, University Park, PA 16802, USA
e-mail: jas58@psu.edu; pmk3@psu.edu

D.F. Romagnolo, O.I. Selmin (eds.), *Mediterranean Diet*, Nutrition and Health,
DOI 10.1007/978-3-319-27969-5_18

in preventing and treating chronic diseases. However, the remarkable progress that has been made in evolving our dietary recommendations (for both nutrients and food-based dietary patterns) has not been coupled to public health benefits, as illustrated by the epidemic of many chronic, yet preventable diseases. Poor nutrition practices are the underlying problem for many nutrition-related chronic diseases. This chapter presents an overview of the health benefits of three recommended dietary patterns, specifically the Dietary Approaches to Stop Hypertension dietary pattern (DASH), the US Department of Agriculture food pattern (USDAFP), and the Mediterranean dietary pattern (MDP). In addition, the short falls (both for nutrients and foods) of the average American diet are discussed. This chapter is a "call to action" to health care professionals and all relevant stakeholders to identify new and innovative strategies for implementing healthier dietary practices to reduce chronic disease risk.

Food-Based Healthy Eating Patterns

Many studies have evaluated how a single nutrient affects health outcomes, e.g., the effect of saturated fat on coronary heart disease (CHD) risk. Interventions that focus on altering just one dietary factor often ignore how the resulting changes in other dietary constituents impact health. For example, only recommending a reduction in saturated fat does not take into consideration what the replacement nutrient is and how different macronutrient substitutions affect CHD. The significance of dietary and lifestyle patterns on health was recognized in the 1960s by Ancel Keys [1]. In the Seven Countries Study, populations from different countries in the Mediterranean region had a lower risk of CHD and stroke than Finland and the USA. There are many countries in the Mediterranean region, each with its own culture, agriculture, and native cuisine. Thus, there are significant differences in food patterns and associated effects on health in these countries. Historically, the island of Crete had the lowest death rates of the region [2]. Generalities of the traditional Crete diet include high olive and olive oil intake; consuming 30 times more fish than people in the USA; vegetables including wild plants such as Purslane, a plant high in n-3 fatty acids; cereals that are unrefined and typically consumed as sourdough bread; fruits, nuts, and legumes (pulses); and moderate amounts of wine. In addition, during Lent, consumption of snails is popular. Interestingly, the n-3 fatty acid content in Greek snails is higher than that of snails found in France. Meat and dairy products come from grass-fed animals that typically are somewhat higher in n-3 fatty acids than grain-fed animals [2]. Egg yolks from Greek-raised free range chickens contain greater amounts of n-3 fatty acids because chickens consume leafy green vegetation, fresh and dried fruits, seeds, insects and occasional worms as they forage [3]. Despite regional differences, traditional cuisines in the Mediterranean region use olive oil as a major fat source [4].

Because the Mediterranean region encompasses a wide geographic area with varied local cuisines, and because globalization is impacting dietary patterns [5] nutrient inadequacies vary among regions and within countries. In the regions where it originated, the MDP has been progressively abandoned (data from 1960 to ~2000) [6]. During this period, a predominant dietary change was an increase in meat consumption by a factor of at least four in Greece, Italy, and Spain [7].

As an example of how dietary changes impact nutrient intake, Castro-Quezada et al. [8] reported that calcium intake, for example, was generally adequate for MDP followers in Spain, Portugal, and Italy. Serra-Majem et al. [9] followed university graduates in Spain (Seguimiento Universidad de Navarra cohort, SUN) and found adequate calcium intake both in those following a traditional MDP and in those following a more Western diet. This study highlighted a possible correlation between higher education and better dietary profiles [10]. However, due to eating a more Westernized diet, adults in the general population currently living in Mediterranean countries often fall short in some nutrient intakes compared to those recommended by the traditional MDP [11]. For example, for calcium intake, data from the European Nutrition and Health Report II indicate that ~44 % of Spanish adults 19–64 years of age fall below the estimated average requirement (EAR). The percentage of adults whose calcium intake falls below the EAR is ~37 % in Greece, ~31 % in Italy, and ~34 % in Portugal. Calcium is one example of the many nutrients that currently are consumed below dietary recommendations, not only in the Mediterranean region but also in other countries. Thus, the objective of this chapter is to discuss how nutrient adequacy for specific nutrients can be achieved by emphasizing consumption of individual foods and food groups that are recommended in the MDP and other healthy eating patterns.

Every 5 years, the USDA and the Department of Health and Human Services issue Dietary Guidelines for Americans (DGA) to provide up-to-date nutrition guidance for population-wide health promotion and disease prevention. The most recent DGA (2010) [12] recommended the DASH, the USDAFP, and the MDP. These dietary patterns have many similarities, including their focus on increasing consumption of plant-based foods and lean proteins while decreasing consumption of refined grains, added sugars, solid fat, saturated fat, trans-fats, and excess alcohol (Fig. 18.1, from Richter et al.) [13]. Importantly, these dietary patterns also have some subtle differences. DASH and USDAFP both emphasize a reduction in dietary sodium but do not emphasize fatty fish consumption. The MDP differs from the DASH and USDAFP by encouraging consumption of extra virgin olive oil (EVOO) and fatty fish, but does not focus on reducing sodium. All three diets differ in the percent of calories from fat, with the MDP allowing the highest fat calories [13].

Evidence supports the effectiveness of these dietary patterns for the prevention of many chronic diseases. Reedy et al. [14] examined the relationships between diet and either all-cause mortality, cardiovascular disease (CVD) or cancer mortality using data from the NIH-AARP Diet and Health Study. More than 424,000 subjects were scored based on adherence to the Healthy Eating Index—2010, an Americanized version of the MDP (aMED), and DASH. All dietary patterns lowered the risk of chronic disease-related mortality, demonstrating the health benefits of different dietary patterns that share core nutritional values. Similarly, Djousse et al. [15] compared the average American diet to the DASH or MDP for more than 19,000 male physicians in the 1997 Physicians Health Study.

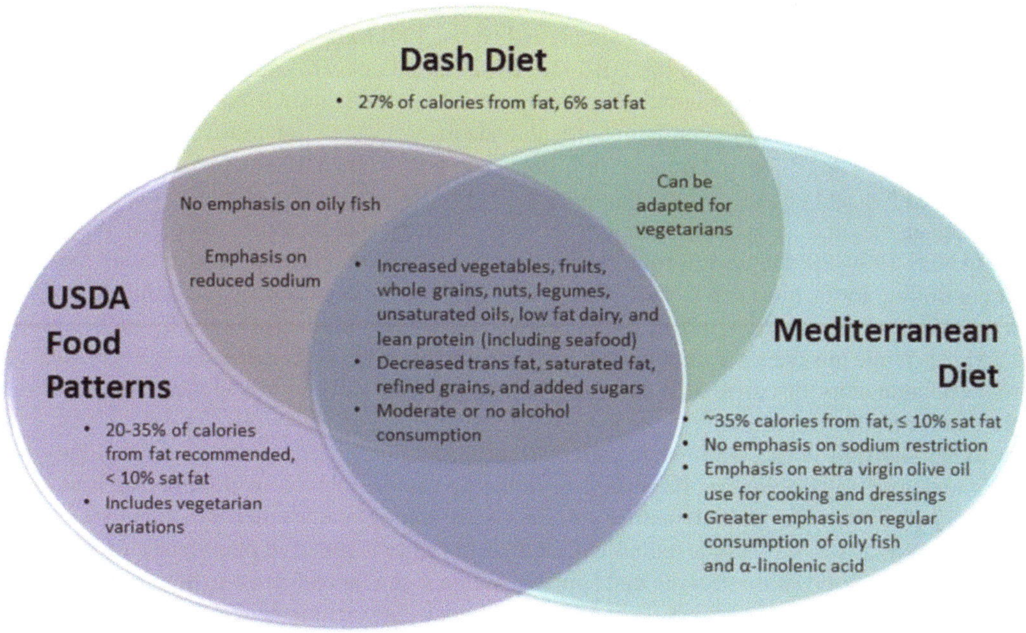

Fig. 18.1 Similarities and unique features of the DASH, USDAFP and MDP

They found both dietary patterns lowered risk of death compared to those not following these healthy eating plans. Specifically, for every doubling of the MED score in their study, the adjusted hazard ratio (HR) for total mortality was 0.81 (95 % CI: 0.77–0.86), and for the DASH score, the HR was equal to 0.81 (95 % CI: 0.71–0.93).

There are other benefits of these healthy eating plans. For example, adherence to the USDAFP, DASH, or MDP also reduced the risk of colorectal cancer [16]. Greater adherence to the MDP as measured by the MedDiet scoring system has also been shown to reduce the rate of cognitive decline in some studies of the elderly [17, 18]; the DASH dietary pattern also has been shown to protect against cognitive decline [19]. Adherence to the MDP also reduces cardio-diabesity, a term describing the relationship among disorders including type 2 diabetes, obesity, metabolic syndrome, and CVD. In a review of epidemiological studies (14 studies related to obesity, 10 to CVD, 9 to metabolic syndrome, and 4 to type 2 diabetes), 33 out of 37 studies showed a strong association between adherence to the MDP and reduced cardio-diabesity risk [20].

The Typical American Dietary Pattern

Many government agencies, health organizations, and individual scientists are voicing concern about the global adoption of the Western/American diet. This is problematic because the typical American diet is associated with many chronic diseases such as diabetes, and obesity/overweight among others that not only decrease lifespan but adversely affect quality of life and greatly impact medical costs. In the USA alone, economic costs attributable to diet-caused cancer, stroke, and diabetes approached ~$71 billion in 1994 [21]. In 2010, the medical cost in the USA related to obesity alone was estimated at $315.8 billion [22]. The typical American diet has many nutrient inadequacies and excesses (including energy intake) that create health problems for consumers. In terms of food-based recommendations, the typical American diet falls short in vegetables, fruits, whole grains, legumes, nuts and seeds, lean meats, low-fat dairy, and seafood [23]. Correcting these imbalances would result in a dietary pattern that is similar to the MDP. However, the MDP in the 1960s provided low to moderate amounts of dairy products typically consumed as yogurt and cheese [24] (most likely full-fat cheese).

At the individual nutrient level, the 2010 DGA [12] raised concerns about inadequate intakes of potassium, fiber, calcium and vitamin D in the typical American diet. Of the nutrients assessed in NHANES 2003–2006, the most common nutrient inadequacies were vitamin B6 (10.5 % of the population), vitamin D (8.1 % of the population), iron (9.5 % of women 12–49 years old and 6.7 % of children aged five and younger), and vitamin C (6 % of the population 6 years and older) [25].

Inadequate magnesium is another dietary shortfall of the typical American diet [26]. An analysis of NHANES 1999–2000 data for adults who were not taking magnesium supplements indicated, after controlling for factors such as age, body mass index (BMI), and exercise, that adults consuming less than the magnesium RDA were 1.5 to 1.8 times more likely to have elevated C-reactive protein (CRP) [27]. While this does not imply causation, the correlation between increased levels of CRP and chronic inflammatory diseases such as CHD [28] suggest that consuming adequate magnesium is important for health promotion.

Another shortfall in the US dietary pattern is an inadequate seafood /omega-3 (n-3) fatty acid intake. Omega-3 fatty acids are important in reducing the prevalence of diseases such as CHD, diabetes, kidney disease, and Alzheimer's disease [29] among many other inflammatory diseases [30]. Omega-3 fatty acids include α-linolenic acid (ALA) that is found in plant-based foods such as canola oil, flaxseed oil, walnuts, kale and spinach. While it can be converted to the longer chain n-3 fatty acids eicosapentaenoic acid (EPA) and possibly docosahexaenoic acid (DHA), the conversion is very inefficient, and thus ALA does not provide the same health benefits as EPA and DHA [31]. Recommendations for n-3 fatty acids range between 250 mg/day [12] and 500 mg/day [32].

Currently, there is no dietary reference intake (DRI) for EPA and DHA [33], although the Institute of Medicine recommends that up to 10 % of the Acceptable Macronutrient Distribution Range (AMDR) for n-3 intake can be provided by EPA/DHA [34]. The intake of total n-3 fatty acids in the USA is approximately 1.6 g/day, but Americans only consume about 100 mg/day of EPA and DHA (NHANES 2011–2012 data) [35]; this indicates Americans are consuming less than 50 % of recently recommended amounts of EPA and DHA (250–500 mg/day). This corresponds to consuming about 1 serving/week of seafood, whereas 2 servings/week are recommended by the 2010 DGA [12].

The typical American diet is high in nutrients as well as foods that increase the risk of chronic diseases [12]. High sodium intake is associated with high blood pressure and CVD [36]. The 2010 DGA [12] recommends a sodium intake of less than 2300 mg/day for most Americans, but suggests an intake of 1500 mg/day for: persons over 51 years of age; African Americans of any age; and any person who has hypertension, diabetes, or chronic kidney disease. The current adequate intake (AI) for sodium is also 1500 mg/day [37]. Current sodium intake for adults is ~3400 mg/day [12], an amount more than twice the AI and approximately 150 % of the maximum recommended intake. Marked sodium reduction can be challenging for many to achieve in the USA because sodium is present in so many foods; more than 70 % of the sodium in the American diet is derived from processed foods [38] and foods eaten away from home [39].

The American diet also exceeds the 2010 DGA [12] recommendation for saturated fat (SFA, typically solid at room temperature). The 2010 DGA [12] recommends consuming less than 10 % of energy intake from SFA. For a 2000 kcal diet, this means fewer than 200 kcal (or fewer than 22 g) of SFA. What nutrients replace these 200 kcal can have a major impact on health. The 2010 DGA [12] recommends replacing SFA with monounsaturated (MUFA) and/or polyunsaturated fatty acids (PUFA). There is strong evidence that CHD risk decreases when SFA are replaced with PUFA; estimates indicate that replacing 1 % of energy present as SFA in a Western (American) diet with PUFA lowers low density lipoprotein (LDL) cholesterol, and will most likely result in a 2–3 % reduction in CHD [40]. Nuts, popular in the MDP, are typically high in MUFA; MUFA consumption, when substituted for SFA, improves blood lipid/lipoprotein profiles and insulin sensitivity [41].

In addition to high levels of SFA, the typical American diet is also high in added sugars and refined grains. The recommended limits for combined solid fat and added sugar (SoFAS) in a 2000 kcal diet is 258 kcal, or 13 % of the energy intake [12]; for a 2400 kcal daily intake, the recommended limit is 330 kcal, or 14 % of the daily intake. While recommended maximum percentages change slightly with caloric intake, daily caloric intakes less than 3000 kcal advocate a maximum of 14 % of kcal from SoFAS. An examination of food sources and their contribution to total energy intake (from NHANES 2005 to 2006), and their energy derived from SoFAS (from NHANES 2003 to 2004) for individuals 2–18 years of age indicated almost 40 % of kcal in a 2000 kcal/day diet were either from solid fats (433 kcal) or added sugars (365 kcal) [42]. The top three foods for this age group were grain-based desserts (138 kcal/day), pizza (136 kcal/day), and sodas (118 kcal/day). Foods contributing the most solid fats included: pizza (50 kcal/day), grain-based desserts (43 kcal/day), whole milk (35 kcal/day), regular cheese (34 kcal/day), and fatty meats (29 kcal/day). Foods contributing the most in added sugars included: soda (116 kcal/day), fruit drinks (55 kcal/day), grain-based desserts (40 kcal/day), dairy-based desserts (29 kcal/day), and candy (25 kcal/day) [42]. Although SoFAS consumption decreased among US children and adolescents between 1994 and 1998 and between 2009 and 2010, mean intakes still exceeded recommended energy intake limits by 18–28 % [43]. The 40 % SoFAS intake noted above [42] most likely resulted in multiple nutrient inadequacies, overweight, or both since the SoFAS calories replaced foods higher in protein, vitamins, minerals, and other essential nutrients.

The 2010 DGA [12] recommends that at least half of all grain products consumed should be whole grains, or that, for a 2000 kcal diet, the intake of refined (enriched) grains is ~ 85 g (3 oz) or less. Refined grains are those where the grain's bran and germ (embryo) are removed during processing [44]. Studies on the health consequences of whole grains and refined grains are mixed. A recent review of

135 studies published between 2000 and 2010 indicates the majority of studies reported no association between the intake of refined grains and CVD, diabetes, weight gain, or overall mortality [45]. Whenever possible, Williams [45] focused on those studies reporting the core-refined grain foods, not grain-based foods with large amounts of SoFAS or sodium such as cakes, cookies, and pizza. Other reviews have reported that consuming whole grains protects against cancer, CVD, diabetes, and obesity [44], while refined grains are often associated with higher levels of fasting insulin [46–48] perhaps due to the lack of fiber and important phytochemicals in refined grains. Diets causing a heightened insulin response are associated with the development of type 2 diabetes [49].

While recommendations are for ~85 g (3 oz) or more of whole grains and 85 g (3 oz) or less of refined grains, NHANES (1999–2002) data indicated that of the total grain servings consumed only 11 % was from whole grains [50]. Based on NHANES 2003–2004 data, the food items contributing the most to the daily intake of refined grains in Americans 2 years old and older are yeast breads (25.9 %), pizza (11.4 %), grain-based desserts (9.9 %), Mexican mixed dishes (8 %), and pasta/pasta dishes (6.7 %) [12].

The 2010 DGA [12] also recommended decreasing trans-fatty acids derived from industrialized sources (hydrogenated oils). Also, the American Heart Association recommended that trans-fats be <1 % of energy intake [51]. Trans-fatty acids are a health risk because they increase LDL cholesterol, decrease high-density lipoprotein (HDL) cholesterol, increase serum triglycerides and reduce LDL particle size [52]. A 2 % increase in energy from trans-fats is associated with a 23 % increase in risk of CVD [53]. While dietary consumption in the USA (aged 2 years or older) has decreased to 1.3 g/day [54], relative to an approximate 3–4 g/day intake noted in the 1980s [55], the amount of industrially produced trans-fats remains highly variable in many US food products [56]. Trans-fats should be removed from all food products with a priority for those foods with the highest levels.

For individuals who consume alcohol, current recommendations suggest moderate intake [12]. This is defined as one drink/day for women, and two drinks/day for men. One drink is defined as 12 fluid ounces (~350 ml) of regular beer, 5 fluid ounces of wine (~150 ml), or 1.5 fluid ounces (~45 ml) of 80 proof (40 % alcohol) distilled spirits; these are equivalent to 0.6 fluid ounces or approximately 17 g of alcohol. NHANES data (2005–2006) indicate that, for adults aged 19 years and older, alcoholic beverages rank fifth (106 kcal/day) among top calorie sources for Americans [12].

A meta-analysis of 34 prospective studies found a J-shaped relationship between the amount of alcohol consumed and mortality in both men and women [57]. The maximum protection was 18 % in women consuming up to two drinks/day; and 17 % in men consuming up to four drinks/day; higher doses were associated with increased mortality. These protective effects were attributed to the action of alcohol on plasma lipoproteins [58]. A meta-analysis of 42 studies found that 30 g of ethanol/day (approximately two drinks) was associated with beneficial increases in HDL cholesterol (3.99 mg/dl) and apolipoprotein A-I (8.82 mg/dl), although triglycerides also increased (5.69 mg/dl) [59]. However, moderate alcohol consumption was also associated with other protective effects. For example, when compared to no or heavy alcohol consumption, moderate drinkers had lower CRP levels [60]. However, binge drinking, even in those who were typically moderate consumers, increased the risk of death from CHD [61] or other diseases such as cancer [62].

Although results of many studies support the health benefits of moderate alcohol consumption, some investigations suggest these benefits are correlative, not causative, effects. Hansel et al. [63] suggested that the lower observed death rate from CHD in moderate drinkers may actually represent social status and general health. Alcohol's benefits may also be clouded by gender and location; a meta-analysis of 28 cohort studies found less protective effects in men living in non-Mediterranean countries [64]. While most studies found no influence of the type of alcohol [65], other studies suggested that distilled spirits had different effects than red wine. Chiva-Blanch et al. [66] studied the effects of consuming red wine, dealcoholized red wine, and gin on plasma lipid profile and glucose metabolism. They found that plasma insulin and measures of insulin resistance decreased with consumption of red wine and dealcoholized red wine (thus presumably due to phytochemicals); lipoprotein (a) decreased with consumption of red wine, while HDL cholesterol, Apolipoprotein A-I and A-II increased with consumption of both red wine and gin (most likely representing the effects of alcohol).

Dietary Patterns and Nutrient Deficiencies

Calcium

Circulating calcium is critical for many functions, including regulation of muscle contraction, neurotransmitter release, vasoconstriction and vasodilation, and cellular signaling [67]. When plasma calcium levels drop, it is replenished by breaking down skeletal reserves. Thus, adequate calcium consumption is essential for bone health. Low calcium consumption in young girls is associated with an increased risk of bone fractures [68], and long-term depletion of skeletal calcium reserves increases the risk of osteoporosis [67]. Low peak bone mass is the major determining factor for developing osteoporosis later in life [69]. Therefore, achieving high peak bone mass during adolescence is important for preventing osteoporosis.

In addition to adequate dietary calcium and vitamin D, bone health requires potassium, magnesium [70], and protein for collagen formation [71]. Diets high in fruits and vegetables have been shown to improve bone health [72], possibly by creating an alkaline environment in the body, whereas grains and excess protein cause an acidic environment [73, 74], leading to calcium loss. Although a meta-analysis did not support this concept [75], a study conducted with rats showed that an acidic milieu induced by diet caused osteoporosis [76]. Bone health may also improve in high fruit/high vegetable diets because a higher level of vitamin C improves collagen formation [77]. Plant-based diets are also higher in vitamin K, another nutrient associated with bone health [78]. Given the importance of fruit and vegetables to bone health, it is not surprising that women following the MDP have greater bone mass [71]. Further statistical analysis of bone mass based on scoring an individual's intake of different MDP components demonstrated that a diet high in fish and olive oil and low in red meat was positively associated with greater lumbar spine bone mineral density [71]. There is also evidence suggesting that the n-3 fatty acids in typical MDP foods such as fish, nuts, seeds, and some plants such as purslane benefit bone metabolism and bone/joint diseases [79].

While calcium-fortified foods and beverages (such as orange juice) can be used as alternative sources to meet calcium requirements, additional nutrients provided by dairy products are difficult to replace in diets of Americans [80]. For example, in 2004, in addition to providing 71 % of the calcium in the US diet, dairy products also supplied 31 % of phosphorous, 14 % of magnesium, 17 % of potassium, and 16 % of zinc [81].

Diets that are low in sodium are associated with reduced calcium excretion and thus a lower osteoporosis risk [82]. While a typical American low-sodium diet decreased urinary calcium loss, a low-sodium DASH diet was also associated with higher serum osteocalcin levels, an indicator of bone formation not evident in the typical American low-sodium diet [82]. Diets high in fruits and vegetables also tend to be higher in potassium and magnesium; potassium is important in acid/base regulation and prevents sodium-induced increases in urinary calcium excretion [82].

Children and adolescents from 9 to 18 years of age should consume 1300 mg calcium daily, while adults 19–50 years of age require 1000 mg/day [37a]. Adults over 51 years of age require 1200 mg/day. For pregnancy and lactation, the calcium RDA for 14–18 years of age is 1300 mg/day, and for women 19–50 years of age it is 1000 mg/day [37a]. Unfortunately, Americans are not consuming the recommended amounts of dietary calcium. Results from the 1999 to 2004 NHANES indicated only 30 % of the US population over 2 years of age consumed adequate calcium [83], while another analysis [84] determined that 40 % of NHANES 1999–2002 participants 19 years of age and older met their daily calcium AI levels. On average, Americans consume only ~75 % of their recommended calcium goal [12]. The groups noted to have inadequate calcium intake are children older than 9 years of age; adolescent girls; adult women and all adults over 51 years of age [12]. Bailey et al. [85] indicated that from 2003 to 2006 in the USA, calcium intakes (from diet alone) were:

- Males 9–13 years: 1074 mg/day (82 % of RDA [37a]).
- Females 9–13 years: 968 mg/day (74 % of RDA).
- Males 14-18 years: 1266 mg/day (97 % of RDA).
- Females 14–18 years: 876 mg/day (67 % of RDA).
- Males 19-30 years: 1209 mg/day (121 % RDA).
- Females 19–30 years: 838 mg/day (83 % of RDA).
- Males 31-50 years: 1118 mg/day (112 % of RDA).
- Females 31–50 years: 864 mg/day (86 % of RDA).
- Males 51–70 years: 951 mg/day (79 % of RDA).
- Females 51–70 years: 788 mg/day (65 % of RDA).

In a review examining MDP followers, Castro-Quezada et al. [8] reported that calcium intake was adequate in Spain, Portugal, and Italy. In the SUN study, Serra-Majem et al. [9] found those in the highest quintile of MDP followers consumed 1409 mg/day, while those in the middle quintile consumed 1194 mg/day. The MDP includes cheese, but also bony fish such as sardines and plenty of vegetables as calcium sources [86]. However, the MDP of Crete in 1960 only provided 826 mg/day of calcium [87].

Calcium intake is also adequate for adults aged 19–50 years of age consuming a 2000 kcal/day DASH dietary pattern (1185 mg/day [88]; 1406 mg/day [89]). The DASH and DASH-Sodium intervention diets meet the majority of calcium requirements by including non-fat dairy (55 %), vegetables (14 %), and whole grains (10 %) [88]. A 2000 kcal USDAFP diet meets the calcium requirements for all adults at 1316 mg/day [89].

All three dietary patterns discussed here provide adequate calcium intakes, but differ in the main food sources supplying calcium. In the DASH and USDAFP, calcium is provided mainly by low-fat dairy products, whereas in the MDP, the primary calcium sources are cheese, bony fish like sardines, and vegetables [86]. Bony fish are not widely consumed in the USA and, thus, recommending them in an MDP for Americans is not a reasonable strategy for increasing calcium consumption.

Magnesium

Magnesium is important for bone health and its effects on many different metabolic processes. Insufficient magnesium intake as well as low plasma magnesium levels are associated with diabetes, metabolic syndrome, hypertension, atherosclerosis, migraine headaches, colon cancer, and asthma [26] among other conditions. The association between magnesium levels and sudden (arrhythmic) cardiac death was evaluated in the Nurses' Health Study over 26 years of follow-up. This study reported that higher magnesium in both diet and plasma was associated with lower risks of sudden cardiac death [90]. A meta-analysis reported that circulating magnesium and dietary magnesium were inversely associated with CVD risk [91]. Higher dietary magnesium intake was also associated with decreased risk of ischemic stroke [92] and type 2 diabetes [93].

Studies have also found that an increase in the calcium–magnesium ratio in the American diet coincided with increased incidence of type 2 diabetes [26]. The association between lower diabetes risk and higher magnesium intake may be due to the role it plays in insulin secretion [94]. Since many of the above chronic diseases are associated with inflammation, it is not surprising that low magnesium levels are also associated with higher levels of C-reactive protein [26]. In a rat model, magnesium-deficient animals had higher plasma interleukin (IL)-1 and IL-6 (indicative of inflammatory status), and tumor necrosis factor (TNF)-α [95]. The RDA for magnesium [96] for the following age groups is:

- Boys and girls 9–13 years of age: 240 mg/day.
- Boys 14–18 years of age 410 mg/day.
- Girls 14–18 years of age 360 mg/day.
- Girls 14–18 years of age during pregnancy 400 mg/day or lactation 360 mg/day.
- Men 19–30 years of age 400 mg/day.
- Women 19–30 years of age 310 mg/day.
- Women 19–30 years of age during pregnancy 350 mg/day or lactation 310 mg/day.
- Men 31–70 years of age 420 mg/day.
- Women 31–70 years of age 320 mg/day.
- Women 31–50 years of age during pregnancy 360 mg/day or lactation 320 mg/day.

Based on NHANES 2001–2002, the percent of males consuming less than their EAR for magnesium was: 55 % of those 19–30 years; 61 % of males 31–50 years; 70 % of males 51–70 years; and 81 % of males over 71 years of age. The percent of women consuming below their EAR was: 64 % of those 19–30 years; 65 % of women 31–50 years; 64 % of women 51–70 years; and 82 % of women over 71 years of age [26]. In 2005–2006, 48 % of the USA population was below the EAR for magnesium [97]. Given the association between low magnesium and cardiac death as well as diabetes, low levels in the elderly are of special concern.

Serra-Majem et al. [9] (SUN study) reported that magnesium consumption increased as adherence to the MDP increased. Those in the highest quintile of MDP adherence had a magnesium intake of 497 mg/day, while individuals in the middle quintile consumed 401 mg/day, an amount adequate for females. In 1960, the Crete MDP provided approximately 483 mg magnesium [87]. Calton [98] reported that the DASH dietary pattern (measured by 3 days of DASH menus) provided 142 % of the RDI for magnesium. Based on a 2000 kcal diet, DASH dietary pattern provides 554 mg magnesium, while the USDAFP provides 380 mg magnesium [89], an amount adequate for females. Assuming that intake increases relative to caloric intake, the higher energy intake of males should provide adequate magnesium in both the MDP (median quintile value) and the USDAFP.

Sources of magnesium in the MDP include vegetables, legumes and nuts. In the DASH dietary pattern, most magnesium is provided by whole grains (29 %), fruits (17 %), vegetables (15 %), low-fat dairy (13 %), and nuts/seeds/legumes (12 %) [88]. Interestingly, magnesium is typically lowest in refined or processed foods, perhaps explaining the decreasing magnesium consumption in the USA [99]. Overall, all three dietary patterns provide adequate amounts of magnesium.

Potassium

Potassium and sodium are closely linked. They are responsible for function of the Na/K pump, and an imbalance is associated with a greater risk of CHD and mortality [100]. A high sodium intake induces endothelium stiffness and decreases nitric oxide synthesis [101], causing vasoconstriction and high blood pressure. Potassium can attenuate these effects by increasing nitric acid release [102]. In a prospective cohort study of more than 12,000 US adults for 14.8 years, potassium was inversely associated with CVD and ischemic heart disease, although the incidence of CVD and ischemic heart disease was better explained by a high Na: K ratio than by potassium alone [100].

The AI for potassium is 4700 mg daily for males and females over the age of 14 years [12]. The AI for pregnant women of any age is also 4700 mg, while lactating women of any age have an AI of 5100 mg [37]. NHANES data from 2005 indicate, however, that less than 3 % of the American population consumes their recommended amount of potassium or higher [83]. The average potassium intake in the USA, based on NHANES 2003–2006, is 2619 mg [80].

MDP, DASH, and USDAFP all provide higher amounts of potassium than current US intakes.

In the SUN study [9], individuals in the highest quintile of MDP adherence consumed 6132 mg/day, while those in the median quintile consumed 4529 mg/day (96 % of recommended intake). While the highest quintile group consumed adequate potassium, the median quintile fell short of recommendations. Estimates of the 1960 Crete diet indicate the population consumed 4504 mg/day [87], almost 96 % of the current recommendation.

According to the 2005 DGA [89], a 2000 kcal DASH diet provides the recommended amount of potassium (4721 mg/day). However, Calton [98] found that sample 3-day DASH menus provided 94 % of the potassium recommendation, while Lin [88] found the DASH dietary pattern provided 4258 mg/day (90.6 % of the recommendation). The primary sources of potassium in the DASH dietary pattern are fruits (33 %), whole grains (17 %), vegetables (16 %), and low-fat dairy (16 %) [88]. The USDAFP diet, based on 2000 kcal provides 4044 mg/day (86 % of the recommendation) [89]. Of these three diet patterns, the MDP provides the most potassium.

Vitamin D

Vitamin D is important for calcium absorption [103] and bone mineralization. Adequate vitamin D intake prevents rickets in children and osteomalacia in adults, and helps prevent some bone fractures [104]. A meta-analysis of 12 randomized controlled trials found vitamin D lowered risk for non-vertebral fractures at doses greater than 10 μg/400 IU [104], while cross-sectional and cohort studies reported that high vitamin D status decreased the risk of falls [105]. Although observational studies reported that low vitamin D status increased the risk of overweight/obesity, type 2 diabetes, and cancer, there is still insufficient evidence to conclude that vitamin D exerts a causative role in prevention of these chronic diseases [105, 106].

The RDA for children and most adults, regardless of gender, is 15 μg (or 600 IU) per day [12], although people over the age of 70 should consume 20 μg (or 800 IU) per day to compensate for changes in skin and sun exposure. Fatty fish such as salmon are high in vitamin D, as are fortified products such as milk and other dairy products. NHANES analysis (2001–2006) indicates 2/3 of the US population had sufficient vitamin D levels (IOM defined as serum 25-hydroxy (25OH)-vitamin D between 50 and 125 nmol/L) while ~25 % of the US population was at risk of vitamin D inadequacy (serum 25OH-vitamin D from 30 to 49 nmol/L); 8 % of the US population were at risk of vitamin D deficiency (serum 25OH-vitamin D less than 30 nmol/L) [107].

Dietary data for vitamin D provide limited information about status because of in vivo synthesis [108]. There is evidence that individuals synthesize >1000 IU daily (25 μg) [109] even when wearing SPF 15 sunscreen. However, other researchers calculated that Caucasian subjects 22–59 years of age synthesized sufficient vitamin D (more than 1200 IU daily, or 30 μg) through sunlight exposure only when the following combination occurred: they were outdoor workers that did not wear sunscreen while at work; more than 30 % of their skin was exposed to sunlight, they took a 2–3 week vacation below 40°N, and only wore sunscreen at beach vacations [110]. By these estimates, it is evident that it is not possible to meet vitamin D needs solely from sunlight and greater attention to dietary sources is necessary.

Another possible source of dietary vitamin D is the metabolized form of 25OH-vitamin D, a compound that is not included in the NHANES diet assessment; this compound is an important contributor to serum vitamin D levels [111]. Taylor et al. [111] reported a potentially meaningful increase in vitamin D intake estimates when 25OH-vitamin D was included in dietary assessment as well as the potency-adjusted value.

Vitamin D content of diets is not often measured. In the SUN study [9], the highest quintile of MDP followers consumed 4.9 µg/day of vitamin D, and those in the median MDP quintile consumed 3.5 µg/day; these levels supplied less than 33 % of the recommended intake. Although both groups spent more than 24 h/week engaging in various physical activities (walking, running, cycling, swimming), given their northern location and recent low estimates of skin production, even individuals who consumed an MDP and spent many hours outside in the sunlight might not have had adequate plasma levels of vitamin D based on dietary vitamin D and sun exposure combined.

Studies showed that sample 3-day DASH menus provided 58 % of the RDA for vitamin D [97]. NHANES analysis indicated that average US intakes were 4.96 µg (33 % of recommended amount) from 2003 to 2006 [80]. Available data suggest that vitamin D intake is low for the MDP and DASH dietary patterns (33 % of recommended intakes), although the adequate serum levels in 80 % of the US population [12] suggests the combination of sun exposure and underestimated 25OH-vitamin D levels may be compensating for low intake levels.

Dietary Fiber

Dietary fiber includes non-digestible carbohydrates and lignin and is categorized as soluble or insoluble, fermentable or non-fermentable, viscous or non-viscous [112]. Fiber-rich foods reportedly induce a feeling of fullness and retain water in the gastrointestinal tract, aiding in laxation [112]. The physical characteristics of dietary fiber also provide other health benefits. For example, water-soluble fibers appear to be most effective in lowering LDL cholesterol, thus decreasing the risk of CHD [112]. Foods high in insoluble fiber significantly lower the risk of type 2 diabetes [113], possibly due to the association of cereal fibers with magnesium and other phytochemicals present in whole grain products [114]. Soluble, viscous fibers slow the absorption of glucose from the gut, lowering the glycemic load of a food and thus the insulin response [115]; this type of fiber also reduces serum cholesterol by binding it in the gastrointestinal tract [116]. Fermentable fibers often act as prebiotics, stimulating the growth of beneficial bacteria in the large intestine [112]. Fermentable fibers are also associated with the synthesis of short chain fatty acids, compounds linked to a decreased risk of some diseases [117]. Indeed, the NIH-AARP Diet and Health Study examined dietary fiber intake in relation to cause-specific mortality in more than 30,000 older people over a 9-year period. Higher dietary fiber intake was associated with lower risk of death from CHD, infectious diseases, and respiratory diseases [118].

The MDP has been reported to protect against type 2 diabetes, and fiber is thought to be one of its protective components. In addition to the effects of insoluble fiber [113], the MDP's protective effect could be due to fiber's satiation properties, resulting in lower obesity rates [119] or creating a lower glycemic index/glycemic load [49]. Other protective attributes of dietary fiber could be due to its association with fruits, vegetables, and whole grains and the beneficial phytochemicals (acting mainly as antioxidants) they contain.

The AI for dietary fiber is 14 g/1000 kcal; men should consume 36 g/day and women should consume 28 g/day [12]. In the USA, adults reportedly consume less than one-half of the AI for dietary fiber; results from 12 cohort epidemiological studies from 1993 to 2000 indicate that men consume 16.7 g/day while women consume 15.6 g/day [120].

During the 1960s in Crete, fiber intake (based on a 2633 kcal diet) was 47 g/day [87]. Serra-Majem et al. [9] (SUN study) found that fiber intake in the highest quintile of MDP followers was 36.9 g/day, while those in the median quintile consumed 26 g fiber/day. The 2005 DGA [89] estimates that a 2000 kcal DASH diet provides 34 g dietary fiber, while the USDAFP diet provides 31 g dietary fiber. The major fiber sources in the DASH diet [88] were whole grains (45 %), fruit (23 %), vegetables (20 %), and nuts/seeds/legumes (5 %). Thus, dietary fiber requirements can be met by following any of these three food patterns discussed in this chapter.

A strategy that has been recommended for increasing fiber intake in the USA is to enrich grain products with fiber that was removed during industrial processing [121]. However, given that nutrients/bioactive components other than the fiber (e.g., magnesium and phytochemicals) [114] may influence chronic diseases/clinical conditions, enriching foods with fiber might have some limitations. In addition, dietary fiber may have a different physical association with starch, lessening the hypoglycemic effect when the fiber is processed [122]. Given that many foods in the MDP are good sources of dietary fiber and are minimally processed, the MDP most easily meets dietary fiber recommendations.

Discussion

The MDP, DASH, and USDAFP meet the nutrient needs for calcium, potassium, magnesium, and fiber. Although these dietary patterns do not provide 100 % of the DRI for vitamin D, they provide higher amounts than current US intakes. While the estimated amounts of vitamin D synthesized via exposure to sunlight are highly variable [109, 110], any dietary inadequacies could be compensated for with adequate sunlight exposure, and better monitored including measures of 25OH-vitamin D [111].

At the food-based level, the abundance of fruits and vegetables in the DASH, USDAFP, and MDP are not only associated with high fiber, calcium, potassium, and magnesium, but also with many beneficial phytochemicals. In a study conducted in Greece's ATTICA region, participants with the highest adherence to the MDP had 11 % higher plasma measures of total antioxidant capacity than those in the lowest adherence group [123]. Although we cannot attribute causation, diets high in phytochemicals/antioxidants may protect against hypertension, CHD, and stroke [124]. Phytochemicals influence a variety of metabolic processes such as inflammation [125–127], a process involved in the pathogenesis of various diseases.

The MDP is high in seafood/ fish/ n-3 fatty acids. In a cross-sectional study examining n-3 consumption as a part of the Prevención con Dieta Mediterránea (PREDIMED) study [128], DHA and EPA were measured in diets and red blood cells in 198 subjects. While participants consumed 44 g of lean fish/day (providing 0.23 g DHA+EPA/day), they also consumed an average of 25 g of fatty fish/day, providing 0.49 g/day DHA+EPA. Participants consumed a variety of other seafood as well (115 g/day), and consumed an average of 0.9 g of DHA+EPA/day, an amount well above the recommended intake. This high fish/n-3 fatty acid consumption explains, in part, the low CHD rates despite the prevalence of risk factors in the population evaluated [128]. In comparison, the DASH recommends 6 oz (170 g) or less of lean meat, poultry and fatty fish daily; while not a specific recommendation, seafood should be considered as a primary source of lean protein.

While the DASH, USDAFP, and MDP all decrease chronic disease risk, the MDP has unique nutrition attributes that distinguish it from the others. Several computer models were used to generate more than 1100 individual, nutritionally adequate diets for adults participating in the French INCA dietary survey [129]. The population was considered to be eating a Western diet. All diets generated needed to meet guidelines for protein, fiber, essential fatty acids, SFA, added sugars, sodium, ten vitamins, and nine minerals. In addition, the computer-generated diets were constrained to make the fewest alterations from the subject's current dietary patterns. The researchers found the models generated fairly consistent food changes for all participants. Most individual's diets were altered by incorporating foods such as unsalted nuts, unrefined grains, legumes, fruits and vegetables, fish and shellfish, while decreasing animal fats, processed meats, and cheese. These computer-generated dietary changes identified the MDP as best for achieving dietary adequacy with the fewest possible changes to the existing diet.

Our understanding of the health benefits of the MDP has been advanced by the PREDIMED study [130]. PREDIMED, a primary intervention trial, assessed the long-term effects of the MDP in individuals who, although initially free of the disease, were at very high risk for CVD. Participants were assigned to one of three groups: MDP supplemented with EVOO (50 ml daily); MDP supplemented with mixed nuts (30 g/day of walnuts, almonds and hazelnuts); or a control diet with advice given on a lower-fat diet. In addition, participants in the two MDP groups significantly increased their fish consumption (by 0.3 servings/week) and legumes (by 0.4 servings/week) compared to the control group. Compared to the lower fat control, after 4.8 years the two MDP diets were associated with a 30 % reduction in cardiovascular events (stroke, myocardial infarction, or death due to such events). Also, both MDPs were associated with lower levels of inflammatory markers, such as C-reactive protein and IL-6 [131].

In addition to reducing CVD, a meta-analysis of ten prospective studies reported that adherence to an MDP was also associated with a 23 % reduced risk of developing type 2 diabetes [132]. In the PREDIMED trial, 418 non-diabetic subjects ranging from 55 to 80 years of age were studied. After a mean follow-up period of 4 years, subjects were scored based on diabetes incidence. The incidence of diabetes was reduced by 52 % in the two MDP groups as compared to the control diet without any significant changes in either body weight or physical activity [133]. Adherence to the MDP does not preclude weight loss; many studies have reported that this dietary pattern was inversely associated with obesity [134].

When the PREDIMED data were analyzed for the development of new cases of metabolic syndrome, the risk did not differ among the treatment and control groups [135]. However, 28 % of the participants who had metabolic syndrome when the study started did not have it by the end of the study. Importantly, participants in either the MDP+nuts or MDP+EVOO treatments had fewer metabolic syndrome criteria than the control group. Both MDP treatment groups decreased central obesity, while the EVOO treatment also decreased fasting glucose [135].

How Can Americans Transition to a Mediterranean Dietary Pattern?

Traditionally, lower fat diets have been recommended to reduce CVD and obesity risk. More recently, however, the 2010 DGA [12] recognized that the MDP is associated with multifaceted health effects, including a decreased risk of CVD. Thus, in addition to the USDAFP, the 2010 DGA [12] recommended both a lower fat DASH dietary pattern and the MDP. Thus, a key question is how can Americans transition to an MDP?

There are two notable differences between the MDP and the average American diet: the MDP is high in MUFA and fruits and vegetables. Meat is also limited in the MDP. One approach for Americans in implementing the MDP is to consume portion-controlled quantities of very lean or lean beef or poultry to reduce saturated fat while including foods high in MUFA such as vegetable oils (e.g., EVOO), avocados and avocado oil (rich in 18:1), and nuts (almonds, hazelnuts, macadamia nuts, pistachios, pecans) in various ways to increase MUFA. In general, total fat intake may remain constant but the fatty acid profile should change to lower SFA and increase MUFA. The development of a simplified exchange list, as utilized in studies by Djuric et al. [136] and Sidahmed et al. [137] (Table 18.1), might be a tool to assist consumers in decreasing SFA and increasing the relative proportion of MUFA as well as the amount and variety of fruits and vegetables. In both studies, fruits and vegetables were increased at the expense of other carbohydrates and exchange lists were used to increase variety in the diet. Olive oil was used to enhance the palatability and acceptance of vegetables.

The 2010 DGA [12] recommends that individuals increase consumption of fruits and vegetables to reduce the risk of chronic diseases. The consumption of fruits and vegetables in the USA is well below recommendations. To encourage changes in consumer behavior, several media campaigns such as the "5 A Day for Better Health" (5 A Day) campaign and, more recently, the "Fruits and Veggies—More Matters" campaign and the 7–13 serving recommendation for fruit and vegetable consumption

Table 18.1 Dietary goals from a modified version of the Mediterranean exchange list

Dietary Goal	Foods	Servings[a]
High MUFA foods	Olive oil (1 tsp), avocado (1/6), macadamia nuts (3, 4), hazelnuts (10), pesto (1 tbsp), olive tapenade (1 tbsp), trail mix with macadamia or hazelnuts (4 tbsp, count as 2 fats and 1 fruit), almond/cashew butter, almonds/cashews (6), canola oil (1 tsp), peanuts (10), peanut butter (2 tsp)	8–10 exchanges per day (5 g per exchange)
High marine omega-3 foods	Tuna, herring, sardines, salmon, mussels, clams, crab, halibut, lobster, scallops, shrimp, sole, tilapia, trout	Twice a week, 3 oz serving size (with limits on fish with higher mercury)
Dark green vegetables	Broccoli, Brussels sprouts, chard, dark green lettuce (kale, spinach), peas* zucchini (with skin)	1–2 servings per day
Orange and yellow vegetables	Baby carrots (4), peppers (red, yellow, orange), carrots (1 med), carrot juice ¼ cup, pumpkin*, tangerines (2), winter squash*, vegetable soup, vegetable juice	1–2 servings per day
Red vegetables	Salsa (1/4 c), spaghetti sauce* (1/4 c), tomatoes, tomato juice (1/2 c), tomato paste (2 tbsp), tomato sauce (1/4 c), tomato soup** (1 c), vegetable juice	1–2 servings per day
Other vegetables	Artichoke, asparagus, baby corn, bamboo shoots, bean sprouts, beets, bok choy, cabbage, cauliflower, celery, corn*, cucumber, eggplant, green beans, green peppers, mushrooms, okra, pea pods, potatoes**, radish, sugar snap peas, water chestnuts	1–2 servings per day
Dark green culinary herbs	Basil, bay leaves, chives, cilantro, dill weed, marjoram, mint, oregano, parsley, peppermint, rosemary, sage, tarragon, thyme	1 serving per day, 1 tablespoon fresh or 1 teaspoon dried
Allium vegetables	Garlic, green onions, leeks, onions, scallions, shallots	Use liberally at least once a day
Fruits	Vitamin C: cantaloupe, grapefruit, guava, kiwi, lemon, orange, mango, papaya, strawberries, tangerine Other: apple, apple sauce, apricot (4), banana, berries, cherries (12), dates (3), figs (2), grapes (15–20), 100 % fruit juice, melon, nectarine, pineapple, plums (2–3), prunes (3), raisins*, peach, pear, star fruit, any other	One serving per day vitamin C fruit and one serving per day other fruit
Whole grains	Barley, brown rice, buckwheat, bulgur, couscous, faro, kamut, oatmeal, polenta, quinoa, wheat berries, whole grain, stone-ground breads, rolls, tortillas, and pasta	At least 3 servings per day
Legumes, nuts, and seeds	Almonds, black-eyed peas, cashews, chickpeas (garbanzo beans), hazelnuts, kidney beans, lentils, lima beans, pecans, pine nuts, pistachios, sesame seeds, sunflower seeds, split peas, walnuts	At least 6 servings per week (3 servings nuts/seeds, 3 servings legumes)

Adapted from: Djuric et al. [136] and Sidahmed et al. [137]
For grains, serving sizes are one ounce equivalents (12 chips or 6 crackers), one slice bread, ½ cup cooked grain, ¾ cup dry cereal, or three cups popcorn
For legumes (beans) ½ cup cooked is a serving, for nuts and seeds 1 oz is a serving
In addition to these recommendations individuals are encouraged to consume two to three exchanges of low-fat dairy foods, and 5–6 oz of lean or very lean meat or other protein, each day, with amounts adjusted to maintain weight
[a]Unless otherwise specified: One serving for fruits and vegetables is defined as one medium, one cup fresh, two cups leafy greens, ½ cup canned or cooked, ½ cup juice (count up to two servings/day for juice, the rest of the goal was to be met from whole foods) or ¼ cup dried. The total fruit and vegetable goal is 7–9 servings/day, depending on baseline energy intake, and variety was defined by use of five exchange groups for vegetables and two exchange groups for fruit. Starred (*) foods were to be counted as both 1 fruit/vegetables exchange and ½ (*) or 1 (**) carbohydrate exchange

have been implemented over the past two decades. The impact of these initiatives remains modest at best, with little effect on increasing daily consumption on a long-term basis [138–141]. Several factors have been identified in both promoting and impeding the increase in fruit and vegetable consumption. Fruits and vegetables are perceived as costly and of less value for the money, particularly due to the potential for rapid spoilage [142]. A longitudinal study of food prices relative to both energy density and nutrient density found that food prices between 2004 and 2008 were positively associated with nutrient density. The mean cost of foods in the top quintile was US $27.20 per 1000 kcal, and these have increased 29.2 % in price over four years. Comparatively, the foods in the bottom quintile of nutrient density cost $3.32 per 1000 kcal and had a 4-year price increase of 16.1 % [143]. Despite the high cost of nutrient-dense foods, a study in Canada found that when women were part of an MDP nutritional intervention, there was no significant increase in daily dietary cost; however, it decreased daily energy density. While participants had increased food costs related to increased intake of vegetables, fruits, legumes, nuts, and seeds, canola/olive oil, whole grains, poultry, and fish, there was a concomitant decrease in money spent on red meat, refined grains, desserts and sweets, and fast food [144].

Other factors influencing increased fruit and vegetable consumption include today's fast paced environment where convenience and preparation time are important. Consumers tend to choose foods that are familiar and easy to use and prepare. Many producers have responded by offering convenient serving size packaging for pre-cut vegetables, steam fresh bags, and pre-portioned stir-fry kits. While fruits are typically consumed raw and require little preparation, vegetables, aside from salads, are often cooked and require some cooking skills as well as knowledge of the different ways in which they can be used. Because some vegetables may be unfamiliar, retailers could assist consumers by offering a wide variety of produce accompanied by recipes and supporting preparation, cooking, selection and storage information. Demonstrations for cooking and tasting vegetable based dishes can enhance familiarity and acceptability, and assist in meal planning.

In the USA, consumption of adequate fruits and vegetables is one of the greatest barriers to achieving nutrient adequacy. However, as discussed herein, there are other barriers as well. These include not consuming adequate amounts of lean proteins, seafood, whole grains, liquid vegetable oils, and low-fat dairy products. Of concern, as well, is that Americans continue to consume too much solid fat, added sugars, sodium, and calories. Efforts are needed to devise and implement innovative strategies to increase awareness of the health benefits of the MDP. Critical to any success in achieving this goal is that the strategies are effective on an individual and population-wide basis

Conclusions

There are many health benefits of an MDP as well as other dietary patterns such as the DASH and USDAFP. We have a good understanding of the health benefits of these dietary patterns. Going forward, the challenge is to identify strategies that effectively modify existing dietary practices of the US population to healthier dietary patterns. Achieving adherence to them will require major changes in the US diet and food behavior. To reach this goal will require a large-scale effort that involves the food and restaurant industries working in collaboration with public health communities and consumers. The MDP is a viable dietary tool to help Americans to reduce the burden of chronic diseases. However, to make the most of this dietary opportunity, all stakeholders should participate in a concerted effort and commit to these dietary and lifestyle changes with dispatch.

References

1. Keys A. Coronary heart disease in seven countries. Circulation. 1970;41(1):186–95.
2. Simopoulos AP. The Mediterranean diets: what is so special about the diet of Greece? The scientific evidence. J Nutr. 2001;131(11):3065S–73.
3. Simopoulos AP, Salem Jr N. n-3 Fatty acids in eggs from range-fed Greek chickens. N Engl J Med. 1989;321:1412–5.
4. Nestle M. Mediterranean diets: historical and research overview. Am J Clin Nutr. 1995;61(6):1313S–20.
5. Brunelle T, Dumas P, Souty F. The impact of globalization on food and agriculture: the case of the diet convergence. J Environ Dev. 2014;23(1):41–65.
6. Alberti-Fidanza A, Fidanza F. Mediterranean adequacy index of Italian diets. Public Health Nutr. 2004;7(07):937–41.
7. Leonhäuser IU, Dorandt S, Willmund E, Honsel J. The benefit of the Mediterranean diet. Eur J Nutr. 2004;43(1):31–8.
8. Castro-Quezada I, Román-Viñas B, Serra-Majem L. The Mediterranean diet and nutritional adequacy: a review. Nutrients. 2014;6(1):231–48.
9. Serra-Majem L, Bes-Rastrollo M, Román-Vinas B, Pfrimer K, Sánchez-Villegas A, Martínez-González MA. Dietary patterns and nutritional adequacy in a Mediterranean country. Br J Nutr. 2009;101(S2):S21–8.
10. Kant AK. Dietary patterns and health outcomes. J Am Diet Assoc. 2004;104(4):615–35.
11. Roman-Vinas B, Ribas Barba L, Ngo J, Gurinovic M, Novakovic R, Cavelaars A, et al. Projected prevalence of inadequate nutrient intakes in Europe. Ann Nutr Metab. 2011;59(2-4):84–95.
12. Dietary Guidelines for Americans. US Department of Agriculture and US Department of Health and Human Services. Dietary Guidelines for Americans. 7th ed. Washington, DC: US Government Printing Office; 2010. December 2010. [Internet, cited 2015 Jan]. Available from: http://www.cnpp.usda.gov/sites/default/files/dietary_guidelines_for_americans/PolicyDoc.pdf.
13. Richter CK, Skulas-Ray AC, Kris-Etherton PM. Recent findings of studies on the Mediterranean diet: what are the implications for current dietary recommendations? Endocrinol Metab Clin North Am. 2014;43(4):963–80.
14. Reedy J, Krebs-Smith SM, Miller PE, Liese AD, Kahle LL, Park Y, et al. Higher diet quality is associated with decreased risk of all-cause, cardiovascular disease, and cancer mortality among older adults. J Nutr. 2014;144(6):881–9.
15. Djousse L, Petrone A, Gaziano JM. Alternate healthy eating index, Mediterranean and DASH dietary patterns and risk of death in the Physician's Health Study. Cardiology. 2014;128:426. Allschwilerstrasse 10, ch-4009 Basel, Switzerland: Karger.
16. Dixon LB, Subar AF, Peters U, Weissfeld JL, Bresalier RS, Risch A, et al. Adherence to the USDA Food Guide, DASH Eating Plan, and Mediterranean Dietary Pattern Reduces Risk of Colorectal Adenoma. J Nutr. 2007;137(11):2443–50.
17. Tangney CC, Kwasny MJ, Li H, Wilson RS, Evans DA, Morris MC. Adherence to a Mediterranean-type dietary pattern and cognitive decline in a community population. Am J Clin Nutr. 2011;93(3):601–7.
18. Lourida I, Soni M, Thompson-Coon J, Purandare N, Lang IA, Ukoumunne OC, et al. Mediterranean diet, cognitive function, and dementia: a systematic review. Epidemiology. 2013;24(4):479–89.
19. Tangney CC. DASH and Mediterranean-type dietary patterns to maintain cognitive health. Curr Nutr Rep. 2014;3(1):51–61.
20. García-Fernández E, Rico-Cabanas L, Rosgaard N, Estruch R, Bach-Faig A. Mediterranean diet and cardiodiabesity: a review. Nutrients. 2014;6(9):3474–500.
21. Frazao E. High costs of poor eating patterns in the United States. In: Frazao E, editor. America's eating habits: changes and consequences. Washington, DC: US Department of Agriculture; 1998. p. 5–32.
22. Cawley J, Meyerhoefer C, Biener A, Hammer M, Wintfeld N. Savings in Medical Expenditures Associated with Reductions in Body Mass Index Among US Adults with Obesity, by Diabetes Status. Pharmacoeconomics. 2015;33(7):707–22.
23. Flock MR, Kris-Etherton PM. Dietary guidelines for Americans 2010: implications for cardiovascular disease. Curr Atheroscler Rep. 2011;13(6):499–507.
24. Willett WC, Sacks F, Trichopoulou A, Drescher G, Ferro-Luzzi A, Helsing E, et al. Mediterranean diet pyramid: a cultural model for healthy eating. Am J Clin Nutr. 1995;61(6):1402S–6.
25. CDC's Second nutrition report: a comprehensive biochemical assessment of the nutrition status of the US population. 2012. [Internet, cited 2015 Jan 11]. Available from: http://www.cdc.gov/nutritionreport/
26. Rosanoff A, Weaver CM, Rude RK. Suboptimal magnesium status in the United States: are the health consequences underestimated? Nutr Rev. 2012;70(3):153–64.
27. King DE, Mainous III AG, Geesey ME, Woolson RF. Dietary magnesium and C-reactive protein levels. J Am Coll Nutr. 2005;24(3):166–71.

28. Ridker PM, Hennekens CH, Buring JE, Rifai N. C-reactive protein and other markers of inflammation in the prediction of cardiovascular disease in women. N Engl J Med. 2000;342(12):836–43.
29. Zivkovic AM, Telis N, German JB, Hammock BD. Dietary omega-3 fatty acids aid in the modulation of inflammation and metabolic health. Calif Agric (Berkeley). 2011;65(3):106.
30. Yates CM, Calder PC, Rainger G. Pharmacology and therapeutics of omega-3 polyunsaturated fatty acids in chronic inflammatory disease. Pharmacol Therapeut. 2014;141(3):272–82.
31. Swanson D, Block R, Mousa SA. Omega-3 fatty acids EPA and DHA: health benefits throughout life. Adv Nutr. 2012;3(1):1–7.
32. Vannice G, Rasmussen H. Position of the academy of nutrition and dietetics: dietary fatty acids for healthy adults. J Acad Nutr Diet. 2014;114(1):136–53.
33. Flock MR, Harris WS, Kris-Etherton PM. Long-chain Omega-3 fatty acids: time to establish a dietary reference intake. Nutr Rev. 2013;71(10):692–707.
34. Kris-Etherton PM, Grieger JA, Etherton TD. Dietary reference intakes for DHA and EPA. Prostaglandins Leukot Essent Fatty Acids. 2009;81(2):99–104.
35. What We Eat in America, NHANES 2011–2012 [Internet, cited 2015 Jan 18]. Available from: http://www.ars.usda.gov/SP2UserFiles/Place/80400530/pdf/1112/Table_1_NIN_GEN_11.pdf
36. Antman EM, Appel LJ, Balentine D, Johnson RK, Steffen LM, Miller EA, et al. Stakeholder discussion to reduce population-wide sodium intake and decrease sodium in the food supply a conference report from the American Heart Association Sodium Conference 2013 Planning Group*. Circulation. 2014;129(25):e660–79. doi:10.1161/CIR.0000000000000051.
37. Institute of Medicine (IOM). Dietary reference intakes (DRIs): recommended dietary allowances and adequate intakes, vitamins. Food and Nutrition Board, Institute of Medicine, National Academies. [Internet, cited 2015 Jan 12]. Available from: http://www.iom.edu/~/media/Files/Activity%20Files/Nutrition/DRIs/New%20Material/2_%20RDA%20and%20AI%20Values_Vitamin%20and%20Elements.pdf
37a. Institute of Medicine of the National Academies. Dietary Reference Intakes for Calcium and Vitamin D. Report Brief 2010. http://iom.nationalacademies.org/~/media/Files/Report%20Files/2010/Dietary-Reference-Intakes-for-Calcium-and-Vitamin-D/Vitamin%20D%20and%20Calcium%202010%20Report%20Brief.pdf
38. Anderson CA, Appel LJ, Okuda N, Brown IJ, Chan Q, Zhao L, et al. Dietary sources of sodium in China, Japan, the United Kingdom, and the United States, women and men aged 40 to 59 years: the INTERMAP study. J Am Diet Assoc. 2010;110(5):736–45.
39. Urban LE, Roberts SB, Fierstein JL, Gary CE, Lichtenstein AH. Sodium, saturated fat, and trans fat content per 1,000 kilocalories: temporal trends in fast-food restaurants, United States, 2000–2013. Prev Chronic Dis. 2014;11:140335. [Internet, cited 2015 Jan 20]. doi:http://dx.doi.org/10.5888/pcd11.140335.
40. Astrup A, Dyerberg J, Elwood P, Hermansen K, Hu FB, Jakobsen MU, et al. The role of reducing intakes of saturated fat in the prevention of cardiovascular disease: where does the evidence stand in 2010? Am J Clin Nutr. 2011;93(4):684–8.
41. Gillingham LG, Harris-Janz S, Jones PJ. Dietary monounsaturated fatty acids are protective against metabolic syndrome and cardiovascular disease risk factors. Lipids. 2011;46(3):209–28.
42. Reedy J, Krebs-Smith SM. Dietary sources of energy, solid fats, and added sugars among children and adolescents in the United States. J Am Diet Assoc. 2010;110(10):1477–84.
43. Slining MM, Popkin BM. Trends in intakes and sources of solid fats and added sugars among US children and adolescents: 1994–2010. Pediatr Obes. 2013;8(4):307–24.
44. Slavin J. Whole grains and human health. Nutr Res Rev. 2004;17(01):99–110.
45. Williams PG. Evaluation of the evidence between consumption of refined grains and health outcomes. Nutr Rev. 2012;70(2):80–99.
46. Giacco R, Costabile G, Della Pepa G, Anniballi G, Griffo E, Mangione A, et al. A whole-grain cereal-based diet lowers postprandial plasma insulin and triglyceride levels in individuals with metabolic syndrome. Nutr Metab Cardiovas Dis. 2014;24(8):837–44.
47. Newby PK, Maras J, Bakun P, Muller D, Ferrucci L, Tucker KL. Intake of whole grains, refined grains, and cereal fiber measured with 7-D diet records and associations with risk factors for chronic disease. Am J Clin Nutr. 2007;86(6):1745–53.
48. Pereira MA, Jacobs DR, Pins JJ, Raatz SK, Gross MD, Slavin JL, et al. Effect of whole grains on insulin sensitivity in overweight hyperinsulinemic adults. Am J Clin Nutr. 2002;75(5):848–55.
49. Biesalski HK. Diabetes preventive components in the Mediterranean diet. Eur J Nutr. 2004;43:i26–30.
50. USDA. Grain consumption by Americans Nutrition Insight 32. United States Department of Agriculture Center for Nutrition Policy and Promotion. [Internet, cited 2015 Jan 20]. 2005. Available from: http://www.cnpp.usda.gov/sites/default/files/nutrition_insights_uploads/Insight32.pdf
51. American Heart Association (AHA) [Internet, cited 2015 Jan 20]. Available from: http://www.heart.org/HEARTORG/Conditions/Cholesterol/PreventionTreatmentofHighCholesterol/Know-Your-Fats_UCM_305628_Article.jsp

52. Dhaka V, Gulia N, Ahlawat KS, Khatkar BS. Trans fats—sources, health risks and alternative approach-a review. J Food Sci Technol. 2011;8(5):534–41.
53. Remig V, Franklin B, Margolis S, Kostas G, Nece T, Street JC. Trans fats in America: a review of their use, consumption, health implications, and regulation. J Am Diet Assoc. 2010;110(4):585–92.
54. Doell D, Folmer D, Lee H, Honigfort M, Carberry S. Updated estimate of trans fat intake by the US population. Food Addit Contam Part A Chem Anal Control Expo Risk Assess. 2012;29(6):861–74.
55. Ascherio A, Hennekens CH, Buring JE, Master C, Stampfer MJ, Willett WC. Trans-fatty acids intake and risk of myocardial infarction. Circulation. 1994;89:94–101.
56. CDC.GOV [Internet]. Trans fats: the Facts [cited 2015 Jan 20]. Available from: http://www.cdc.gov/nutrition/everyone/basics/fat/transfat.html
57. di Castelnuovo A, Costanzo S, Bagnardi V, Donati MB, Iacoviello L, de Gaetano G. Alcohol dosing and total mortality in men and women: an updated meta-analysis of 34 prospective studies. Arch Intern Med. 2006;166(22):2437–45.
58. De Oliveira E Silva ER, Foster D, McGee Harper M, Seidman CE, Smith JD, Breslow JL, Brinton EA. Alcohol consumption raises HDL cholesterol levels by increasing the transport rate of apolipoproteins A-I and A-II. Circulation. 2000;102:2347–52.
59. Rimm EB, Williams P, Fosher K, Criqui M, Stampfer MJ. Moderate alcohol intake and lower risk of coronary heart disease: meta-analysis of effects on lipids and haemostatic factors. BMJ. 1999;319(7224):1523–8.
60. Albert MA, Glynn RJ, Ridker PM. Alcohol consumption and plasma concentration of C-reactive protein. Circulation. 2003;107(3):443–7.
61. Roerecke M, Rehm J. Irregular heavy drinking occasions and risk of ischemic heart disease: a systematic review and meta-analysis. Am J Epidemiol. 2010;171(6):633–44.
62. Boffetta P, Hashibe M. Alcohol and cancer. Lancet Oncol. 2006;7(2):149–56.
63. Hansel B, Thomas F, Pannier B, Bean K, Kontush A, Chapman MJ, et al. Relationship between alcohol intake, health and social status and cardiovascular risk factors in the urban Paris-Ile-De-France Cohort: is the cardioprotective action of alcohol a myth? Eur J Clin Nutr. 2010;64(6):561–8.
64. Corrao G, Rubbiati L, Bagnardi V, Zambon A, Poikolainen K. Alcohol and coronary heart disease: a meta-analysis. Addiction. 2000;95(10):1505–23.
65. Mukamal KJ, Conigrave KM, Mittleman MA, Camargo Jr CA, Stampfer MJ, Willett WC, et al. Roles of drinking pattern and type of alcohol consumed in coronary heart disease in men. N Engl J Med. 2003;348(2):109–18.
66. Chiva-Blanch G, Urpi-Sarda M, Ros E, Valderas-Martinez P, Casas R, Arranz S, et al. Effects of red wine polyphenols and alcohol on glucose metabolism and the lipid profile: a randomized clinical trial. Clin Nutr. 2013;32(2):200–6.
67. del Valle HB, Yaktine AL, Taylor CL, Ross AC, editors. Dietary reference intakes for calcium and vitamin D. Washington, DC: National Academies Press; 2011.
68. Goulding A, Cannan R, Williams SM, Gold EJ, Taylor RW, Lewis-Barned NJ. Bone mineral density in girls with forearm fractures. J Bone Miner Res. 1998;13:143–8.
69. Loro ML, Sayre J, Roe TF, Goran MI, Kaufman FR, Gilsanz V. Early identification of children predisposed to low peak bone mass and osteoporosis later in life 1. J Clin Endocrin Metab. 2000;85(10):3908–18.
70. Tucker KL, Hannan MT, Chen H, Cupples LA, Wilson PW, Kiel DP. Potassium, magnesium, and fruit and vegetable intakes are associated with greater bone mineral density in elderly men and women. Am J Clin Nutr. 1999;69(4):727–36.
71. Kontogianni MD, Melistas L, Yannakoulia M, Malagaris I, Panagiotakos DB, Yiannakouris N. Association between dietary patterns and indices of bone mass in a sample of Mediterranean women. Nutrition. 2009;25(2):165–71.
72. New SA. Intake of fruit and vegetables: implications for bone health. Proc Nutr Soc. 2003;62(04):889–99.
73. Remer T, Manz F. Potential renal acid load of foods and its influence on urine pH. J Am Diet Assoc. 1995;95(7):791–7.
74. Barzel US, Massey LK. Excess dietary protein can adversely affect bone. J Nutr. 1998;128(6):1051–3.
75. Fenton TR, Lyon AW, Eliasziw M, Tough SC, Hanley DA. Meta-analysis of the effect of the acid-Ash hypothesis of osteoporosis on calcium balance. J Bone Miner Res. 2009;24(11):1835–40.
76. Barzel US, Jowsey J. The effects of chronic acid and alkali administration on bone turnover in adult rats. Clin Sci. 1969;36:517–24.
77. Simon JA, Hudes ES. Relation of ascorbic acid to bone mineral density and self-reported fractures among US adults. Am J Epidemiol. 2001;154(5):427–33.
78. Jie KS, Bots ML, Vermeer C, Witteman JCM, Grobbee DE. Vitamin K status and bone mass in women with and without aortic atherosclerosis: a population-based study. Calcif Tissue Int. 1996;59(5):352–6.
79. Watkins BA, Li Y, Lippman HE, Seifert MF. Omega-3 polyunsaturated fatty acids and skeletal health. Exp Biol Med (Maywood). 2001;226(6):485–97.

80. Fulgoni III VL, Keast DR, Auestad N, Quann EE. Nutrients from dairy foods are difficult to replace in diets of Americans: food pattern modeling and an analyses of the National Health and Nutrition Examination Survey 2003-2006. Nutr Res. 2011;31(10):759–65.
81. Hiza HAB, Bente L. Nutrient content of the US Food Supply, 1909–2004: a summary report. USDA, Washington, DC. 2007. [Internet, cited 2015 Jan 5]. Available from: http://www.cnpp.usda.gov/sites/default/files/nutrient_content_of_the_us_food_supply/FoodSupply1909-2000.pdf
82. Lin PH, Ginty F, Appel LJ, Aickin M, Bohannon A, Garnero P, et al. The DASH Diet and sodium reduction improve markers of bone turnover and calcium metabolism in adults. J Nutr. 2003;133(10):3130–6.
83. Nicklas TA, O'Neil CE, Fulgoni III VL. The role of dairy in meeting the recommendations for shortfall nutrients in the American diet. J Am Coll Nutr. 2009;28(suppl):73S–81.
84. Ma J, Johns RA, Stafford RS. Americans are not meeting current calcium recommendations. Am J Clin Nutr. 2007;85(5):1361–6.
85. Bailey RL, Dodd KW, Goldman JA, Gahche JJ, Dwyer JT, Moshfegh AJ, et al. Estimation of total usual calcium and Vitamin D intakes in the United States. J Nutr. 2010;140(4):817–22.
86. Simopoulos AP. The Mediterranean food guide: Greek column rather than an Egyptian pyramid. Nutr Today. 1995;30(2):54–61.
87. Kafatos A, Verhagen H, Moschandreas J, Apostolaki I, Westerop JJV. Mediterranean diet of Crete: foods and nutrient content. J Am Diet Assoc. 2000;100(12):1487–93.
88. Lin PH, Aickin M, Champagne C, Craddick S, Sacks FM, McCarron P, et al. Food group sources of nutrients in the dietary patterns of the DASH-sodium trial. J Am Diet Assoc. 2003;103(4):488–96.
89. Dietary Guidelines for Americans. US Department of Health and Human Services, US Department of Agriculture. 2005 [Internet, cited 2015 Jan 5]. Available from: http://www.health.gov/dietaryguidelines/dga2005/document/html/chapter2.htm
90. Chiuve SE, Korngold EC, Januzzi JL, Gantzer ML, Albert CM. Plasma and dietary magnesium and risk of sudden cardiac death in women. Am J Clin Nutr. 2011;93(2):253–60.
91. Del Gobbo LC, Imamura F, Wu JH, de Oliveira Otto MC, Chiuve SE, Mozaffarian D. Circulating and dietary magnesium and risk of cardiovascular disease: a systematic review and meta-analysis of prospective studies. Am J Clin Nutr. 2013;98(1):160–73.
92. Larsson SC, Orsini N, Wolk A. Dietary magnesium intake and risk of stroke: a meta-analysis of prospective studies. Am J Clin Nutr. 2012;95(2):362–6.
93. Hata A, Ninomiya T, Mukai N, Hirakawa Y, Hata J, Ozawa M, et al. Magnesium intake decreases type 2 diabetes risk through the improvement of insulin resistance and inflammation: the Hisayama Study. Diabet Med. 2013;30(12):1487–94.
94. Reis MA, Reyes FG, Saad MJ, Velloso LA. Magnesium deficiency modulates the insulin signaling pathway in liver but not muscle of rats. J Nutr. 2000;130(2):133–8.
95. Weglicki WB, Phillips TM, Freedman AM, Cassidy MM, Dickens BF. Magnesium-deficiency elevates circulating levels of inflammatory cytokines and endothelin. Mol Cell Biochem. 1992;110(2):169–73.
96. Dietary reference intakes for calcium, phosphorus, magnesium, vitamin D, and fluoride. National Academy of Sciences. Institute of Medicine. Food and Nutrition Board. 1997. [Internet, cited 2015 Jan 5]. Available from: http://www.nal.usda.gov/fnic/DRI//DRI_Calcium/190-249.pdf
97. Moshfegh A, Goldman JD, Ahuja J, Rhodes D, LaComb R. (2009) What we eat in America, NHANES 2005-6: usual nutrient intakes from food and water compared to 1997 dietary reference intakes for vitamin D, calcium, phosphorus, and magnesium. U.S. Department of Agriculture, Agricultural Research Service pp. 1–24.
98. Calton JB. Prevalence of micronutrient deficiency in popular diet plans. J Int Soc Sports Nutr. 2010;7:24.
99. Marier JR. Magnesium content of the food supply in the modern-day world. Magnesium. 1985;5(1):1–8.
100. Yang Q, Liu T, Kuklina EV, Flanders WD, Hong Y, Gillespie C, et al. Sodium and potassium intake and mortality among US adults: prospective data from the Third National Health and Nutrition Examination Survey. Arch Intern Med. 2011;171(13):1183–91.
101. Fels J, Oberleithner H, Kusche-Vihrog K. Ménage à Trois: aldosterone, sodium and nitric oxide in vascular endothelium. Biochim Biophys Acta. 2010;1802(12):1193–202.
102. Büssemaker E, Hillebrand U, Hausberg M, Pavenstädt H, Oberleithner H. Pathogenesis of hypertension: interactions among sodium, potassium, and aldosterone. Am J Kidney Dis. 2010;55(6):1111–20.
103. Van Cromphaut SJ, Dewerchin M, Hoenderop JG, Stockmans I, Van Herck E, Kato S, et al. Duodenal calcium absorption in vitamin d receptor–knockout mice: functional and molecular aspects. Proc Natl Acad Sci U S A. 2001;98(23):13324–9.
104. Thacher TD, Clarke BL. Vitamin D insufficiency. Mayo Clin Proc. 2011;86(1):50–60.
105. Rosen CJ, Adams JS, Bikle DD, Black DM, Demay MB, Manson JE, et al. The nonskeletal effects of vitamin D: an endocrine society scientific statement. Endocr Rev. 2012;33(3):456–92.

106. Mitri J, Muraru MD, Pittas AG. Vitamin D and type 2 diabetes: a systematic review. Eur J Clin Nutr. 2011;65(9):1005–15.
107. Looker AC, Johnson CL, Lacher DA, Pfeiffer CM, Schleicher RL, Sempos CT. Vitamin D status: United States, 2001–2006. NCHS Data Brief No. 59 March 2011 US Department Of Health and Human Services, Centers for Disease Control and Prevention National Center for Health Statistics. 2011. [Internet, cited 2015 Jan 22]. Available from: http://www.cdc.gov/nchs/data/databriefs/db59.pdf
108. Webb AR. Who, what, where and when—influences on cutaneous vitamin D synthesis. Prog Biophys Mol Biol. 2006;92(1):17–25.
109. Lim HW, Gilchrest BA, Cooper KD, Bischoff-Ferrari HA, Rigel DS, Cyr WH, et al. Sunlight, tanning booths, and vitamin D. J Am Acad Dermatol. 2005;52(5):868–76.
110. Godar DE, Pope SJ, Grant WB, Holick MF. Solar UV doses of adult Americans and vitamin D3 production. Dermatoendocrinol. 2011;3(4):243.
111. Taylor CL, Patterson KY, Roseland JM, Wise SA, Merkel JM, Pehrsson PR, et al. Including food 25-hydroxyvitamin D in intake estimates may reduce the discrepancy between dietary and serum measures of vitamin D status. J Nutr. 2014;144(5):654–9.
112. Slavin J. Fiber and prebiotics: mechanisms and health benefits. Nutrients. 2013;5(4):1417–35.
113. Meyer KA, Kushi LH, Jacobs DR, Slavin J, Sellers TA, Folsom AR. Carbohydrates, dietary fiber, and incident type 2 diabetes in older women. Am J Clin Nutr. 2000;71(4):921–30.
114. Salas-Salvadó J, Martinez-Gonzalez MA, Bullo M, Ros E. The role of diet in the prevention of type 2 diabetes. Nutr Metab Cardiovasc. 2011;21:B32–48.
115. Dikeman CL, Fahey Jr GC. Viscosity as related to dietary fiber: a review. Crit Rev Food Sci. 2006;46(8):649–63.
116. Jenkins DJ, Kendall CW, Axelsen M, Augustin LS, Vuksan V. Viscous and nonviscous fibres, nonabsorbable and low glycaemic index carbohydrates, blood lipids and coronary heart disease. Curr Opin Lipidol. 2000;11(1):49–56.
117. Macfarlane GT, Macfarlane S. Fermentation in the human large intestine: its physiologic consequences and the potential contribution of prebiotics. J Clin Gastroenterol. 2011;45:S120–7.
118. Park Y, Subar AF, Hollenbeck A, Schatzkin A. Dietary fiber intake and mortality in the NIH-AARP Diet and Health Study. Arch Intern Med. 2011;171(12):1061–8.
119. Schröder H. Protective mechanisms of the Mediterranean diet in obesity and type 2 diabetes. J Nutr Biochem. 2007;18(3):149–60.
120. Anderson JW, Baird P, Davis Jr RH, Ferreri S, Knudtson M, Koraym A, et al. Health benefits of dietary fiber. Nutr Rev. 2009;67(4):188–205.
121. Clemens R, Kranz S, Mobley AR, Nicklas TA, Raimondi MP, Rodriguez JC, et al. Filling America's fiber intake gap: summary of a roundtable to probe realistic solutions with a focus on grain-based foods. J Nutr. 2012;142(7):1390S–401.
122. Riccardi G, Clemente G, Giacco R. Glycemic index of local foods and diets: the Mediterranean experience. Nutr Rev. 2003;61(s5):S56–60.
123. Pitsavos C, Panagiotakos DB, Tzima N, Chrysohoou C, Economou M, Zampelas A, et al. Adherence to the Mediterranean diet is associated with total antioxidant capacity in healthy adults: the ATTICA study. Am J Clin Nutr. 2005;82(3):694–9.
124. Boeing H, Bechthold A, Bub A, Ellinger S, Haller D, Kroke A, et al. Critical review: vegetables and fruit in the prevention of chronic diseases. Eur J Nutr. 2012;51(6):637–63.
125. Macready AL, George TW, Chong MF, Alimbetov DS, Jin Y, Vidal A, et al. Flavonoid-rich fruit and vegetables improve microvascular reactivity and inflammatory status in men at risk of cardiovascular disease—FLAVURS: a randomized controlled trial. Am J Clin Nutr. 2014;99(3):479–89. Erratum in: doi: 10.3945/ajcn.114.091884. *Am J Clin Nutr.* **100**(2),733.
126. Kelley DS, Rasooly R, Jacob RA, Kader AA, Mackey BE. Consumption of Bing sweet cherries lowers circulating concentrations of inflammation markers in healthy men and women. J Nutr. 2006;136(4):981–6.
127. Watzel B, Kulling SE, Moseneder J. A 4-week intervention with high intake of carotenoid-rich vegetables and fruit reduces plasma C-reactive protein in healthy, non-smoking men. Am J Clin Nutr. 2005;82:1052–8.
128. Sala-Vila A, Harris WS, Cofán M, Pérez-Heras AM, Pintó X, Lamuela-Raventós RM, et al. Determinants of the Omega-3 index in a Mediterranean population at increased risk for CHD. Br J Nutr. 2011;106(03):425–31.
129. Maillot M, Issa C, Vieux F, Lairon D, Darmon N. The shortest way to reach nutritional goals is to adopt Mediterranean food choices: evidence from computer-generated personalized diets. Am J Clin Nutr. 2011. doi:10.3945/ajcn.111.016501.
130. Estruch R, Ros E, Salas-Salvadó J, Covas MI, Corella D, Arós F, et al. Primary prevention of cardiovascular disease with a Mediterranean diet. N Engl J Med. 2013;368(14):1279–90.
131. Salas-Salvadó J, Garcia-Arellano A, Estruch R, Marquez-Sandoval F, Corella D, Fiol M, et al. Components of the Mediterranean-type food pattern and serum inflammatory markers among patients at high risk for cardiovascular disease. Eur J Clin Nutr. 2007;62(5):651–9.

132. Koloverou E, Esposito K, Giugliano D, Panagiotakos D. The effect of Mediterranean diet on the development of type 2 diabetes mellitus: a meta-analysis of 10 prospective studies and 136,846 participants. Metabolism. 2014;63(7):903–11.
133. Salas-Salvadó J, Bulló M, Babio N, Martínez-González MÁ, Ibarrola-Jurado N, Basora J, et al. Reduction in the incidence of Type 2 diabetes with the Mediterranean diet results of the PREDIMED-Reus nutrition intervention randomized trial. Diabetes Care. 2011;34(1):14–9.
134. Martínez-González MA, García-Arellano A, Toledo E, Salas-Salvado J, Buil-Cosiales P, Corella D, et al. A 14-item Mediterranean diet assessment tool and obesity indexes among high-risk subjects: the PREDIMED trial. PLoS One. 2012;7(8):e43134.
135. Babio N, Toledo E, Estruch R, Ros E, Martínez-González MA, Castañer O, et al. Mediterranean diets and metabolic syndrome status in the PREDIMED randomized trial. Can Med Assoc J. 2014;186(17):E649–57.
136. Djuric Z, Vanloon G, Radakovich K, Dilaura NM, Heilbrun LK, Sen A. Design of a Mediterranean exchange list diet implemented by telephone counseling. J Am Diet Assoc. 2008;108(12):2059–65.
137. Sidahmed E, Cornellier ML, Ren J, Askew LM, Li Y, Talaat N, et al. Development of exchange lists for Mediterranean and Healthy Eating Diets: implementation in an intervention trial. J Hum Nutr Diet. 2014;27: 413–25. doi:10.1111/jhn.12158.
138. Grimm KA, Scanlon KS, Moore LV, Grummer-Strawn LM. State-specific trends in fruit and vegetable consumption among adults. United States, 2000–2009. Morb Mortal Wkly Rep. 2010;59(35):1125–30.
139. Erinosho TO, Moser RP, Oh AY, Nebeling LC, Yaroch AL. Awareness of the Fruits and Veggies-More Matters campaign, knowledge of the fruit and vegetable recommendation, and fruit and vegetable intake of adults in the 2007 Food Attitudes and Behaviors (FAB) Survey. Appetite. 2012;59(1):155–60.
140. Stables GJ, Subar AF, Patterson BH, Dodd K, Heimendinger J, Van Duyn MA, Nebeling L. Changes in vegetable and fruit consumption and awareness among US adults: results of the 1991 and 1997 5 A Day for Better Health Program surveys. J Am Diet Assoc. 2002;102(6):809–17.
141. Krebs-Smith SM, Heimendinger J, Patterson BH, Subar AF, Kessler R, Pivonka E. Psychosocial factors associated with fruit and vegetable consumption. Am J Health Promot. 1995;10(2):98–104.
142. Rekhy R, McConchie R. Promoting consumption of fruit and vegetables for better health. Have campaigns delivered on the goals? Appetite. 2014;79:113–23.
143. Monsivais P, Mclain J, Drewnowski A. The rising disparity in the price of healthful foods: 2004–2008. Food Policy. 2010;35(6):514–20.
144. Goulet J, Lamarche B, Lemieux S. A nutritional intervention promoting a Mediterranean food pattern does not affect total daily dietary cost in North American women in free-living conditions. J Nutr. 2008;138(1):54–9.

Chapter 19
Building the Mediterranean Pyramid: Part A—Mediterranean Recipes

Ornella I. Selmin and Donato F. Romagnolo

Key Points

- In this chapter, we provide a compilation of selected recipes from the Mediterranean region (PART A). For each recipe, we cataloged information on the ingredients, quantities, and preparation.
- The recipes presented in this chapter are not intended as a medical recommendation, but as examples of dishes that can be prepared without specific culinary training. We are aware that among Mediterranean countries differences exist about cooking methods and exclusion of certain foods and wine based on cultural and religious customs.
- Extra-virgin olive oil was the preferred vegetable oil for dressing due to its wide use in Mediterranean countries. Unfortunately, because of space limitation not all pertinent Mediterranean recipes could be presented.
- We refer the reader to Chap. 20 for PART B of building the Mediterranean Pyramid in which we provide a nutritional assessment of these recipes and their use with other foods to balance a weekly food pyramid.

Keywords Mediterranean pyramid • Foods • Mediterranean recipes • Dish preparation

Introduction

In this chapter, we provide a compilation of selected recipes from the Mediterranean region. The recipes were a part of the instructional material used for the Mediterranean Diet & Health Study Abroad Program of The University of Arizona, Tucson, AZ [1]. This program provides an overview of

---

The recipes are from the instructional material prepared by La Cucina di Antonia Polese, Verona, Italy for the Mediterranean Diet & Health Study Abroad Program of The University of Arizona, Tucson, AZ [1]; and Vicente Sanchez of Casa Vicente, Tucson, AZ for the Research Frontiers in Nutritional Sciences Conference on "Health Benefits of the Mediterranean Diet, Bringing Science to the Plate," January 29–30, 2015, Department of Nutritional Sciences, The University of Arizona [2].

O.I. Selmin, Ph.D. (✉) • D.F. Romagnolo, Ph.D., M.Sc.
Department of Nutritional Sciences, The University of Arizona, Shantz Bldg, Tucson, AZ 85721, USA
e-mail: selmin@u.arizona.edu; donato@u.arizona.edu

D.F. Romagnolo, O.I. Selmin (eds.), *Mediterranean Diet*, Nutrition and Health,
DOI 10.1007/978-3-319-27969-5_19

(1) how dietary patterns and foods associated with the Mediterranean diet modify the risk of chronic diseases including obesity, diabetes and cancer; (2) the impact of foods in the Mediterranean diet on regulation of metabolic pathways; (3) how agriculture and food preparation contribute to culture and healthy living; and (4) how inclusion of Mediterranean foods in the Western diet can improve quality of life and reduce morbidity/mortality associated with chronic diseases. Also, recipe information was gathered from the Research Frontiers in Nutritional Sciences Conference on "Health Benefits of the Mediterranean Diet, Bringing Science to the Plate," January 29–30, 2015, Department of Nutritional Sciences, The University of Arizona. The agenda of the conference included several speakers who are contributors to this volume [2].

Mediterranean Recipes

For each recipe, we cataloged information on the ingredients, quantities, and preparation. Specific quantities for table salt were not included in the recipe as salt use may vary depending on individual preference and region as well as sodium dietary intake requirements (DRI) [3].

Vegetable-Pesto Pasta

For 6–8 people. Preparation time: 20–30 min; cooking time: 10–12 min.
Ingredients and directions:

- Pasta: 225 g penne pasta.
- Vegetables: Two vine tomatoes, half yellow pepper, one clove of garlic, and one pinch of red pepper; 30 ml extra-virgin olive oil; 15 g of toasted pine nuts; two basil leaves. Blanch the tomatoes, remove the skin and seeds and cut into cubes. Wash the peppers, remove the skin, and cut into small cubes. Stir together for 15 min in a bowl the tomatoes, bell pepper, garlic cloves cut in half, a pinch of red pepper and cover with olive oil. Set aside until pasta is ready. Remove the garlic and add the toasted pine nuts.
- Pesto: 15 g of fresh leaves of basil; half clove of garlic; 15 g of toasted pine nuts; 15 g of parmesan or pecorino cheese. Place all ingredients in a blender or a food processor and process until finely chopped and blended.
- Cook pasta "al dente" in salted water. After draining, dress pasta with the pesto sauce. Add the vegetables, garnish with basil leaves, and serve.
- Variation: if preferred, pasta could be dressed with pesto sauce only if the meal includes other vegetable dish.

Minestrone of Cereals and Legumes

For 6–8 people. Preparation time: 30 min; cooking time: 40 min.
Ingredients and directions:

- 200 g pearl barley; 100 g of dried pinto beans; 50 g of lentils; 100 g of pumpkin; 60 g of cabbage; 100 g of cauliflower; two potatoes; one leek; one carrot; one onion; one stalk of celery; one clove of garlic; one bay leaf and three sage leaves; one sprig of rosemary; 2.5 L of water; extra-virgin olive oil; salt and freshly ground pepper.

- Soak the beans in water for about 12 h (e.g., overnight). Wash the barley in cold water and boil in salted water for about 25–30 min. Drain the beans and add them to cold water without salt, and boil them for 20–30 min or until cooked. Then, set aside. Peel, wash, and chop celery, carrot, and onion and sauté in a pan with two tablespoons of extra-virgin olive oil. Add the chopped vegetables, lentils, bay leaf, water, and cook for about 40 min. Add beans and cook for another 5 min. Season with salt and pepper.
- Take two tablespoons of soup, pass them through the vegetables mill and add them to the rest of the preparation. Complete with the addition of barley and chopped herbs. Serve with a drizzle of extra-virgin olive oil and freshly ground pepper.
- Variation: pasta (little egg pasta, i.e., maltagliati, farro (*Triticum* sp.) could be added to the minestrone soup.

Bread with Olive Oil, Garlic and Tomato (Similar to Italian Bruschetta and Spanish Pan Con Tomate)

For 6–8 people. Preparation time: 15–20 min.

Ingredients and directions:

- Six slices of bread (~250 g total) (i.e., French baguette, Greek, Italian ciabatta, grain bread); four ripe tomatoes; one clove of garlic; extra-virgin olive oil (45 ml); salt and pepper.
- Blanch the tomatoes in boiling salted water for a few seconds; drain and pass under running cold water. Remove the skin and seeds and cut into small cubes, then place them in a colander and sprinkle with salt. Toast the slices of bread, rub with a clove of garlic; cover with the diced tomato and with extra-virgin olive oil.

Braised Lentils

For 6–8 people. Preparation time: 10–15 min; cooking time: 40 min.

Ingredients and directions:

- Ingredients: 300 g of lentils; one small onion; one carrot (medium); one stalk of celery; one clove of garlic; one bay leaf; two ripe tomatoes (medium); 300 ml vegetable broth; one sprig of rosemary; two sage leaves; one sprig of thyme; four tablespoons of extra-virgin olive oil; salt and pepper;
- Clean, wash, and soak the lentils for about 10 min. Drain and toast lentils in a large pan with oil. Add the finely chopped vegetables, bay leaf, tomatoes (after removing the skin and seeds), and add the vegetable broth. Cook for 30/40 min with the lid on. Season with salt and pepper and add the chopped herbs.
  Variation: add small egg pasta or cereal (e.g,. rice, farro—*Triticum* sp., ~20 g/person).

Rice with Shrimps and Vegetable Leaves (i.e., Radicchio, Cichorium *sp.; Spinach, or Dandelions)*

For 6–8 people. Preparation time: 25 min; cooking time: 18 min.
Ingredients and directions:

- Ingredients: 350 g rice; 300 g shrimp; 100 g of red radicchio; 1 L of water (or shrimp broth if available); one onion; one carrot; one celery; one bay leaf; one sprig of thyme; one clove of garlic; one shallot or onion; one teaspoon of curry; half cup (~115 ml) of white wine; 20 ml extra-virgin olive oil; salt and pepper.
- Shell the shrimp, wash thoroughly and set aside the shells. In a saucepan, put one tablespoon (~15 ml) of olive oil, onion, carrot, and celery cut into small pieces, add the herbs and the shells of shrimp, brown, deglaze with the wine, let it evaporate and cover with hot water. Add a little salt and cook for about half an hour, strain and keep warm.
- In a frying pan with two tablespoons of oil, cook for a few minutes the red radicchio, cut into strips and set aside. In the same pan, cook for a few minutes the shrimps with olive oil, garlic previously crushed, curry, salt and pepper.
- In a saucepan, saute` the shallots in a little oil, add the rice and toast, pour a bit at a time the hot broth and continue cooking until the rice is "al dente," Add the radicchio and shrimps, season with salt and pepper, and toss with olive oil. Serve warm.
- Variation: replace radicchio with spinach or dandelions.

Flan of Leeks and Onions

For 6–8 people. Preparation time: 10 min; cooking time: 40 min.
Ingredients and directions:

- 3–4 tablespoons of bread crumbs; two white onions; 400 g leeks, trimmed; two egg yolks; 50 ml heavy cream; 50 ml whole milk; four tablespoons grated Parmesan cheese; two tablespoons extra-virgin olive oil; salt and pepper.
- Prepare a buttered and dusted with breadcrumbs mold (~22 × 16 cm), and keep it in the fridge until ready to use. Clean, wash, and slice the onions, wash the leeks and cut into rounds. Add onions and leeks in a pan, with the olive oil, a few tablespoons of water, and salt. Cook (low-heat) for 20–25 min (do not need to brown).
- Place the onions and leeks in a colander and let drain while cooling down. In a bowl, beat the egg yolks, the cream and milk, a tablespoon of grated Parmesan cheese, salt and pepper.
- Place on the mold the drained onions and leeks, sprinkle with remaining cheese, and then pour the mixture of egg yolks and cream/milk. Bake in oven at 170 °C for 15–20 min. Serve the flan warm.

Egg Pasta and Beans

For 6–8 people: preparation time: 20 min; cooking time: 1 h.

Ingredients and directions: 500 g of dried pinto beans; 2 L of water; one carrot; one onion; one stalk of celery; 120 g of fresh egg pasta; six tablespoons extra-virgin olive oil; fresh rosemary; salt; six tablespoons Parmesan cheese, and freshly ground pepper.

- Soak the beans for 12 h (e.g., overnight). Drain the soaked beans and place in a pot with about 2 L of cold water without salt, and cook over low heat for about 40–50 min; add salt only at the end.
- Chop carrot, onion, celery and fry in a pan with a little olive oil.
  When the beans are cooked, pass one half through a mill and pour the puree over the sauce, season with salt and pepper. Cook the pasta, drain it and add it to the sauce. Add the leftover beans and olive oil and mix. Serve the pasta adding on top freshly ground pepper, Parmesan cheese, and chopped rosemary.

Couscous with Vegetables

For 6–8 people: preparation time: 20 min; cooking time: 1 h.

Ingredients and directions: 300 g of whole wheat pre-cooked couscous; four tablespoons of extra-virgin olive oil; 200 g of zucchini; 150 g of cannellini (white kidney, Greek fasolia) beans; three carrots; one pepper (1/2 yellow and 1/2 red); ten cherry tomatoes; 30 g of raisins; 30 g of toasted pine nuts; one teaspoon saffron; one tablespoon of parsley.

- Put the beans to soak in warm water for 3 h, drain and boil them in unsalted water. Wash very well the raisins and soak them in water.
- In a saucepan, boil 350 ml (~1/3 of L) of lightly salted water, pour it over the couscous, add two tablespoons of extra-virgin olive oil, and stir occasionally.
- Dissolve the saffron in a ladle of hot water, add to the couscous, and stir to mix it.
- Clean and wash the zucchini, cut off the green and reduce it into cubes; cook for a few min in a pan with one tablespoon of extra-virgin olive oil; add salt and pepper. In the same pan, brown the carrots and peppers and add them to the couscous with the cooked beans.
- Wash the tomatoes and cut them in half; remove the seeds, and add the sliced tomatoes to the couscous.
- Drain the raisins and mix them with the couscous. Add the pine nuts and garnish with chopped parsley, one tablespoon of extra-virgin olive oil and let rest (1–2 h) until serving.
- Variation: if you decide to prepare the couscous yourself, bring water to boil, remove from the stove, add the couscous and cover the pan. Let sit and mix a few times until ready.

Mediterranean Sea Bass

For 6–8 people. Preparation time: 10 min; cooking time: 30 min.

Ingredients and directions: one sea bass, ~0.5 kg; 100 g cherry tomatoes; ten olives; 0.5 tablespoon salted capers; oregano; 2.5 tablespoons of extra-virgin olive oil; two bay leaves; fennel bunch to decorate; salt and pepper.

- Scale the fish with a knife or other tool. After cleaning and rinsing the fish, dry with paper towels. Rub the fish with salt, both inside and outside. Place the fish in the middle of a sheet of baking paper.
- Sprinkle with oregano and spread over the fish tomatoes, olives, capers (desalted) and one tablespoon of olive oil.
- Close the foil and bake in preheated oven at 200 °C for about 30 min. Serve warm, decorate with herbs and dress with extra-virgin olive oil.

Polenta and Sardines

For 6–8 people. Preparation time: 40 min; cooking time: 40 min.

Ingredients and directions: 220 g corn flour; 1 L water; one tablespoon chive; 250 g sardine fillets; 150 ml milk; one tablespoon extra-virgin olive oil; 200 g finely chopped onion; 20 g pine nuts; 20 g raisins; 100 ml white vinegar; 100 ml dry white wine; salt and pepper.

- Pour the flour slowly into boiling salted water, cook for about 40 min mixing frequently. Then, add the chopped chives and mix. Pour the polenta on a baking dish and let it cool, then turn it upside down on a cutting board.
- With a round pastry cutter, cut the polenta in squared pieces 3 cm high and 6 cm wide, and place the pieces in a greased pan. With a spoon, carve the top of each polenta piece to create a cup-like groove.
- Cut the sardine fillets into strips, soak them in milk for 30 min, drain, dry on paper towel, dust with flour, and fry in extra-virgin olive oil for a few min, then put them in a baking dish.
- Saute` the onion with a tablespoon of extra-virgin olive oil; then add the vinegar and wine and reduce slowly. Turn off the heat. Add the pine nuts and raisins, mix. Fill the top of each piece of polenta with the sardine fillets. Cover with the onion/pine nuts/raisin sauce. Heat in the oven for 10 min, then serve on a bed of vegetable leaves (e.g., green lettuce).

Shell Seafood Au Gratin

For 6–8 people. Preparation time: 25 min; cooking time: 10 min.

Ingredients and directions: 150 g swordfish; 100 g fresh tuna; 75 g peeled shrimps; 50 g fresh salmon; 60 ml of dry white wine; two tablespoons vegetable broth; one slice of bread for crumbs; one tablespoon grated Parmesan cheese; half tablespoon chopped parsley; one clove of garlic (minced); 1.5 tablespoons extra-virgin olive oil; salt and pepper; large scallop shells.

- Cut swordfish, salmon and shrimp into small pieces and transfer them into a bowl.
  Drizzle with half tablespoon of olive oil, salt, pepper and let rest in the refrigerator for 30 min.
  Mix the bread crumbs, Parmesan cheese, garlic, parsley, salt, and pepper.
- Oil the empty shells with a kitchen brush, place one piece of each fish in each shell; sprinkle with a tablespoon of vegetable broth; sprinkle with flavored bread and drizzle with extra-virgin olive oil. Bake at 200 °C for 8–10 min.

Roast in Pistachio Crust with Herbs

For 6–8 people. Preparation time: 15 min; Cooking time: 20–30 min.

Ingredients and directions: 300 g pork tenderloin; 1.5 tablespoons extra-virgin olive oil; half carrot; half onion; half stem celery; half clove garlic; salt and pepper. For the pistachio mix: 30 g fresh peeled pistachios; 15 g toasted pine nuts; 10 g blanched almonds; half tablespoon rosemary; half tablespoon thyme; salt and pepper.

- Chop the pistachios, pine nuts and almonds with herbs (rosemary, thyme); salt and pepper and place the mixture on a sheet of parchment paper.
- Wash and dry the meat, lightly rub with garlic and wrap it in the chopped herbs.

- In a saucepan, brown the fillet with extra-virgin olive oil, add the vegetables and cook for about 20 min.
- Serve the sliced tenderloin at room temperature with the reduced juices (or with a balsamic vinaigrette–extra-virgin olive oil mix).
- Variation: replace the pork tenderloin with lean lamb tenderloin.

Chicken with Olives and Nuts

For 6–8 people; Preparation time, 15 min; cooking time 20–30 min.

Ingredients and directions: 250 chicken breast; half carrot; half onion; half celery stalk; half sprig parsley; half sprig thyme; three bay leaves; 60 g green and black olives; 20 g capers; lemon juice (~half a lemon); half teaspoon mustard; 15 g toasted pine nuts; 1.5 tablespoons chopped hazelnuts; salt and pepper.

- Prepare a vegetable broth with about a liter of water, flavored with the vegetables and the bouquet garnish (parsley, thyme, bay leaves, salt) and when the broth boils, dip the chicken breasts. Cook for about 15 min at low-medium heat making sure that the water does not come to a boil, turn off and leave the chicken breast in the broth for another 20 min.
- After removing the chicken from the water, let it cool down and cut it into thin slices.
- Prepare the sauce: whisk together extra-virgin olive oil, four tablespoons of broth, lemon juice, mustard, salt and pepper; season the chicken with the sauce, add the olives cut into quarters, and the capers washed and dried. Sprinkle the chicken with toasted pine nuts and chopped hazelnuts, and serve on a bed of green lettuce or endives.

Spanish Paella

For eight people. Preparation time, 30–45 min; cooking time, 45–50 min.

Ingredients and directions: 25 ml extra-virgin olive oil; two chicken thighs; 1.5 garlic cloves; half onion; half red pepper; half green pepper; one tomato; 100 g squids; 0.75 L water; 2.0 g turmeric yellow powder; 0.5 g saffron; 175 g rice (e.g., Arborio); 60 g green peas; 60 g green beans; 75 g clams with shell; 75 g mussels with shell; 120 shrimps; 15 g pimento in strings; one lemons; salt and pepper.

- In a Paella pan (~30–50 cm diameter) prepare a Spanish "sofrito": heat the extra-virgin olive oil. Add the chicken thighs, previously salted and peppered, and cook on high fire until golden. Lower the heat and add the garlic to roast. When the chopped garlic is yellow-golden, add the chopped onion and the red and green peppers. Stir to roast. When the onion becomes golden, add the chopped tomatoes and mix.
- In half a cup of hot water, dissolve the saffron and the turmeric and add to the sofrito and mix. Then, add the chopped squid and green beans and stir at medium-high heat.
- Add the water, mix, and salt (to taste) and bring to boiling temperature. Add the rice and mix.
- Then, add the green peas and mix; follow with mussels, clams, and shrimps with mixing. Cook for ~20–25 min then let rest for ~5 min. Decorate with pimento and lemon slices. Serve warm.
- Variation: replace cooking water with fat-free chicken or vegetable broth. Some regional Spanish recipes may include other meats in addition to chicken.

Crudites with Olive, Mustard, and Citronette Sauce

For six people. Preparation time: 15–20 min. Cooking time: 0 min.

Ingredients and directions: two carrots; two heads of Belgian endive; one red pepper; one yellow pepper; 15 cherry tomatoes; two fennels, five stalks of celery; one head of red radicchio (or other *Cichorium* sp.).

- Wash all the vegetables and cut them into strips. Browse and wash the leaves of radicchio. In a large plate, put all the vegetables inside the leaves of radicchio and serve with the sauces.
- *Olive sauce*: 250 g green and black olives; one clove of garlic; 50 g anchovy fillets; 25 g salted capers; 80 ml extra-virgin olive oil; juice and zest of half lemon; salt and pepper.
- Blend all the ingredients.
- *Mustard vinaigrette*: 100 g olive oil; 15 g mustard seeds; four tablespoons white vinegar; salt and pepper.
- *Citronette*: 100 ml extra-virgin olive oil; 50 ml lemon juice; salt and pepper. Mix all the ingredients.

Seasonal Vegetables "Au Gratin"

For 6–8 people. Preparation time: 15 min; cooking time: 30 min.

Ingredients and directions: one yellow pepper; one red pepper; two medium potatoes; three ripe tomatoes; one eggplant; two white onions or two leeks; four tablespoons of breadcrumbs; 60 g parmesan or pecorino cheese; one tablespoon oregano; one tablespoon extra-virgin olive oil; salt and pepper.

- Wash the peppers and cut into strips. Peel the potatoes, wash and cut into slices (1/5 in. thick). Wash and slice the tomatoes, eggplant, and onions (1/2 in. thick). Mix the breadcrumbs with cheese and oregano.
- Oil a sheet of baking paper covering an oven plate, and arrange the vegetables slightly crossed. Sprinkle with flavored bread, add salt, pepper and drizzle with a little olive oil.
  Place the plate in an oven pre-heated to 180 °C and bake for about 30 min, until the vegetables are tender and have formed a golden crust on the surface. Serve warm.

Sweet and Sour Pumpkin Dessert

For six people. Preparation time: 15 min; cooking time 30 min.

Ingredients and directions: 60 g sugar; 100 ml apple vinegar; one clove (1/4 tsp ground); 500 g peeled pumpkin; one tablespoon extra-virgin olive oil; one tablespoon thyme; 20 g raisins; 15 g toasted pine nuts; salt and pepper.

- Cook the sugar at low-medium heat with a tablespoon of water, vinegar, and the clove. When starting to caramelize, add the remaining apple vinegar and continue cooking until obtaining a syrup-like sauce.
- Cut the pumpkin into cubes, season with two tablespoons of olive oil, a pinch of thyme, salt and pepper.
- In a large skillet cook the pumpkin and at the end pour the sweet and sour sauce, add the pine nuts, raisins, stir and season with salt and pepper. Let stand covered for 2–3 h.

Lemon Cream with Berries

For eight people. Preparation time: 5 min; cooking time: 8 min.

Ingredients and directions: 500 ml heavy cream; 80 g sugar; juice of two lemons; 75 g fresh strawberries; 75 g fresh raspberries; 75 g fresh blueberries; one tablespoon powdered sugar; lemon zest.

- Warm up the cream with the sugar and the lemon zest. Cool down and add the lemon juice. Mix and pour into individual bowls. Store in the fridge for at least 3–4 h. Garnish with berries and powdered sugar before serving.

Rustic Pie with Extra-virgin Olive Oil

For ten people. Preparation time: 15 min; cooking time: 35 min.

Ingredients and directions: 10 g raisins; 125 g flour; 4 g teaspoon of baking powder; 10 g toasted pine nuts; 60 ml extra-virgin olive oil; 80 g sugar; one lemon (juice and zest); one large egg; salt; half tablespoon powdered sugar.

- Preheat the oven to 180 °C (350 °F); Soak, wash and dry the raisins. Sift flour with baking powder, then add the raisins, pine nuts, and a pinch of salt. Add the extra-virgin olive oil, sugar, lemon juice and zest in a bowl and whisk until emulsified. Add the egg yolks and beat until mixture is fluffy. Add to the flour mix.
- Beat the egg whites with a teaspoon of lemon and add them to the flour mixture, pour it into a baking pan (12–14 in. in diameter, ~25–30 cm) and bake for about 30 min.
  Turn out the cake and let it cool on a wire rack. Sprinkle with powdered sugar.

Olive Oil and Almonds Cookies

Preparation time: 15 min; cooking time: 15 min.

Ingredients and directions to prepare 24 cookies: 250 g flour; 100 g of sugar; 60 ml of extra-virgin olive oil; 100 g peeled and chopped almonds; two eggs.

- Arrange the flour and salt on a work surface, slowly add all ingredients and knead. Shape the dough into a loaf. Lay on a baking sheet covered with parchment paper and bake for 7–8 min at 180 °C (350 °F). Remove the paper and allow to cool down; cut the loaf diagonally to obtain cookies ~¾ in. thick.
- Put the cookies back in the oven and bake at the same temperature for 5–6 min.

Summary and Conclusions

We refer the reader to Chap. 20 (PART B) for an assessment of the nutritional contribution of each recipe and their potential use to balance a weekly Mediterranean food pyramid for a target individual with different lifestyle (sedentary, active, very active). The recipes presented in this chapter are not intended as a medical recommendation, but as working examples of dishes that can be prepared without specific culinary training. Figure 19.1 presents examples of various recipes. We regret that because of space limitation not all pertinent recipes are included.

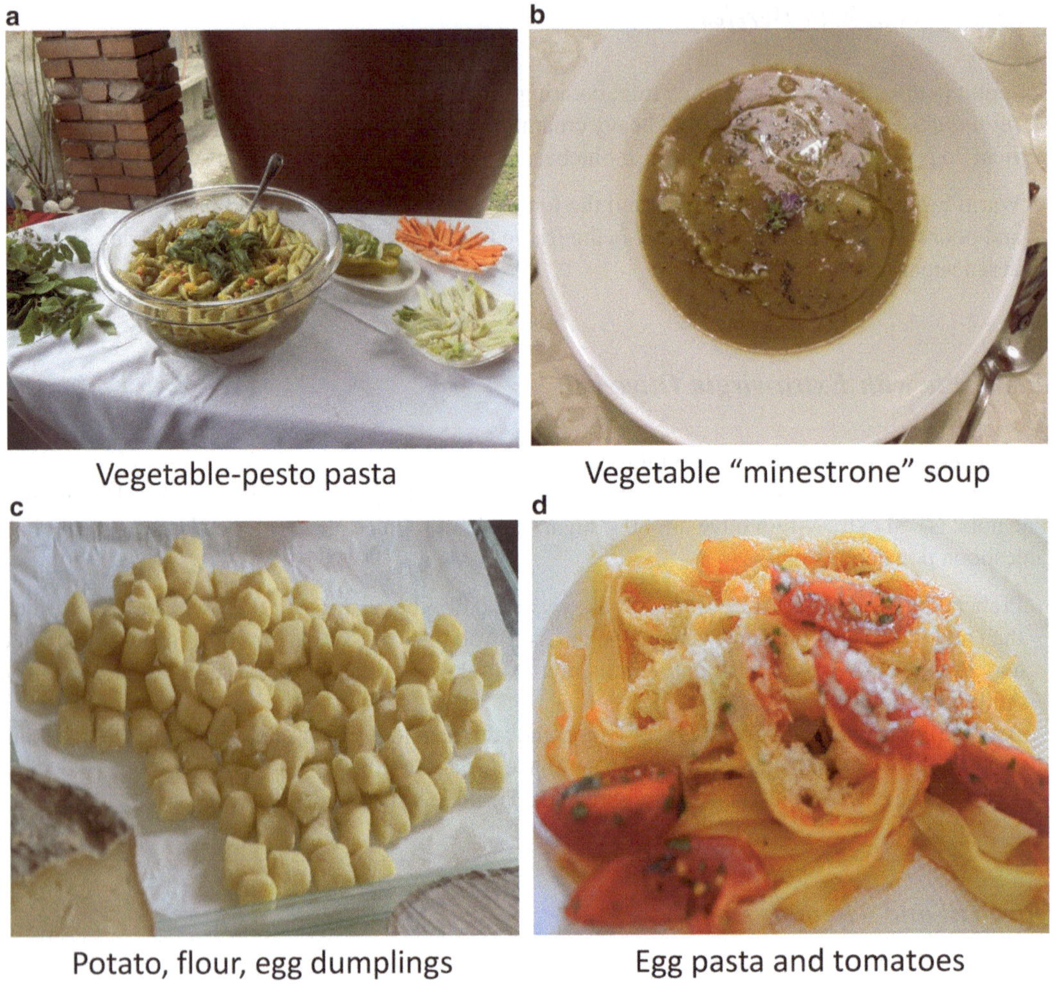

Fig. 19.1 Examples of common Mediterranean dishes. (**a**) Vegetable-pesto pasta; (**b**) Minestrone of cereals and legumes; (**c**) potato, flour, and egg dumplings; (**d**) egg pasta with tomatoes; (**e**) rice with shrimp and vegetables; (**f**) flan of leek and onions; (**g**) bread with herbs and salmon; (**h**) couscous with tomatoes and herbs; (**i**) Mediterranean sea bass with tomatoes; (**j**) polenta and sardines; (**k**) shell seafood au gratin; (**l**) roast in pistachio crust with herbs; (**m**) chicken with olives and nuts; (**n**) rice (Spanish) paella; (**o**) crudites (with olive, mustard or citronette sauce); (**p**) seasonal vegetables "au gratin"; (**q**) aged cheese; (**r**) lemon cream with berries; (**s**) rustic pie with extra-virgin olive oil and berries; (**t**) pumpkin flowers

These dishes may be served, as is often the case in Mediterranean countries, as separate courses, which enhances tasting of food flavors and enriches the gathering around the table with family and friends. It also helps organizing meals into smaller portion sizes while increasing food variety, for example for lunch a traditional meal may include pasta or other cereal grain dish with vegetable or fish, a salad, and some fruits; whereas dinner may include fish, chicken or other meats or aged cheese with salad and fruits and wine if desirable and culturally acceptable. In the Mediterranean region, extra-virgin olive oil is the preferred vegetable oil for dressing, so when using other vegetable oils one should consider the loss of phenolic compounds normally found in extra-virgin olive oil. These dishes are often accompanied with various servings of cheese and wine.

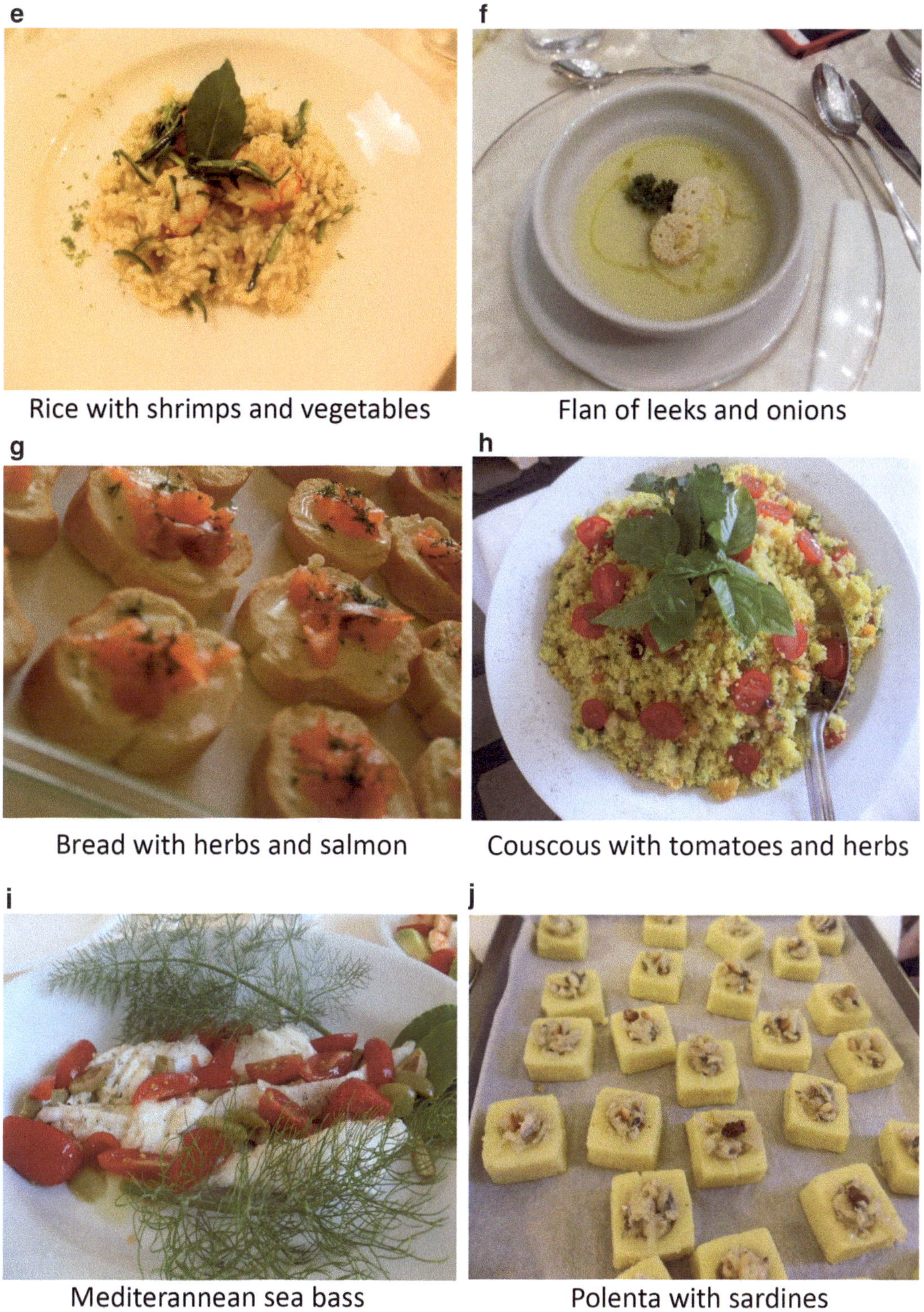

Fig. 19.1 (continued)

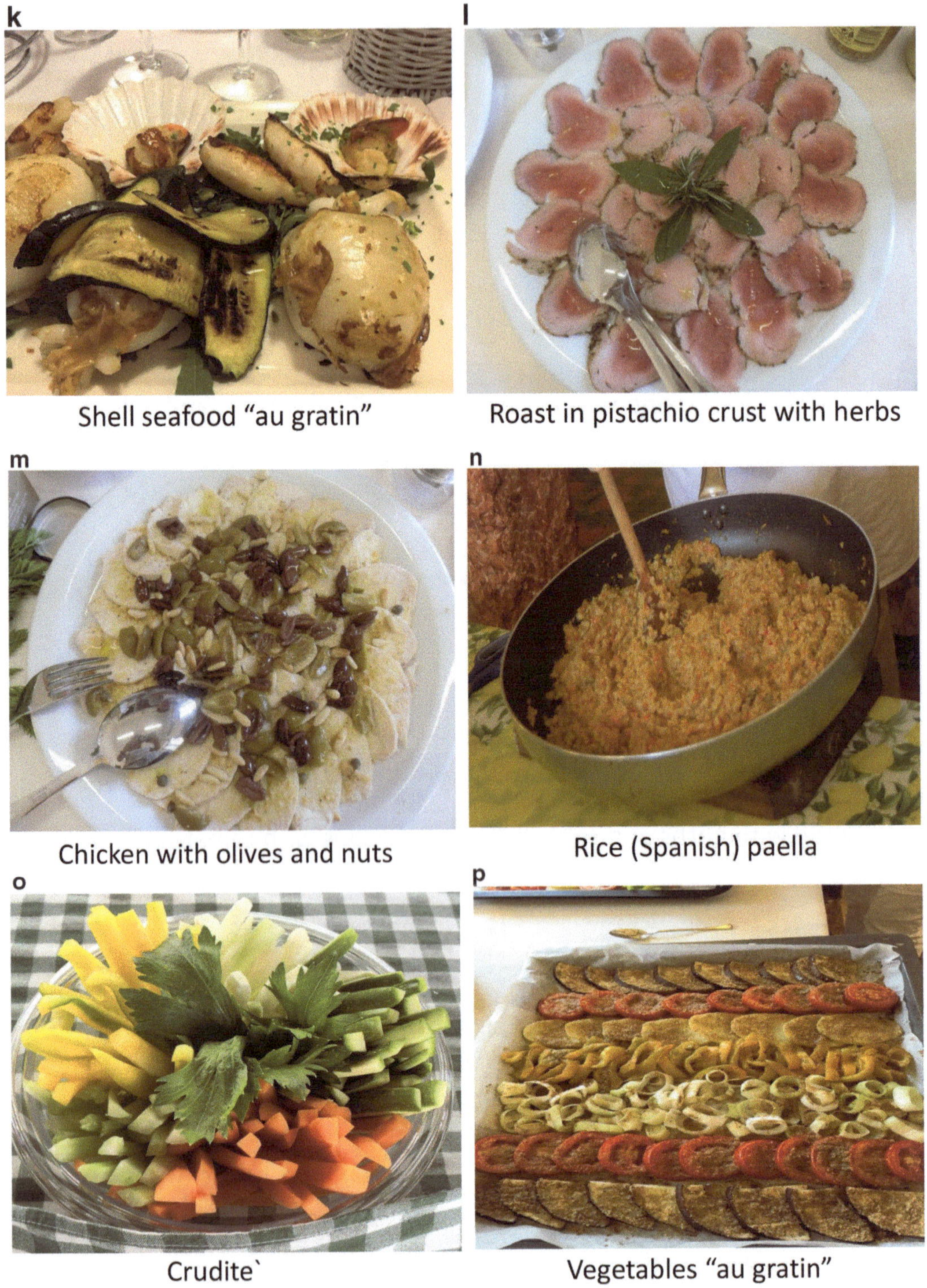

Fig. 19.1 (continued)

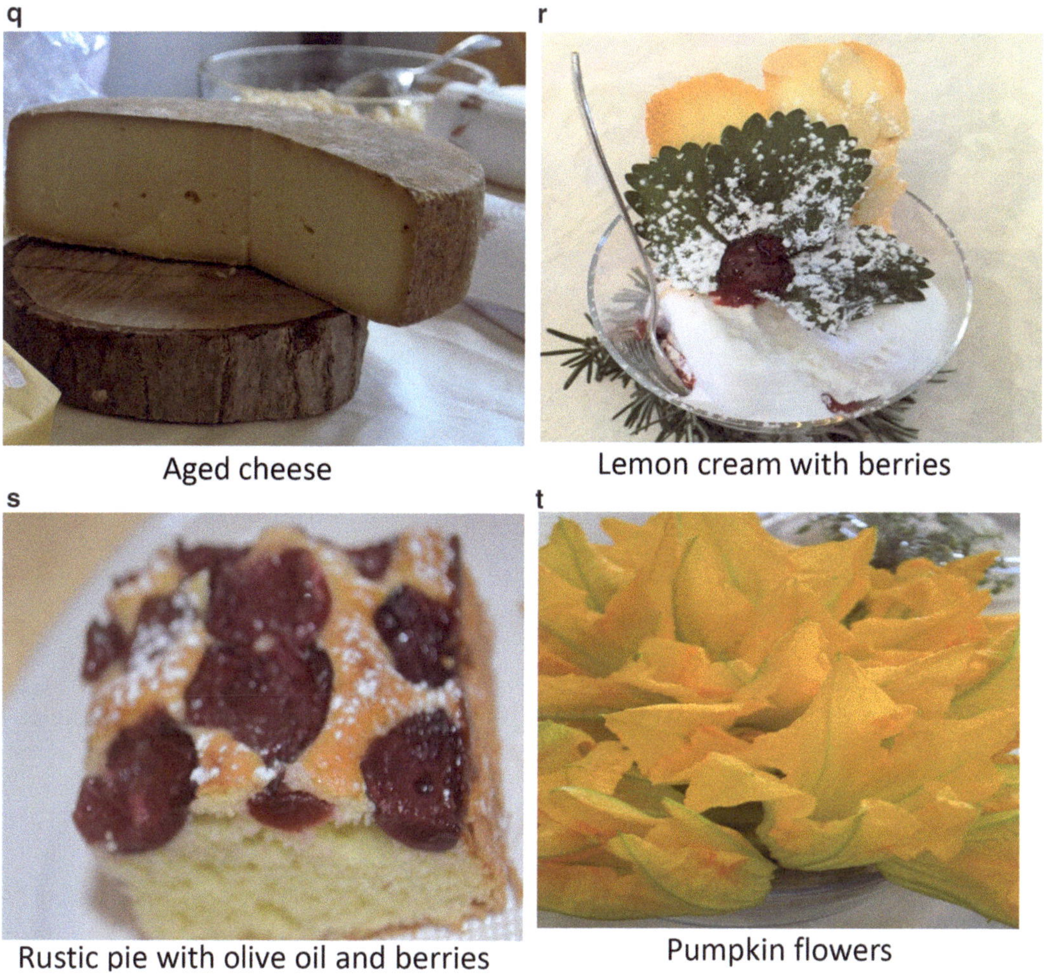

Fig. 19.1 (continued)

References

1. Mediterranean Diet & Health Study Abroad Program of The University of Arizona, Tucson, AZ. Available at: http://nutrition.cals.arizona.edu/mediterranean-diet-and-health. Accessed 13 Oct 2015.
2. Research Frontiers in Nutritional Sciences Conference, "Health Benefits of the Mediterranean Diet, Bringing Science to the Plate", January 29–30, 2015, Department of Nutritional Sciences, The University of Arizona, Tucson, AZ. Available at: http://nutrition.cals.arizona.edu/nutrition-schedule.
3. U.S. Department of Agriculture. Dietary Reference Intake Calculator for Healthcare Professionals. http://fnic.nal.usda.gov/fnic/interactiveDRI/dri_results.php. Accessed 10 Sep 2015.

Chapter 20
Building the Mediterranean Pyramid: Part B—Balancing the Plate

Donato F. Romagnolo, Kelly A. Jackson, Patricia L. Sparks, and Ornella I. Selmin

Key Points

- The traditional Mediterranean diet finds its roots in the diverse cultures and traditions of the countries bordering the Mediterranean Sea. Foundational elements of the Mediterranean pyramid can be found in those of the 1960' in Crete, much of Greece and Southern Italy.
- Completing the traditional Mediterranean pyramid is wine, usually consumed in moderation with meals, although not by all Mediterranean populations, regular physical activity, in the past mostly associated to agricultural activities; and opportunities for conviviality and social interactions.
- Overlapping in food recommendations across different cultures suggests that even people who reside in non-Mediterranean countries could include into their lifestyle Mediterranean-like foods that complement ethnic dishes and improve health. In Chap. 19, we compiled examples of Mediterranean recipes with information about ingredients and preparation.
- In this chapter, we present estimates of nutrients composition for those recipes and their inclusion into a weekly food program following some of the dietary guidelines of the Mediterranean diet. Opportunities exist for inclusion into modern diets of a diverse list of foods and for balancing our plates through adoption of a Mediterranean-like pyramid approach.

Keywords Mediterranean diet • Balancing the plate • Food pyramid • Healthy eating and lifestyle

Introduction

The traditional Mediterranean diet finds its roots in the diverse cultures and traditions of the countries bordering the Mediterranean Sea. The fact that foods and dietary habits vary considerably among populations facing the Mediterranean basin makes it difficult to develop specific nutrition standards for food choices, intakes, and recipes. This is complicated further by vast differences in lifestyle and physical activity (e.g., sedentary, active, very active). Foundational elements of the Mediterranean

D.F. Romagnolo, Ph.D., M.Sc. (✉) • K.A. Jackson, M.S., R.D. • P.L. Sparks, Ph.D. • O.I. Selmin, Ph.D.
Department of Nutritional Sciences, The University of Arizona, Shantz Bldg, Tucson, AZ 85721-0038, USA
e-mail: donato@u.arizona.edu; kjackson@email.arizona.edu; psparks@email.arizona.edu; selmin@u.arizona.edu

D.F. Romagnolo, O.I. Selmin (eds.), *Mediterranean Diet*, Nutrition and Health,
DOI 10.1007/978-3-319-27969-5_20

pyramid are those of the 1960' in Crete, much of Greece and Southern Italy and include from top (used sparingly) to bottom (used more often) [1]:

1. Red meat (a few times in small amount/month).
2. Sweets, a few times/week; more often fresh fruit as dessert.
3. A maximum of four eggs/week or lower.
4. Poultry, a few times/week.
5. Fish, a few times/week.
6. Cheese and yogurt, daily.
7. Olive oil, as primary dietary fat, daily and often in combination with fresh salads.
8. Vegetables, fruits, beans, other legumes and nuts; herbs and spices, daily.
9. Bread, pasta, rice, couscous, polenta, bulgur (*Durum* sp.) wheat, other grains and potatoes, daily.

Completing the traditional Mediterranean pyramid is wine, depending on religious and cultural beliefs, usually consumed in moderation with meals; regular physical activity; and opportunities for conviviality and social interactions.

Prior to industrialization, limited processing and commercial exchange favored consumption of locally produced foods and seasonality of dishes often tied to religious and cultural events. Overall, the traditional Mediterranean diet would provide less than ~7–8 % energy as saturated fat with total fat mainly from olive oil, contributing on average ~25–35 % energy, with upper levels approaching ~35–40 %. Results of early epidemiological studies informed that adoption of a Mediterranean-like diet and lifestyle was associated with improved health and longevity [2]. As discussed throughout this volume, however, considerable changes in dietary choices have contributed in Western and even Mediterranean countries to the growing prevalence of overweight/obesity and related diseases (i.e., diabetes). These trends beg the question of what major changes in food intake and behavior have occurred during the last three decades that contributed to the overweight and obesity epidemics in modernized communities.

Data from the US Census Bureau [3] about consumption of major food commodities and commercially available fruits and vegetable from 1980 to 2009 revealed that consumption of eggs and total red meat (beef, veal, lamb and mutton, and pork) actually decreased by ~9 % and 16 %, respectively (Fig. 20.1a). Conversely, during the same period there has been an increase in the consumption of flour and cereal products (~35 %), and total dairy products (~12 %). Consumption of total vegetables and fish and shellfish increased by ~15 % and 27 % respectively (Fig. 20.1b), whereas there have been no major changes in consumption of total fruits and butter. Interestingly, there have been major increases in the consumption of poultry (~70 %); total cheese (~87 %) (mozzarella cheese consumption nearly tripled from 3 to ~11 lb/capita); salad and cooking oils (~145 %); high-fructose corn syrup (~165 %); and non-frozen yogurt (~413 %). These data suggest there has been a major increase in the intake of high-energy density foods (mainly fats and sugars) compared to fish, fruits, and vegetable, whose consumption had not changes or increased slightly, with no impactful changes in intake of total red meat and eggs. Specifically, the per capita consumption of salad and cooking oils increased from ~21.0 lb in 1980 to ~52.0 lb in 2009. For high-fructose corn syrup, consumption increased from 19.0 lb in 1980 to ~50 lb in 2009. Thus, compared to 1980, higher intakes of cooking oils and high-fructose contributed in 2009 to an increase of ~350 kcal/day (~250–300 kcal/day from cooking oils, ~38 g/day and ~100 kcal/day from high-fructose corn syrup, ~38 g/day at ~2.8 kcal/g). These estimates approach the energy intake data from the National Health and Nutrition Examination Survey (NHANES) indicating that between 1971 and 2000, the average total energy consumption among US adults increased by ~22 % in women, from 1542 to 1886 kcal/day (+344 kcal), and by 10 % in men from 2450 to 2693 kcal/day (+243 kcal/day), with a large percentage (~30 %) of adults engaging in no aerobic leisure-time physical activity [4] (Fig. 20.2). Clearly, the increased energy intakes associated with reduced physical activity represent major risk factors for overweight, obesity, and other chronic diseases (i.e., cardiovascular, diabetes, and cancer).

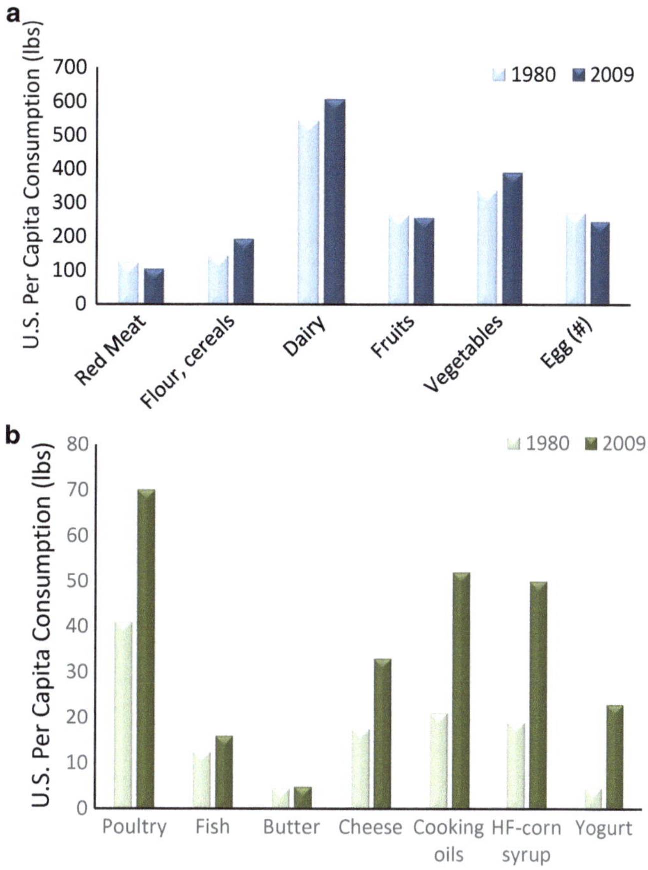

Fig. 20.1 Changes in US consumption of major foods commodities and commercially available fruits and vegetables from 1980 to 2009 [3]

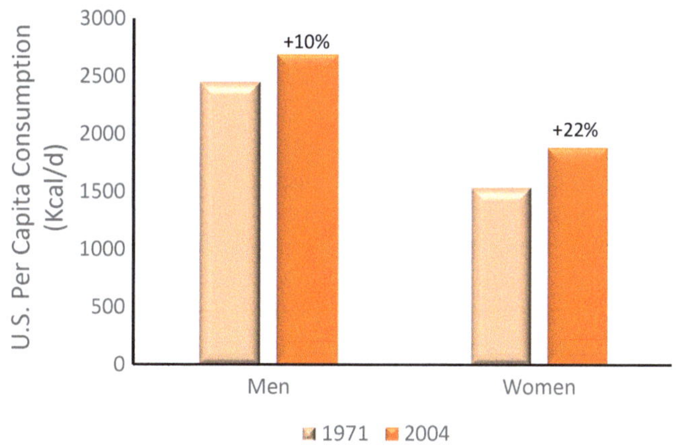

Fig. 20.2 Changes in US per capita energy consumption from 1971 to 2004 [4]

During the last three decades, changes in agricultural activities and globalization of food supplies have modified food behavior not only in Western societies but also in traditional Mediterranean communities. Interestingly, the Mediterranean pyramid shares various characteristics with other ethnic dietary patterns (i.e., Asian) that recommend low levels of refined sugars and processed grains; high intake of fruits and vegetables, nuts, and legumes; plant oils other than olive oil (i.e., peanut oil);

limited dairy products and red meat while poultry and eggs appear more often [5]. This suggests that populations residing in Western countries could include into their diets foods that complement various healthy ethnic diets and customs (i.e., Indo-Mediterranean [6]). This approach may afford some flexibility when preparing meals while maintaining traditional and local heritages, and enjoying eating tasty meals.

In recognition of the societal changes that have occurred during the last three decades within Mediterranean countries and advances in nutrition and health research, a new Mediterranean Diet Pyramid for today's lifestyle was released in 2011 [7]. This was a multinational effort that involved various research institutions and public health agencies in countries around the Mediterranean region as well as international nutrition and health organizations. The next section describes the nutritional components of various Mediterranean recipes and their inclusion into a Mediterranean Pyramid.

Balancing the Plate

Nutritional Assessment of Mediterranean Recipes

In Chap. 19, we presented various examples of Mediterranean recipes with information about ingredients and preparation. As a follow-up, we first estimated the macronutrient composition for each recipe (Table 20.1). Recipes with foods that contribute to the base of the Mediterranean pyramid (i.e., pasta, rice, cereals, couscous, and bread dishes) tend to have higher energy content from carbohydrates ranging from 44 to 63 %. Conversely, for fish and meat-based recipes, a higher percentage of energy is derived from fat and protein (~40–60 %). For most recipes, monounsaturated fatty acids, mainly from olive oil, contribute the highest energy of total fat except for dairy-based recipes for which saturated fat contributes ~50 % of energy. Expectedly, vegetables-based recipes provide the highest fiber/serving (e.g., braised lentils, ~17 g/serving; crudites and couscous with vegetables, ~9 g/serving). The recipes that contribute the highest total cholesterol/serving (~80 mg) include shrimp- and dairy-based desserts. We are aware that nutrition parameters for recipes are estimates and actual composition may vary based on many factors including chemical composition of ingredients, regional plant varieties, agricultural practices (i.e., irrigation), harvesting and processing techniques, storage and cooking methods, and portion sizes. For example, variations in fatty acid profile from olive oil should be considered due to tree variety, age of olives, and processing [8]. Spain, Italy, and Greece produce most of the olive produced in the Mediterranean region and significant variability exists in fatty acid composition and phenolic compounds. A good quality olive oil should have at least ~73 % oleic acid and less than ~10 % linoleic acid producing an oleic/linoleic acid ratio greater than 7 [9]. According to standards set by the International Olive Council (OIC) [10], the percentage of the various fatty acids should be within the following ranges: monounsaturated fatty oleic acid (18:1) from 55 to 83 %; palmitic (16:0), stearic (18:0), and arachidic (20:0) acid from ~7.5 to 20 %, 0.5–5.0 %, and <0.6 % respectively; linoleic (18:2), linolenic (18:3), and gadoleic (20:1) acid from 3.5 to 21 %, and <1.0 %, and <0.4 %, respectively. Therefore, even in Mediterranean-like diets some provisions need to be made for the intake of both saturated (e.g., 16:0 and 18:0) and polyunsaturated (18:2; 18:3) fatty acids from olive oil and olive consumption in addition to those coming from dairy foods. Also, the concentration of phenolic compounds in olive oil can vary greatly. For example, total phenols were reported to vary from ~242 mg/kg in the variety Arbequina to ~550–600 mg/kg in the Cornicabra and Picual varieties [11].

Table 20.1 Macronutrient composition of selected Mediterranean recipes presented in Chap. [19]

Recipes and servings		Energy (kcal)	Fat (g)	SFA (g)	PUFA (g)	MUFA (g)	Chol. (mg)	Protein (g)	Carbohydrates (g)	Fiber (g)
Vegetable pesto pasta[a]	6 people	232.0	9.3	1.4	2.5	4.5	1.7	7.0	31.0	1.9
	8 people	174.0	7.0	1.0	1.8	3.4	1.3	5.2	23.2	1.5
	% kcal		34.0	5.0	9.0	17.0	–	11.0	54.0	–
Minestrone of cereals and legumes[b]	6 people	197.0	6.5	1.0	1.4	3.8	–	5.0	32.0	5.4
	8 people	147.0	4.9	0.7	1.0	2.9	–	3.8	24.0	4.1
	% kcal		29.0	14.6	21.1	59.2	–	8.1	62.6	–
Bread, olive oil, garlic, and tomato[c]	6 people	176.0	8.2	1.3	1.3	5.3	–	4.0	22.0	1.6
	8 people	132.0	6.2	1.0	1.0	4.0	–	2.9	16.4	1.2
	% kcal		41.0	6.0	6.0	26.0	–	9.0	50.0	–
Braised lentils[d]	6 people	272.0	9.1	1.4	1.3	6.7	–	14.0	34.0	16.5
	8 people	204	7.4	1.0	1.0	5.0	–	11.0	26.0	13.4
	% kcal		32.0	1.4	13.1	68.5	–	18.0	50.0	–
Rice with shrimp and radicchio[e]	6 people	188.0	6.0	1.0	1.0	3.7	80.0	11.0	21.0	1.6
	8 people	141.0	4.5	0.8	0.8	2.8	60.0	8.3	15.4	1.2
	% kcal		28.7	16.3	16.5	61.0	–	24.0	44.0	–
Flan of leeks and onions[f]	6 people	147.0	10.5	3.8	1.0	5.2	76.0	3.7	11.0	1.4
	8 people	110.0	7.9	2.9	0.7	3.9	57.0	2.8	8.0	1.0
	% kcal		63.0	37.0	9.3	49.5	–	10.0	27.0	–
Egg pasta and beans[g]	6 people	318.0	22.0	3.5	5.0	12.5	10.5	8.0	24.0	4.7
	8 people	239.0	16.3	2.6	3.7	9.5	8.0	6.0	18.0	3.7
	% kcal		60.0	16.0	23.0	58.0	–	10.0	30.0	–
Couscous with vegetables[h]	6 people	295.0	13.0	1.6	3.0	7.5	–	10.0	37.3	9.2
	8 people	221.0	9.8	1.2	2.3	5.6	–	7.4	28.0	6.9
	% kcal		38.5	12.3	22.0	59.0	–	11.5	50.3	–
Mediterranean sea bass[i]	6 people	185.0	11.0	1.9	2.2	6.3	41.5	19.0	2.1	0.7
	8 people	139.0	8.3	1.5	1.7	4.7	31.0	14.2	1.6	0.6
	% kcal		52.6	17.1	20.0	57.0	–	43.5	3.6	–
Polenta and sardines[j]	6 people	310.0	12.0	2.5	3.0	5.2	37.0	14.2	34.0	3.3
	8 people	232.0	9.0	1.9	2.3	3.9	27.5	10.6	25.0	2.5
	% kcal		33.6	21.0	25.7	43.8	–	18.0	43.2	–
Shell seafood "au gratin"[k]	6 people	127.0	5.6	1.1	1.0	3.15	41.0	14.0	2.9	0.2
	8 people	96.0	4.2	0.8	0.7	2.4	30.5	10.5	2.2	0.1
	% kcal		39.0	8.0	7.0	22.0	–	46.0	9.0	–
Roast, pistachio crust, herbs[l]	6 people	145.5	9.3	1.4	2.2	5.0	32.5	12.5	3.5	1.1
	8 people	109.5	9.5	1.1	1.7	3.7	24.5	9.7	2.6	0.9
	% kcal		55.0	9.0	13.0	30.0	–	35.0	10.0	–

(continued)

Table 20.1 (continued)

Recipes and servings		Energy (kcal)	Fat (g)	SFA (g)	PUFA (g)	MUFA (g)	Chol. (mg)	Protein (g)	Carbohydrates (g)	Fiber (g)
Chicken with olives and nuts[m]	6 people	189.0	14.3	2.0	2.2	9.1	39.2	13.3	2.7	1.0
	8 people	141.0	10.5	1.5	1.7	6.8	30.0	9.8	2.0	0.8
	% kcal		64.0	13.5	15.4	64.0	–	21.0	4.7	–
Spanish paella[n]	8 people	162.0	7.3	1.5	1.3	3.8	62.5	12.2	12.0	2.0
	% kcal		40.0	21.0	18.3	53.0	–	31.0	28.0	–
Vegetables[o]	6 people	71.0	0.7	0.2	0.3	–	–	3.7	15.0	9.0
	% kcal		6.0	26.0	50.0	–	–	11.0	58.0	–
Olives[p]	6 people	182.0	18.2	2.6	2.0	13.0	3.4	3.0	3.4	1.5
	% kcal		87.0	12.0	9.0	62.0	–	7.0	6.0	–
Mustard[p]	6 people	161.0	17.4	2.3	11.3	75.6	–	0.6	1.0	0.4
	% kcal		96.0	13.0	2.0	70.0	–	1.0	3.0	–
Vinaigrette[p]	6 people	150.0	17.0	2.3	1.8	12.0	–	–	1.0	–
	% kcal		98.0	14.0	10.0	72.0	–	–	2.0	–
Seasonal vegetables "au gratin"[q]	6 people	200.5	7.0	2.5	1.0	3.0	7.0	7.6	30.0	6.5
	8 people	150.0	5.3	1.8	0.7	2.3	5.0	5.6	22.3	4.8
	% kcal		30.0	10.0	4.0	14.0	–	13.0	56.0	–
Sweet, sour pumpkin dessert[r]	6 people	111.0	4.0	0.5	6.5	13.0	–	1.3	19.0	7.3
	% kcal		33.0	4.0	9.0	17.0	–	3.0	64.0	–
Lemon cream with berries[s]	8 people	271.0	23.4	14.5	0.9	6.8	86.0	1.6	21.0	1.3
	% kcal		76.0	47.0	3.0	22.0	–	2.0	22.0	–
Rustic pie, extra-virgin olive oil[t]	10 people	153.5	7.5	1.1	1.1	4.8	32.2	2.5	19.5	0.5
	% kcal		43.0	7.0	7.0	28.0	–	6.0	50.0	–
Olive oil, almond cookies[u]	Cookie	104.0	5.0	0.6	0.8	3.2	17.5	2.5	13.0	0.8
	% kcal		41.0	5.0	7.0	26.0	–	9.0	50.0	–
Aged cheese[v] (cow, goat)	30 g serving	118–136	7.8–10.7	4.9–7.4	0.2	2.2–2.5	20–31	9.0–11.0	0.7–1.0	–

[a]High in complex carbohydrates and medium/high in calories (174–232 kcal/serving); medium in protein and fat (mainly monounsaturated from olive oil)

[b]Medium in calories (197 kcal/serving); low content of protein and fiber (~5.5 g/serving)

[c]Medium calories (132–176 kcal/serving). Fats are low mainly monounsaturated fatty acids from olive oil; low in fiber if not grain bread

[d]Medium/high calories (204–272 kcal/serving); medium protein, and fiber (~16 g)

[e]Medium calories (~141–188 kcal/serving)

[f]Medium calories (110–147 kcal) and fat content mainly from monounsaturated

[g]High calories (~239–320 kcal/serving) and medium fat (16.3–22.0 g/serving) mainly from monounsaturated

[h]High calories (221.0–295.0 kcal/serving); medium fat (9.8–13.0 g/serving) mainly from monounsaturated, and low/medium fiber (~6.9–9.2 g/serving)

[i]Medium-calories (139–185 kcal/serving); medium/high in protein (14–19.0 g/serving) and low/medium in fat (8.3–11.0 g/serving, ~50 % from monounsaturated mainly from olive oil)

[j]High calories (232–310.0 kcal/serving); medium protein (10.6–14.2 g/serving)

Table 20.1 (continued)

[k]Medium calories (96–127 kcal/serving) and low fat (4.2–5.6 g/serving); medium protein (10.5–14.0 g/serving) and low in fiber (<0.5 g/serving)
[l]Medium calories (109–145.5 kcal) and fat (~9.5 g) mainly monounsaturated; and medium/high in protein (9.7–12.5 g)
[m]Medium calories (141–189 kcal), protein (~9.8–13.3 g), and fat (10.5–14.3 g/serving). Low in carbohydrates (2.0–2.7 g/serving)
[n]Medium calories (162 kcal), low fat (7.3 g), and low carbohydrates (12 g/serving)
[o]Low calories (71 kcal); medium in fiber (~10 g)
[p]Medium calories (~150–180 kcal/serving), medium in fat (17–18 g/serving) mostly monounsaturated
[q]Medium/high calories (150–200 kcal) and medium carbohydrates (22–30 g)
[r]Low calories (~110 kcal) and carbohydrates (19 g); low fat (4 g) and protein (1.3 g)
[s]High calories (271 kcal) and fat (23 g); low in protein (~1.6 g) and fiber (~1.3 g)
[t]Medium calories (153 kcal) and carbohydrates (~20 g); low in protein (2.5 g) and fiber (<1 g)
[u]Medium in calories (~105 kcal/cookie)
[v]Aged cow parmesan, goat cheese

Building the Pyramid

Based on the nutritional information of the various recipes and foods listed in Table 20.1, we developed a weekly food pyramid following the 14-item food questionnaire criteria used to evaluate adherence to a Mediterranean diet by patients enrolled in the "PREvencion con DIeta MEDiterranea (PREDIMED) trial [12] (Box 20.1). A 1-point increase in this 14-point Mediterranean diet adherence questionnaire was associated with a 12.5 % decrease in cardiovascular disease incidence (also see Chap. 1). To meet the constraints of the PREDIMED study, we created serving units for breakfast (low and high protein), vegetable, fruits, aged cheese, and mixed nuts (30 g/day, 3 servings/week) which were used to balance daily nutrient requirements for a food pyramid (Box 20.2). Often a Mediterranean meal would include small quantities of soft or aged cow, sheep, or goat cheese either with pasta, a salad, e.g., arugula and parmesan cheese as is the case for the Italian cuisine; or feta cheese and olives in a salad in Greece. For example, for the hard Italian cheeses Parmigiano Reggiano and Grana Padano (3.9 kcal/g), the fat content ranges from 24 to 28 %, of which ~81 % is saturated, whereas the remaining (~7–8 %) is mostly monounsaturated. These cheeses have a high content in protein (~33–36 %). Other popular soft cheeses (i.e., French Brie, Camembert) have a similar caloric content (~3.5 kcal/g), with fat and protein ranging from 25 to 30 % and 17 to 22 %, respectively [13]. As an example and to meet nutritional goals, the weekly food pyramid included the consumption of 30 g/day of hard parmesan/goat cheese. Mixed nuts were included as a rich source of MUFA, which approach 24 % (g/100) in pistachios, peanuts, and brazil nuts; 28–30 % in cashews and almonds; 41 % in pecans; 46 % in hazelnuts, and ~60 % in macadamia nuts. Also, we included 1 glass of wine/day except for day 6 (2 glasses) and day 7 (1.5 glasses) to meet the wine requirement (≥7 glasses/week) of the PREDIMED questionnaire [12] (Box 20.1).

Table 20.2 summarizes daily and weekly values for macronutrients and some micronutrients (vitamin D) and minerals (calcium, sodium, and potassium) for the food pyramid built using the recipes and foods listed in Table 20.1 and Box 20.2. Overall, energy from total fat ranged from ~23 to 40 % with an average value for the week of 33 %. Average energy from SFA was 7 % and only on day 6 it approached ~11.0 %. Average energy from PUFA and MUFA was 5.2 % and 18.5 %, respectively, whereas average energy contribution from protein and carbohydrates was ~12.0 % and ~60.0 % respectively. Average fiber was ~50 g/day. These values for macronutrients were within range or above minimum requirements suggested to be adequate for meeting nutritional goals when adopting Mediterranean food choices [14, 15]. We also compared the average nutrition parameters of the pyramid to the USDA DRI goals for a male individual, 40 years of age, body weight 68 kg, height 175 cm; BMI = 22.2; and with different physical activities (sedentary, active, and very active) [16] (Table 20.2).

Table 20.2 Nutrient composition of weekly dietary pyramid built using recipes presented in Chap. 19

Weekly pyramid	Energy (kcal)	Fat (g)	SFA (g)	PUFA (g)	MUFA (g)	Chol. (mg)	Prot. (g)	Carbohydrates (g)	Fiber (g)	Vit. D (μg)	Ca (mg)	Na (mg)	K (mg)
Day 1	2430	99.6	19.0	17.0	59.0	55.8	67.0	326.6	50.0	9.6	996.7	2137	5307
	% kcal	36.8	7.0	6.3	21.8	–	12.1	59.1	–	–	–	–	–
Day 2	2476	82.1	16.1	11.9	47.9	139.8	68.0	365.2	44.0	1.0	958.0	2033	5781
	% kcal	28.4	4.3	4.5	17.4	–	10.8	67.95					
Day 3	2486	113.0	23.5	18.8	66.5	110.0	67.9	304.7	54.4	1.4	1060	2110	4659
	% kcal	40.0	8.5	6.8	24.1	–	12.0	53.9	–	–	–	–	–
Day 4	2436	85.4	17.0	14.0	49.4	78.6	67.2	351.0	46.8	2.2	1017	1828	5460
	% kcal	31.5	6.2	5.2	18.3	–	12.0	63.4	–	–	–	–	–
Day 5	2537	91.3	17.9	16.5	45.6	66.9	70.2	368.1	52.2	1.4	1035	1568	4987
	% kcal	32.4	6.4	5.8	16.1	–	12.1	63.8	–	–	–	–	–
Day 6	2487	100.8	30.2	11.9	55.4	211.2	65.5	324.5	42.8	1.7	1057	2257	4882
	% kcal	36.5	10.9	4.3	20.0	–	11.6	57.4	–	–	–	–	–
Day 7	2426	61.7	16.1	9.3	32.6	149.5	67.7	307.8	56.4	2.5	1394	2044	6217
	% kcal	22.9	6.0	3.5	12.0	–	12.3	55.8	–	–	–	–	–
Average:	2468	90.6	20.0	14.2	51.0	116.0	67.6	335.0	49.5	2.8	1074	1996	5327
% kcal		33.0	7.0	5.2	18.5	116.0	12.0	60.0					
Maillot [14, 15]	(%) kcal	20–35	≤10	6–11	15–20	<300	10–20	50–75	≥30.0			2500[a]	

DRI [16]:													
Sedentary	2307	51–90	[b]	[c]	[c]	[d]	54	260–375[e]	38	15.0[f]	1000[g]	<2300[h]	4700
Active	2814	63–109	[b]	[c]	[c]	[d]	54	317–457	38	15.0	1000	<2300	4700
Very active	3280	73–128	[b]	[c]	[c]	[d]	54	369–533	38	15.0	1000	<2300	4700

[a]Maximum 2759 mg for men; 2365 mg for women

[b]Target values were calculated using the DRI for a male subject, 40 years of age, body weight, 68 kg; BMI = 22.2, and various physical activities (sedentary; active; very active) [16]

[c]As low as possible while consuming a nutritionally adequate diet (REF). Levels of monounsaturated plus polyunsaturated of ~20–30 % energy reduced the risk of cardiovascular disease [17, 18]

[d]As low as possible while consuming a nutritionally adequate diet [16]

[e]Based on DRI contributing ~50–71.5 % total energy [16]. Carbohydrates are from recipes only and do not include beverages, sodas, or any other source of sweetened food or drink

[f]Vitamin D levels from simple foods only and do not take into account supplemental vitamin D from fortified foods (e.g., milk) or production from sun exposure

[g]Calcium levels from foods only

[h]Sodium values are from foods only and do not included added table salt

Box 20.1: 14-Item Questionnaire of Mediterranean Diet Adherence

	Criteria for diet adherence
1. Use of olive oil as main culinary fat	Yes
2. Olive oil consumption	≥4 tbsp/day
3. Number of vegetable servings (~200 g/serving)	≥2/day
4. Number of fruit units	≥3/day
5. Servings of red meat (1 serving = 100–150 g)	<1/day
6. Servings of butter, margarine, or cream (1 serving = 12 g)	<1/day
7. Sweet or carbonated beverages	<1/day
8. Wine drinks	≥7 glasses/week
9. Servings of legumes (1 serving, ~150 g)	≥3/week
10. Servings of fish or shellfish (1 serving, 100–150 g of fish; 4–5 units or 200 of shellfish)	≥3/week
11. Consumption of commercial (not homemade) sweets or pastries	<3/week
12. Serving of nuts	≥3 week
13. Consume preferentially chicken	Yes
14. Consume vegetable, pasta, rice, and other dishes prepared with sauces made with tomatoes, onions, leeks, garlic and olive oil	≥2/week

Box 20.2: Food Pyramid

	Daily dishes
Day 1	**Breakfast** : grain bagel/toast with preserve, whole yogurt, fruit salad, coffee. **Lunch**: vegetable pasta, fruit, mixed nuts (30 g). **Dinner**: minestrone, bread and olives, vegetables, sea bass, potatoes, wine (1 glass), grated parmesan cheese with minestrone or end of meal (~30 g).
Day 2	**Breakfast**: grain bagel/toast with preserve, whole yogurt, fruit salad, coffee. **Lunch**: rice with shrimps, potatoes, vegetables, fruits. **Dinner**: minestrone soup, pan con tomate, roast with pistacchio, potatoes, vegetables, rustic pie, wine (1 glass), hard parmesan/goat cheese with main course or end of meal (~30 g).
Day 3	**Breakfast**: grain bagel/toast with preserve, whole yogurt, fruit salad, coffee. **Lunch**: egg pasta and beans, vegetables, fruit, mixed nuts (30 g). **Dinner**: flan of leeks, bread with olives and garlic, vegetables, braised lentils, wine (1 glass), hard parmesan/goat cheese with main course or end of meal (~30 g).
Day 4	**Breakfast**: grain bagel/toast with preserve, whole yogurt, fruit salad, coffee. **Lunch**: couscous with vegetables, vegetables, fruits. **Dinner**: polenta and sardines, bread with olives, potatoes, vegetables, olive oil cookie, wine (1 glass), hard parmesan/goat cheese with main course or end of meal (~30 g).
Day 5	**Breakfast**: grain bagel/toast with preserve, whole yogurt, fruit salad, coffee. **Lunch** : shell seafood, vegetables, fruits. **Dinner**: bread with olives, pasta with vegetables, potatoes, vegetables, fruits, wine (1 glass), hard parmesan/goat cheese (~30 g) with main course or end of meal.
Day 6	**Breakfast**: grain bagel/toast with preserve, whole yogurt, fruit salad, coffee. **Lunch**: chicken with olives and nuts, vegetables, fruits. **Dinner**: pan con tomate or bruschetta, paella, vegetables, lemon cream with fruits, wine (2 glasses), hard cheese (~30 g) with paella or end of meal.
Day 7	**Breakfast**: grain bagel/toast with preserve and egg, whole yogurt, fruit salad, coffee. **Lunch**: crudite' with olives, fruits. **Dinner**: bread with olives, vegetables "au gratin" and potatoes, fruits, wine (1.5 glass), hard parmesan/goat cheese (~30 g) with vegetables or end of meal.

Average pyramid values for daily energy (2468 kcal/day), fat (90.6 g/day), carbohydrates (335.0 g/day), fiber (49.5 g/day), calcium (1074 mg/day), sodium (1996 mg/day), and potassium (5327) fell within or met the DRI requirements targets. It should be noted that recipes used to build the weekly food pyramid did not include table salt, which should be used with a reference target of <2.300 mg/day. Average levels of MUFA plus PUFA (~24 %) fell within the range of 20–30 % found to be associated with a reduced risk of cardiovascular diseases [17, 18]. Average protein (~68 g/day) was above the 54 g/day calculated DRI but below the maximum recommended level (~15 % energy from protein) [15]. On the other hand, a protein intake moderately higher than current recommendations (0.8 g/kg body weight/day, ~13 % energy) has been suggested as a strategy to provide health benefits for adults and aging populations [19] as well as assist with body weight/fat loss [20]. In comparison, the average protein intake in the USA is ~98 g/day for men, and 68 g/day for women, mainly consumed during the evening meals. Distributing protein consumption over the various daily meals may improve protein utilization. Conversely, average vitamin D levels from foods (2.8 μg/day) were well below the DRI requirements of 15 μg/day. Only on day 1 of the food pyramid vitamin D levels approached ~10 μg/day primarily from fish (sea bass recipe) further reinforcing the concept that food pyramids rich in fish and fish oils may provide higher, albeit not sufficient, daily levels of vitamin D to support endogenous vitamin production through skin exposure to ultraviolet light or supplementation via supplements or fortified foods and milk. The inadequacy of the food pyramid presented in Table 20.2 to satisfy vitamin D requirements is in keeping with findings of studies of nutrient intakes in Europe showing mean intakes for both males and females below estimated average requirements [21]. Similarly, estimates from NHANES confirmed the average vitamin D intake levels in the USA from foods was well below the recommended DRI levels and ranged from ~150 to 300 IU/day (~3.8–7.5 μg/day) [22]. Finally, energy from alcohol in wine ranged from ~130 to 200 kcal/day, which was below the recommended level of <10 % energy/day [15]. Calculations were extended to a male 60 years of age, and a female (40 and 60 years of age) with different BMI and physical activities (sedentary, active, very active).

Summary and Conclusions

Foundational elements of the Mediterranean pyramid have been associated to improved health and longevity. During the last three decades, the average total energy consumption among US adults has increased for both men and women, with a large percentage of adults engaging in no aerobic leisure-time physical activity. We estimated the macronutrient, vitamin D, and mineral composition of various Mediterranean recipes and used these to assemble a Mediterranean food pyramid based on criteria of Mediterranean diet adherence. In general, Mediterranean recipes and foods organized into a weekly food pyramid helped to meet the requirements for selected target DRI including energy and macronutrients (fat, carbohydrate, protein, and fiber); and for selected minerals (calcium, sodium, and potassium). A major contributor to energy is MUFA from olive oil and nuts. Concerns exist about the quality of olive oil commercially available. For example, in the USA imported extra-virgin olive oil often fails OIC and USDA qualitative standards [23]. Large variations in fatty acid and phenols composition may reduce olive oil grade and health benefits of olive oil consumption. In addition, requirements for vitamin D may not be met through foods and recipes only. Thus endogenous production induced via *UV* exposure and/or dietary supplementation may be necessary to achieve minimum vitamin D goals. Strategies useful to alleviate inadequacies in vitamin D include the intake (≥3 times/week) of fish-based recipes, adequate sun exposure, and possibly, supplemental doses. Clearly, the usefulness of Mediterranean recipes and food pyramids in meeting nutrient requirements is influenced by various factors including physical activity, body weight, height, gender, and age (Table 20.3). These factors need to be considered in order to maximize the health benefits of a Mediterranean diet and lifestyle.

Table 20.3 Examples of USDA Dietary Reference Intakes for males and females of different age, body weight, and physical activity

	Normal-Weight (63.4 kg, 20 kg/m²)			Overweight (85.55 kg, 27 kg/m²)			Obese (105 kg, 33 kg/m²)		
	Sedentary	Active	Very active	Sedentary	Active	Very active	Sedentary	Active	Very active
	Male (178 cm, 40 years)								
Total calories (kcal/day)	2250	2742	3195	2602	3182	3716	2912	3570	4175
Carbohydrates (g/day)	253–366	306–446	359–519	293–423	358–517	418–604	328–473	402–580	470–678
Total fiber (g/day)	38	38	38	38	38	38	38	38	38
Protein (g/day)	51	51	51	68	68	68	84	84	84
Fat (g/day)	50–87	61–107	71–124	58–101	71–124	83–144	65–113	79–139	93–162
Total water (L/day)	3.7	3.7	3.7	3.7	3.7	3.7	3.7	3.7	3.7
Vitamin C (mg/day)	90	90	90	90	90	90	90	90	90
Vitamin D (mcg/day)	15	15	15	15	15	15	15	15	15
Calcium (mg/day)	1000	1000	1000	1000	1000	1000	1000	1000	1000
Sodium (g/day)	1.5	1.5	1.5	1.5	1.5	1.5	1.5	1.5	1.5
Potassium (g/day)	4.7	4.7	4.7	4.7	4.7	4.7	4.7	4.7	4.7
	Male (178 cm, 60 years)								
Total calories (kcal/d)	2059	2552	3005	2411	2991	3525	2721	3379	3984
Carbohydrates (g/day)	232–335	287–415	338–488	271–392	337–486	397–573	306–442	380–549	448–647
Total fiber (g/day)	30	30	30	30	30	30	30	30	30
Protein (g/day)	51	51	51	68	68	68	84	84	84
Fat (g/day)	46–80	57–99	67–117	54–94	66–116	78–137	60–106	75–131	89–155
Total water (L/day)	3.7	3.7	3.7	3.7	3.7	3.7	3.7	3.7	3.7
Vitamin C (mg/day)	90	90	90	90	90	90	90	90	90
Vitamin D (mcg/day)	15	15	15	15	15	15	15	15	15
Calcium (mg/day)	1000	1000	1000	1000	1000	1000	1000	1000	1000
Sodium (g/day)	1.3	1.3	1.3	1.3	1.3	1.3	1.3	1.3	1.3
Potassium (g/day)	4.7	4.7	4.7	4.7	4.7	4.7	4.7	4.7	4.7

Total calories (kcal/day)	1745	2195	2496	1932	2433	2767	2063	2600	2957
Carbohydrates (g/day)	196–284	247–357	281–406	217–314	274–395	311–450	232–335	292–422	333–481
Total fiber (g/day)	25	25	25	25	25	25	25	25	25
Protein (g/day)	42	42	42	58	58	58	69	69	69
Fat (g/day)	39–68	49–85	55–97	43–75	54–95	61–108	46–80	58–101	66–115
Total water (L/day)	2.7	2.7	2.7	2.7	2.7	2.7	2.7	2.7	2.7
Vitamin C (mg/day)	75	75	75	75	75	75	75	75	75
Vitamin D (mcg/day)	15	15	15	15	15	15	15	15	15
Calcium (mg/day)	1000	1000	1000	1000	1000	1000	1000	1000	1000
Sodium (g/day)	1.5	1.5	1.5	1.5	1.5	1.5	1.5	1.5	1.5
Potassium (g/day)	4.7	4.7	4.7	4.7	4.7	4.7	4.7	4.7	4.7
	Female (162 cm, 60 years)								
Total calories (kcal/day)	1607	2057	2357	1794	2295	2629	1925	2461	2819
Carbohydrates (g/day)	181–261	231–334	265–383	202–292	258–373	296–427	217–313	277–400	317–458
Total fiber (g/day)	21	21	21	21	21	21	21	21	21
Protein (g/day)	42	42	42	58	58	58	69	69	69
Fat (g/day)	36–62	46–80	52–92	40–70	51–89	58–102	43–75	55–96	63–110
Total water (L/day)	2.7	2.7	2.7	2.7	2.7	2.7	2.7	2.7	2.7
Vitamin C (mg/day)	75	75	75	75	75	75	75	75	75
Vitamin D (mcg/day)	15	15	15	15	15	15	15	15	15
Calcium (mg/day)	1200	1200	1200	1200	1200	1200	1200	1200	1200
Sodium (g/day)	1.3	1.3	1.3	1.3	1.3	1.3	1.3	1.3	1.3
Potassium (g/day)	4.7	4.7	4.7	4.7	4.7	4.7	4.7	4.7	4.7

References

1. Willett WC, Sacks F, Trichopoulou A, Drescher G, Ferro-Luzzi A, Helsing E, Trichopoulos D. Mediterranean diet pyramid: a cultural model for healthy eating. Am J Clin Nutr. 1995;61(6 Suppl):1402S–6. Review. PubMed.
2. Trichopoulou A, Kouris-Blazos A, Wahlqvist ML, Gnardellis C, Lagiou P, Polychronopoulos E, Vassilakou T, Lipworth L, Trichopoulos D. Diet and overall survival in elderly people. BMJ. 1995;311(7018):1457–60.
3. US Census Bureau, Statistical Abstract of the United States: 2012. Health and Nutrition. Available at: http://www.census.gov/. Accessed 15 Sep 2015
4. National Health and Nutrition Examination Survey (NHANES). United States, 1971–2000. Trends in Intake of Energy and Macronutrients -United States, 1971–2000. Available at: http://www.cdc.gov/mmwr/preview/mmwrhtml/mm5304a3.htm
5. US Department of Agriculture, Ethnic/Cultural Food Pyramids. http://fnic.nal.usda.gov/dietary-guidance/past-food-pyramid-materials/ethniccultural-food-pyramids. Accessed 6 Sep 2015
6. Singh RB, Dubnov G, Niaz MA, Ghosh S, Singh R, Rastogi SS, Manor O, Pella D, Berry EM. Effect of an Indo-Mediterranean diet on progression of coronary artery disease in high risk patients (Indo-Mediterranean Diet Heart Study): a randomised single-blind trial. Lancet. 2002;360(9344):1455–61.
7. Bach-Faig A, Berry EM, Lairon D, Reguant J, Trichopoulou A, Dernini S, Medina FX, Battino M, Belahsen R, Miranda G, Serra-Majem L, Mediterranean Diet Foundation Expert Group. Mediterranean diet pyramid today. Science and cultural updates. Public Health Nutr. 2011;14:2274–84.
8. Ranalli A, Ferrante ML, De Mattia G, Costantini N. Analytical evaluation of virgin olive oil of first and second extraction. J Agric Food Chem. 1999;47(2):417–24.
9. León L, Uceda M, Jiménez A, Martín LM, Rallo L. Variability of fatty acid composition in olive (Olea europaea L.) progenies. Spanish J Agric Res. 2004;2:353–9.
10. International Olive Council. Available at: http://www.internationaloliveoil.org/. Visited on 15 Sep 2015.
11. Alvarruiz A, Álvarez-Ortí M, Mateos B, Sena E, Pardo JE. Quality and composition of virgin olive oil from varieties grown in Castilla-La Mancha (Spain). J Oleo Sci. 2015;64(10):1075–82.
12. Martínez-González MA, García-Arellano A, Toledo E, Salas-Salvadó J, Buil-Cosiales P, Corella D, Covas MI, Schröder H, Arós F, Gómez-Gracia E, Fiol M, Ruiz-Gutiérrez V, Lapetra J, Lamuela-Raventos RM, Serra-Majem L, Pintó X, Muñoz MA, Wärnberg J, Ros E, Estruch R, PREDIMED Study Investigators. A 14-item Mediterranean diet assessment tool and obesity indexes among high-risk subjects: the PREDIMED trial. PLoS One. 2012;7(8):e43134.
13. Hinrichs J. Mediterranean milk and milk products. Eur J Nutr. 2004;43 Suppl 1:I/12–7.
14. Maillot M, Issa C, Vieux F, Lairon D, Darmon N. The shortest way to reach nutritional goals is to adopt Mediterranean food choices: evidence from computer-generated personalized diets. Am J Clin Nutr. 2011;94(4):1127–37. doi:10.3945/ajcn.111.016501. Epub 2011 Sep 7. Erratum in: Am J Clin Nutr. 2011 Dec;94(6):1655.
15. Varela-Moreiras G, Ruiz E, Valero T, Avila JM, del Pozo S. The Spanish diet: an update. Nutr Hosp. 2013;28 suppl 5:13–20.
16. United States Department of Agriculture. Dietary Reference Intakes. Available at: http://fnic.nal.usda.gov/dietary-guidance/dietary-reference-intakes. Accessed 15 Sep 2015
17. Leren P. The Oslo Diet-Heart Study. Circulation. 1970;42:935–42.
18. Deol P, Evans JR, Dhahbi J, Chellappa K, Han DS, Spindler S, Sladek FM. Soybean oil is more obesogenic and diabetogenic than coconut oil and fructose in mouse: potential role for the liver. PLoS One. 2015;10(7):e0132672.
19. Arentson-Lantz E, Clairmont S, Paddon-Jones D, Tremblay A, Elango R. Protein: a nutrient in focus. Appl Physiol Nutr Metab. 2015;40(8):755–61.
20. Skov AR, Toubro S, Rønn B, Holm L, Astrup A. Randomized trial on protein vs carbohydrate in ad libitum fat reduced diet for the treatment of obesity. Int J Obes Relat Metab Disord. 1999;23(5):528–36.
21. Roman Viñas B, Ribas Barba L, Ngo J, Gurinovic M, Novakovic R, Cavelaars A, de Groot LC, van't Veer P, Matthys C, Serra ML. Projected prevalence of inadequate nutrient intakes in Europe. Ann Nutr Metab. 2011;59(2–4):84–95.
22. Bailey RL, Dodd KW, Goldman JA, Gahche JJ, Dwyer JT, Moshfegh AJ, Sempos CT, Picciano MF. Estimation of total usual calcium and vitamin D intakes in the United States. J Nutr. 2010;140(4):817–22.
23. Frankel EN, Mailer RJ, Shoemaker CF, Wang SC, Flynn JD. Tests indicate that imported "extra virgin" olive oil often fails international and USDA standards. UC Davis Olive Center, July 2010. Robert Mondavi Institute for Wine and Food Science, University of California, Davis.

Appendix: 2015 Dietary Guidelines for Americans

The information provided in this Appendix was obtained from the U.S. Department of Agriculture (http://www.cnpp.usda.gov/dietaryguidelines/) as a resource to the readers who wishes to integrate the material presented in this volume about the Mediterranean diet and lifestyle with the 2015 Dietary Recommendations for Americans issued by the U.S. Departments of Agriculture and Human and Health Services. This is the eighth edition since 1980.

Appendix A: Dietary Guidelines and Recommendations

BOX 1: 2015-2020 Dietary Guidelines for Americans: Overarching Guidelines[1]

1. **Follow a healthy eating pattern across the lifespan.**
   All food and beverage choices matter. Choose a healthy eating pattern at an appropriate calorie level to help achieve and maintain a healthy body weight, support nutrient adequacy, and reduce the risk of chronic disease.
2. **Focus on variety, nutrient density, and amount.**
   To meet nutrient needs within calorie limits, choose a variety of nutrient-dense foods across and within all food groups in recommended amounts.
3. **Limit calories from added sugars and saturated fats and reduce sodium intake.**
   Consume an eating pattern low in added sugars, saturated fats, and sodium. Cut back on foods and beverages higher in these components to amounts that fit within healthy eating patterns.
4. **Shift to healthier food and beverage choices.**
   Choose nutrient-dense foods and beverages across and within all food groups in place of less healthy choices. Consider cultural and personal preferences to make these shifts easier to accomplish and maintain.
5. **Support healthy eating patterns for all.**
   Everyone has a role in helping to create and support healthy eating patterns in multiple settings nationwide, from home to school to work to communities.

[1]Source: Adapted from U.S. Department of Agriculture, Center for Nutrition Policy and Promotion. 2015-2020 Dietary Guidelines for Americans. 8th Edition. Available at: http://www.cnpp.usda.gov/2015-2020-dietary-guidelines-americans.

D.F. Romagnolo, O.I. Selmin (eds.), *Mediterranean Diet*, Nutrition and Health,
DOI 10.1007/978-3-319-27969-5

BOX 2: 2015-2020 Dietary Guidelines for Americans: Key Recommendations[1]

Consume a healthy eating pattern that accounts for all foods and beverages within an appropriate calorie level

1. A healthy eating pattern includes:

- A variety of vegetables from all of the subgroups—dark green, red and orange, legumes (beans and peas), starchy, and other;
- Fruits, especially whole fruits;
- Grains, at least half of which are whole grains;
- Fat-free or low-fat dairy, including milk, yogurt, cheese, and/or fortified soy beverages;
- A variety of protein foods, including seafood, lean meats and poultry, eggs, legumes (beans and peas), and nuts, seeds, and soy products;
- Oils

2. A healthy eating pattern limits:

- Saturated fats and *trans* fats, added sugars, and sodium.
- Key recommendations that are quantitative are provided for several components of the diet that should be limited. These components are of particular public health concern in the United States, and the specified limits can help individuals achieve healthy eating patterns within calorie limits:
  - Consume less than 10 percent of calories per day from added sugars
  - Consume less than 10 percent of calories per day from saturated fats
  - Consume less than 2,300 milligrams (mg) per day of sodium
- If alcohol is consumed, it should be consumed in moderation—up to one drink per day for women and up to two drinks per day for men—and only by adults of legal drinking age.

Americans of all ages—children, adolescents, adults, and older adults—should meet the *Physical Activity Guidelines for Americans* to help promote health and reduce the risk of chronic disease

1. ***Americans should aim to achieve and maintain a healthy body weight.***
2. ***The relationship between diet and physical activity contributes to calorie balance and managing body weight.***
   - Meet the *Physical Activity Guidelines for Americans.*

[1]Source: Adapted from U.S. Department of Agriculture, Center for Nutrition Policy and Promotion. 2015-2020 Dietary Guidelines for Americans. 8th Edition. Available at: http://www.cnpp.usda.gov/2015-2020-dietary-guidelines-americans.

Appendix B: Physical Activity

BOX 3a: Physical Activity for Americans: Definitions[1]

Physical Activity	Definition
Moderate-intensity	Aerobic activity that increases a person's heart rate and breathing to some extent. On a scale relative to a person's capacity, moderate-intensity activity is usually a 5 or 6 on a 0 to 10 scale. Brisk walking, dancing, swimming, or bicycling on a level terrain are examples.
Vigorous-intensity	Aerobic activity that greatly increases a person's heart rate and breathing. On a scale relative to a person's capacity, vigorous-intensity activity is usually a 7 or 8 on a 0 to 10 scale. Jogging, singles tennis, swimming continuous laps, or bicycling uphill are examples.
Muscle-strengthening	Physical activity, including exercise that increases skeletal muscle strength, power, endurance, and mass. It includes strength training, resistance training, and muscular strength and endurance exercises.
Bone-strengthening	Physical activity that produces an impact or tension force on bones, which promotes bone growth and strength. Running, jumping rope, and lifting weights are examples.

[1]Source: Adapted from U.S. Department of Agriculture, Center for Nutrition Policy and Promotion. 2015-2020 Dietary Guidelines for Americans. 8th Edition. Available at: http://www.cnpp.usda.gov/2015-2020-dietary-guidelines-americans.

BOX 3b: Physical Activity for Americans: Recommendations[1]

Age	Recommendations
6 to 17 years	***Children and adolescents should do 60 minutes (1 hour) or more of physical activity daily*** ➢ Aerobic: Most of the 60 or more minutes a day should be either moderate or vigorous-intensity aerobic physical activity, and should include vigorous-intensity physical activity at least 3 days a week. ➢ Muscle-strengthening: as part of their 60 or more minutes of daily physical activity, children and adolescents should include muscle-strengthening physical activity on at least 3 days of the week. ➢ Bone-strengthening: as part of their 60 or more minutes of daily physical activity, children and adolescents should include bone-strengthening physical activity on at least 3 days of the week. ➢ It is important to encourage young people to participate in physical activities that are appropriate for their age, that are enjoyable, and that offer variety.
18 to 64 years	***All adults should avoid inactivity*** ➢ Some physical activity is better than none, and adults who participate in any amount of physical activity gain some health benefits. ➢ For substantial health benefits, adults should do at least 150 minutes (2 hours and 30 minutes) a week of moderate-intensity, or 75 minutes (1 hour and 15 minutes) a week of vigorous-intensity aerobic physical activity, or an equivalent combination of moderate- and vigorous-intensity aerobic activity. Aerobic activity should be performed in episodes of at least 10 minutes, and preferably, it should be spread throughout the week. ➢ For additional and more extensive health benefits, adults should increase their aerobic physical activity to 300 minutes (5 hours) a week of moderate-intensity, or 150 minutes a week of vigorous-intensity aerobic physical activity, or an equivalent combination of moderate- and vigorous-intensity activity. Additional health benefits are gained by engaging in physical activity beyond this amount. ➢ Adults should also include muscle-strengthening activities that involve all major muscle groups on 2 or more days a week.
65 years and older	***Older adults should follow the adult guidelines*** ➢ When older adults cannot meet the adult guidelines, they should be as physically active as their abilities and conditions will allow. ➢ Older adults should do exercises that maintain or improve balance if they are at risk of falling. ➢ Older adults should determine their level of effort for physical activity relative to their level of fitness. ➢ Older adults with chronic conditions should understand whether and how their conditions affect their ability to do regular physical activity safely.

[1]Source: Adapted from U.S. Department of Agriculture, Center for Nutrition Policy and Promotion. 2015-2020 Dietary Guidelines for Americans. 8th Edition. Available at: http://www.cnpp.usda.gov/2015-2020-dietary-guidelines-americans.

BOX 3c: U.S. Physical Activity Resources[1]	
Source	Link
Dietary Guidelines for Americans	www.dietaryguidelines.gov
Physical Activity Guidelines for Americans	www.health.gov/paguidelines
MyPlate	www.choosemyplate.gov
SuperTracker	www.supertracker.usda.gov
U.S. Department of Health and Human Services	www.hhs.gov
Office of Disease Prevention and Health Promotion	www.health.gov
Healthy People	www.healthypeople.gov
Healthfinder	www.healthfinder.gov
Food and Drug Administration	www.fda.gov
Centers for Disease Control and Prevention	www.cdc.gov
National Institutes of Health	www.nih.gov
Rethinking Drinking Alcoholic beverage calculators	http://rethinkingdrinking.niaaa.nih.gov/ToolsResources/CalculatorsMain.asp
President's Council on Fitness, Sports & Nutrition	www.fitness.gov
U.S. Department of Agriculture (USDA)	www.usda.gov
Center for Nutrition Policy and Promotion	www.cnpp.usda.gov
Food and Nutrition Service	www.fns.usda.gov
Food and Nutrition Information Center	http://fnic.nal.usda.gov
National Institute of Food and Agriculture	www.nifa.usda.gov
Let's Move!	www.letsmove.gov
U.S. National Physical Activity Plan[a]	www.physicalactivityplan.org

[1]Source: Adapted from U.S. Department of Agriculture, Center for Nutrition Policy and Promotion. 2015-2020 Dietary Guidelines for Americans. 8th Edition. Available at: http://www.cnpp.usda.gov/2015-2020-dietary-guidelines-americans.

Appendix C: Caloric Needs and Food Groups

BOX 4a: Estimated Caloric Needs Per Day Ranked by Age and Physical Activity: Males[1]

Age	Sedentary[a]	Moderately-Active[b]	Active[c]	Age	Sedentary	Moderately-Active	Active
2	1,000	1,000	1,000	17	2,400	2,800	3,200
3	1,000	1,400	1,400	18	2,400	2,800	3,200
4	1,200	1,400	1,600	19-20	2,600	2,800	3,000
5	1,200	1,400	1,600	21-25	2,400	2,800	3,000
6	1,400	1,600	1,800	26-30	2,400	2,600	3,000
7	1,400	1,600	1,800	31-35	2,400	2,600	3,000
8	1,400	1,600	2,000	36-40	2,400	2,600	2,800
9	1,600	1,800	2,000	41-45	2,200	2,600	2,800
10	1,600	1,800	2,200	46-50	2,200	2,400	2,800
11	1,800	2,000	2,200	51-55	2,200	2,400	2,800
12	1,800	2,200	2,400	56-60	2,200	2,400	2,600
13	2,000	2,200	2,600	61-65	2,000	2,400	2,600
14	2,000	2,400	2,800	66-70	2,000	2,200	2,600
15	2,200	2,600	3,000	71-75	2,000	2,200	2,600
16	2,400	2,800	3,200	76 and up	2,000	2,200	2,400

[1]Source: Adapted from U.S. Department of Agriculture, Center for Nutrition Policy and Promotion. 2015-2020 Dietary Guidelines for Americans. 8th Edition. Available at: http://www.cnpp.usda.gov/2015-2020-dietary-guidelines-americans; [a]Sedentary means a lifestyle that includes only the physical activity of independent living; [b]Moderately active means a lifestyle that includes physical activity equivalent to walking about 1.5-3 miles/day at 3-4 miles/hour, in addition to the activities of independent living; [c]Active means a lifestyle that includes physical activity equivalent to walking >3 miles/day at 3-4 miles/hour, in addition to the activities of independent living.

BOX 4b: Estimated Caloric Needs Per Day Ranked by Age and Physical Activity: Females Not Pregnant or Breastfeeding[1]

Age	Sedentary[a]	Moderately-Active[b]	Active[c]	Age	Sedentary	Moderately-Active	Active
2	1,000	1,000	1,000	17	1,800	2,000	2,400
3	1,000	1,200	1,400	18	1,800	2,000	2,400
4	1,200	1,400	1,400	19-20	2,000	2,200	2,400
5	1,200	1,400	1,600	21-25	2,000	2,200	2,400
6	1,200	1,400	1,600	26-30	1,800	2,000	2,400
7	1,200	1,600	1,800	31-35	1,800	2,000	2,200
8	1,400	1,600	1,800	36-40	1,800	2,000	2,200
9	1,400	1,600	1,800	41-45	1,800	2,000	2,200
10	1,400	1,800	2,000	46-50	1,800	2,000	2,200
11	1,600	1,800	2,000	51-55	1,600	1,800	2,200
12	1,600	2,000	2,200	56-60	1,600	1,800	2,200
13	1,600	2,000	2,200	61-65	1,600	1,800	2,000
14	1,800	2,000	2,400	66-70	1,600	1,800	2,000
15	1,800	2,000	2,400	71-75	1,600	1,800	2,000
16	1,800	2,000	2,400	76 and up	1,600	1,800	2,000

[1]Source: Adapted from U.S. Department of Agriculture, Center for Nutrition Policy and Promotion. 2015-2020 Dietary Guidelines for Americans. 8th Edition. Available at: http://www.cnpp.usda.gov/2015-2020-dietary-guidelines-americans; [a]Sedentary means a lifestyle that includes only the physical activity of independent living; [b]Moderately active means a lifestyle that includes physical activity equivalent to walking about 1.5-3 miles/day at 3-4 miles/hour, in addition to the activities of independent living; [c]Active means a lifestyle that includes physical activity equivalent to walking >3 miles/day at 3-4 miles/hour, in addition to the activities of independent living.

BOX 5a: Foods in Each Group and Subgroup[1]

Food Group	Subgroup Description
Vegetables	**Dark-green vegetables:** ➢ All fresh, frozen, and canned dark-green leafy vegetables and broccoli, cooked or raw. For example, broccoli, spinach, romaine, kale, collard, turnip, and mustard greens. **Red and orange vegetables:** ➢ All fresh, frozen, and canned red and orange vegetables or juice, cooked or raw. For example, tomatoes, tomato juice, red peppers, carrots, sweet potatoes, winter squash, and pumpkin. **Legumes (beans and peas):** ➢ All cooked from dry or canned beans and peas. For example, kidney beans, white beans, black beans, lentils, chickpeas, pinto beans, split peas, and edamame (green soybeans). Does not include green beans or green peas. **Starchy vegetables:** ➢ All fresh, frozen, and canned starchy vegetables. For example, white potatoes, corn, green peas, green lima beans, plantains, and cassava. **Other vegetables:** ➢ All other fresh, frozen, and canned vegetables, cooked or raw. For example, iceberg lettuce, green beans, onions, cucumbers, cabbage, celery, zucchini, mushrooms, and green peppers.
Fruits	**All fresh, frozen, canned, and dried fruits and fruit juices**: For example, oranges and orange juice, apples and apple juice, bananas, grapes, melons, berries, and raisins.
Grains	**Whole grains**: ➢ All whole-grain products and whole grains used as ingredients. For example, whole-wheat bread, whole-grain cereals and crackers, oatmeal, quinoa, popcorn, and brown rice. **Refined grains:** ➢ All refined-grain products and refined grains used as ingredients. For example, white breads, refined grain cereals and crackers, pasta, and white rice. Refined grain choices should be enriched.
Dairy	**All milk, including lactose-free and lactose-reduced products and fortified soy beverages (soymilk), yogurt, frozen yogurt, dairy desserts, and cheeses.** ➢ Most choices should be fat-free or low-fat. Cream, sour cream, and cream cheese are not included due to their low calcium content.
Protein Foods	**All seafood, meats, poultry, eggs, soy products, nuts, and seeds.** ➢ Meats and poultry should be lean or low-fat and nuts should be unsalted. Legumes (beans and peas) can be considered part of this group as well as the vegetable group, but should be counted in one group only.

[1]Source: Adapted from U.S. Department of Agriculture, Center for Nutrition Policy and Promotion. 2015-2020 Dietary Guidelines for Americans. 8th Edition. Available at: http://www.cnpp.usda.gov/2015-2020-dietary-guidelines-americans.

BOX 5b: Quantity Equivalent for Each Food Group[1]

Food Group	Quantity Equivalent
Vegetables and Fruits	1 cup-equivalent is 1 cup raw or cooked vegetable or fruit;1 cup vegetable or fruit juice; 2 cups leafy salad greens; ½ cup dried fruit or vegetable.
Grains	1 ounce-equivalent is ½ cup cooked rice, pasta, or cereal; 1 ounce dry pasta or rice; 1 medium (1 ounce) slice bread; 1 ounce of ready-to-eat cereal (about 1 cup of flaked cereal).
Dairy	1 cup-equivalent is:1 cup milk, yogurt, or fortified soymilk; 1½ ounces natural cheese such as cheddar cheese or 2 ounces of processed cheese.
Protein Foods	1 ounce-equivalent is 1 ounce lean meat, poultry, or seafood; 1 egg; ¼ cup cooked beans or tofu; 1 tbsp peanut butter; ½ ounce nuts or seeds.

[1]Source: Adapted from U.S. Department of Agriculture, Center for Nutrition Policy and Promotion. 2015-2020 Dietary Guidelines for Americans. 8th Edition. Available at: http://www.cnpp.usda.gov/2015-2020-dietary-guidelines-americans.

Appendix D: Healthy US-Style Eating Pattern

BOX 6a: Healthy US-Style Eating Pattern. Food Group: Vegetables, Fruits, Grains, and Dairy (1000 to 2,200 Calorie Level)[1]

Calorie Level of Pattern[a]	1,000	1,200	1,400	1,600	1,800	2,000	2,200
Food Group[b]	Daily Amount[c] of Food From Each Group (vegetable foods subgroup are amounts/week)						
Vegetables	1 c-eq	1½ c-eq	1½ c-eq	2 c-eq	2½ c-eq	2½ c-eq	3 c-eq
Dark-green vegetables (c-eq/wk)	½	1	1	1½	1½	1½	2
Red and orange vegetables (c-eq/wk)	2½	3	3	4	5½	5½	6
Legumes (beans and peas) (c-eq/wk)	½	½	½	1	1½	1½	2
Starchy vegetables (c-eq/wk)	2	3½	3½	4	5	5	6
Other vegetables (c-eq/wk)	1½	2½	2½	3½	4	4	5
Fruits	1 c-eq	1 c-eq	1½ c-eq	1½ c-eq	1½ c-eq	2 c-eq	2 c-eq
Grains	3 oz-eq	4 oz-eq	5 oz-eq	5 oz-eq	6 oz-eq	6 oz-eq	7 oz-eq
Whole grains[d] (oz-eq/day)	1½	2	2½	3	3	3	3½
Refined grains (oz-eq/day)	1½	2	2½	2	3	3	3½
Dairy	2 c-eq	2½ c-eq	2½ c-eq	3 c-eq	3 c-eq	3 c-eq	3 c-eq

[1]Source: Adapted from U.S. Department of Agriculture, Center for Nutrition Policy and Promotion. 2015-2020 Dietary Guidelines for Americans. 8th Edition. Available at: http://www.cnpp.usda.gov/2015-2020-dietary-guidelines-americans;

[a] Food intake patterns at 1,000, 1,200, and 1,400 calories are designed to meet the nutritional needs of 2-8-year-old children. Patterns from 1,600 to 3,200 calories are designed to meet the nutritional needs of children 9 years and older and adults. If a child 4-8 years of age needs more calories and, therefore, is following a pattern at 1,600 calories or more, his/her recommended amount from the dairy group should be 2.5 cups/day. Children 9 years and older and adults should not use the 1,000-, 1,200-, or 1,400-calorie patterns.

[b] Foods in each group and subgroup are those listed in BOX 5a.

[c] Food group amounts are shown in cup-(c) or ounce-equivalents (oz-eq). Oils are shown in grams (g). Quantity equivalents for each food group are listed in BOX 5b.

[d] Amounts of whole grains in the Patterns for children are less than the minimum of 3 oz-equivalent in all Patterns recommended for adults.

BOX 6b: Healthy US-Style Eating Pattern. Food Group: Vegetables, Fruits, Grains, and Dairy (2,000 to 3,200 Calorie Level)[1]

Calorie Level of Pattern[a]	2,000	2,200	2,400	2,600	2,800	3,000	3,200
Food Group[b]	Daily Amount[c] of Food From Each Group (vegetable foods subgroup are amounts/week)						
Vegetables	2½ c-eq	3 c-eq	3 c-eq	3½ c-eq	3½ c-eq	4 c-eq	4 c-eq
Dark-green vegetables (c-eq/wk)	1½	2	2	2½	2½	2½	2½
Red and orange vegetables (c-eq/wk)	5½	6	6	7	7	7½	7½
Legumes (beans and peas) (c-eq/wk)	1½	2	2	2½	2½	3	3
Starchy vegetables (c-eq/wk)	5	6	6	7	7	8	8
Other vegetables (c-eq/wk)	4	5	5	5½	5½	7	7
Fruits	2 c-eq	2 c-eq	2 c-eq	2 c-eq	2½ c-eq	2½ c-eq	2½ c-eq
Grains	6 oz-eq	7 oz-eq	8 oz-eq	9 oz-eq	10 oz-eq	10 oz-eq	10 oz-eq
Whole grains[d] (oz-eq/day)	3	3½	4	4½	5	5	5
Refined grains (oz-eq/day)	3	3½	4	4½	5	5	5
Dairy	3 c-eq	3 c-eq	3 c-eq	3 c-eq	3 c-eq	3 c-eq	3 c-eq

[1]Source: Adapted from U.S. Department of Agriculture, Center for Nutrition Policy and Promotion. 2015-2020 Dietary Guidelines for Americans. 8th Edition. Available at: http://www.cnpp.usda.gov/2015-2020-dietary-guidelines-americans;

[a] Food intake patterns at 1,000, 1,200, and 1,400 calories are designed to meet the nutritional needs of 2-8-year-old children. Patterns from 1,600 to 3,200 calories are designed to meet the nutritional needs of children 9 years and older and adults. If a child 4-8 years of age needs more calories and, therefore, is following a pattern at 1,600 calories or more, his/her recommended amount from the dairy group should be 2.5 cups/day. Children 9 years and older and adults should not use the 1,000-, 1,200-, or 1,400-calorie patterns.

[b] Foods in each group and subgroup are those listed in BOX 5a.

[c] Food group amounts are shown in cup-(c) or ounce-equivalents (oz-eq). Oils are shown in grams (g). Quantity equivalents for each food group are listed in BOX 5b.

[d] Amounts of whole grains in the Patterns for children are less than the minimum of 3 oz-equivalent in all Patterns recommended for adults.

BOX 6c: Healthy US-Style Eating Pattern. Food Group: Protein Foods and Oils (1,000 to 2,200 Calorie Level)[1]

Calorie Level of Pattern[a]	1,000	1,200	1,400	1,600	1,800	2,000	2,200
Food Group[b]	Daily Amount[c] of Food From Each Group (Protein foods subgroup are amounts/week)						
Protein Foods	2 oz-eq	3 oz-eq	4 oz-eq	5 oz-eq	5 oz-eq	5½ oz-eq	6 oz-eq
Seafood (oz-eq/wk)	3	4	6	8	8	8	9
Meats, poultry, eggs (oz-eq/wk)	10	14	19	23	23	26	28
Nuts seeds, soy products (oz-eq/wk)	2	2	3	4	4	5	5
Oils	15 g	17 g	17 g	22 g	24 g	27 g	29 g

BOX 6d: Healthy US-Style Eating Pattern. Food Group: Protein Foods and Oils (2,000 to 3,200 Calorie Level)[1]

Calorie Level of Pattern[a]	2,000	2,200	2,400	2,600	2,800	3,000	3,200
Food Group[b]	Daily Amount[c] of Food From Each Group (Protein foods subgroup are amounts/week)						
Protein Foods	5½ oz-eq	6 oz-eq	6½ oz-eq	6½ oz-eq	7 oz-eq	7 oz-eq	7 oz-eq
Seafood (oz-eq/wk)	8	9	10	10	10	10	10
Meats, poultry, eggs (oz-eq/wk)	26	28	31	31	33	33	33
Nuts seeds, soy products (oz-eq/wk)	5	5	5	5	6	6	6
Oils	27 g	29 g	31 g	34 g	36 g	44 g	51 g

[1]Source: Adapted from U.S. Department of Agriculture, Center for Nutrition Policy and Promotion. 2015-2020 Dietary Guidelines for Americans. 8th Edition. Available at: http://www.cnpp.usda.gov/2015-2020-dietary-guidelines-americans;

[a] Food intake patterns at 1,000, 1,200, and 1,400 calories are designed to meet the nutritional needs of 2-8-year-old children. Patterns from 1,600 to 3,200 calories are designed to meet the nutritional needs of children 9 years and older and adults. If a child 4-8 years of age needs more calories and, therefore, is following a pattern at 1,600 calories or more, his/her recommended amount from the dairy group should be 2.5 cups/day. Children 9 years and older and adults should not use the 1,000-, 1,200-, or 1,400-calorie patterns.

[b] Foods in each group and subgroup are those listed in BOX 5a.

[c] Food group amounts are shown in cup-(c) or ounce-equivalents (oz-eq). Oils are shown in grams (g). Quantity equivalents for each food group are listed in BOX 5b.

BOX 6e: Healthy US-Style Eating Pattern. Limits on Calories for Other Uses (1,000 to 3,200 Calorie Level)[1]

Calorie Level of Pattern[a]	1,000	1,200	1,400	1,600	1,800	2,000	2,200
Limit on Calories for Other Uses, calories (% of calories)[b,c]	150 (15%)	100 (8%)	110 (8%)	130 (8%)	170 (9%)	270 (14%)	280 (13%)
Calorie Level of Pattern[a]	2,000	2,200	2,400	2,600	2,800	3,000	3,200
Limit on Calories for Other Uses, calories (% of calories)[b,c]	270 (14%)	280 (13%)	350 (15%)	380 (15%)	400 (14%)	470 (16%)	610 (19%)

[1]Source: Adapted from U.S. Department of Agriculture, Center for Nutrition Policy and Promotion. 2015-2020 Dietary Guidelines for Americans. 8th Edition. Available at: http://www.cnpp.usda.gov/2015-2020-dietary-guidelines-americans;

[a] Food intake patterns at 1,000, 1,200, and 1,400 calories are designed to meet the nutritional needs of 2-8-year-old children. Patterns from 1,600 to 3,200 calories are designed to meet the nutritional needs of children 9 years and older and adults. If a child 4-8 years of age needs more calories and, therefore, is following a pattern at 1,600 calories or more, his/her recommended amount from the dairy group should be 2.5 cups/day. Children 9 years and older and adults should not use the 1,000-, 1,200-, or 1,400-calorie patterns.

[b] All foods are assumed to be in nutrient-dense forms, lean or low-fat and prepared without added fats, sugars, refined starches, or salt. If all food choices to meet food group recommendations are in nutrient-dense forms, a small number of calories remain within the overall calorie limit of the Pattern (i.e., limit on calories for other uses). The number of these calories depends on the overall calorie limit in the Pattern and the amounts of food from each food group required to meet nutritional goals.

Nutritional goals are higher for the 1,200- to 1,600-calorie Patterns than for the 1,000-calorie Pattern, so the limit on calories for other uses is lower in the 1,200- to 1,600-calorie Patterns. Calories up to the specified limit can be used for added sugars, added refined starches, solid fats, alcohol, or to eat more than the recommended amount of food in a food group.

The overall eating Pattern also should not exceed the limits of less than 10% of calories from added sugars and less than 10% of calories from saturated fats. At most calorie levels, amounts that can be accommodated are less than these limits.

For adults of legal drinking age who choose to drink alcohol, a limit of up to 1 drink/day for women and up to 2 drinks/day for men within limits on calories for other uses applies (see BOX 11 for additional information on alcoholic drink-equivalents); and calories from protein, carbohydrate, and total fats should be within the Acceptable Macronutrient Distribution Ranges (AMDRs).

[c]Values are rounded.

Appendix E: Healthy Mediterranean-Style Eating Pattern

BOX 7a: Healthy Mediterranean-Style Eating Pattern. Food Group: Vegetables, Fruits, Grains, and Dairy (1,000 to 2,200 Calorie Level)[1]

Calorie Level of Pattern[a]	1,000	1,200	1,400	1,600	1,800	2,000	2,200
Food Group[b]	Daily Amount[c] of Food From Each Group (vegetable foods subgroup are amounts/week)						
Vegetables	1 c-eq	1½ c-eq	1½ c-eq	2 c-eq	2½ c-eq	2½ c-eq	3 c-eq
Dark-green vegetables (c-eq/wk)	½	1	1	1½	1½	1½	2
Red and orange vegetables (c-eq/wk)	2½	3	3	4	5½	5½	6
Legumes (beans and peas) (c-eq/wk)	½	½	½	1	1½	1½	2
Starchy vegetables (c-eq/wk)	2	3½	3½	4	5	5	6
Other vegetables (c-eq/wk)	1½	2½	2½	3½	4	4	5
Fruits	1 c-eq	1 c-eq	1½ c-eq	2 c-eq	2 c-eq	2½ c-eq	2½ c-eq
Grains	3 oz-eq	4 oz-eq	5 oz-eq	5 oz-eq	6 oz-eq	6 oz-eq	7 oz-eq
Whole grains[d] (oz-eq/day)	1½	2	2½	3	3	3	3½
Refined grains (oz-eq/day)	1½	2	2½	2	3	3	3½
Dairy	2 c-eq	2½ c-eq	2½ c-eq	2 c-eq	2 c-eq	2 c-eq	2 c-eq

[1]Source: Adapted from U.S. Department of Agriculture, Center for Nutrition Policy and Promotion. 2015-2020 Dietary Guidelines for Americans. 8th Edition. Available at: http://www.cnpp.usda.gov/2015-2020-dietary-guidelines-americans;

[a] Food intake patterns at 1,000, 1,200, and 1,400 calories are designed to meet the nutritional needs of 2-8-year-old children. Patterns from 1,600 to 3,200 calories are designed to meet the nutritional needs of children 9 years and older and adults. If a child 4-8 years of age needs more calories and, therefore, is following a pattern at 1,600 calories or more, his/her recommended amount from the dairy group should be 2.5 cups/day. Children 9 years and older and adults should not use the 1,000-, 1,200-, or 1,400-calorie patterns.

[b] Foods in each group and subgroup are those listed in BOX 5a.

[c] Food group amounts are shown in cup-(c) or ounce-equivalents (oz-eq). Oils are shown in grams (g). Quantity equivalents for each food group are listed in BOX 5b.

[d] Amounts of whole grains in the Patterns for children are less than the minimum of 3 oz-equivalent in all Patterns recommended for adults.

BOX 7b: Healthy Mediterranean-Style Eating Pattern. Food Group: Vegetables, Fruits, Grains, and Dairy (2,000 to 3,200 Calorie Level)[1]

Calorie Level of Pattern[a]	2,000	2,200	2,400	2,600	2,800	3,000	3,200
Food Group[b]	Daily Amount[c] of Food From Each Group (vegetable foods subgroup are amounts/week)						
Vegetables	2½ c-eq	3 c-eq	3 c-eq	3½ c-eq	3½ c-eq	4 c-eq	4 c-eq
Dark-green vegetables (c-eq/wk)	1½	2	2	2½	2½	2½	2½
Red and orange vegetables (c-eq/wk)	5½	6	6	7	7	7½	7½
Legumes (beans and peas) (c-eq/wk)	1½	2	2	2½	2½	3	3
Starchy vegetables (c-eq/wk)	5	6	6	7	7	8	8
Other vegetables (c-eq/wk)	4	5	5	5½	5½	7	7
Fruits	2½ c-eq	2½ c-eq	2½ c-eq	2½ c-eq	3 c-eq	3 c-eq	3 c-eq
Grains	6 oz-eq	7 oz-eq	8 oz-eq	9 oz-eq	10 oz-eq	10 oz-eq	10 oz-eq
Whole grains[d] (oz-eq/day)	3	3½	4	4½	5	5	5
Refined grains (oz-eq/day)	3	3½	4	4½	5	5	5
Dairy	2 c-eq	2 c-eq	2½ c-eq	2½ c-eq	2½ c-eq	2½ c-eq	2½ c-eq

[1]Source: Adapted from U.S. Department of Agriculture, Center for Nutrition Policy and Promotion. 2015-2020 Dietary Guidelines for Americans. 8th Edition. Available at: http://www.cnpp.usda.gov/2015-2020-dietary-guidelines-americans;

[a] Food intake patterns at 1,000, 1,200, and 1,400 calories are designed to meet the nutritional needs of 2-8-year-old children. Patterns from 1,600 to 3,200 calories are designed to meet the nutritional needs of children 9 years and older and adults. If a child 4-8 years of age needs more calories and, therefore, is following a pattern at 1,600 calories or more, his/her recommended amount from the dairy group should be 2.5 cups/day. Children 9 years and older and adults should not use the 1,000-, 1,200-, or 1,400-calorie patterns.

[b] Foods in each group and subgroup are those listed in BOX 5a.

[c] Food group amounts are shown in cup-(c) or ounce-equivalents (oz-eq). Oils are shown in grams (g). Quantity equivalents for each food group are listed in BOX 5b.

[d] Amounts of whole grains in the Patterns for children are less than the minimum of 3 oz-equivalent in all Patterns recommended for adults.

BOX 7c: Healthy Mediterranean-Style Eating Pattern. Food Group: Protein Foods and Oils (1,000 to 2,200 Calorie Level)[1]

Calorie Level of Pattern[a]	1,000	1,200	1,400	1,600	1,800	2,000	2,200
Food Group[b]	Daily Amount[c] of Food From Each Group (protein foods subgroup are amounts/week)						
Protein Foods	2 oz-eq	3 oz-eq	4 oz-eq	5½ oz-eq	6 oz-eq	6½ oz-eq	7 oz-eq
Seafood (oz-eq/wk)[d]	3	4	6	11	15	15	16
Meats, poultry, eggs (oz-eq/wk)	10	14	19	23	23	26	28
Nuts, seeds, soy products (oz-eq/wk)	2	2	3	4	4	5	5
Oils	15 g	17 g	17 g	22 g	24 g	27 g	29 g

BOX 7d: Healthy Mediterranean-Style Eating Pattern. Food Group: Protein Foods and Oils (2,000 to 3,200 Calorie Level)[1]

Calorie Level of Pattern[a]	2,000	2,200	2,400	2,600	2,800	3,000	3,200
Food Group[b]	Daily Amount[c] of Food From Each Group (protein foods subgroup are amounts/week)						
Protein Foods	6½ oz-eq	7 oz-eq	7½ oz-eq	7½ oz-eq	8 oz-eq	8 oz-eq	8 oz-eq
Seafood (oz-eq/wk)[d]	15	16	16	17	17	17	17
Meats, poultry, eggs (oz-eq/wk)	26	28	31	31	33	33	33
Nuts, seeds, soy products (oz-eq/wk)	5	5	5	5	6	6	6
Oils	27 g	29 g	31 g	34 g	36 g	44 g	51 g

[1]Source: Adapted from U.S. Department of Agriculture, Center for Nutrition Policy and Promotion. 2015-2020 Dietary Guidelines for Americans. 8th Edition. Available at: http://www.cnpp.usda.gov/2015-2020-dietary-guidelines-americans; [a] Food intake patterns at 1,000, 1,200, and 1,400 calories are designed to meet the nutritional needs of 2-8-year-old children. Patterns from 1,600 to 3,200 calories are designed to meet the nutritional needs of children 9 years and older and adults. If a child 4-8 years of age needs more calories and, therefore, is following a pattern at 1,600 calories or more, his/her recommended amount from the dairy group should be 2.5 cups/day. Children 9 years and older and adults should not use the 1,000-, 1,200-, or 1,400-calorie patterns; [b] Foods in each group and subgroup are those listed in BOX 5a; [c] Food group amounts are shown in cup-(c) or ounce-equivalents (oz-eq). Oils are shown in grams (g). Quantity equivalents for each food group are listed in BOX 5b; [d]The U.S. Food and Drug Administration (FDA) and the U.S. Environmental Protection Agency (EPA) provide joint guidance regarding seafood consumption for women who are pregnant or breastfeeding and young children. For more information, see the FDA or EPA websites www.FDA.gov/fishadvice; www.EPA.gov/fishadvice.

BOX 7e: Healthy Mediterranean-Style Eating Pattern. Limits on Calories for Other Uses[1]

Calorie Level of Pattern[a]	1,000	1,200	1,400	1,600	1,800	2,000	2,200
Limit on Calories for Other Uses, calories (% of calories)[b,c]	150 (15%)	100 (8%)	110 (8%)	140 (9%)	160 (9%)	260 (13%)	270 (12%)
Calorie Level of Pattern[a]	2,000	2,200	2,400	2,600	2,800	3,000	3,200
Limit on Calories for Other Uses, calories (% of calories)[b,c]	260 (13%)	270 (12%)	300 (13%)	330 (13%)	350 (13%)	430 (14%)	570 (18%)

[1]Source: Adapted from U.S. Department of Agriculture, Center for Nutrition Policy and Promotion. 2015-2020 Dietary Guidelines for Americans. 8th Edition. Available at: http://www.cnpp.usda.gov/2015-2020-dietary-guidelines-americans;

[a] Food intake patterns at 1,000, 1,200, and 1,400 calories are designed to meet the nutritional needs of 2-8-year-old children. Patterns from 1,600 to 3,200 calories are designed to meet the nutritional needs of children 9 years and older and adults. If a child 4-8 years of age needs more calories and, therefore, is following a pattern at 1,600 calories or more, his/her recommended amount from the dairy group should be 2.5 cups/day. Children 9 years and older and adults should not use the 1,000-, 1,200-, or 1,400-calorie patterns.

[b] All foods are assumed to be in nutrient-dense forms, lean or low-fat and prepared without added fats, sugars, refined starches, or salt. If all food choices to meet food group recommendations are in nutrient-dense forms, a small number of calories remain within the overall calorie limit of the Pattern (i.e., limit on calories for other uses).

The number of these calories depends on the overall calorie limit in the Pattern and the amounts of food from each food group required to meet nutritional goals. Nutritional goals are higher for the 1,200- to 1,600-calorie Patterns than for the 1,000-calorie Pattern, so the limit on calories for other uses is lower in the 1,200- to 1,600-calorie Patterns. Calories up to the specified limit can be used for added sugars, added refined starches, solid fats, alcohol, or to eat more than the recommended amount of food in a food group.

The overall eating Pattern also should not exceed the limits of less than 10% of calories from added sugars and less than 10% of calories from saturated fats. At most calorie levels, amounts that can be accommodated are less than these limits.

For adults of legal drinking age who choose to drink alcohol, a limit of up to 1 drink/day for women and up to 2 drinks/day for men within limits on calories for other uses applies (see BOX 11 for additional information on alcoholic drink-equivalents); and calories from protein, carbohydrate, and total fats should be within the Acceptable Macronutrient Distribution Ranges (AMDRs).

[c]Values are rounded.

Appendix F: Healthy Vegetarian Eating Pattern

BOX 8a: Healthy Vegetarian Eating Pattern. Food Group: Vegetables, Fruits, Grains, and Dairy (1,000 to 2,000 Calorie Level)[1]

Calorie Level of Pattern[a]	1,000	1,200	1,400	1,600	1,800	2,000
Food Group[b]	Daily Amount[c] of Food From Each Group (vegetable foods subgroup are amounts/week)					
Vegetables	1 c-eq	1½ c-eq	1½ c-eq	2 c-eq	2½ c-eq	2½ c-eq
Dark-green vegetables (c-eq/wk)	½	1	1	1½	1½	1½
Red and orange vegetables (c-eq/wk)	2½	3	3	4	5½	5½
Legumes (beans and peas) (c-eq/wk)[d]	½	½	½	1	1½	1½
Starchy vegetables (c-eq/wk)	2	3½	3½	4	5	5
Other vegetables (c-eq/wk)	1½	2½	2½	3½	4	4
Fruits	1 c-eq	1 c-eq	1½ c-eq	1½ c-eq	1½ c-eq	2 c-eq
Grains	3 oz-eq	4 oz-eq	5 oz-eq	5½ oz-eq	6½ oz-eq	6½ oz-eq
Whole grains[e] (oz-eq/day)	1½	2	2½	3	3½	3½
Refined grains (oz-eq/day)	1½	2	2½	2½	3	3
Dairy	2 c-eq	2.5 c-eq	2.5 c-eq	3 c-eq	3 c-eq	3 c-eq

[1]Source: Adapted from U.S. Department of Agriculture, Center for Nutrition Policy and Promotion. 2015-2020 Dietary Guidelines for Americans. 8th Edition. Available at: http://www.cnpp.usda.gov/2015-2020-dietary-guidelines-americans;

[a] Food intake patterns at 1,000, 1,200, and 1,400 calories are designed to meet the nutritional needs of 2-8-year-old children. Patterns from 1,600 to 3,200 calories are designed to meet the nutritional needs of children 9 years and older and adults. If a child 4-8 years of age needs more calories and, therefore, is following a pattern at 1,600 calories or more, his/her recommended amount from the dairy group should be 2.5 cups/day. Children 9 years and older and adults should not use the 1,000-, 1,200-, or 1,400-calorie patterns.

[b] Foods in each group and subgroup are those listed in BOX 5a.

[c] Food group amounts are shown in cup-(c) or ounce-equivalents (oz-eq). Oils are shown in grams (g). Quantity equivalents for each food group are listed in BOX 5b.

[d] About half of total legumes are shown as vegetables, in cup-eq, and half as protein foods, in oz-eq. Total legumes in the Patterns, in cup-eq, is the amount in the vegetable group plus the amount in protein foods group (in oz-eq) divided by 4.

[e] Amounts of whole grains in the Patterns for children are less than the minimum of 3 oz-equivalent in all Patterns recommended for adults.

BOX 8b: Healthy Vegetarian Eating Pattern. Food Group: Vegetables, Fruits, Grains, and Dairy (2,200 to 3,200 Calorie Level)[1]

Calorie Level of Pattern[a]	2,200	2,400	2,600	2,800	3,000	3,200
Food Group[b]	Daily Amount[c] of Food From Each Group (vegetable foods subgroup are amounts/week)					
Vegetables	3 c-eq	3 c-eq	3½ c-eq	3½ c-eq	4 c-eq	4 c-eq
Dark-green vegetables (c-eq/wk)	2	2	2½	2½	2½	2½
Red and orange vegetables (c-eq/wk)	6	6	7	7	7½	7½
Legumes (beans and peas) (c-eq/wk)[d]	2	2	2½	2½	3	3
Starchy vegetables (c-eq/wk)	6	6	7	7	8	8
Other vegetables (c-eq/wk)	5	5	5½	5½	7	7
Fruits	2 c-eq	2 c-eq	2 c-eq	2½ c-eq	2½ c-eq	2½ c-eq
Grains	7½ oz-eq	8½ oz-eq	9½ oz-eq	10½ oz-eq	10½ oz-eq	10½ oz-eq
Whole grains[e] (oz-eq/day)	4	4½	5	5½	5½	5½
Refined grains (oz-eq/day)	3½	4	4½	5	5	5
Dairy	3 c-eq	3 c-eq	3 c-eq	3 c-eq	3 c-eq	3 c-eq

[1]Source: Adapted from U.S. Department of Agriculture, Center for Nutrition Policy and Promotion. 2015-2020 Dietary Guidelines for Americans. 8th Edition. Available at: http://www.cnpp.usda.gov/2015-2020-dietary-guidelines-americans;

[a] Food intake patterns at 1,000, 1,200, and 1,400 calories are designed to meet the nutritional needs of 2-8-year-old children. Patterns from 1,600 to 3,200 calories are designed to meet the nutritional needs of children 9 years and older and adults. If a child 4-8 years of age needs more calories and, therefore, is following a pattern at 1,600 calories or more, his/her recommended amount from the dairy group should be 2.5 cups/day. Children 9 years and older and adults should not use the 1,000-, 1,200-, or 1,400-calorie patterns.

[b] Foods in each group and subgroup are those listed in BOX 5a.

[c] Food group amounts are shown in cup-(c) or ounce-equivalents (oz-eq). Oils are shown in grams (g). Quantity equivalents for each food group are listed in BOX 5b.

[d] About half of total legumes are shown as vegetables, in cup-eq, and half as protein foods, in oz-eq. Total legumes in the Patterns, in cup-eq, is the amount in the vegetable group plus the amount in protein foods group (in oz-eq) divided by 4.

[e] Amounts of whole grains in the Patterns for children are less than the minimum of 3 oz-equivalent in all Patterns recommended for adults.

BOX 8c: Healthy Vegetarian-Style Eating Pattern. Food Group: Protein Foods, Oils and Total Legumes (1,000 to 2,000 Calorie Level)[1]

Calorie Level of Pattern[a]	1,000	1,200	1,400	1,600	1,800	2,000
Food Group[b]	Daily Amount[c] of Food From Each Group (protein foods subgroup and total legumes are amounts/week)					
Protein Foods	1 oz-eq	1½ oz-eq	2 oz-eq	2½ oz-eq	3 oz-eq	3½ oz-eq
Eggs (oz-eq/wk)	2	3	3	3	3	3
Legumes (beans and peas) (oz-eq/wk)[d]	1	2	4	4	6	6
Soy products (oz-eq/wk)	2	3	4	6	6	8
Nuts and seeds (oz-eq/wk)	2	2	3	5	6	7
Oils	15 g	17 g	17 g	22 g	24 g	27 g
Total Legumes (beans and peas) (c-eq/wk)	1	1	1½	2	3	3

[1]Source: Adapted from U.S. Department of Agriculture, Center for Nutrition Policy and Promotion. 2015-2020 Dietary Guidelines for Americans. 8th Edition. Available at: http://www.cnpp.usda.gov/2015-2020-dietary-guidelines-americans;

[a] Food intake patterns at 1,000, 1,200, and 1,400 calories are designed to meet the nutritional needs of 2-8-year-old children. Patterns from 1,600 to 3,200 calories are designed to meet the nutritional needs of children 9 years and older and adults. If a child 4-8 years of age needs more calories and, therefore, is following a pattern at 1,600 calories or more, his/her recommended amount from the dairy group should be 2.5 cups/day. Children 9 years and older and adults should not use the 1,000-, 1,200-, or 1,400-calorie patterns.

[b] Foods in each group and subgroup are those listed in BOX 5a.

[c] Food group amounts are shown in cup-(c) or ounce-equivalents (oz-eq). Oils are shown in grams (g). Quantity equivalents for each food group are listed in BOX 5b.

[d] About half of total legumes are shown as vegetables, in cup-eq, and half as protein foods, in oz-eq. Total legumes in the Patterns, in cup-eq, is the amount in the vegetable group plus the amount in protein foods group (in oz-eq) divided by 4.

BOX 8d: Healthy Vegetarian-Style Eating Pattern. Food Group: Protein Foods, Oils and Total Legumes (2,200 to 3,000 Calorie Level)[1]

Calorie Level of Pattern[a]	2,200	2,400	2,600	2,800	3,000	3,200
Food Group[b]	Daily Amount[c] of Food From Each Group (protein foods subgroup and total legumes are amounts/week)					
Protein Foods	3½ oz-eq	4 oz-eq	4½ oz-eq	5 oz-eq	5½ oz-eq	6 oz-eq
Eggs (oz-eq/wk)	3	3	3	4	4	4
Legumes (beans and peas) (oz-eq/wk)[d]	6	8	9	10	11	12
Soy products (oz-eq/wk)	8	9	10	11	12	13
Nuts and seeds (oz-eq/wk)	7	8	9	10	12	13
Oils	29 g	31 g	34 g	36 g	44 g	51 g
Total Legumes (beans and peas) (c-eq/wk)	3½	4	5	5	6	6

[1]Source: Adapted from U.S. Department of Agriculture, Center for Nutrition Policy and Promotion. 2015-2020 Dietary Guidelines for Americans. 8th Edition. Available at: http://www.cnpp.usda.gov/2015-2020-dietary-guidelines-americans;

[a] Food intake patterns at 1,000, 1,200, and 1,400 calories are designed to meet the nutritional needs of 2-8-year-old children. Patterns from 1,600 to 3,200 calories are designed to meet the nutritional needs of children 9 years and older and adults. If a child 4-8 years of age needs more calories and, therefore, is following a pattern at 1,600 calories or more, his/her recommended amount from the dairy group should be 2.5 cups/day. Children 9 years and older and adults should not use the 1,000-, 1,200-, or 1,400-calorie patterns.

[b] Foods in each group and subgroup are those listed in BOX 5a.

[c] Food group amounts are shown in cup-(c) or ounce-equivalents (oz-eq). Oils are shown in grams (g). Quantity equivalents for each food group are listed in BOX 5b.

[d] About half of total legumes are shown as vegetables, in cup-eq, and half as protein foods, in oz-eq. Total legumes in the Patterns, in cup-eq, is the amount in the vegetable group plus the amount in protein foods group (in oz-eq) divided by 4.

BOX 8e: Healthy Vegetarian-Style Eating Pattern. Limits on Calories for Other Uses (1,000 to 3,200 Calorie Level)[1]

Calorie Level of Pattern[a]	1,000	1,200	1,400	1,600	1,800	2,000
Limit on Calories for Other Uses, calories (% of calories)[b,c]	190 (19%)	170 (14%)	190 (14%)	180 (11%)	190 (11%)	290 (15%)
Calorie Level of Pattern[a]	2,200	2,400	2,600	2,800	3,000	3,200
Limit on Calories for Other Uses, calories (% of calories)[b,c]	330 (15%)	390 (16%)	390 (15%)	400 (14%)	440 (15%)	550 (17%)

[1]Source: Adapted from U.S. Department of Agriculture, Center for Nutrition Policy and Promotion. 2015-2020 Dietary Guidelines for Americans. 8th Edition. Available at: http://www.cnpp.usda.gov/2015-2020-dietary-guidelines-americans;

[a] Food intake patterns at 1,000, 1,200, and 1,400 calories are designed to meet the nutritional needs of 2-8-year-old children. Patterns from 1,600 to 3,200 calories are designed to meet the nutritional needs of children 9 years and older and adults. If a child 4-8 years of age needs more calories and, therefore, is following a pattern at 1,600 calories or more, his/her recommended amount from the dairy group should be 2.5 cups/day. Children 9 years and older and adults should not use the 1,000-, 1,200-, or 1,400-calorie patterns.

[b] All foods are assumed to be in nutrient-dense forms, lean or low-fat and prepared without added fats, sugars, refined starches, or salt. If all food choices to meet food group recommendations are in nutrient-dense forms, a small number of calories remain within the overall calorie limit of the Pattern (i.e., limit on calories for other uses).

The number of these calories depends on the overall calorie limit in the Pattern and the amounts of food from each food group required to meet nutritional goals. Nutritional goals are higher for the 1,200- to 1,600-calorie Patterns than for the 1,000-calorie Pattern, so the limit on calories for other uses is lower in the 1,200- to 1,600-calorie Patterns. Calories up to the specified limit can be used for added sugars, added refined starches, solid fats, alcohol, or to eat more than the recommended amount of food in a food group.

The overall eating Pattern also should not exceed the limits of less than 10% of calories from added sugars and less than 10% of calories from saturated fats. At most calorie levels, amounts that can be accommodated are less than these limits.

For adults of legal drinking age who choose to drink alcohol, a limit of up to 1 drink/day for women and up to 2 drinks/day for men within limits on calories for other uses applies (see Box 11 for additional information on alcoholic drink-equivalents); and calories from protein, carbohydrate, and total fats should be within the Acceptable Macronutrient Distribution Ranges (AMDRs).

[c]Values are rounded.

Appendix G: Nutritional Goals

BOX 9a. Nutritional Goals Ranked by Gender and Age Based on Dietary Reference Intakes: Macronutrients[1]

	Source of goal [a]	Child 1-3	Female 4-8	Male 4-8	Female 9-13	Male 9-13	Female 14-18	Male 14-18
Calorie level(s) assessed		1,000	1,200	1,400, 1,600	1,600	1,800	1,800	2,200, 2,800, 3,200
Macronutrients								
Protein, g	RDA	13	19	19	34	34	46	52
Protein, % kcal	AMDR	5-20	10-30	10-30	10-30	10-30	10-30	10-30
Carbohydrate, g	RDA	130	130	130	130	130	130	130
Carbohydrate, % kcal	AMDR	45-65	45-65	45-65	45-65	45-65	45-65	45-65
Dietary Fiber, g	14g/ 1,000 kcal	14	16.8	19.6	22.4	25.2	25.2	30.8
Added sugars, % kcal	DGA	<10%	<10%	<10%	<10%	<10%	<10%	<10%
Total fat, % kcal	AMDR	30-40	25-35	25-35	25-35	25-35	25-35	25-35
Saturated fat, % kcal	DGA	<10%	<10%	<10%	<10%	<10%	<10%	<10%
Linoleic acid, g	AI	7	10	10	10	12	11	16
Linolenic acid, g	AI	0.7	0.9	0.9	1	1.2	1.1	1.6

[1]Source: Adapted from U.S. Department of Agriculture, Center for Nutrition Policy and Promotion. 2015-2020 Dietary Guidelines for Americans. 8th Edition. Available at: http://www.cnpp.usda.gov/2015-2020-dietary-guidelines-americans;
[a] RDA = Recommended Dietary Allowance, AI = Adequate Intake, UL = Tolerable Upper Intake Level, AMDR = Acceptable Macronutrient Distribution Range, DGA = *2015-2020 Dietary Guidelines* recommended limit; 14 g fiber per 1,000 kcal = basis for AI for fiber.

BOX 9b. Nutritional Goals Ranked by Gender and Age Based on Dietary Reference Intakes: Macronutrients[1]

	Source of goal [a]	Female 19-30	Male 19-30	Female 31-50	Male 31-50	Female 51+	Male 51+
Calorie level(s) assessed		2,000	2,400, 2,600, 3,000	1,800	2,200	1,600	2,000
Macronutrients							
Protein, g	RDA	46	56	46	56	46	56
Protein, % kcal	AMDR	10-35	10-35	10-35	10-35	10-35	10-35
Carbohydrate, g	RDA	130	130	130	130	130	130
Carbohydrate, % kcal	AMDR	45-65	45-65	45-65	45-65	45-65	45-65
Dietary Fiber, g	14g/ 1,000 kcal	28	33.6	25.2	30.8	22.4	28
Added sugars, % kcal	DGA	<10%	<10%	<10%	<10%	<10%	<10%
Total fat, % kcal	AMDR	20-35	20-35	20-35	20-35	20-35	20-35
Saturated fat, % kcal	DGA	<10%	<10%	<10%	<10%	<10%	<10%
Linoleic acid, g	AI	12	17	12	17	11	14
Linolenic acid, g	AI	1.1	1.6	1.1	1.6	1.1	1.6

[1]Source: Adapted from U.S. Department of Agriculture, Center for Nutrition Policy and Promotion. 2015-2020 Dietary Guidelines for Americans. 8th Edition. Available at: http://www.cnpp.usda.gov/2015-2020-dietary-guidelines-americans;
[a] RDA = Recommended Dietary Allowance, AI = Adequate Intake, UL = Tolerable Upper Intake Level, AMDR = Acceptable Macronutrient Distribution Range, DGA = *2015-2020 Dietary Guidelines* recommended limit; 14 g fiber per 1,000 kcal = basis for AI for fiber.

BOX 10a. Nutritional Goals Ranked by Gender and Age Based on Dietary Reference Intakes: Minerals[1]

	Source of goal[a]	Child 1-3	Female 4-8	Male 4-8	Female 9-13	Male 9-13	Female 14-18	Male 14-18
Calorie level(s) assessed		1,000	1,200	1,400, 1,600	1,600	1,800	1,800	2,200, 2,800, 3,200
Minerals								
Calcium, mg	RDA	700	1,000	1,000	1,300	1,300	1,300	1,300
Iron, mg	RDA	7	10	10	8	8	15	11
Magnesium, mg	RDA	80	130	130	240	240	360	410
Phosphorus, mg	RDA	460	500	500	1,250	1,250	1,250	1,250
Potassium, mg	AI	3,000	3,800	3,800	4,500	4,500	4,700	4,700
Sodium, mg	UL	1,500	1,900	1,900	2,200	2,200	2,300	2,300
Zinc, mg	RDA	3	5	5	8	8	9	11
Copper, mcg	RDA	340	440	440	700	700	890	890
Manganese, mg	AI	1.2	1.5	1.5	1.6	1.9	1.6	2.2
Selenium, mcg	RDA	20	30	30	40	40	55	55

[1]Source: Adapted from U.S. Department of Agriculture, Center for Nutrition Policy and Promotion. 2015-2020 Dietary Guidelines for Americans. 8th Edition. Available at: http://www.cnpp.usda.gov/2015-2020-dietary-guidelines-americans;

[a] RDA = Recommended Dietary Allowance, AI = Adequate Intake, UL = Tolerable Upper Intake Level, AMDR = Acceptable Macronutrient Distribution Range, DGA = *2015-2020 Dietary Guidelines* recommended limit; 14 g fiber per 1,000 kcal = basis for AI for fiber.

BOX 10b. Nutritional Goals Ranked by Gender and Age Based on Dietary Reference Intakes: Minerals[1]

	Source of goal[a]	Female 19-30	Male 19-30	Female 31-50	Male 31-50	Female 51+	Male 51+
Calorie level(s) assessed		2,000	2,400, 2,600, 3,000	1,800	2,200	1,600	2,000
Minerals							
Calcium, mg	RDA	1,000	1,000	1,000	1,000	1,200	1,000[b]
Iron, mg	RDA	18	8	18	8	8	8
Magnesium, mg	RDA	310	400	320	420	320	420
Phosphorus, mg	RDA	700	700	700	700	700	700
Potassium, mg	AI	4,700	4,700	4,700	4,700	4,700	4,700
Sodium, mg	UL	2,300	2,300	2,300	2,300	2,300	2,300
Zinc, mg	RDA	8	11	8	11	8	11
Copper, mcg	RDA	900	900	900	900	900	900
Manganese, mg	AI	1.8	2.3	1.8	2.3	1.8	2.3
Selenium, mcg	RDA	55	55	55	55	55	55

[1]Source: Adapted from U.S. Department of Agriculture, Center for Nutrition Policy and Promotion. 2015-2020 Dietary Guidelines for Americans. 8th Edition. Available at: http://www.cnpp.usda.gov/2015-2020-dietary-guidelines-americans;

[a] RDA = Recommended Dietary Allowance, AI = Adequate Intake, UL = Tolerable Upper Intake Level, AMDR = Acceptable Macronutrient Distribution Range, DGA = *2015-2020 Dietary Guidelines* recommended limit; 14 g fiber per 1,000 kcal = basis for AI for fiber.

[b] Calcium RDA for males ages 71+ years is 1,200 mg.

BOX 11a. Nutritional Goals Ranked by Gender and Age Based on Dietary Reference Intakes: Vitamins[1]

	Source of goal[a]	Child 1-3	Female 4-8	Male 4-8	Female 9-13	Male 9-13	Female 14-18	Male 14-18
Calorie level(s) assessed		1,000	1,200	1,400, 1,600	1,600	1,800	1,800	2,200, 2,800, 3,200
Vitamins								
Vitamin A, mg RAE	RDA	300	400	400	600	600	700	900
Vitamin E, mg AT	RDA	6	7	7	11	11	15	15
Vitamin D, IU	RDA	600	600	600	600	600	600	600
Vitamin C, mg	RDA	15	25	25	45	45	65	75
Thiamin, mg	RDA	0.5	0.6	0.6	0.9	0.9	1	1.2
Riboflavin, mg	RDA	0.5	0.6	0.6	0.9	0.9	1	1.3
Niacin, mg	RDA	6	8	8	12	12	14	16
Vitamin B_6, mg	RDA	0.5	0.6	0.6	1	1	1.2	1.3
Vitamin B_{12}, mcg	RDA	0.9	1.2	1.2	1.8	1.8	2.4	2.4
Choline, mg	AI	200	250	250	375	375	400	550
Vitamin K, mcg	AI	30	55	55	60	60	75	75
Folate, mcg DFE	RDA	150	200	200	300	300	400	400

[1]Source: Adapted from U.S. Department of Agriculture, Center for Nutrition Policy and Promotion. 2015-2020 Dietary Guidelines for Americans. 8th Edition. Available at: http://www.cnpp.usda.gov/2015-2020-dietary-guidelines-americans;

[a] RDA = Recommended Dietary Allowance, AI = Adequate Intake, UL = Tolerable Upper Intake Level, AMDR = Acceptable Macronutrient Distribution Range, DGA = *2015-2020 Dietary Guidelines* recommended limit; 14 g fiber per 1,000 kcal = basis for AI for fiber.

BOX 11b. Nutritional Goals Ranked by Gender and Age Based on Dietary Reference Intakes: Vitamins[1]

	Source of goal[a]	Female 19-30	Male 19-30	Female 31-50	Male 31-50	Female 51+	Male 51+
Calorie level(s) assessed		2,000	2,400, 2,600, 3,000	1,800	2,200	1,600	2,000
Vitamins							
Vitamin A, mg RAE	RDA	700	900	700	900	700	900
Vitamin E, mg AT	RDA	15	15	15	15	15	15
Vitamin D, IU	RDA	600	600	600	600	600[b]	600[b]
Vitamin C, mg	RDA	75	90	75	90	75	90
Thiamin, mg	RDA	1.1	1.2	1.1	1.2	1.1	1.2
Riboflavin, mg	RDA	1.1	1.3	1.1	1.3	1.1	1.3
Niacin, mg	RDA	14	16	14	16	14	16
Vitamin B_6, mg	RDA	1.3	1.3	1.3	1.3	1.5	1.7
Vitamin B_{12}, mcg	RDA	2.4	2.4	2.4	2.4	2.4	2.4
Choline, mg	AI	425	550	425	550	425	550
Vitamin K, mcg	AI	90	120	90	120	90	120
Folate, mcg DFE	RDA	400	400	400	400	400	400

[1]Source: Adapted from U.S. Department of Agriculture, Center for Nutrition Policy and Promotion. 2015-2020 Dietary Guidelines for Americans. 8th Edition. Available at: http://www.cnpp.usda.gov/2015-2020-dietary-guidelines-americans;

[a]RDA = Recommended Dietary Allowance, AI = Adequate Intake, UL = Tolerable Upper Intake Level, AMDR = Acceptable Macronutrient Distribution Range, DGA = *2015-2020 Dietary Guidelines* recommended limit; 14 g fiber per 1,000 kcal = basis for AI for fiber.

[b]Vitamin D RDA for males and females ages 71+ years is 800 IU.

BOX 12: Alcoholic Drink-Equivalents of Selected Beverages[1]

Drink Description	Drink-Equivalent[a,b]
Beer, beer coolers, and malt beverages	
12 fl oz at 4.2% alcohol[c]	0.8
12-16 fl oz at 5% alcohol (reference beverage)	1.0-1.3
12 fl oz at 7-9% alcohol	1.4-1.8
Wine	
5-9 fl oz at 12% alcohol (reference beverage)	1.0-1.8
5 fl oz at 15-17% alcohol	1.3-1.4
Distilled Spirits	
1.5 fl oz 80 proof distilled spirits (40% alcohol) (reference beverage)	1
Mixed drink with more than 1.5 fl oz 80 proof distilled spirits (40% alcohol)	> 1[d]

[1]Source: Adapted from U.S. Department of Agriculture, Center for Nutrition Policy and Promotion. 2015-2020 Dietary Guidelines for Americans. 8th Edition. Available at: http://www.cnpp.usda.gov/2015-2020-dietary-guidelines-americans.

[a] One alcoholic drink-equivalent is defined as containing 14 grams (0.6 fl oz) of pure alcohol. The following are reference beverages that are one alcoholic drink-equivalent: 12 fluid ounces of regular beer (5% alcohol), 5 fluid ounces of wine (12% alcohol), or 1.5 fluid ounces of 80 proof distilled spirits (40% alcohol). Drink-equivalents are not intended to serve as a standard drink definition for regulatory purposes.

[b] To calculate drink-equivalents, multiply the volume in ounces by the alcohol content in percent and divide by 0.6 ounces of alcohol per drink-equivalent. For example: 16 fl oz beer at 5% alcohol: (16 fl oz)(0.05)/0.6 fl oz = 1.3 drink-equivalents.

[c] Light beer represents a substantial proportion of alcoholic beverages consumed in the United States. Light beer is approximately 4.2% alcohol or 0.8 alcoholic drink-equivalents in 12 fluid ounces.

[d] Depending on factors, such as the type of spirits and the recipe, one mixed drink can contain a variable number of drink-equivalents.

BOX 13a. Food Sources of Potassium Ranked by Amount and Energy[1]

Food	Standard Portion Size	Calories in Standard Portion[a]	Potassium in Standard Portion (mg)[a]	Calories per 100 grams[a]	Potassium per 100 grams (mg)[a]
Potato, baked, flesh and skin	1 medium	163	941	94	544
Prune juice, canned	1 cup	182	707	71	276
Carrot juice, canned	1 cup	94	689	40	292
Passion-fruit juice, yellow or purple	1 cup	126-148	687	51-60	278
Tomato paste, canned	¼ cup	54	669	82	1,014
Beet greens, cooked from fresh	½ cup	19	654	27	909
Adzuki beans, cooked	½ cup	147	612	128	532
White beans, canned	½ cup	149	595	114	454
Plain yogurt, nonfat	1 cup	127	579	56	255
Tomato puree	½ cup	48	549	38	439
Sweet potato, baked in skin	1 medium	103	542	90	475
Salmon, Atlantic, wild, cooked	3 ounces	155	534	182	628
Clams, canned	3 ounces	121	534	142	628

[1]Source: Adapted from U.S. Department of Agriculture, Center for Nutrition Policy and Promotion. 2015-2020 Dietary Guidelines for Americans. 8th Edition. Available at: http://www.cnpp.usda.gov/2015-2020-dietary-guidelines-americans;

[a]Source: U.S Department of Agriculture, Agricultural Research Service, Nutrient Data Laboratory. 2014. USDA National Nutrient Database for Standard Reference, Release 27. Available at: http://www.ars.usda.gov/nutrientdata.

BOX 13b. Food Sources of Potassium Ranked by Amount and Energy[1]

Food	Standard Portion Size	Calories in Standard Portion[a]	Potassium in Standard Portion (mg)[a]	Calories per 100 grams[a]	Potassium per 100 grams (mg)[a]
Pomegranate juice	1 cup	134	533	54	214
Plain yogurt, low-fat	8 ounces	143	531	63	234
Tomato juice, canned	1 cup	41	527	17	217
Orange juice, fresh	1 cup	112	496	45	200
Soybeans, green, cooked	½ cup	127	485	141	539
Chard, swiss, cooked	½ cup	18	481	20	549
Lima beans, cooked	½ cup	108	478	115	508
Mackerel, various types, cooked	3 ounces	114-171	443-474	134-201	521-558
Vegetable juice, canned	1 cup	48	468	19	185
Chili with beans, canned	½ cup	144	467	112	365
Great northern beans, canned	½ cup	150	460	114	351
Yam, cooked	½ cup	79	456	116	670
Halibut, cooked	3 ounces	94	449	111	528

[1]Source: Adapted from U.S. Department of Agriculture, Center for Nutrition Policy and Promotion. 2015-2020 Dietary Guidelines for Americans. 8th Edition. Available at: http://www.cnpp.usda.gov/2015-2020-dietary-guidelines-americans;
[a]Source: U.S Department of Agriculture, Agricultural Research Service, Nutrient Data Laboratory. 2014. USDA National Nutrient Database for Standard Reference, Release 27. Available at: http://www.ars.usda.gov/nutrientdata.

BOX 13c. Food Sources of Potassium Ranked by Amount and Energy[1]

Food	Standard Portion Size	Calories in Standard Portion[a]	Potassium in Standard Portion (mg)[a]	Calories per 100 grams[a]	Potassium per 100 grams (mg)[a]
Tuna, yellowfin, cooked	3 ounces	111	448	130	527
Acorn squash, cooked	½ cup	58	448	56	437
Snapper, cooked	3 ounces	109	444	128	522
Soybeans, mature, cooked	½ cup	149	443	173	515
Tangerine juice, fresh	1 cup	106	440	43	178
Pink beans, cooked	½ cup	126	430	149	508
Chocolate milk (1%, 2% and whole)	1 cup	178-208	418-425	71-83	167-170
Amaranth leaves, cooked	½ cup	14	423	21	641
Banana	1 medium	105	422	89	358
Spinach, cooked from fresh or canned	½ cup	21-25	370-419	23	346-466
Black turtle beans, cooked	½ cup	121	401	130	433
Peaches, dried, uncooked	¼ cup	96	399	239	996
Prunes, stewed	½ cup	133	398	107	321

[1]Source: Adapted from U.S. Department of Agriculture, Center for Nutrition Policy and Promotion. 2015-2020 Dietary Guidelines for Americans. 8th Edition. Available at: http://www.cnpp.usda.gov/2015-2020-dietary-guidelines-americans;
[a]Source: U.S Department of Agriculture, Agricultural Research Service, Nutrient Data Laboratory. 2014. USDA National Nutrient Database for Standard Reference, Release 27. Available at: http://www.ars.usda.gov/nutrientdata.

BOX 13d. Food Sources of Potassium Ranked by Amount and Energy[1]

Food	Standard Portion Size	Calories in Standard Portion[a]	Potassium in Standard Portion (mg)[a]	Calories per 100 grams[a]	Potassium per 100 grams (mg)[a]
Rockfish, Pacific, cooked	3 ounces	93	397	109	467
Rainbow trout, wild or farmed, cooked	3 ounces	128-143	381-383	150-168	448-450
Skim milk (nonfat)	1 cup	83	382	34	156
Refried beans, canned, traditional	½ cup	106	380	89	319
Apricots, dried, uncooked	¼ cup	78	378	241	1162
Pinto beans, cooked	½ cup	123	373	143	436
Lentils, cooked	½ cup	115	365	116	369
Avocado	½ cup	120	364	160	485
Tomato sauce, canned	½ cup	30	364	24	297
Plantains, slices, cooked	½ cup	89	358	116	465
Kidney beans, cooked	½ cup	113	357	127	403
Navy beans, cooked	½ cup	128	354	140	389

[1]Source: Adapted from U.S. Department of Agriculture, Center for Nutrition Policy and Promotion. 2015-2020 Dietary Guidelines for Americans. 8th Edition. Available at: http://www.cnpp.usda.gov/2015-2020-dietary-guidelines-americans;
[a]Source: U.S Department of Agriculture, Agricultural Research Service, Nutrient Data Laboratory. 2014. USDA National Nutrient Database for Standard Reference, Release 27. Available at: http://www.ars.usda.gov/nutrientdata.

BOX 14a. Food Sources of Calcium Ranked by Amount and Energy[1]

Food	Standard Portion Size	Calories in Standard Portion[a]	Calcium in Standard Portion (mg)[a]	Calories per 100 grams[a]	Calcium per 100 grams (mg)[a]
Fortified ready-to-eat cereals[b]	¾-1¼ cup	70-197	137-1,000	234-394	455-3,333
Past. processed Amer. cheese	2 ounces	210	593	371	1,045
Parmesan cheese, hard	1.5 ounces	167	503	392	1,184
Plain yogurt, nonfat	8 ounces	127	452	56	199
Romano cheese	1.5 ounces	165	452	387	1,064
Almond milk (all flavors)[b]	1 cup	91-120	451	38-50	188
Past. processed Swiss cheese	2 ounces	189	438	334	772
Tofu, raw, regular, with Ca sulfate	½ cup	94	434	76	350
Gruyere cheese	1.5 ounces	176	430	413	1,011
Plain yogurt, low-fat	8 ounces	143	415	63	183
Vanilla yogurt, low-fat	8 ounces	193	388	85	171
Past. Amer. cheese food	2 ounces	187	387	330	682
Fruit yogurt, low-fat	8 ounces	238	383	105	169
Orange juice, calcium fortified[b]	1 cup	117	349	47	140
Soymilk (all flavors)[b]	1 cup	109	340	45	140
Ricotta cheese, part skim	½ cup	171	337	138	272
Swiss cheese	1.5 ounces	162	336	380	791
Evaporated milk	½ cup	170	329	135	261

[1]Source: Adapted from U.S. Department of Agriculture, Center for Nutrition Policy and Promotion. 2015-2020 Dietary Guidelines for Americans. 8th Edition. Available at: http://www.cnpp.usda.gov/2015-2020-dietary-guidelines-americans; [a]Source: U.S Department of Agriculture, Agricultural Research Service, Nutrient Data Laboratory. 2014. USDA National Nutrient Database for Standard Reference, Release 27. Available at: http://www.ars.usda.gov/nutrientdata; [b]Calcium fortified.

BOX 14b. Food Sources of Calcium Ranked by Amount and Energy[1]

Food	Standard Portion Size	Calories in Standard Portion[a]	Calcium in Standard Portion (mg)[a]	Calories per 100 grams[a]	Calcium per 100 grams (mg)[a]
Sardines, canned in oil, drained	3 ounces	177	325	208	382
Provolone cheese	1.5 ounces	149	321	351	756
Monterey cheese	1.5 ounces	159	317	373	746
Mustard spinach (tendergreen), raw	1 cup	33	315	22	210
Muenster cheese	1.5 ounces	156	305	368	717
Low-fat milk (1%)	1 cup	102	305	42	125
Mozzarella cheese, part-skim	1.5 ounces	128	304	301	716
Skim milk (nonfat)	1 cup	83	299	34	122
Reduced fat milk (2%)	1 cup	122	293	50	120
Colby cheese	1.5 ounces	167	291	394	685
Low-fat chocolate milk (1%)	1 cup	178	290	71	116
Cheddar cheese	1.5 ounces	173	287	406	675
Rice drink[b]	1 cup	113	283	47	118
Whole buttermilk	1 cup	152	282	62	115
Whole chocolate milk	1 cup	208	280	83	112
Whole milk	1 cup	149	276	61	113
Reduced fat chocolate milk (2%)	1 cup	190	273	76	109
Ricotta cheese, whole milk	½ cup	216	257	174	207

[1]Source: Adapted from U.S. Department of Agriculture, Center for Nutrition Policy and Promotion. 2015-2020 Dietary Guidelines for Americans. 8th Edition. Available at: http://www.cnpp.usda.gov/2015-2020-dietary-guidelines-americans; [a]Source: U.S Department of Agriculture, Agricultural Research Service, Nutrient Data Laboratory. 2014. USDA National Nutrient Database for Standard Reference, Release 27. Available at: http://www.ars.usda.gov/nutrientdata; [b]Calcium fortified.

BOX 15a. Food Sources of Vitamin D Ranked by Amount and Energy[1]

Food	Standard Portion Size	Calories in Standard Portion[a]	Vitamin D in Standard Portion (μg)[a,b]	Calories per 100 grams[a]	Vitamin D per 100 grams (μg)[a,b]
Salmon, sockeye, canned	3 ounces	142	17.9	167	21.0
Trout, rainbow, farmed, cooked	3 ounces	143	16.2	168	19.0
Salmon, chinook, smoked	3 ounces	99	14.5	117	17.1
Swordfish, cooked	3 ounces	146	14.1	172	16.6
Sturgeon, mixed species, smoked	3 ounces	147	13.7	173	16.1
Salmon, pink, canned	3 ounces	117	12.3	138	14.5
Fish oil, cod liver	1 tsp	41	11.3	902	250
Cisco, smoked	3 ounces	150	11.3	177	13.3
Salmon, sockeye, cooked	3 ounces	144	11.1	169	13.1
Salmon, pink, cooked	3 ounces	130	11.1	153	13.0
Sturgeon, mixed species, cooked	3 ounces	115	11.0	135	12.9
Whitefish, mixed species, smoked	3 ounces	92	10.9	108	12.8
Mackerel, Pacific and jack, cooked	3 ounces	171	9.7	201	11.4
Salmon, coho, wild, cooked	3 ounces	118	9.6	139	11.3
Mushrooms, UV light, grilled	½ cup	18	7.9	29	13.1
Tuna, light, canned in oil, drained	3 ounces	168	5.7	198	6.7
Halibut, Atlantic/Pacific, cooked	3 ounces	94	4.9	111	5.8

[1]Source: Adapted from U.S. Department of Agriculture, Center for Nutrition Policy and Promotion. 2015-2020 Dietary Guidelines for Americans. 8th Edition. Available at: http://www.cnpp.usda.gov/2015-2020-dietary-guidelines-americans; [a]Source: U.S Department of Agriculture, Agricultural Research Service, Nutrient Data Laboratory. 2014. USDA National Nutrient Database for Standard Reference, Release 27. Available at: http://www.ars.usda.gov/nutrientdata; [b]1 μg of vitamin D is equivalent to 40 IU.

BOX 15b. Food Sources of Vitamin D Ranked by Amount and Energy[1]

Food	Standard Portion Size	Calories in Standard Portion[a]	Vitamin D in Standard Portion (μg)[a,b]	Calories per 100 grams[a]	Vitamin D per 100 grams (μg)[a,b]
Herring, Atlantic, cooked	3 ounces	173	4.6	203	5.4
Sardine, canned in oil, drained	3 ounces	177	4.1	208	4.8
Rockfish/Pacific, mix. spec. cooked	3 ounces	93	3.9	109	4.6
Whole milk[c]	1 cup	149	3.2	61	1.3
Whole chocolate milk[c]	1 cup	208	3.2	83	1.3
Tilapia, cooked	3 ounces	109	3.1	128	3.7
Flatfish (flounder and sole), cooked	3 ounces	73	3.0	86	3.5
Reduced fat chocolate milk (2%)[c]	1 cup	190	3.0	76	1.2
Yogurt (various types and flavors)[c]	8 ounces	98-254	2.0-3.0	43-112	0.9-1.3
Milk (non-fat, 1% and 2%)[c]	1 cup	83-122	2.9	34-50	1.2
Soymilk[c]	1 cup	109	2.9	45	1.2
Low-fat chocolate milk (1%)[c]	1 cup	178	2.8	71	1.1
Fort. ready-to-eat cereals (various)[c]	⅓-1¼ cup	74-247	0.2-2.5	248-443	0.8-8.6
Orange juice, fortified[c]	1 cup	117	2.5	47	1.0

[1]Source: Adapted from U.S. Department of Agriculture, Center for Nutrition Policy and Promotion. 2015-2020 Dietary Guidelines for Americans. 8th Edition. Available at: http://www.cnpp.usda.gov/2015-2020-dietary-guidelines-americans; [a]Source: U.S Department of Agriculture, Agricultural Research Service, Nutrient Data Laboratory. 2014. USDA National Nutrient Database for Standard Reference, Release 27. Available at: http://www.ars.usda.gov/nutrientdata; [b]1 μg of vitamin D is equivalent to 40 IU; [c] Vitamin D fortified.

BOX 15c. Food Sources of Vitamin D Ranked by Amount and Energy[1]

Food	Standard Portion Size	Calories in Standard Portion[a]	Vitamin D in Standard Portion (μg)[a,b]	Calories per 100 grams[a]	Vitamin D per 100 grams (μg)[a,b]
Almond milk (all flavors)[c]	1 cup	91-120	2.4	38-50	1.0
Rice drink[c]	1 cup	113	2.4	47	1.0
Pork, cooked (various cuts)	3 ounces	122-390	0.2-2.2	143-459	0.2-2.6
Mushrooms, morel, raw	½ cup	10	1.7	31	5.1
Margarine (various)[c]	1 Tbsp	75-100	1.5	533-717	10.7
Mushrooms, Chanterelle, raw	½ cup	10	1.4	38	5.3
Egg, hard-boiled	1 large	78	1.1	155	2.2

[1]Source: Adapted from U.S. Department of Agriculture, Center for Nutrition Policy and Promotion. 2015-2020 Dietary Guidelines for Americans. 8th Edition. Available at: http://www.cnpp.usda.gov/2015-2020-dietary-guidelines-americans; [a]Source: U.S Department of Agriculture, Agricultural Research Service, Nutrient Data Laboratory. 2014. USDA National Nutrient Database for Standard Reference, Release 27. Available at: http://www.ars.usda.gov/nutrientdata; [b]1 μg of vitamin D is equivalent to 40 IU; [c]Vitamin D fortified.

BOX 16a. Food Sources of Fiber Ranked by Amount and Energy[1]

Food	Standard Portion Size	Calories in Standard Portion[a]	Dietary Fiber in Standard Portion (g)[a]	Calories per 100 grams[a]	Dietary Fiber per 100 grams (g)[a]
High fiber bran ready-to-eat cereal	⅓ – ¾ cup	60-81	9.1-14.3	200-260	29.3-47.5
Navy beans, cooked	½ cup	127	9.6	140	10.5
Small white beans, cooked	½ cup	127	9.3	142	10.4
Yellow beans, cooked	½ cup	127	9.2	144	10.4
Shredded wheat, ready cereals	1-1 ¼ cup	155-220	5.0-9.0	321-373	9.6-15.0
Cranberry (roman) beans, cooked	½ cup	120	8.9	136	10.0
Adzuki beans, cooked	½ cup	147	8.4	128	7.3
French beans, cooked	½ cup	114	8.3	129	9.4
Split peas, cooked	½ cup	114	8.1	116	8.3
Chickpeas, canned	½ cup	176	8.1	139	6.4
Lentils, cooked	½ cup	115	7.8	116	7.9
Pinto beans, cooked	½ cup	122	7.7	143	9.0
Black turtle beans, cooked	½ cup	120	7.7	130	8.3
Mung beans, cooked	½ cup	106	7.7	105	7.6
Black beans, cooked	½ cup	114	7.5	132	8.7
Artichoke, globe or French, cooked	½ cup	45	7.2	53	8.6
Lima beans, cooked	½ cup	108	6.6	115	7.0

[1]Source: Adapted from U.S. Department of Agriculture, Center for Nutrition Policy and Promotion. 2015-2020 Dietary Guidelines for Americans. 8th Edition. Available at: http://www.cnpp.usda.gov/2015-2020-dietary-guidelines-americans; [a]Source: U.S Department of Agriculture, Agricultural Research Service, Nutrient Data Laboratory. 2014. USDA National Nutrient Database for Standard Reference, Release 27. Available at: http://www.ars.usda.gov/nutrientdata.

BOX 16b. Food Sources of Fiber Ranked by Amount and Energy[1]

Food	Standard Portion Size	Calories in Standard Portion[a]	Dietary Fiber in Standard Portion (g)[a]	Calories per 100 grams[a]	Dietary Fiber per 100 grams (g)[a]
Great northern beans, canned	½ cup	149	6.4	114	4.9
White beans, canned	½ cup	149	6.3	114	4.8
Kidney beans, all types, cooked	½ cup	112	5.7	127	6.4
Pigeon peas, cooked	½ cup	102	5.6	121	6.7
Cowpeas, cooked	½ cup	99	5.6	116	6.5
Wheat bran flakes ready-to-eat cereal (various)	¾ cup	90-98	4.9-5.5	310-328	16.9-18.3
Pear, raw	1 medium	101	5.5	57	3.1
Pumpkin seeds, whole, roasted	1 ounce	126	5.2	446	18.4
Baked beans, canned, plain	½ cup	119	5.2	94	4.1
Soybeans, cooked	½ cup	149	5.2	173	6.0
Plain rye wafer crackers	2 wafers	73	5.0	334	22.9
Avocado	½ cup	120	5.0	160	6.7
Broadbeans (fava beans), cooked	½ cup	94	4.6	110	5.4
Pink beans, cooked	½ cup	126	4.5	149	5.3
Apple, with skin	1 medium	95	4.4	52	2.4
Green peas, cooked (fresh, frozen, canned)	½ cup	59-67	3.5-4.4	69-84	4.1-5.5

[1]Source: Adapted from U.S. Department of Agriculture, Center for Nutrition Policy and Promotion. 2015-2020 Dietary Guidelines for Americans. 8th Edition. Available at: http://www.cnpp.usda.gov/2015-2020-dietary-guidelines-americans; [a]Source: U.S Department of Agriculture, Agricultural Research Service, Nutrient Data Laboratory. 2014. USDA National Nutrient Database for Standard Reference, Release 27. Available at: http://www.ars.usda.gov/nutrientdata.

BOX 16c. Food Sources of Fiber Ranked by Amount and Energy[1]

Food	Standard Portion Size	Calories in Standard Portion[a]	Dietary Fiber in Standard Portion (g)[a]	Calories per 100 grams[a]	Dietary Fiber per 100 grams (g)[a]
Refried beans, canned	½ cup	107	4.4	90	3.7
Chia seeds, dried	1 Tbsp	58	4.1	486	34.4
Bulgur, cooked	½ cup	76	4.1	83	4.5
Mixed vegetables, cooked from frozen	½ cup	59	4.0	65	4.4
Raspberries	½ cup	32	4.0	52	6.5
Blackberries	½ cup	31	3.8	43	5.3
Collards, cooked	½ cup	32	3.8	33	4.0
Soybeans, green, cooked	½ cup	127	3.8	141	4.2
Prunes, stewed	½ cup	133	3.8	107	3.1
Sweet potato, baked in skin	1 medium	103	3.8	90	3.3
Figs, dried	¼ cup	93	3.7	249	9.8
Pumpkin, canned	½ cup	42	3.6	34	2.9
Potato, baked, with skin	1 medium	163	3.6	94	2.1
Popcorn, air-popped	3 cups	93	3.5	387	14.5
Almonds	1 ounce	164	3.5	579	12.5
Pears, dried	¼ cup	118	3.4	262	7.5
Whole wheat spaghetti, cooked	½ cup	87	3.2	124	4.5

[1]Source: Adapted from U.S. Department of Agriculture, Center for Nutrition Policy and Promotion. 2015-2020 Dietary Guidelines for Americans. 8th Edition. Available at: http://www.cnpp.usda.gov/2015-2020-dietary-guidelines-americans; [a]Source: U.S Department of Agriculture, Agricultural Research Service, Nutrient Data Laboratory. 2014. USDA National Nutrient Database for Standard Reference, Release 27. Available at: http://www.ars.usda.gov/nutrientdata.

BOX 16d. Food Sources of Fiber Ranked by Amount and Energy[1]

Food	Standard Portion Size	Calories in Standard Portion[a]	Dietary Fiber in Standard Portion (g)[a]	Calories per 100 grams[a]	Dietary Fiber per 100 grams (g)[a]
Parsnips, cooked	½ cup	55	3.1	71	4.0
Sunflower seed kernels, dry roasted	1 ounce	165	3.1	582	11.1
Orange	1 medium	69	3.1	49	2.2
Banana	1 medium	105	3.1	89	2.6
Guava	1 fruit	37	3.0	68	5.4
Oat bran muffin	1 small	178	3.0	270	4.6
Pearled barley, cooked	½ cup	97	3.0	123	3.8
Winter squash, cooked	½ cup	38	2.9	37	2.8
Dates	¼ cup	104	2.9	282	8.0
Pistachios, dry roasted	1 ounce	161	2.8	567	9.9
Pecans, oil roasted	1 ounce	203	2.7	715	9.5
Hazelnuts or filberts	1 ounce	178	2.7	628	9.7
Peanuts, oil roasted	1 ounce	170	2.7	599	9.4
Whole wheat paratha bread	1 ounce	92	2.7	326	9.6
Quinoa, cooked	½ cup	111	2.6	120	2.8

[1]Source: Adapted from U.S. Department of Agriculture, Center for Nutrition Policy and Promotion. 2015-2020 Dietary Guidelines for Americans. 8th Edition. Available at: http://www.cnpp.usda.gov/2015-2020-dietary-guidelines-americans; [a]Source: U.S Department of Agriculture, Agricultural Research Service, Nutrient Data Laboratory. 2014. USDA National Nutrient Database for Standard Reference, Release 27. Available at: http://www.ars.usda.gov/nutrientdata.

Index

D.F. Romagnolo, O.I. Selmin (eds.), *Mediterranean Diet*, Nutrition and Health,
DOI 10.1007/978-3-319-27969-5

MIX
Papier aus verantwortungsvollen Quellen
Paper from responsible sources
FSC® C105338

If you have any concerns about our products,
you can contact us on
ProductSafety@springernature.com

In case Publisher is established outside the EU,
the EU authorized representative is:
Springer Nature Customer Service Center GmbH
Europaplatz 3, 69115 Heidelberg, Germany

Printed by Libri Plureos GmbH
in Hamburg, Germany